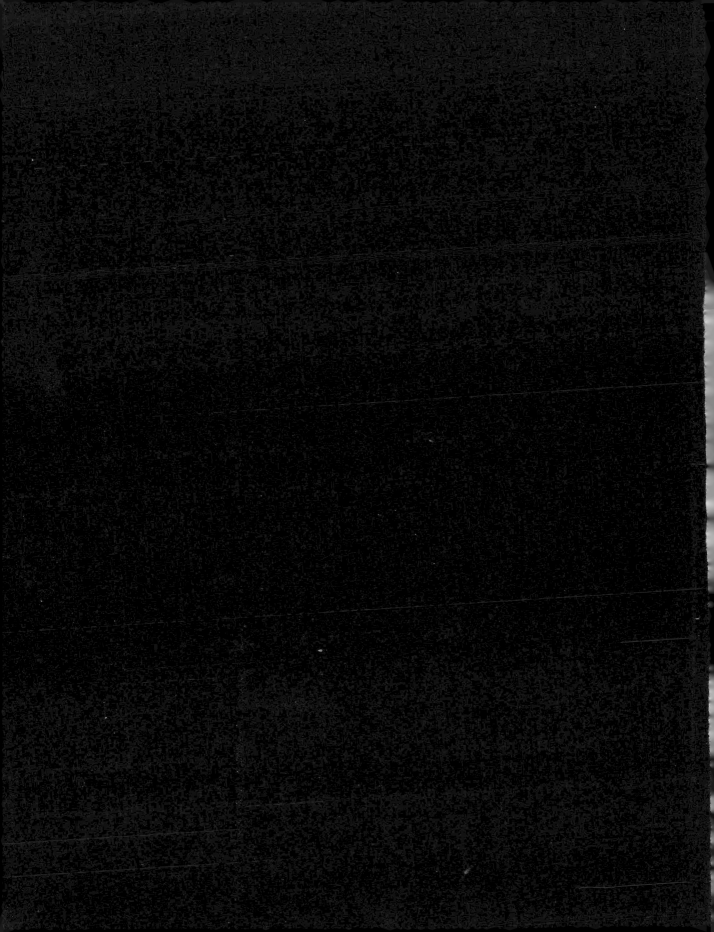

The Lumbar Spine and Back Pain

The Lumbar Spine and Back Pain

EDITED BY

Malcolm I. V. Jayson MD, FRCP

Professor of Rheumatology,
Rheumatic Diseases Centre, University of Manchester,
Hope Hospital, Salford, UK

With an Introduction by

Allan St J. Dixon

Consultant Physician,
Royal National Hospital for
Rheumatic Diseases, Bath, UK

THIRD EDITION

CHURCHILL LIVINGSTONE
EDINBURGH LONDON MELBOURNE AND NEW YORK 1987

CHURCHILL LIVINGSTONE
Medical Division of Longman Group UK Limited

Distributed in the United States of America by
Churchill Livingstone Inc., 1560 Broadway, New York,
N.Y. 10036, and by associated companies, branches
and representatives throughout the world.

First edition 1976
Second edition 1980
Third edition 1987
  Reprinted 1987

ISBN 0 443 03642 X

British Library Cataloguing in Publication Data
The Lumbar spine and back pain.—3rd ed.
   1. Vertebrae, Lumbar—Diseases   2. Spinal
cord—Diseases
   I. Jayson, Malcolm I. V.
   617'.375   RD768

Library of Congress Cataloging in Publication Data
The Lumbar spine and back pain.
   Includes bibliographies and index.
   1. Backache.   2. Vertebrae, Lumbar—Diseases.
3. Intervertebral disk—Diseases.   I. Jayson,
Malcolm I. V.   [DNLM: 1. Backache.
2. Spine—physiopathology.   WE 720 L957]
RD768.L85   1986   617'.56   86–17563

Printed and bound in Great Britain by
William Clowes Limited, Beccles and London

Preface

Back pain is an immense problem. Despite being a major cause of pain, suffering and disability, the subject has been relatively neglected by the medical profession. The lack of interest was partly due to the great difficulties in achieving a precise diagnosis. Treatment has often been on an empirical basis rather than based on a fundamental understanding of the underlying problem.

In recent years increasing attention has been paid to the back pain problem and we are no longer satisfied with simply treating the symptom without proper understanding of the underlying disorder. With critical thought and new investigational tools the whole subject has become a fascinating area of study.

In this third edition I have concentrated on the same objectives as in the first and second editions. We need to understand the structure and function of the spine, what goes wrong, how lesions produce back pain, how to assess the severity of the problem, the relation of symptoms and disability to psychological factors, and the indications and values for various forms of treatment. No special attention has been paid to inflammatory causes of back pain such as ankylosing spondylitis or metabolic bone disease, neoplasms and so on, as these do not present the same conceptual problems and the objectives of treatment are relatively well defined. The authors have all brought their chapters up to date and there has been considerable expansion in the scope of problems that have been covered with many new contributors.

I must thank all my authors for their hard work. I hope that this book will stimulate further interest and research and contribute towards improved management of this complex and painful problem.

M.I.V.J.

Contributors

John A. D. Anderson MD, FFCM, MFOM
Professor of Community Medicine, Guy's
Hospital Medical School, London, UK

Gunnar B. J. Andersson MD, PhD
Professor of Orthopedic Surgery, Rush-
Presbyterian-St Luke's Medical Center, Chicago,
Illinois, USA

Nagi Antoun MB, BCh, MRCP(UK), FRCR
Department of Diagnostic Radiology, University
of Manchester, Medical School, Manchester, UK

Shirley Ayad PhD
Research Associate, Department of Biochemistry,
University of Manchester Medical School,
Manchester, UK

Elizabeth M. Badley DPhil, MSc
Deputy Director, Arthritis and Rheumatism
Council, Epidemiology Research Unit, Stopford
Building, University of Manchester, Manchester,
UK

Neil I. Chafetz MD
University of California, San Francisco, USA

Philip J. Clements MD
Associate Physician, The Arthritis & Back Pain
Center, Santa Monica; Associate Professor of
Medicine (Adjunct series), UCLA, California,
USA

Allan St J. Dixon MD, FRCP
Consultant Physician, Royal National Hospital for
Rheumatic Diseases, Upper Borough Walls, Bath
UK

Harry K. Genant MD
Professor of Radiology Medicine and Orthopaedic
Surgery, University of California, San Francisco,
USA

Thurman Gillespy MD
University of California, San Francisco, USA

Vijay K. Goel PhD
Assistant Professor, Department of Biomedical
Engineering, University of Iowa, Iowa City,
Iowa, USA

David W. L. Hukins BSc PhD
Senior Lecturer, Department of Medical
Biophysics, University of Manchester,
Manchester, UK

J. Erik Hult MS
Biomechanics Research Laboratory, Department
of Surgery, Yale Medical School, New Haven,
Connecticut, USA

Ian Isherwood MRCP, FRCR, FFRRCSI (Hon)
Professor of Diagnostic Radiology, University of
Manchester, Manchester, UK

Malcolm I.V. Jayson MD, FRCP
Professor of Rheumatology, Rheumatic Diseases
Centre, University of Manchester, Hope Hospital,
Salford, UK

Y. King Liu PhD
Professor and Director, Center for Materials
Research, Department of Biomedical Engineering,
University of Iowa, Iowa City, Iowa, USA.

Chris J. Main PhD
Department of Clinical Psychology, Salford
Health Authority; Honorary Research Fellow
Rheumatic Diseases Centre, University of
Manchester, Hope Hospital, Salford, UK

Iain W. McCall MB, ChB, FRCR
Consultant Radiologist, Robert Jones & Agnes
Hunt Orthopaedic Hospital, Oswestry,
Shropshire, UK

John A. McCulloch MD, FRCS (C)
Associate Professor of Orthopaedics, Northeastern
Ohio Universities College of Medicine,
Rootstown, Ohio, USA

J. M. H. Moll DM, PhD, FRCP
Consultant Physician in Rheumatology; Head,
Sheffield Centre for Rheumatic Diseases, Nether
Edge Hospital, Sheffield, UK

Vert Mooney MD
Professor and Chairman, Department of
Orthopaedic Surgery, University of Texas, Health
Science Center, Dallas, USA

Alf L. Nachemson MD, PhD
Professor of Orthopaedic Surgery, University of
Goteborg; Department of Orthopaedics, Sahlgren
Hospital, Goteborg, Sweden

Martin A. Nelson MD, BS, FRCS
Consultant Orthopaedic Surgeon, Department of
Orthopaedics, Leeds General Infirmary; Senior
Lecturer in Orthopaedics, University of Leeds,
Leeds, UK

Manohar M. Panjabi PhD, DrTech
Professor of Surgery and Director of
Biomechanics, Department of Surgery, Yale
Medical School, New Haven, Connecticut, USA

Richard W. Porter MD, FRCS, FRCSE
Consultant Orthopaedic Surgeon, Doncaster
Royal Infirmary, Doncaster, UK

Albert B. Schultz PhD
Vennema Professor of Mechanical Engineering
and Applied Mechanics, University of Michigan,
Ann Arbor, Michigan, USA

Hugh A. Smythe MD, FRCP(C)
Professor and Head, Rheumatic Diseases Unit,
Wellesley Hospital and University of Toronto,
Toronto, Canada

Robert L. Swezey MD FACP
Medical Director, The Arthritis & Back Pain
Center, Santa Monica; Clinical Professor of
Medicine, UCLA, California, USA

Barrie Vernon-Roberts MD, PhD, FRCPath,
FRCPA
Professor and Chairman, Department of
Pathology, University of Adelaide; Head of
Division of Tissue Pathology, Institute of Medical
and Veterinary Science, Adelaide, South Australia

Gordon Waddell BSc, MD, FRCS(Ed)
Consultant Orthopaedic Surgeon, Western
Infirmary, Glasgow, UK

Jacqueline B. Weiss DSc
Reader in Medical Biochemistry, Department of
Rheumatology, University of Manchester Medical
School, Manchester, UK

Augustus A. White III MD, DMedSci
Professor of Orthopaedic Surgery, Harvard
Medical School, Boston, Massachusetts, USA

Philip H. N. Wood MB, FRCP, FFCM
Director, Arthritis and Rheumatism Council,
Epidemiology Research Unit; Honorary Professor
of Community Medicine, University of
Manchester; Honorary Regional Specialist in
Community Medicine, North Western Regional
Health Authority, Manchester, UK

Verna Wright MD, FRCP
Professor of Rheumatology, University of Leeds,
Leeds, UK

Barry Wyke MD
Research Professor of Neurology, Royal College
of Surgeons, Lincoln's Inn Fields, London, UK

Contents

Introduction

Since the first edition of this book was planned ten years ago, much has changed in the field of the lumbar spine and back pain. Third and fourth generation computerised axial tomography scanning systems have been developed, illuminating changes in the anatomy of the living back, which previously could only be guessed at. Nuclear magnetic resonance imaging is just round the corner. Science has undoubtedly advanced and the main problem facing doctors now is the delivery of some of the benefits of those advances to patient-sufferers. There are 139 joints in the spine and numerous bursae, all of them equipped with sensitive pain nerve endings. We are now beginning to bridge the gap between the common clinical back pain syndromes and their underlying pathological anatomy.

Indeed back troubles are so common, that the reader is likely to be well aware from his own unpleasant experience just what they feel like. It is a doubtful compliment to point out that he is in interesting company. The skeleton of the thirty foot long gigantosaurus at the British Museum (Natural History) reveals that spinal disease existed all those millions of years ago. But what of it? – he shares our common vertebrate inheritance. It is not of much comfort to anyone off work because of a painful back, to know that of all rheumatic complaints, back troubles are the greatest cause of lost time in industry, and it suggests that he is but a single statistic in a sum total so large that by implication he must accept it. Indeed many students of back pain think that the changes of spinal ageing are so inevitable as to be regarded as normal and by implication unpreventable.

In his role as sufferer from back pain, the reader will want evidence of a more positive and optimistic attitude. Such an attitude is not hard to justify since death itself has a normal and natural association with ageing. Science cannot prevent death but death has

been delayed and postponed for up to twenty years for most of us, so why not postpone and delay back disease? A few lucky people live to vigorous old age without any spinal problems at all. If nature can do this for a few, why not the many? Can research really be powerless in the face of the question, 'How can one prevent or delay degenerative disease of the spine?' Put like this the task becomes familiar and it is a truism that modern science is such that if a question can be clearly put, technology can almost certainly answer it.

In 1976 a Back Pain Working Party, representing a range of therapists and researchers concerned with back pain was set up by the Department of Health. Out of moutains of evidence only ten carefully controlled trials of treatment existed in the world literature at that time. These uniformly concluded that the benefits, if any, of the various manipulations, injections, applications and immobilisations used traditionally were at best temporary in their effect. Since one treatment did not differ markedly from another or from no treatment at all, the studies could be regarded as exercises in the natural history of back pain. The outstanding finding was of the high frequency of spontaneous improvement or recovery. Even chronic low back pain sufferers, culled from hospital orthopaedic out patient referrals, showed a 60–70% 'cure' or improvement if carefully followed for twelve months or more. Only for surgical removal of a prolapsed intervertebral disc which had been pressing on a nerve root was there scientifically acceptable evidence of a benefit caused by that particular treatment. The Working Party drew attention to the increasing problem of back pain in children and adolescents, a group not normally identified with back pain. It recommended that heterodox treatments were worthy of investigation by the method of the controlled trial, not forgetting that perceived benefit, even if significant, might not necessarily be the result of the therapist's manoeuvres nor even support his theories. The placebo effect of the various forms of manipulation and of the laying on of hands is very strong.

One of the important effects of the scientific study of lumbar spine and back pain is the removal of traditional myths. One of these myths is the 'slipped disc'. Discs do not 'slip' in the way that most laymen and not a few doctors imagine, like orange pips squeezed between the finger and thumb. Discs can not even hurt since they contain no nerve endings capable of registering pain. Only the surrounding structures can hurt. Because the vast majority of painful spinal conditions are never operated on, nor cause death, the source and site of pain can not usually be verified by direct observation.

Back pain is as much a problem of pain as a problem of the back, hence the study of back pain is both a job for the anatomist and for the neuro-physiologist (as in Ch. 4). Because the normal anatomy can become diseased and the disease state can often heal, the anatomist and neuro-physiologist must also be concerned with the remarkable powers of healing, repair, regeneration and compensatory overgrowth that the body can deploy in order to restore reasonable function. Not least amongst these is the concept of differences in pain threshold, whereby a miner may be able to keep at work when one of his office-bound relatives with apparently similar radiological back disturbances is unable to do so. Nor will any serious study of low back pain be able to ignore the problems of motivation. The industrial and politicial questions raised in the introduction to the first edition of this book included problems of pre-employment screening, problems such as 'should people with unilateral sacralisation be denied to work in the docks?' Can an equitable system of compensation for job related back injury be worked out? Is it possible to agree a legal limit to the weight that a worker could be asked lift? In contrast, the television coverage of the 1984 Olympics reminded us what enormous weights can be safely handled by trained athletes. We have still not applied these lessons to lifting at work. Yet the social climate is now much more favourable to the introduction of legislation to protect the worker from back injury. The Health & Safety & Welfare At Work provisions are effective and have force. Paradoxically we may now find that embalmed in new laws are provisions

which by the time they are enacted are scientifically out of date as the study of training programmes for prevention of back injury advances. The study of the treatment of back pain has paradoxically been retarded by the relatively benign nature of most instances of back pain and the tendency to spontaneous recovery. Only one or two in every thousand incidents of back pain that occur in the population become so severe that they lead to hospital style investigation or to operation. Because of this, heterodox treatments of all sorts have flourished and seem successful. Each therapist has his own theory ranging from the plausible to those which can only be described as systematised delusions. In the past, this has tended to frighten off scientific workers capable of applying strict disciplines and critical attitudes to their work but in the ten years since this book was first published, there has been considerable change. The need for this change has become apparent from various sources but primarily from epidemiologists who have counted the cost in numbers of people who lose time from work because of episodes of back pain. They have compared the consequential loss to the economy with a very small investment into back pain research. Specialist scientific societies have been set up and have spear-headed the study of back pain and much has been achieved. But there is still little evidence that the American rheumatological community regards the study of back pain as part of its work judging from the official journal of the American Rheumatism Association. In some countries there are two sorts of rheumatologist. There are the classical rheumatologists who view the cure of rheumatoid arthritis and of systemic lupus as their crock of gold at the other end of an immunological rainbow. There are also the 'back-necks-and-shoulders' rheumatologists who in some countries are more or less synonymous with rehabilitationists and physical medicine specialists. However, in many countries in Europe, back pain is closely associated with orthopaedic surgery, an association now historically inappropriate in that back pain is relatively rarely operated on and the majority of treatments are medical. Thus in many parts of the world, the community response to the back pain problem is inappropriate, and it is the function of this book to help redress the situation.

1987   A.St J.D.

Unit equivalents

The following SI units are used in this book and are given with their imperial equivalents:

Unit of length: metre
1 m (= 1000 mm = 100 cm) = 39.4 in

Unit of mass: kilogram
1 kg = 2.205 lb

Unit of force: newton
(A newton is defined as the force necessary to give a mass of 1 kg an acceleration of 1 m/s^2)
10 N = 2.25 lbf

Unit of pressure: pascal
1 Pa = 1 N/m^2
1 MPa = 10^6 Pa = 145 lbf/in^2

Philip H. N. Wood and Elizabeth M. Badley

Epidemiology of back pain

INTRODUCTION

Any epidemiological appraisal has to begin with an examination of the nature of the condition of interest. The previous (second) edition of this book included a lengthy essay on understanding back pain;[1] no major new insights have been acquired since then, so there would be little point in going over the ground again. Similarly, limitations in routinely available data on the problem were also reviewed,[2] and these difficulties scarcely merit recapitulation.

On this occasion we shall begin by making explicit what epidemiology can contribute to different classes of reader, followed by a few brief remarks on types of aetiology. We shall then discuss spondylosis and other abnormalities, before turning to non-specific back troubles and a review of the community burden.

Contribution of epidemiology

Insights from epidemiology have a bearing on most aspects of clinical activity. The frequency and characteristics of occurrence of individual syndromes provide a background for diagnosis. Comparative data on similar conditions indicate probabilities for differential diagnosis. Appreciation of natural history and outcomes guides the development of prognosis. Finally, management is enlightened by knowledge of specific impairments and features such as a family history.

The import is somewhat different for biomedical scientists. Understanding of pathological processes and possible aetiological determinants has to be related to what is known about the specifics of occurrence of an individual syndrome. An epidemiological viewpoint therefore establishes a context and has value for exposing ideas to falsification, because viable hypotheses must be capable of taking account of all the features associated with a particular occurrence.

Health care planning is more concerned with measures of the community burden. As soon as initiatives for control are contemplated, it is necessary to draw on more specific epidemiological insights as well. For instance, appreciation of the interplay of influences associated with development of a particular syndrome may indicate factors that could be manipulated as a means of prevention. Alternatively, the attributes of persons affected may be used as a basis for identifying populations at risk, such as by screening, so that education or other prophylactic initiatives may be concentrated where they will show greatest return.

Types of aetiology

It is customary to differentiate between certain broad classes of aetiology. In the first place, there are inflammatory disorders that affect the axial skeleton. These include ankylosing spondylitis and a number of rather similar spondylarthropathies. Also to be thought of are infections, such as brucellosis and tuberculosis. Second, there are various developmental abnormalities of the spine. Third, there are a host of other specific diseases that may be associated with back pain, notably osteoporosis. Lastly, there are so-called mechanical or degenerative disorders. Most of this chapter will be concerned with the latter, but some comment on associations with other diseases is called for.

There is an embarrassing abundance of pathological states that can give rise to back pain.

Unfortunately we have no good indication of the relative frequency of all these different conditions as the source of people's complaints. For example, although we think of back pain as an obvious feature of osteoporosis, what proportion of all back pain is in fact attributable to this disorder? The underlying difficulty is that, even if such conditions are identified, this does not necessarily mean that whatever may be detected is responsible for the individual's complaint — a point to which we shall return.

What is important to recognize is that confounding often occurs, i.e. uncertainty about which explanation to accept for an individual's symptoms. Having said that, we shall refer to the various pathological causes only when they illustrate particular difficulties for the drawing of inferences. This will allow us to devote most of our attention to the biggest class of spinal problem: back pain that is not associated with an underlying 'disease'.

SPONDYLOSIS

We propose to consider evidence on structural changes related to the spine separately, deferring the more general problem of 'non-specific' back pain for discussion later. In this context we shall use the term spondylosis as a generic descriptor for 'degenerative' processes in the spine, whether these are in the apophyseal joints or related to intervertebral discs.

Obstacles to understanding

A series of interrelated features combine to retard appreciation of the nature of anatomical features associated with back pain. Much of the difficulty can be attributed to how observations are regarded and how evidence is interpreted. One influence is really psychological, the notion of 'degeneration' and a wearing-out of parts scarcely encouraging optimism about the possibilities for arrest or reversal of the underlying process. Such views derive largely from patterns of occurrence with age. At this stage it suffices to say that the case for regarding most spinal disorders as being degenerative or attributable to ageing is certainly open to serious question.

The most extensive parts of our knowledge are based on observations of structural changes either directly, in morbid anatomical specimens, or indirectly through the medium of shadows on X-ray plates. Apart from levels of detail, such as that fibrillation of cartilage may be observed pathologically but cannot be identified radiographically, the two sources of evidence have yielded broadly compatible findings. However, this line of reasoning glosses over a number of aspects. A concatenation of features tends to be treated as a whole, neglecting the fact that some may be fundamental, whereas others are only associated or confounding. For example, osteophytes probably fall in the latter category.[3] Moreover, what is observed to be similar structurally could nevertheless reflect just a common end-expression of a number of different processes. This leads us to suggest that what can be regarded as regularity at the micro level may have deflected attention away from important locus-specific differences.

Another aspect, and clinically the most important, is that significant discontinuities in the evidence get neglected. Specific structural abnormalities are relatively easy to study, and they have been productive of useful biomedical concepts. These concepts tend to be linked to clinical problems on the basis of the observation that severe structural changes in the spine are often associated with symptoms. This leads to a common clinical syllogism:[4]

1. 'degenerative' changes cause symptoms;
2. this patient has 'degenerative' changes;
3. therefore this patient's symptoms are due to the 'degenerative' changes.

Although this is frequently a reasonable guide, the vulnerability of the conclusion is that the first premise does not state that all degenerative changes always cause symptoms. In other words, available biomedical concepts have a limited applicability in the elucidation of an individual's subjective problems. This is because there is an appreciable discordance between clinical problems and evidence of underlying abnormalities such as may be revealed by radiographs. The discordance is illustrated in Table 1.1. A major, but by no means exclusive, part of the problem is attributable to the fact that most structural changes are irreversible, whereas symptoms in any one individual tend to be inconstant. The latter is a feature that also makes clinical trials

Table 1.1 Discordance between symptom experience and evidence of structural change (derived from Lawrence[14])

Complaint	Radiographic findings	Concordance* (complaint with X-ray changes) (%)	Discordance† (X-ray changes without complaint) (%)
Cervicobrachial pain	Cervical DD	50	35
Back–hip–sciatic pain	Lumbar DD	59	45

*Equivalent to sensitivity of radiographic changes as a criterion
†Equivalent to complement of specificity, derived by subtracting latter from 100

more difficult, because non-therapeutic variation is greater.

Our terminology is undoubtedly unsatisfactory and confusing. This is largely a reflection of the crudity of nosological distinctions, and appreciable heterogeneity is almost certainly being concealed at present. Underlying the problems with nomenclature has been poverty of clinical observation. For example, there has been a dearth of careful and detailed natural history studies, and this means that we are still uncertain about how uniformly progressive these disorders are, and at what rate they progress. Basic biological changes have also not been adequately established, such as the possibility that symptom expression may alter with age.[5]

The other important implication concerns the use we make of concepts and how far we extend their application. On one plane it may be very helpful to regard back pain as emanating from disturbances of the intervertebral disc. However, for many other purposes it is more profitable to examine form and alignment, such as stenosis of the spinal canal, and for yet others to concentrate on patterns of use and overuse, including the influence of posture and habitual activities.

Characteristics

There is a dearth of information available on arthrosis of the diarthrodial interfacetal joints, in both the clinical and the epidemiological literature. Despite considerable detail in a report on the relationship between symptoms and radiographic changes,[6] even in his meticulous monograph Lawrence[7] makes little more than passing mention of the condition, other than to note that it can frequently be observed in women with generalized osteoarthrosis.

The explanation probably lies with the fact that commonly available lateral radiographs of the spine are less satisfactory for detecting apophyseal abnormalities than they are for revealing intervertebral disc degeneration.

Disc degeneration (DD) is characterized by the triad of disc space narrowing, osteophytes on the vertebral bodies, and sclerosis of the vertebral endplates, as described by Friberg & Hirsch.[8] Standards for radiographic gradings have been developed,[9] although it has been noted[7] that intra-observer variation over time can still be an appreciable problem. Frykholm[10] described osteophytes in two locations — ventral (anterior) spurs, especially thoracolumbar, which do not seem to be related to DD; and lipping, either marginal or affecting the entire circumference, observable throughout the spine and presumed to be the consequence of DD with disc collapse. The latter can also result in subluxation of corresponding interfacetal joints, leading to secondary osteophyte formation at these sites. However, it is difficult to pursue the epidemiology of these relationships with the limited radiographs available from population studies.

There is a paradox concerning interpretation of X-ray findings related to DD. It is understandable that great weight should be attached to the most obvious features, osteophytes. On the other hand, symptoms usually arise from an articular segment that is vulnerable to instability because of DD, and yet the presence of osteophytes generally indicates that stabilization has probably begun to occur.[11] This contrast offers a likely explanation for the fall-off in incidence of many back complaints with age (Fig. 1.1), despite the fact that radiographic abnormalities tend to show a sustained increase in extent and severity. More generally, it probably accounts for much of the discordance between symptoms and

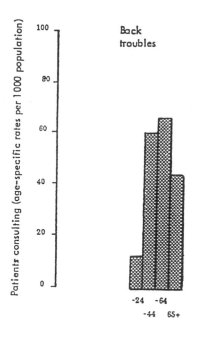

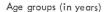

Fig. 1.1 Age-specific incidence rates for back troubles in general practice (derived from OPCS data[13])

structural evidence of degeneration in the spine[12] (Table 1.1).

Epidemiology

The most extensive work on DD has been carried out by Lawrence,[14] who has also reviewed the whole field,[7] including the differential affection of individual segments of the spine. In summary, the prevalence of DD increases with age, and after the age of 60 years it is rare to find a completely normal spine on radiographic investigation. Frequency estimates obviously depend on the severity of changes to which attention is paid, although the patterns of progression with age are parallel for different grade thresholds. The age composition of samples studied also influences overall measures of frequency in the population. Taking all these factors into account the more recent work by Julkunen[15] appears to be broadly in accord with Lawrence's estimates, and an overall figure for the prevalence of DD in a population of adults is of the order of 45%.

The role of heavy manual work in encouraging multiple DD, especially as may be seen in the lumbar region in coalminers, appears to depend on both its nature (and particularly exposure to injury) and its duration. Sedentary workers exhibit frequencies of involvement of the cervical spine that are similar to those encountered in people engaged in physically more taxing pursuits, but in the former the severity of changes is only minimal. There is also evidence of variability in predisposition to DD. Ochronosis provides an obvious but uncommon clinical example. Paleopathological evidence[16] reinforces variation in the frequency of DD, both between different segments of the spine and as regards the upper and lower margins of the vertebral bodies. Such variation is most likely to represent not ethnic or geographical differences but differential stress related mainly to habitual patterns of use. Only infrequently are antecedent causes identifiable, such as adolescent kyphosis, scoliosis, tuberculous infection, spondylolysis or spondylolisthesis, and spinal osteochondrosis.[17]

Familial aggregation has been described by Lawrence, and Bull[18] observed both concordance in twins and relative freedom from cervical spondylosis in certain other families. However, until inherited influences on properties such as disc metabolism have been identified, the results from genetic studies are not straightforward for interpretation. Families do differ in attributes such as habitual postures and mannerisms (i.e. patterns of use), but these could be related to cultural assimilation (unconscious mimicry, etc.) as much as to genetic factors. There is insufficient evidence to establish the characteristics of those in whom spondylosis is associated with development of myelopathy, and so the role of constitutional factors in regard to this complication is indeterminate.

OTHER ABNORMALITIES

Reviews of evidence on back pain usually identify specific abnormalities of structure that are assumed to be relevant. However, a general caution should be noted. Many of these conditions have been implicated on the basis of guilt by association, i.e. with back pain. This may be a productive starting point, but all too often the essential sequel has been neglected — to establish whether such conditions are necessary and sufficient causes of the complaints presented. The challenge arises because we are not confronted by unique associations. Instead we observe what appear to be increases in risk, that given lesions seem to be more common in those with backache. It is the extent and nature of this risk that requires elucidation. As one of us has noted,[19] to resolve this problem it is necessary to study a group of people with a particular lesion, record their complaints and then relate the findings to symptom experience in a comparable group of people without the lesion. With a few notable exceptions such testimony is largely lacking, although the work of Magora[20,21] is exemplary.

What is particularly worrying is that not only does available evidence tend to be unsatisfactory, which retards research enquiry, but also that this does not deter people from prescriptive infringement of individual liberty. This is most evident in regard to pre-employment screening, because anatomical abnormalities are the easiest features to detect radiographically. On the basis of currently inadequate knowledge, curtailing the individual's freedom of choice when he or she is seeking employment would appear to be scientifically and ethically unjustifiable in many instances.

Identification criteria for ankylosing hyperostosis (AH) have been suggested.[7,22] Whether the condition represents a unique 'degenerative' disorder[23] or just a particular variety of spondylosis[24] is controversial. Epidemiological work by Julkunen[22,25,26] has helped to clarify the status of the condition. However, it is perplexing to find lack of apophyseal and peripheral involvement cited in this work as a distinguishing feature of what is referred to as DISH (diffuse idopathic skeletal hyperostosis). Differences in distributional characteristics and linked features indicate that AH is distinct from spondylosis — the former occurs later in life (AH is six to ten times less frequent than spondylosis, although the ratio of the former relative to the latter increases with age[15]), is unrelated to strenuous work, is associated with diabetes mellitus[15] and has a lower risk in regard to future cardiovascular disease.[27]

Conditions such as spina bifida occulta and transitional vertebra, especially sacralization of L5, are probably more common than has been realized.[26,27] However, the evidence does not support the view that these anomalies have a meaningful relation to back complaints. A whole host of theories about the pathogenesis of associated pain therefore become suspect.[26] The same also appears to be true of spondylolysis and spondylolisthesis.[28] The situation is even less satisfactory in regard to scoliosis, as we have discussed elsewhere.[29] All one can conclude is that the extent of the contribution these different conditions make, both to DD and to back pain, has yet to be established.

Spinal stenosis is as much a functional as a structural abnormality. It represents disproportion between the cross-sectional areas of the spinal canal and associated tunnels and foramina on the one hand and of the nervous structures disposed within them on the other. The result can be compression of the latter, and interference with the blood supply. A variety of lesions may give rise to the condition.[30] Pulsed echo ultrasound offers an acceptable means for large-scale investigation and has been used in the study of patients and selected samples of children and of adults in particular occupational groups.[31] More evidence is required, especially on alterations over time, because observed trends in measurements such as oblique diameters could reflect cohort effects as much as changes associated with age. The concept of spinal stenosis appears to represent one factor of significance in certain clinical syndromes, though it is probably less relevant in older patients and in those with root entrapment.[31]

OTHER BACK TROUBLES

Physicians are generally happier if they can find so-called objective evidence to support a diagnostic conclusion. At the same time the tradition of medical practice encourages identification of an underlying pathological state, even if only by inference. Unfortunately, back pain cannot easily be constrained in this manner. Associated physical signs tend to be non-specific and are as likely to represent the consequence of the complaint, such as limitation of spinal mobility, as they are to provide an independent clue to the origin of the problem.

Such a state of affairs can encourage further investigation, especially by the use of radiographs. However, the symptom discordance already indicated (Table 1.1) suggests that too often it is not possible to make very much of the findings. This would suggest that radiography has a limited role in clinical practice, and it has been argued that routine X-rays should be reserved for those patients who have not recovered from their back complaints within three months.[32]

A more general point is that, although an array of different conditions may give rise to pain in the back, these are insufficiently differentiated to allow an epidemiologist to make any significant contribution. This is an example of the dependence of less-specialized disciplines on being presented with clearly defined problems by clinical medicine.[33] One is therefore limited to evidence of two types. The first is frequency measures derived from health service utilization and the uptake of benefits, which we shall discuss later. The second is circumstantial evidence, what we referred to above as guilt by association, relating to the overall influence of various factors on the heterogeneity of conditions concealed by the term non-specific back pain. Before considering this evidence, though, there is one other 'lesion' that has to be taken into account.

Disc prolapse

Much of the literature on back complaints is confused by references to prolapse of the inter-vertebral discs (PID). Although these structures undoubtedly may prolapse, herniate, or in other ways be displaced, the difficulty lies in establishing both when this may have happened and whether it is clinically significant. In severe cases there may be little doubt, especially when contrast radiography can be used to demonstrate the lesion. However, there are many sources of uncertainty — criteria for identification are notable more for their vagaries and lack of uniformity in application than anything else; the source of pain is often not explored systematically, particularly as regards differentiation between articular, dural and neurological origins, and confirmatory evidence cannot be derived from plain radiography. In particular, narrowing of the disc space on its own has never been established as having a relationship to symptoms.[34]

The result is loose usage of the term disc prolapse by both practitioners and the public. Whereas the former often mislead themselves, for reasons such as we have noted or perhaps to conceal ignorance, the latter may wish for more prestigious diagnostic

status or may even seek secondary gain, such as through social security benefits or compensation. Serious and provocative challenges to the validity of the concept[35,36] have unfortunately not succeeded in stemming this tide.

Recognizing this terminological carelessness, we are not satisfied that reports supposedly concerned with epidemiological aspects of disc prolapse in fact contribute any enlightenment on this condition. We prefer to acknowledge these uncertainties and to consider all that has been so ascribed in the more general context of non-specific back pain. However, for those interested, a recent review has pursued a specific focus on disc prolapse.[28]

Unfortunately, the confusion extends to other areas of unspecialized research as well. For example, work on intradiscal pressures[37] is of interest in its own right in regard to the biology of discs. However, attempts to apply these insights to clinical problems suffer from the weaknesses we have discussed — i.e. to what extent can symptoms be ascribed or otherwise related to lesions that are only postulated, however plausible the inferences may appear to be? Underlying this is another difficulty, that the relationship between disc prolapse and DD has not been adequately elucidated, so that one is often compelled to resort to generic designation of disc lesions. In fact much of the evidence, such as that on the mechanical properties of lumbar spine segments,[38] would suggest that DD is of much more general importance than uncomplicated prolapse.

Occurrence of back pain

Estimates of prevalence for what is usually a relatively short-lived but nevertheless very common complaint are not particularly enlightening. More graphic is the appreciation Hult developed[39,40] that 60% of a sample of men up to age 69 years had at some time suffered from symptoms related to the lower back, and that the proportion increased to 80% when attention was focused on those involved in physically demanding occupations.

Recent work employing the same concept of lifetime incidence has yielded similar results.[41] The same report revealed that more than a quarter of those not admitting to such a history nevertheless had experienced time off work with low back pain, so that even these impressive figures represent an underestimate. This reinforces the caution needed in interpreting responses to questionnaires.[42] From a similar baseline of lifetime incidence, a prospective study[43] established a one-year incidence of first attacks of low back pain of 11% in 30-year-olds, the rate decreasing to 6% or less in older decades. As is often found, recurrences were commoner in those who had experienced back pain both recently and more frequently in the past.

Confronted with such enormity one has to seek means of reducing the problem to comprehensible dimensions. At a crude level, two aspects deserve more attention, relating to location and duration. Unfortunately it is not always clear from the literature to what extent these distinctions have been made. As a result there are often taxing difficulties over comparability between estimates from different sources. The first aspect is the more straightforward of the two. For some purposes it is useful to treat the spine or the back as a whole, perhaps especially when documenting the community burden. However, for aetiological or control-oriented enquiries it is essential to differentiate between the functional and anatomical regions of the spine.

The most important distinction requires separation of cervical from lumbar involvement, particularly as the former may give rise to complaints that can be difficult to distinguish from parts of soft-tissue syndromes. Lumbar disorders outnumber cervical by a factor of two to one,[44] and so it is not surprising that the bulk of the literature is devoted to lumbosacral problems. However, even under the topic of low back pain there is generally insufficient differentiation between lumbago and sciatica, distinctions which the concept of disc prolapse has unhelpfully tended to blur. Both the thoracic region[45] and the sacro-iliac joint also have to be considered; the latter is a not uncommon source of low backache.[46]

For the other aspect we have found it useful to employ a very simple taxonomy[47] that allows us to identify the broad areas to which published work appears to relate, so that constraints upon inference from one set of observations to another are made evident. This scheme differentiates between three types of problem:

1. *Transient* back pain, the evanescent twinges that everyone probably experiences at some time in their lives. The hallmark is brevity, a passing awareness of

discomfort or perhaps sharper sensations related to the back. By their very universality such symptoms make up much the biggest class of back pain. However, it is unlikely that this order of complaint is usually presented to a doctor, so that it tends to be outside our professional experience and to be neglected in consideration of the problem. Nevertheless the context has to be taken note of because enquiries about symptom experience may well tap an unknown part of this reservoir of discomfort, and this may be especially relevant to retrospective studies of lumbar symptomatology (as is documented in some of the studies reviewed above).

2. *Acute* back pain is probably what most readily comes to mind. The key distinction concerns duration: symptoms present for sufficient time to compel most sufferers to take note of them; the range probably extends from some hours to a few weeks. The onset of complaints may be dramatic, as with the hexenschuss or witch's blow, or it may be gradual. The symptoms may be confined to the lumbar region (lumbago), or they may also radiate to other areas, or they may be present only in the lower limbs (sciatica). Finally, the severity of suffering may extend from the mild to the severe, and relief may be afforded differentially by support, warmth[48] or other factors. Although reflected by measures such as consultations with general practitioners and certified incapacity for work, these sources are almost certainly not exhaustive because it is unlikely that all people with acute back pain seek medical advice. Problems in interpretation arise partly because of overlap between this category and more transient experiences when pursuing anamnestic enquiries, recall of durations being notoriously variable. However, a more particular difficulty stems from the fact that most research reports emanate from hospital-based doctors, and the selectivity of referral for specialist help will not be the same across the wide spectrum of back pain. Thus until clinical nosography has provided us with greater discriminatory power between different syndromes, and the criteria by which these may be identified have been applied rigorously, considerable caution is needed in determining how applicable the findings in one study may be in another context.

3. *Chronic* back pain is the minority class, including all those who suffer for periods in excess of a few weeks. Although the critical distinction between

acute and chronic is largely a function of duration, there are other important differences in the nature of the difficulties encountered by this group. Of particular note are the influence on everyday life[47] and the tendency to be neglected because fewer people are affected by chronic back pain. Unfortunately what is perhaps the key question — whether chronic backs are such from the beginning or whether they progress from unfavourable response to an acute back — is difficult to answer because of the uncertain applicability of many clinical and research findings. Differentiation between acute and chronic backs is also complicated by uncertainty about the significance of episodic or recurrent complaints, particularly in aetiological terms.

Characteristics

In patients attending a referral clinic for the first time, it was not possible to identify information that had useful predictive value in regard to outcome,[32] apart from a tendency for those who came to radiculography to have shorter histories and for those who became chronic attenders to have longer ones. However, when lifetime experience in the population was considered, where the cumulated incidence of lumbago, sciatica and intermittent claudication of the cauda equina was 56, 24 and 6% respectively,[49] the situation was a little more positive. The X-ray findings still had relatively little discriminatory value, and abnormalities revealed by contrast radiography were not necessarily associated with a poor prognosis. What did emerge was that a poor outlook was related more to the frequency of attacks than their duration; in one group the recurrence rate was as high as 50%.

Experience in general practice is not dissimilar, the unfavourable omens being more than three previous episodes, gradual onset of symptoms, referral of pain distal to the femur, and delays in reporting complaints exceeding a month.[50] Another study indicated that a history of back pain lasting more than one week and limitation of straight-leg raising were harbingers of a poor outcome four weeks after initial consultation.[51] The relationship to pain radiating down the leg was not so clear. A past history of back pain was not related to the outcome of the episode studied, but was linked to the risk of recurrence over the following year. A population-based survey[43] supported the suggestion that gradual onset or exacerbation was associated with a worse prognosis for recurrence, as was a history of pain radiating down to the leg.

These features appear to be relied upon quite frequently in primary care assessments.[52] However, whilst it seems that reasonable consistency in reporting the timing and location of pain is achieved,[42,53] the same may not be true for all aspects of a clinical examination.[51,53] Relationships to age may require clarification. Figure 1.1 depicted the crude pattern observed in consultations with general practitioners and reflected the maximal burden of complaints in the middle years of life. When this is translated into lifetime experience, symptoms are usually first experienced in the earlier part of adulthood. Surgical treatment is most commonly undertaken for those between the ages of 35 and 45 years, but durations of incapacity for work tend to increase progressively with age.

A syndrome that appears to have attracted relatively little attention is the association of dull backache with skin hyperaesthesia, a tender spot, and limitation of spinal movement.[54] Various other phenomena have been investigated for their association with back pain — electromyographic recordings,[55,56] muscle strength,[57] capillary resistance,[58] nerve entrapment,[59] pregnancy,[60] and how various biomechanical properties, already referred to, may influence clinical decision-making.[61] The principal influence of comorbidity, such as chronic bronchitis, appears to be on symptom exacerbation with coughing rather than on developing back pain in the first place.

We shall discuss psychological factors shortly but, whatever part they may play, the affected individual is commonly regarded as being able to make personal contributions to recovery. Self-care initiatives depend on knowledge and understanding, so that patient education is important;[62] this is an important feature in 'back schools'. It is sometimes asserted that acute back complaints are more disabling than chronic problems[49] but we have tried to display the limitations in such a view.[47] Certainly it is chronic backache that is often an important cause of premature retirement[63] and of problematic medical assessments for purposes such as workmen's compensation.[64] Hadler[65] has exposed three moot issues that underlie the latter, and concludes that the law requires an inference of causality that is generally beyond medical determination. In regard to sickness absence, the longer the incapacity for work related to back complaints, the less is the likelihood of a return to gainful employment.[66]

Individual factors

In his comprehensive review, Andersson[67] comments that data on individual factors are even more confusing to interpret than are those on occupational influences. This difficulty notwithstanding, some comments are called for. Symptom experience seems to be similar in the two sexes, despite reports that disc prolapse appears to be observed more frequently in men. Male chauvinism might account for the discrepancy, although Kelsey & Ostfeld[68] have offered a more charitable explanation, that women may be willing to wait for improvement from conservative therapy while men are more anxious to return to work quickly.

Although some studies have suggested that the risk of developing back pain is increased in those who are tall and heavy,[69] no consistent relationship with anthropometric characteristics is evident in the bulk of reported work. Body disposition is influenced not only by structural abnormalities, already considered, but also by habitual postures. Standing height shows circadian fluctuations,[70] but longer-term trends in the loss of height with age could bear some relationship to back pain. Such shrinkage is commonly attributed to reduction in intervertebral disc spaces, but the erectness required of long-serving military personnel is associated with less height loss,[71] and whether such veterans experience less back pain does not seem to have been studied.

Physical fitness is related to activity and occupation, which we shall discuss shortly. However, one aspect that is more appropriately considered at this juncture is back mobility, which has been studied quite extensively and in different contexts. The latter have included development during adolescence,[72,73] cadaveric specimens,[74,75] screening for ankylosing spondylitis,[76-78] and more generally in regard to back pain.[79-84] Overall it is difficult to assess whether spinal mobility has aetiological significance, apart from evidence on dynamic aspects of back movement, although it has been suggested that a hypermobile back may be a risk factor for back pain in men.[85]

The same prospective study has indicated that good isometric endurance of the musculature of the back may lessen the risk of developing low back pain.[85] Subjects with persistent or recurring back pain had weaker back muscles and reduced flexibility/elasticity of the back and hamstrings, thought to be a residue from previous back troubles. Inevitably these findings raise questions about the role of back muscle endurance training in the prevention of symptomatic complaints.

Crown[86] has carried out a helpful systematic review of psychological aspects of back pain. There is some indication that significant life events in the preceding three months are experienced more frequently by those destined to develop backache than by those who do not,[87] and the complaint is encountered with greater frequency in those with broken marriages.[88] It has been suggested that so-called non-organic physical signs may be useful as a simple clinical screen to identify patients requiring more detailed psychological assessment.[89] Certainly, psychological variables appear to influence the 'reliability' of proffered information.[90] An interrelationship between spinal mobility and ability to cope with pain has been demonstrated, and this seems to influence recovery of normal motion.[91]

People suffering from backache are more likely to manifest features of anxiety[92,93] and a history of psychiatric problems,[94] although when screened by standard instruments and compared with other patients those with acute back pain did not show an excess of current psychiatric illness.[94] Earlier work was much concerned with low back pain as a possible expression of an underlying depressive state, loss of libido and appetite being useful discriminators for this condition.[95] The origins of such depression are uncertain, especially in regard to poor response to treatment, although Stevenson[96] has argued that it may be a primary result of back injury rather than a reaction to treatment failure.

Some of these threads have been brought together in a report suggesting that it is possible to identify three subgroups.[97] One group had little restriction of movement in the back, an insidious onset of pain and a history of psychiatric illness, and also generally tended to be of lower social class. Another was characterized by general restriction of movement, and the third had little restriction but a sudden onset and was of higher social class.

Other influences

Data on incapacity for work show an increase in sickness absence from back troubles over time, but this is more likely to reflect secular changes in society rather than indicating a real increase in the occurrence of these complaints. Geographical comparisons have been few, and they are difficult to interpret because cultural influences on the expression of discomfort tend to vary pari passu. However, it is interesting that, as industrialization increases in Africa, back pain appears to emerge as a problem on the same scale as in Western Europe and North America.

The topic investigated most abundantly has been the relationship between back pain and bodily activity, especially as determined at the workplace. Certainly there is much in the characteristics of occurrence of backache to suggest that mechanical factors are important. However, the mediation of such influences, and even their magnitude, remain to be elucidated. Many simplistic explanations have been offered, but most founder on neglected inconsistencies in the data. To illustrate this, heavy lifting, twisting and trauma are commonly stated as causes of low back pain (sources cited in [43]), but in a study of patients claiming work-related causes a physician was able to confirm this in only about one-third of cases.[98]

The prima facie case rests on the generally greater frequency of back pain in blue- as opposed to white-collar workers[40,99] and the very striking differences in absences from work due to back disorders in heavy and light industry, the ratio between the two being five to one.[100] However, similar sources yield data that are not easy to reconcile with a simple mechanical load hypothesis, such as the anomalous duration of intervertebral disc morbidity in insurance and banking.[101] Another example is that, although nurses claim their backache is precipitated by activities at work, the overall prevalence of the complaint is similar in teachers, who customarily do not lift heavy people in bed.[102] Only a part of the discrepancies is likely to be related to the fact that the severity of back pain tends to be greater when mechanical loading of the spine is increased.

Mechanical forces cannot be regarded as a uniform stress because the conditions of loading may vary. Two major types of situation have to be considered, but within these are also important subvarieties. Dynamic loading is the more obvious condition. A physiological example is afforded by pregnancy, multiparity being encountered more frequently among women with back pain than in those without.[103] However, there is some evidence that at least some of the back complaints associated with pregnancy can be avoided by instruction on back care.[104]

The more common image is heavy physical work, and especially if this involves lifting — which itself tends to be associated with twisting and bending. This is the foundation for campaigns of instruction in manual handling and lifting, although satisfactory evidence on the protective effect is not available.[105] More generally, physical work characterized by high energy demand is not consistently associated with back troubles.

We have already noted not only a relationship between dynamic loading and DD, but also how injury may play a part. The whole notion of injury to the back tends to be ill-defined, and inevitably it is also coloured by possibilities of fault and compensation. Slipping appears to be much more important than tripping as a cause of lumbosacral injury,[106] and falls are associated with longer absences from work and higher rates of recurrence of back pain.[107] However, the importance of what can perhaps be regarded as cultural factors is highlighted by the influence of repetitive work. There is a greater frequency of backache among assembly-line workers than in their colleagues employed in offices at the same plant,[108] although this only mirrors increases in sickness absence in general under such circumstances of work.

The other major class of condition is static loading, and this is influenced by posture. Backache appears to occur with increased frequency in those with sedentary occupations and in people in whom postures at work involve bending over. Prolonged sitting may be compounded by vibration, such as in vehicle driving,[109-111] but as with so much else the findings are not wholly consistent. For example, tractor drivers show no higher prevalence of low back pain than do non-driving farmworkers.[110] Whereas insufficient physical exercise may increase the risk of developing back troubles so, too, does the other extreme in certain sporting activities.[112,113]

Table 1.2 Measures of the frequency of experiences with back disorders (expressed as ratios per thousand population at risk for the year 1978* — from Wood[114])

Disorder	ICD rubric (8th revn)	GP consultations (home population)		Sickness incapacity certifications† (insured population)		Hospital attendances (home population)				Impaired persons (adults, >16 yr)		Deaths (home population)
		Consultations	Episodes	Spells	Days lost	outpatients New	Total	admissions	operations ‖	All degrees	Severe and v. severe	
Back troubles		81.7	43.7	20.68	738	8.5	33.5	0.86	0.07	2.00	0.20	0.0025
Sciatica	353	3.3	1.7	2.79	115	—	—	0.06	—	0.34	0.01	0.00002
Lumbago	717.0	15.3	9.1	3.56	72	—	—	—	—	—	—	0.002
Spondylosis	713.1	13.7	7.6	—	—	—	—	—	—	—	—	—
Displaced i-v disc	725	17.5	6.4	3.79	277	—	—	0.3	—	1.66	0.19	0.0002
Vertebrogenic pain	728 ex 728.9	10.9	5.4	3.54	120	—	—	0.5	—	—	—	0.0003
Other back pain	728.9	21.0	13.5	7.00	154	—	—	—	—	—	—	—
MUSCULOSKELETAL DISORDERS		310.1	74.3	71.17	3082	25.14	101.54	8.58	4.52	30.44	5.14	0.3
ALL DISEASES AND CONDITIONS (all medical and surgical conditions)		3009.6	1808.6‡ (571.7)	429.41	15191	157.07	691.45	89.7§	40.88	77.99	12.66	11.93

*Sizes of populations for computation of national experience in England and Wales — multiply rate shown by home population, $49.1 \times 49.1 \times 10^3$; insured population, 23.3×10^3. (All population figures are quoted in thousands.)

†Injury incapacity not included

‡Rate for episodes for all diseases & conditions inflated by persons with more than one episode, due to different causes; rate in parentheses is for patients consulting and is more useful for comparison with rates shown

§Hospital admissions for all diseases & conditions exclude maternity and those to psychiatric hospitals

‖Laminotomy and laminectomy (condensed operation list 0C2) for back troubles; all operations on musculoskeletal system includes list codes 002 and 093—106 (excluding amputations)

—Not separately identifiable in primary data source

A synthesis

How is one to seek enlightenment from this welter of information? A recurring theme is the notion that back pain is an epiphenomenon of cultural evolution of the human species. However, there is no agreement on what characteristic of this process might be implicated. It is likely that the complaint represents the resultant of a complex interplay of factors, such as has been reviewed by Wood.[1]

Within the heterogeneity of problems one can suggest at least two broad types of origin for common back pains, based on different patterns of occurrence with age.[47] Some individuals are affected in early maturity; their complaints may often be labelled as the disc syndrome, and it is in these people that the search for precipitating circumstances, especially mechanical factors, may well be most profitable. The other type of back pain tends to become progressively more of a problem with increasing age, and is often rather loosely designated as being degenerative. It is difficult to assess the importance of these considerations until better delineation of syndromes is possible.

THE COMMUNITY BURDEN

The impact of back pain was discussed in our earlier review,[2] and few of the estimates quoted then can be updated. Table 1.2 presents a summary of what information is available, the greatest loss being up-to-date data on incapacity for work which, since responsibility for benefits has been transferred to employers, are no longer strictly comparable.

Table 1.2 displays a greater variety of diagnostic labels than were reported in the previous edition of this book, but the broad patterns are much as we discussed before.[2] Overall back complaints were responsible for just under 5% of all time lost from work due to any cause of sickness. To offer an estimate for the cost of these absences to the economy as a whole has been rendered almost meaningless, due to the effects of both inflation and mounting unemployment.

The longest spells off work were experienced by those labelled as having a displaced disc followed, in descending order, by sciatica, vertebrogenic pain, other back pain and lumbago. Referral patterns to hospital do not appear to have altered. The new statistics introduced into Table 1.2 relate to mortality. Most of the deaths recorded are attributed to spondylosis rather than to the other, and much commoner, types of back disorder.

CONCLUSION

The amount of research effort devoted to investigation of back complaints is certainly increasing, as should be evident from the bibliography (as well as from the appearance of a third edition of this book). However, there is a disparate quality to much of this work, as we have indicated in our discussion. Certainly the magnitude of the problem, revealed by the various statistics, merits sustained commitment. In addition, it is to be hoped that more initiative will be directed to resolving inconsistencies in the evidence; at present these constitute a serious obstacle to deriving practical conclusions from work that has been done.

REFERENCES

1   Wood P H N 1980 Understanding back pain. In: Jayson M I V (ed) The lumbar spine and back pain, 2nd edn. Pitman Medical, Tunbridge Wells, ch 1, p 1–27
2   Wood P H N, Badley E M 1980 Epidemiology of back pain. In: Jayson M I V (ed) The lumbar spine and back pain, 2nd edn. Pitman Medical, Tunbridge Wells, ch 2, p 29–55
3   Wood P H N 1986 The basis of rheumatological practice, including nomenclature and classification. In: Scott J T (ed) Copeman's textbook of the rheumatic diseases, 6th edn. Churchill Livingstone, Edinburgh, ch 2

4   Wood P H N 1976 Osteoarthrosis in the community. In: Wright V (ed) Osteoarthrosis. Clin. Rheum. Dis. 2, ch 1, p 495–507
5   Acheson R M 1982 Heberden oration 1981: epidemiology and the arthritides. Ann. Rheum. Dis. 41: 325–334
6   Lawrence J S, Bremner J M, Bier F 1966 Osteoarthrosis: prevalence in the population and relationship between symptoms and X-ray changes. Ann. Rheum. Dis. 25: 1–24
7   Lawrence J S 1977 Rheumatism in populations. Heinemann Medical, London
8   Friberg S, Hirsch C 1948 Anatomical studies on lumbar disc degeneration. Acta Orthop. Scand. 17: 224–230

9   Atlas of standard radiographs of arthritis 1963 The epidemiology of chronic rheumatism, vol 2. Blackwell Scientific, Oxford

10   Frykholm R 1951 Lower cervical vertebrae and intervertebral discs: surgical anatomy and pathology. Acta Chir. Scand. 101: 345–359

11   Kellgren J H 1977 The anatomical source of back pain. Rheum. Rehab. 16: 3–12

12   Torgerson W R, Dotter W E 1976 Comparative roentgenographic study of the asymptomatic and symptomatic lumbar spine. J. Bone Jt Surg. 58A: 850–853

13   Office of Population Censuses and Surveys (OPCS) 1974 Morbidity statistics from general practice, second national study 1970–1971. The Royal College of General Practitioners, Office of Population Censuses and Surveys, and Department of Health and Social Security. Studies on Medical and Population Subjects No 26. HMSO, London

14   Lawrence J S 1969 Disc degeneration: its frequency and relationship to symptoms. Ann. Rheum. Dis. 28: 121–137

15   Julkunen H, Aromaa A, Knekt P 1981 Diffuse idiopathic skeletal hyperostosis (DISH) and spondylosis deformans as predictors of cardiovascular diseases and cancer. Scand. J. Rheum. 10: 241–248

16   Stewart T D 1966 Some problems in human palaeopathology. In: Jarcho S (ed) Human palaeopathology. Yale University Press, New Haven, p 43–55

17   Stoddard A, Osborn J F 1979 Scheuermann's disease or spinal osteochondrosis, its frequency and relationship with spondylosis. J. Bone Jt Surg. 61B: 56–58

18   Bull J, El Gamnal T, Pophan M 1969 A possible genetic factor in cervical spondylosis. Br. J. Radiol. 42: 9–16

19   Wood P H N 1972 Radiology in the diagnosis of arthritis and rheumatism. Trans. Soc. Occup. Med. 22: 69–73

20   Magora A, Schwartz A 1978 Relation between the low back pain syndrome and X-ray findings: 2 transitional vertebra (mainly sacralization). Scand. J. Rehab. Med. 10: 135–145

21   Magora A, Schwartz A 1980 Relation between the low back pain syndrome and X-ray findings: 3 spina bifida occulta. Scand. J. Rehab. Med. 12: 9–15

22   Julkunen H, Heinonen O P, Pyorala K 1971 Hyperostosis of the spine in an adult population, its relation to hyperglycaemia and obesity. Ann. Rheum. Dis. 30: 605–612

23   Forestier J, Lagier R 1971 Ankylosing hyperostosis of the spine. Clin. Orth. Rel. Res. 74: 65–83

24   Ott V R, Schwenkenbecher H, Iser H 1963 Die Spondylose bei Diabetes mellitus. Zeitschrift fur Rheumaforsch 22: 278–290

25   Julkunen H, Heinonen O P, Knekt P, Maatela J 1975 The epidemiology of hyperostosis of the spine together with its symptoms and related mortality in a general population. Scand. J. Rheum. 4: 23–27

26   Julkunen H, Knekt P, Aromaa A, Maatela J 1979 Heart disease and diffuse idiopathic skeletal hyperostosis in Finland. Abstracts of IX European Congress of Rheumatology, Wiesbaden, 385

27   Julkunen H, Knekt P, Aromaa A 1981 Spondylosis deformans and diffuse idiopathic skeletal hyperostosis (DISH) in Finland. Scand. J. Rheum. 10: 193–203

28   Kelsey J L, White A A 1980 Epidemiology and impact of low-back pain. Spine 5: 133–142

29   Wood P H N, Badley E M 1986 Epidemiology of individual rheumatic disorders. In: Scott J T (ed) Copeman's textbook of the rheumatic diseases, 6th edn. Churchill Livingstone, Edinburgh, ch 3

30   Critchley E M R 1982 Lumbar spinal stenosis. Br. Med. J. 284: 1588–1589

31   Porter R W, Hibbert C, Wellman P 1980 Backache and the lumbar spinal canal. Spine 5: 99–105

32   Currey H L F, Greenwood R M, Lloyd G G, Murray R S 1979 A prospective study of low back pain. Rheum. Rehab. 18: 94–104

33   Himsworth H 1969 Administration and the structure of scientific knowledge. Br. Med. J. 4: 517–522. (see also Himsworth H 1970 The development and organization of scientific knowledge. Heinemann, London)

34   Troup J D G 1965 Relation of lumbar spine disorders to heavy manual work and lifting. Lancet 1: 857–861

35   Troup J D G 1961 The significance of disc lesions. Lancet 2: 43–45

36   Strange F G St C 1966 Debunking the disc. Proc. Roy. Soc. Med. 59: 952–956

37   Nachemson A 1975 Towards a better understanding of low-back pain: a review of the mechanics of the lumbar disc. Rheum. Rehab. 14: 129–143

38   Nachemson A L, Schultz A B, Berkson M H 1979 Mechanical properties of human lumbar spine motion segments: influences of age, sex, disc level and degeneration. Spine 4: 1–8

39   Hult L 1954 Cervical, dorsal, and lumbar spinal syndromes. Acta Orth. Scand. Suppl 24: 174–175

40   Hult L 1954 The Munkfors investigation. Acta Orth. Scand. Suppl 16

41   Svensson H-O, Andersson G B J 1982 Low back pain in forty to forty-seven year old men: 1 frequency of occurrence and impact on medical services. Scand. J. Rehab. Med. 14: 47–53

42   Biering-Sørensen F, Hilden J 1984 Reproducibility of the history of low-back trouble. Spine 9: 280–286

43   Biering-Sørensen F 1983 A prospective study of low back pain in a general population: occurrence, recurrence and aetiology. Scand. J. Rehab. Med. 15: 71–79

44   Fry J 1972 Soft tissue rheumatism and the 'acute back' in general practice. In: Weber J C P (ed) Back pain and soft tissue rheumatism, Colloquium Proceedings No 1. Advisory Services (Clinical and General), London, p 8

45   Editorial 1976 Thoracic discs are different. Br. Med. J. 1: 608

46   Davis P, Lentle B C 1978 Evidence for sacroiliac disease as a common cause of low backache in women. Lancet 2: 496–497

47   Wood P H N, Badley E M 1980 Back pain in the community. In: Grahame R (ed) Low back pain. Clinics in Rheumatic Diseases 6: ch 1, p 3–16

48   Dixon A St J, Owen-Smith B D, Harrison R A 1972 Cold sensitive non-specific low back pain: a comparative trial of treatment. Clin. Trials J. 9: 16–21

49   Hasue M, Fujiwara M 1979 Epidemiologic and clinical studies of long-term prognosis of low-back pain and sciatica. Spine 4: 150–155

50   Pedersen P A 1981 Prognostic indicators in low back pain. J. Roy. Coll. Gen. Pract. 31: 209–216

51   Roland M O, Morrell D C, Morris R W 1983 Can general practitioners predict the outcome of episodes of back pain? Br. Med. J. 286: 523–525

52   Hull F M 1982 Diagnosis and prognosis of low back pain in three countries. J. Roy. Coll. Gen. Pract. 32: 352–356

53   Waddell G, Main C J, Morris E W, Venner R M, Rae P S, Sharmy S H, Galloway H 1982 Normality and reliability in the clinical assessment of backache. Br. Med. J. 284: 1519–1523

54   Glover J R 1960 Back pain and hyperaesthesia. Lancet 1: 1165–1169

55   Jayasinghe W J, Harding R H, Anderson J A D, Sweetman B J 1978 An electromyographic investigation of postural fatigue in low back pain — a preliminary study. Electrom. Clin. Neurophys. 18: 191–198

56   Sweetman B J, Page S, McMaster G W, Ellam S, Anderson J A D 1980 EMG correlates of low back pain work factor observations. In: Stott F D, Raftery E B, Goulding L (eds) ISAM 1979, proceedings of the third international symposium on ambulatory monitoring. Academic Press, London, p 433–439

57   Karvonen M J, Viitasalo J T, Komi P V, Nummi J, Jarvinen T 1980 Back and leg complaints in relation to muscle strength in young men. Scand. J. Rehab. Med. 12: 53–59

58   Sweetman B J, Anderson J A D 1975 Capillary resistance and back pain. Rheum. Rehab. 14: 1–6

59   Kirkaldy-Willis W H, Hill R J 1979 A more precise diagnosis for low-back pain. Spine 4: 102–109

60   Mantle M J, Greenwood R M, Currey H L F 1977 Backache in pregnancy. Rheum. Rehab. 16: 95–101

61   Pope M H, Wilder D G, Stokes I A F, Frymoyer J W 1979 Biomechanical testing as an aid to decision making in low-back pain patients. Spine 4: 135–140

62   Kvien T K, Nilsen H, Vik P 1981 Education and self-care of patients with low back pain. Scand. J. Rheum. 10: 318–320

63   Damlund M, Goth S, Hasle P, Munk K 1982 Low-back pain and early retirement among Danish semi-skilled constructive workers. Scand. J. Work Env. Health 8 Suppl 1: 100–104

64   Lehmann T R, Brand R A 1982 Disability in the patient with low back pain. Orth. Clin. N. Am. 13: 559–568

65   Hadler N M 1978 Legal ramifications of the medical definition of back disease. Ann. Int. Med. 89: 992–999

66   McGill C M 1968 Industrial back problems, a control program. J. Occup. Med. 10: 174–178

67   Andersson G B J 1981 Epidemiologic aspects on low-back pain in industry. Spine 6: 53–60

68   Kelsey J L, Ostfeld A M 1975 Demographic characteristics of persons with acute herniated lumbar intervertebral disc. J. Chron. Dis. 28: 37–50

69   Hrubec Z, Nashold B S Jr 1975 Epidemiology of lumbar disc lesions in the military in World War II. Am. J. Epid. 102: 366–376

70   Wood P H N, Badley E M 1983 An epidemiological appraisal of bone and joint disease in the elderly. In: Wright V (ed) Bone and joint disease. Churchill Livingstone, Edinburgh, ch 1, p 1–22

71   Lipscomb F M, Parnell R W 1954 The physique of Chelsea Pensioners. J. Roy. Army Med. Corps 100: 247–255

72   van Adrichem J A M, van der Korst J K 1973 Assessment of the flexibility of the lumbar spine, a pilot study in children and adolescents. Scand. J. Rheum. 2: 87–91

73   Moran H M, Hall M A, Barr A, Ansell B M 1979 Spinal mobility in the adolescent. Rheum. Rehab. 18: 181–185

74   Hilton R C, Ball J, Benn R T 1979 In-vitro mobility of the lumbar spine. Ann. Rheum. Dis. 38: 378–383

75   Taylor J, Twomey L 1980 Sagittal and horizontal plane movement of the human lumbar vertebral column in cadavers and in the living. Rheum. Rehab. 19: 223–232

76   Macrae I F, Wright V 1969 Measurement of back movement. Ann. Rheum. Dis. 28: 584–589

77   Moll J M H, Wright V 1971 Normal range of spinal mobility, an objective clinical study. Ann. Rheum. Dis. 30: 381–386

78   Hart F D, Strickland D, Cliffe P 1974 Measurement of spinal mobility. Ann. Rheum. Dis. 33: 136–139

79   Loebl W Y 1967 Measurement of spinal posture and range of spinal movement. Ann. Phys. Med. 9: 103–110

80   Troup J D G, Hood C A, Chapman A E 1968 Measurements of the sagittal mobility of the lumbar spine and hips. Ann. Phys. Med. 9: 308–321

81   Sweetman B J, Anderson J A D, Dalton E R 1974 The relationship between little-finger mobility, lumbar mobility, straight-leg raising and low back pain. Rheum. Rehab. 13: 161–165

82   Anderson J A D, Sweetman B J 1975 A combined flexi-rule/hydrogoniometer for measurement of lumbar spine and its sagittal movement. Rheum. Rehab. 14: 173–179

83   Kiernan P J 1981 Monitoring spinal movement relating to back pain. Rheum. Rehab. 20: 143–147

84   Lankhorst G J, van de Stadt R J, Vogelaar T W, van der Korst J K, Prevo A J H 1982 Objectivity and repeatability of measurements in low back pain. Scand. J. Rehab. Med. 14: 21–26

85   Biering-Sørensen F 1984 Physical measurements as risk indicators for low-back trouble over a one-year period. Spine 9: 106–119

86   Crown S 1978 Psychological aspects of low back pain. Rheum. Rehab. 17: 114–124

87   Rose H J 1975 The lives of patients before presentation with pain in the neck or back. J. Roy. Coll. Gen. Pract. 25: 771–772

88   Westrin C G, Hirsch C, Lindegard B 1972 The personality of the back patient. Clin. Orth. Rel. Res. 87: 209–216

89   Waddell G, McCulloch J A, Kummel E, Venner R M 1980 Nonorganic physical signs in low-back pain. Spine 5: 117–125

90   Westrin C G 1974 The reliability of auto-anamnesis, a study of statements regarding low back trouble. Scand. J. Soc. Med. 2: 23–35

91   Pope M H, Rosen J C, Wilder D G, Frymoyer J W 1980 The relation between biomechanical and psychological factors in patients with low-back pain. Spine 5: 173–178

92   Gilchrist I C 1976 Psychiatric and social factors related to low-back pain in general practice. Rheum. Rehab. 15: 101–107

93 Frymoyer J W, Pope M H, Costanza M C, Rosen J C, Goggin J E, Wilder D G 1980 Epidemiologic studies of low-back pain. Spine 5: 419–423

94 Gilchrist I C 1983 Psychological aspects of acute low back pain in general practice. J. Roy. Coll. Gen. Pract. 33: 417–419

95 Forrest A J, Wolkind S N 1974 Masked depression in men with low back pain. Rheum. Rehab. 13: 148–153

96 Stevenson H G 1970 Back injury and depression — a medico-legal problem. Med. J. Aus. 1: 1300–1302

97 Gilchrist I C 1983 Different groups of patients with low back pain. J. Roy. Coll. Gen. Pract. 33: 420–423

98 Magora A 1972 Investigation of the relation between low back pain and occupation: 3 Physical requirements — sitting, standing and weight lifting. Ind. Med. 41: 5–9

99 Svensson H-O 1982 Low back pain in forty to forty-seven year old men — ii socio-economic factors and previous sickness absence. Scand. J. Rehab. Med. 14: 55–60

100 Troup J D G 1968 The function of the lumbar spine. PhD thesis, University of London

101 Wood P H N, McLeish C L 1974 Statistical appendix. Digest of data on the rheumatic diseases: 5 Morbidity in industry, and rheumatism in general practice. Ann. Rheum. Dis. 33: 93–105

102 Cust G, Pearson J C G, Mair A 1972 The prevalence of low back pain in nurses. Intern. Nursing Review 19: 169–179

103 Frymoyer J W, Pope M H, Costanza M C, Rosen J C, Goggin J E, Wilder D G 1980 Epidemiologic studies of low-back pain. Spine 5: 419–423

104 Mantle M J, Holmes J, Currey H L F 1981 Backache in pregnancy II: prophylactic influence of back care classes. Rheum. Rehab. 20: 227–232

105 Glover J R 1971 Occupational health research and the problem of back pain. Trans. Soc. Occup. Med. 21: 2–12

106 Manning D P, Shannon H S 1981 Slipping accidents causing low-back pain in a gearbox factory. Spine 6: 70–72

107 Troup J D G, Martin J W, Lloyd D C E F 1981 Back pain in industry, a prospective survey. Spine 6: 61–69

108 Bergquist-Ullmann M, Larsson V 1977 Acute low back pain in industry. Acta Orth. Scand. Suppl 170

109 Kelsey J L, Hardy R J 1975 Driving of motor vehicles as a risk factor for acute herniated lumbar intervertebral disc. Am. J. Epidem. 102: 63–73

110 Auquier L, Henrard J C, Siaud J R 1981 Enquête contrôlée sur le rachis lombaire des tractoristes. In: Peyron J G (ed) Epidemiologie de l'arthrose, Symposium, Paris, 1980. Ciba Geigy, Pimart, Paris, p 172–179

111 Buckle P W, Kember P A, Wood A D, Wood S N 1980 Factors influencing occupational back pain in Bedfordshire. Spine 5: 254–258

112 Kelsey J L 1975 An epidemiological study of the relationship between occupations and acute herniated lumbar intervertebral discs. Intern. J. Epidem. 4: 197–205

113 Billings R A, Burry H C, Jones R 1977 Low back injury and sport. Rheum. Rehab. 16: 236–240

114 Wood P H N, Badley E M 1985 Musculoskeletal system. In: Holland W W (ed) Oxford textbook of public health. Oxford University Press, London, ch 15 (in press)

Back pain and occupation

INTRODUCTION

The control of infectious diseases, particularly in developed countries, has altered patterns of morbidity and focused attention on non-communicable diseases. Back pain is an important component of non-infectious morbidity, particularly in relation to sickness absence, job changes and early retirement among the working population. Concurrently, industry has become concentrated into large units where many workers carry out repetitive tasks as members of a team. It follows therefore that in addition to work loss and sickness absence there may be further reduction of output caused by a fall in work speeds. Sickness costs and those for early retirements nowadays cannot be measured solely in terms of compensation payments to the individual; they must also include the cost of losses from reorganization of staff and the deprivation effects on teams due to absence of a key member or the member's reduced efficiency through disability.[1]

Definition of syndromes

The problem of semantics, which used to bedevil research into rheumatic diseases as a whole, has been resolved to some extent in relation to the arthritides and many rare but nevertheless important diseases of connective tissue. In the field of back pain, however, chaos still reigns with rheumatologists, neurologists, orthopaedic surgeons, neurosurgeons, gynaecologists and psychiatrists, to say nothing of general physicians and surgeons all trying to classify according to their own nomenclatures. Many studies have been conducted in Britain under the auspices of the Arthritis and Rheumatism Council in Manchester,[2-6] Edinburgh[7-10] and at

Guy's Hospital.[11-13] These findings and reports from elsewhere in Europe, Japan and North America[14-19] confirm that the problem is substantial among the working population.

Unfortunately, the lack of standard definitions in these various studies means that comparisons are unreliable. Thus, classifications based entirely on a single criterion (e.g. structural defect, site of pain or disease label) are almost bound to result in a sizeable residue of 'other unspecified conditions'.[20]

Problems of surveys

Epidemiological aspects of back pain have already been considered in detail in Chapter 1; however, from an occupational point of view there are three areas of particular difficulty:

1. Intermittency of pain

Point prevalence studies in industry tend to be of limited value because of the intermittency of pain. Retrospective studies, usually depending on absence records or memory, tend to be unreliable, while cohort (prospective) studies may be costly to plan and follow through, particularly at a time of economic recession when large numbers of the work force may be forcibly retired — especially those with a history of repeated sickness absence such as may apply to employees with chronic pain.

2. Location of pain

The back extends from the neck to the coccyx. Low back pain (perhaps more accurately called lumbosacral pain) occurs below the 12th rib and above the gluteal folds, while upper back pain, sometimes divided into cervical and dorsal, is found between the occiput and the bottom of the rib cage: the term 'shoulder girdle pain' bridges the overlap between the lower cervical and upper dorsal vertebrae. All these areas, either singly or in combination, are involved in the performance of most work tasks and, though workers in heavy industry may make more demands on their backs in terms of muscular effort, there are others such as light sedentary jobs and housework where prolonged stooping or awkward posture may affect several regions of the back at the same time.

3. Diagnostic labels

The latest version of the International Classification of Diseases (ICD)[21] is substantially better than its predecessors in that conditions such as sciatica and lumbar neuralgia, which were previously classified with neurological conditions, have now been placed with other vertebrogenic syndromes in the rubrics relating to rheumatic diseases. As far as occupational factors are concerned, perhaps the most important groups excluded from the rheumatic section at the present time are those relating to congenital defects and acute injury; thus, unless a clear indication is given that the condition is *chronic*, such diagnoses as lumbosacral strain may have to be identified separately in routinely presented medical statistics. There also remains difficulty in distinguishing lumbosacral from cervicoscapular pain in cases diagnosed as having disc disease; there is also a problem in identifying those with back pain from among those diagnosed as having unspecified osteoarthorosis without engaging in a specially mounted study.[22]

RELATIONSHIPS BETWEEN BACK PAIN AND OCCUPATION

Against the foregoing background, this chapter will consider possible relationships between back pain and occupational factors under four main headings:

1. *Diagnosis*: Which disease and syndromes should be included under the heading of 'low back pain'?
2. *Effects*: To what extent are sickness absence, change of job, premature retirement and other manifestations due to the low back pain to which they are attributed?
3. *Cause*: Is there any relationship between the measurable effects of back pain in an occupational group and causal agents or risk factors in the working conditions of that group?
4. *Prevention and control*: Can environmental control at the place of work, health education, personnel selection or rehabilitation reduce the incidence of low back pain or limit the effects among those already afflicted?

DIAGNOSIS

The nomenclature of back pain is difficult to systematize.[23] One diagnostic problem relates to so-called non-articular rheumatism which makes up such a high proportion of pains in the back. Even in the Middle Ages many of the pains ascribed to rheumatism were acknowledged to be referred from painful lesions of the spinal joints.[24] Many modern rheumatologists share this view: some believe there is a relationship between surface pain and hyper-aesthesia of the skin, on the one hand, and nipping of the synovial membranes or tension of ligaments on the other.[25] Sensory fibres similar to those found in other joints exist in capsules of the discs themselves and of the intervertebral joints and also in the ligamentum flavum,[26,27] and Kellgren[28] has demarcated outlines of painful areas related to nerve roots caused by injections of hypertonic saline. A popular concept in Europe is that muscular rheumatism of the neck and back is probably separate from disc degeneration in the first instance but that the former moves progressively towards the latter as time passes.[29] This idea is supported in some measure by industrial surveys in Britain[8] and the United States[18] and if accepted can probably be applied also to low back pain.

Disease labels

While it must be admitted that some clearcut syndromes have emerged in recent years in relation to the nosology of low back pain, there has also been a tendency for disease labels to proliferate; many such labels merely indicate the site of pain, while others do not even achieve this. However well defined syndromes such as *fibrositis* may appear to some observers,[30] the term is still used loosely on sickness absence certificates to indicate vague pain in different parts of the body, thus converting the label into a diagnostic scrap-heap.[31] Accordingly, terms such as pain of undetermined diagnosis (PUD), although unsatisfactory to both clinician and epidemiologist, probably lead to less confusion in the long run than the use of labels which sound scientific but are applied inaccurately. Unfortunately, pain remains a subjective phenomenon, and the number who admit to having had back pain at some time in their lives can be raised to 100% if the specificity of criteria for inclusion is broad enough.[32]

Prevalence

Statistical information published by government departments does not give a detailed breakdown of all diagnoses associated with low back pain.[21,23,33] Specific surveys are also difficult to compare in the absence of agreed semantics. However, a guide to the size of the problem based on one study of males in Britain from a range of occupations is shown in Figure 2.1.[12] Back pain was recorded in 30%, and low back (lumbosacral) pain either as disc disease or PUD in 76% of these (i.e. 23% of the sample).

Figure 2.2 shows how the prevalence of rheumatic complaints as a whole was found to increase up to the age of 55 and fall away slightly thereafter. Disc disease also increases with age, while low back PUD is less consistent, the prevalence rates falling off in later life. Lumbosacral pain as a whole has a fairly steady prevalence rate between the ages of 25 and 65 years in this group of workers. However, absolute increases in prevalence of other rheumatic diseases (particularly osteoarthrosis) over the age of 50 mean that, whereas lumbosacral pain accounts for 70% of rheumatic pains in those under 20, and 67% among the 25–30 age bracket, the proportion falls to 43% in men over 55 years of age. It is clear from these observations that any attempt to relate back pain to occupation must make allowance for differences that may exist in the ages of the working groups being studied.

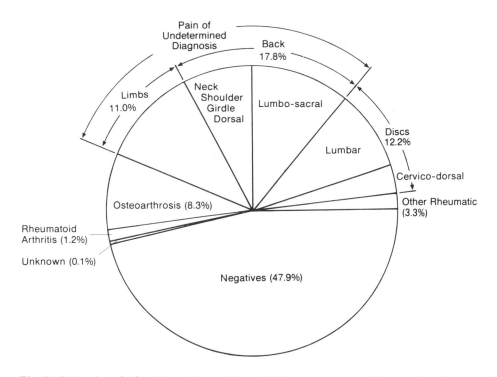

Fig. 2.1 Back pain and other rheumatic complaints in 2684 male employees. 44 men had multiple complaints

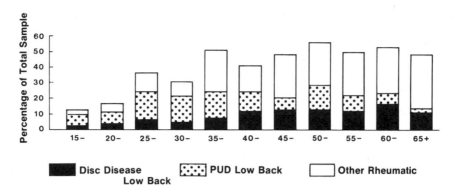

Fig. 2.2 Positives and lumbosacral pain by age (2684 male manual workers)

EFFECTS OF BACK PAIN

Sickness absence

Sickness absence is probably the most important effect of back pain in the working population, and brief reference has already been made to this in relation to Western Europe[12,14] and North America.[18]

In a review of the impact of musculoskeletal disorders on the population of the United States using data from the social security administration[34] and the National Center for Health Statistics,[35] Kelsey and others emphasized the importance of low back pain as a cause of limitation of activity and the award of disability allowances.[36] Impairments of the back and spine were recorded as the most frequent causes of limitation of activity in persons of less than 45 years of age and ranked third after heart disease and arthritis and rheumatism in those aged between 45 and 64 years. It was estimated that a total of eight million people in the United States had impairments arising from disorders of the back and spine and that displacement of intervertebral discs accounted for about 5% of those granted disability allowances.

In Canada an initial report that about 12 000 claims in respect of low back pain were accepted annually by the Workman's Compensation Board[37] was subsequently amended[38] to 48 839 low back injuries reported in a year.

Chaffin[39] looked specifically at back pain caused by overexertion and injury. He claimed that 27% of all industrial injury and illness leading to compensation were due to overexertion from lifting, pushing, carrying or a combination of these and that

some industries had much higher rates than others. Thus machine metal workers and those working in knitting mills, chemical industries and motor tyre manufacturing, as well as those employed in health and social services, had higher than average records of injuries being ascribed to overexertion, sprains and strains.

Although back pain occurs with dramatic suddenness in some cases, it is more often a long drawn-out process with intermittent absence over many years.[23] This can be illustrated by comparing routinely collected data with that available from special studies. Thus insurance certificates were used by Wood and his colleagues[5,6] to calculate work loss in the United Kingdom attributable to back pain. They reported an annual loss of 747 days per 1000 employed males, a figure that included some industrial injuries. Part of these data had to be estimated or obtained specially from the Department of Health and Social Security (DHSS), as it is not customary to break down some of the rubrics of the ICD in routine presentation of statistics relating to sickness absence. It is also clear that some widely-embracing diagnostic labels used on sickness certificates do not give an immediate indication of whether or not back pain is a significant feature. It seems possible, therefore, that routine use of the ICD will result in an underestimate of lost days.

In order to assess the size of these errors a detailed study of sickness absence was carried out prospectively in Edinburgh on a cohort of 1249 manual workers over a period of one year. This indicated that certificates for disc disease and identifiable back pain accounted for 77.5 per cent of the 2132 days of absence (1707 days per 1000 men) in which back pain was a demonstrable cause of sickness absence (Table 2.1).

often a cause. In Ontario, 10% of men with low back pain receiving workmen's compensation had been disabled for more than six weeks,[43] while 21 out of 23

Table 2.1 Annual sickness absence (certificated) among 1249 mixed manual workers

Cause of absence	Men (rate/1000)	Spells (rate/1000)	Days (rate/1000)
Disc disease	29 (23.2)	73 (58.4)	903 (723.0)
Other identifiable back pain	38 (30.4)	40 (32.0)	749 (599.7)
Other rheumatic complaints	14	19	480
a. Masking back pain	(11.2)	(15.2)	(384.3)
b. *Not* back pain	15 (12.0)	20 (16.0)	484 (387.5)
Other diagnoses			
a. Men with back pain in the past year	108 (86.5)	174 (139.3)	5 254 (4 206.6)
b. Men without back pain in the past year	344 (275.4)	440 (352.3)	11 708 (9 373.9)
Total sickness absence	517* (413.9)	766 (613.3)	19 578 (15 674.9)

*31 men with rheumatic absence had other illnesses as well.

Further possibilities of under-recording relate to the former '3-day rule' (by which benefit in the UK was not paid until absence had lasted at least 3 days) and the current policy of self-certification for periods of up to 7 days. In relation to this possible source of error, a study of 6892 postmen showed that uncertificated absence from back pain at all sites computed over a period of one year added a further 508 days to the certificated total of 11 446, thus raising the annual total from 1661 to 1735 days per 1000 postmen in the study.[40]

Even allowing for the fact that these sickness surveys relate to manual workers and that the pattern of absence is different in the non-manual group[41,42] it would seem reasonable to conclude that on a national basis more than half the absence ascribed to rheumatic complaints as a whole is likely to be due to back pain. This would mean a probable loss in the UK of something in excess of 15 million work days per annum from this cause, with an equivalent loss of 60 million work days in the USA.

Long-term handicap

Chronic absence is likely to lead to prolonged or permanent unemployment, and low back pain is

men with back pain at all sites in Edinburgh who had been out of work for at least three months ascribed their long unemployment to this cause.[44] Unfortunately, reliability is suspect in such studies since the size of payments may depend on the history. Fear of sanctions is more likely to lead to inaccuracy than ignorance, since most disabled people have a reasonably accurate knowledge of their diagnosis, even though they may be uncertain of the underlying pathological processes.[45]

By no means all sickness absence results in long-term handicap (particularly the component which is uncertificated). However, it would seem reasonable to infer that hospital admission, work absence of six weeks or more, or pain lasting at least a year which has either been continuous or of increasing severity and for which medical advice has been sought during that year would qualify in this respect. Table 2.2 shows how these criteria for low back pain were applied and recorded in the 2684 manual workers described above.

Substitution

Periods of absence which are ascribed to a disease need not always be caused by that disease. Thus, doctor, patient, or both may be influenced by previous episodes. Mild back pain which in another individual would be accepted as part of a systematic disorder, such as a viral infection, may be designated as 'lumbago' in someone with a history of this disorder, thus giving an exaggerated picture of absence from this cause. However, it is possible to infer the extent to which back pain may have been used as a substitute for more general sickness absence rates of those known to have back pain and those claiming that they have never had this affliction.

Figure 2.3 shows the weeks of absence over a one-year period for employed men in five age groups. Sickness rates for illnesses other than 'rheumatism' in men with back pain are either similar to or slightly higher than the equivalent rates for those free from rheumatic complaints up to the age of 45 years. Above that age, and particularly in the age group 55–65. the reverse applies, a change that may possibly have been caused by some substitution in those recognized as having chronic back pain.

However, the total absence is higher at all ages for those with back pain than for those without.

Findings such as these have been noted in several occupations.[7,9,41,46] In addition, it is known that factors other than substitution affect sickness absence, particularly when this absence is ascribed to a chronic disease: these include length of service and prolonged nightshift work.[47-49] It is also well known that retrospective studies of sickness absence without the back-up of certificates result in gross inaccuracy because of memory failure on the part of workers.[50]

Demands for medical care

About half those with low back pain limit their care to self-treatment. Furthermore the requirement to support sickness absence (from low back pain or any other cause) by a medical certificate after seven days of absence means that consultations with general practitioners are often made solely for this purpose. Hospital referral, on the other hand, suggests a more

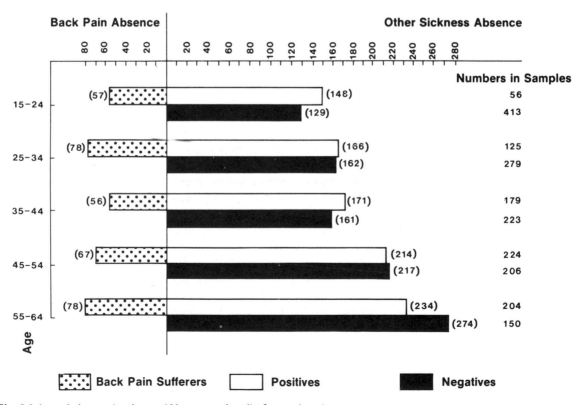

Fig. 2.3 Annual absence (weeks per 100 men employed) of manual workers

serious level of incapacity, while hospital admission may reasonably be deemed to be associated with substantial handicap, as has already been discussed (see Table 2.2). Table 2.3 shows the proportions of those with low back pain who reported self-treatment, visited their general practitioner or had hospital contacts during a year of study. It also shows, as would be expected, that such demands for medical care are more frequently made by those with disc disease than with vague back pains.

Table 2.2 Low back pain (2684 mixed manual workers)

Hospital admission	33
Absence 6/52 +	42
Severe symptoms 1 year + consultation	44
(Continuous pain 23	
Increasing severity 21)	
Two of above criteria	27
Three of above criteria	5
	151 (5.6%)

Change of job

Prolonged or repeated absences can force a man to change jobs, particularly manual workers in inclement conditions. Change can be made within the same industry;[7,8] this is likely to be easier in large industrial concerns than among smaller workforces, since the former have scope for absorbing their own disabled staff. However, suggestion or auto-suggestion has to be considered in relation to retrospective surveys concerned with change of employment. It is more creditable to ascribe change to a physical disability such as low back pain, which fulfils the criteria of medical respectability,[51] rather than admit that emotional, intellectual or social inadequacy might be the dominant factor in bringing about the change. Obviously there is a psychological component in all work situations, and it is well nigh impossible to measure the extent to which back pain, without obvious deformity, may lead to a change of job in any particular individual. Matched-pair studies in a naval dockyard,[8] suggest that the number of employees who change are comparable among those with and without back pain.

By contrast,[7] face workers in a coal mine with back pain, particularly those with disc disease, reported a higher rate of changing jobs (either within the colliery or elsewhere) than those who have never had back pain.

CAUSES OF BACK PAIN

Occupational trauma

Some colourful descriptions for painful conditions of the back, such as maltsman's monkey or weaver's bottom, have occupations incorporated in their titles. These lesions and others can be brought on by repetitive movements commonly, though not exclusively, associated with work; others can result from overindulgence in hobbies or sports after prolonged periods of inactivity. In addition, it is generally accepted that violent trauma may damage cartilage and cause osteoarthrosis,[52] whence it is but a short step to postulating that prolonged heavy manual work may encourage the development of degenerative changes in the joints. Furthermore, if these changes are part of the process of ageing, it would be fair to assume that they might occur at an earlier age among those doing heavy manual work,[53] though other predisposing factors are known to play a part in the aetiology.[54]

Table 2.3 Demands for medical care due to disc disease and PUD of the low back (2684 male manual workers)

	Disc disease	PUD	Total %
	%	%	
Self-treatment	122 (51.3)	95 (25.4)	217 (35.5)
Attended GP's surgery	109 (45.8)	115 (30.7)	224 (36.6)
Attended hospital	94 (39.5)	41 (11.0)	135 (22.1)
Admitted to hospital	30 (12.6)	3 (0.8)	33 (5.4)
Total affected	238 (100)	374 (100)	612 (100)

Acute trauma

Every clinician encountering patients with back pain knows that there are episodes of incapacity that can be attributed to acute injuries, twists or sprains. An unexpectedly heavy weight may result in acute trauma if supporting musculature is caught off guard. A similar result may follow if someone tries to lift an unduly heavy object with his or her back in a position of undue vulnerability, (e.g. with legs straight and back fully flexed).[55] Analysis of 130 referrals to a back-pain clinic revealed that there were 59 (46%) with a history of precipitating injury or short-term overindulgence in unaccustomed activity in association with their first attack.[56] However, there are obvious pitfalls. Patients from industry need a history of precipitating injury to qualify for higher benefit rates and compensation; even when this is not a feature, most patients like to have a clear starting point to their problem and tend to identify a causal injury. By way of contrast, minor trauma resulting in transitory discomfort will be forgotten almost at once, thus making it difficult to estimate the number of negative controls when trying to conduct a retrospective study to clarify this point.

The importance of acute trauma as a cause of chronic low back pain remains a matter of doubt in many cases, and the view of Rowe[57] that only about 4% of back pain patients have symptoms induced by immediate trauma may well be nearer the truth than many authorities would like to believe.

Stresses and strains

The distinction between spinal osteoarthrosis and degenerative disc disease is more dependent on nosology than on generally accpepted criteria. Those suffering from generalized osteoarthrosis may have spinal manifestations, particularly when associated with heavy lifting or injuries.[3] It has also been suggested that head loads might account for a relatively higher prevalence of cervical disc disease in a Jamaican as opposed to an English population, particularly as lumbar disc disease was similar in the two groups.[58]

Complex forces operate on lumbar discs during rotational movements and lifting weights while in the stooping position, and the difficulties of measuring the real pressure, for instance on disc L4/5, when a man is doing heavy manual work, are considerable.[59,60] Also, accurate measurements of the effects of prolonged effort on the different components of an intervertebral disc and its related vertebrae, to say nothing of the apophyseal joints, require complex techniques.[61,62] Normal radiological films are of little help; for instance, one study[63] indicated no difference in the X-ray appearances of discs in the recumbent and upright positions in 24 of 35 patients with definite disc disease. This is hardly surprising, since a weight of 100 kg on vertebrae can compress the space of a healthy disc by about 1 mm and cause lateral bulging of 0.5 mm;[26] for damaged discs the figures were 1.5–2 mm compression and 1 mm lateral bulging. These changes are unlikely to be discernible by radiology except under artificially controlled conditions. However, modern techniques hold out hope of demonstrating degenerative changes including minifractures.[64,65] Cineradiology has also been used and is helpful in showing apophyseal malalignments in the cervical region.[66] Disc bulging or compression is less obvious in the lumbar region, and in any event the use of this technique for research purposes, particularly in the lower back, raises ethical questions of dosage.

Chaffin and co-workers[39,67-70] have evolved a technique for calculating what they call lifting strength ratios (LSR) based on each weight lifted in the job and the predicted lifting strength of large/strong men in various postures. They have shown that back pain has a higher incidence rate among those who are required to lift weights in manual materials handling which make maximum demands in terms of lifting strength. They have also stressed the importance of load position in relation to the weight-bearing axis of the body.

The methods and calculations of this technique are impressive, as are the correlations between back pain and high LSR. However, the difficulty of relating laboratory measurements to the working situation and also the problem of compounding variables discussed earlier in this section may be factors which have enabled many employers to evade the issue in terms of adapting tasks to suit the workforce.

It may be that other ways of considering muscular strain with consequent back pain which can be applied in the working situation will have to be used in combination with the calculation of LSR to drive home the point. Such techniques might include the study of changes in intra-abdominal pressure using balloons, or in more modern terms, radio pills to postulate that pressure changes might be related to effort by the lumbar as well as by the abdominal muscles[71,72] — particularly as it has been shown[73] that intradiscal pressure on lifting a load varies with the posture of the trunk and the position of the load in relation to the axis of the spine. However, cautious interpretation is necessary because abnormal tension on the walls of a viscus can cause backache associated with dyspepsia.

Posture

With correct posture it is possible to carry weights considerably in excess of the maximum recommended by the International Labour Office,[74] particularly if the individual is in training through regular experience as, for instance, meat porters and jute stackers, who frequently carry weights of 100 kg or more for short distances. At the other end of the scale, lifting an unexpectedly light weight when the spinal musculature has been braced for a heavy one can also result in severe back pain and prolonged incapacity.

Stooping alone without any lifting requirement may also cause sudden pain, though it is difficult to assess the extent to which this happens in a subject who does not have predisposing degenerative changes, even though these may not be discernible by present-day methods of investigation.

Studies of e.m.g. tracings using intramuscular electrodes introduced by hollow needles[75,76] and surface electrodes[77] indicate that prolonged stooping, especially if this is oblique to the sagittal axis of the spine, causes changes in EMG patterns of the antigravity muscles. If, as seems reasonable, these changes are an indication of muscle fatigue, then the forces acting against gravity will become increasingly directed at the other spinal tissues such as ligaments which are more vulnerable to stretching and subsequent laxity. Under such circumstances this may lead to minor malalignments of the apophyseal joints, resulting in osteoarthrosis and chronic backache in the long term, while transient nipping of synovial tissue may also cause acute episodes of pain.

Vibration

The jarring effects of substandard suspension may be relevant in those whose occupations require higher than average exposures to this hazard. This issue has been studied in general terms by Griffin and colleagues,[78] while claims have also been made that vibration may be relevant to the production of back-pain problems in tractor drivers.[79–81] In support of this idea Stayner and others[82] have studied vibration simulation as an aid to tractor design.

Types of work and back pain

Various surveys suggest that men whose jobs make the greatest demands on the lower back in terms of muscular effort have a relatively high prevalence of disc disease. Similar findings can be demonstrated for rheumatic complaints in general, but not for PUD of the back. Stooping for long periods has also been shown to be associated with a high prevalence of back pain spasm in relation to disc disease rather more than PUD; however, prolonged standing shows no such correlation.[83] Those in sedentary occupations also tend to have a higher prevalence of all types of back pain than those whose jobs involve standing or walking about. Further, this trend is not confined to those with disc disease, nor is it clear whether those with back pain elect to do sedentary work or that the easy life itself (possibly in a poorly designed chair) contributes to the onset.[12]

Back pain is also slightly commoner among indoor as opposed to outdoor workers,[8] but this may be an artefact caused either by self-selection or by enforced change from outdoor to indoor environment at a much earlier date by those starting to have chronic back pain.

One of the problems of trying to relate back pain to occupational activities is that there are often several hazards associated with particular jobs. Thus, coal miners[7,18,19] have to undertake heavy lifting and may also have to adopt awkward postures while doing so.

Stooping is also a feature of some agricultural tasks. In the case of outdoor workers, such as those engaged in the manual picking of brussel sprouts, there may be the added factor of exposure to cold and damp. However, even without such exposure (as in glasshouse workers), it has been shown that strawberry pickers who stoop have significantly more back pain than in those who stand, such as aubergine (eggplant) pickers.[84]

Many tractor drivers have to face inclement working conditions, but they also have to contend with vibration problems as discussed above. However, in addition other factors may contribute to the overall increased incidence of back pain among such workers.[85] Thus access to the cab may result in stretching lesions of spinal ligaments.[86] Also, spinal rotation may cause chronic strain, as when the work requires the driver to look behind him for long periods from a seat which does not swivel.[87] Even without these factors the positioning of pedals and the strength required for their operation have been suggested as potential hazards in relation to the onset of back pain.[88]

The extent to which posture while driving other vehicles such as cars or lorries contributes to back pain is also difficult to assess. However, age-specific complaint rates in postmen drivers are higher than among those with no driving commitments.[89] Also at the clinical level, it is well recognized that long car journeys can precipitate attacks and aggravate chronic pain, particularly if the front seat has limited capacity for adjustment and the relative size of driver and cabin space are such that undue flexion of knees and hips is required, or it is necessary to stretch in order to reach pedals and gear lever.

Housewives form yet another important occupational group who have multiple risk factors. They have to lift many and varied weights, often unassisted and without the protection of safety officers or trade union officials. They also have to stand for long periods at work surfaces which are seldom designed for individual requirements as far as heights are concerned. It is difficult to assess the size of the disability problem in housewives, since, being uninsured, they do not have spells of certificated sickness. Furthermore, it is logistically much more difficult to carry out surveys involving direct observation techniques on cohorts of housewives than it is to observe factory or office workers.

Even if it were possible to limit the risk factors associated with the job, there is a further difficulty associated with using industrial groups to study diseases in relation to physical requirements. Unfortunately for epidemiologists and ergonomists, not all workers with the same designated occupation perform tasks in the same way in terms of such factors as posture or load-carrying. A possible way to overcome this difficulty is to link studies of back pain with job analyses based on personal observations of men in their working situations.[12]

However, continuous direct observation of individual workers is not only very expensive but is likely to lead to changes in working patterns and habits on the part of those being observed. Furthermore, minor changes in forward or lateral adjustments of the relative position of loads to the axis of the spine may well pass unnoticed by the human observer and, as mentioned above, the resulting changes in posture may lead to alterations in intradiscal pressure and e.m.g. activity. There are also ethical and logistic difficulties in using intradiscal manometry or needle electrodes for recording e.m.g.s at the workbench.

Accordingly, continuous observation using less direct methods has been develloped so that tasks within a job profile which may be potentially hazardous can be identified and, where necessary, modified. Several instrumental methods of measuring movement and muscular effort of the lower back are available. One such is depicted in Figure 2.4.

Surface electrodes are placed over the two lumbar masses and the inclinometers over the sacrum

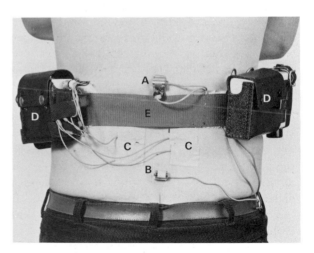

Fig. 2.4 Device for ambulatory recording of posture and effort by low back while at work; **A** dual inclinometer measuring antero-postero and lateral flexion at T12; **B** inclinometer measuring antero-postero flexion over sacrum; **C** paired surface electrodes measuring e.m.g. of lumbar muscles; **D** slow-running tape-recorders in parallel; **E** belt for supporting recorders; antenna for recording transmissions from intra-abdominal radio pill is carried on front of belt.

(measuring hip flexion) and the upper lumbar spine — the difference between the readings being a measure of lumbar flexion. Simultaneous recordings of intra-abdominal pressure are obtained from a swallowed radio pressure pill.[90] This apparatus can be worn for a full work shift of 8 hours and continuous readings recorded on slow-running tape-recorders, with subsequent analysis of readings by computer.[91,92] Examples are shown in Figure 2.5.

Less direct methods of gauging differences between jobs may also be obtained by assessing limb activities through the use of pedometers or actimeters attached to the limbs.[93]

Conclusions about the cause of back pain in relation to occupation

Although there is reasonable agreement that frank injury, malalignment or deformity may predispose to disc degeneration in some cases, the possibility that heavy work without injury might cause disc changes is disputed by many observers.[19,94–96] In other words, the relationship between trauma and disc disease is less clearcut than for osteoarthrosis of the limbs.

In spite of these reservations, many observers accept that the comparatively high prevalence of disc

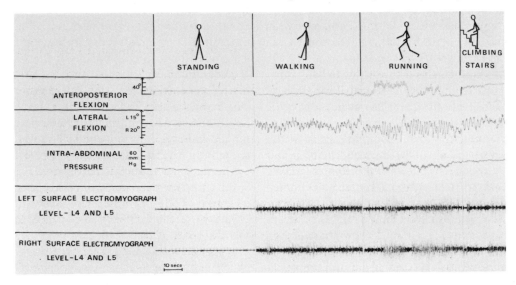

Fig. 2.5a Normal activities of stance and gait

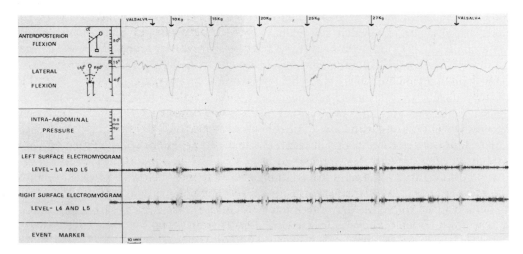

Fig. 2.5b Valsalva and weight-lifting 10–27 kg

disease among those who have been engaged in heavy manual work and its onset at an earlier age are strong presumptive evidence of a causal relationship. Less certain are the links between muscular effort at work and the onset of PUD, even though it seems reasonable to assume that, if these pains are precursors of osteoarthrosis/disc disease, then it should be possible to demonstrate a relationship between heavy work and the prevalence of PUD.

However controversial the relationship between occupation and the spinal changes associated with back pain, there is general agreement about sickness absence. Published results from the survey units of the Arthritis and Rheumatism Council in Edinburgh and Manchester, and other sources, particularly in Scandinavia, the United States and Canada and Japan, to which reference has been made,[2-19,34-39] all indicate that sickness absence ascribed to back pain is substantially higher in jobs associated with heavy physical effort than among workers performing light tasks.

Evidence published about complaint rates is far from conclusive, and when complaints are standardized for age distribution among different groups of workers, then the correlations become even more tenuous. However, jobs involving heavy muscular effort by the back over long periods and sudden or unexpected movements in circumstances where the spinal muscles are untrained or unprepared can be regarded as likely risk factors in the onset of back pain. Prolonged stooping or other awkward posture (including possibly sitting in unsuitable chairs) may well be additional factors, though the evidence is less convincing.

PREVENTION AND CONTROL OF LOW BACK PAIN IN RELATION TO OCCUPATION

Many of the studies mentioned so far have suggested that back pain is occupationally linked. It seems logical, therefore, to consider how its onset may be prevented or delayed. Should a school-leaver be compelled to attend a course on posture and lifting techniques? Should a man with spondylolisthesis be advised to keep away from coalmining? Can we identify all the changes that will predict a serious outcome unless evasive action is taken?

In theoretical terms it should be possible to prevent at least some of the disastrous consequences of low back pain in the working population by one of two techniques: primary prevention, which implies action to ensure that a disease does not occur, and secondary prevention, which seeks to identify symptoms or presymptomatic changes including predisposing conditions at a stage where therapeutic action will be effective. In practical terms, however, the two stages in the preventive process tend to become blurred in relation to most painful conditions of the back. Furthermore, neither method on its own is entirely effective, nor are the two when taken in combination.

Primary prevention: maximum loads

Regulations about weight-lifting are often rather indecisive, centring round the generalization that no one should be required to handle a load of such a weight that it is likely to cause injury. However, specific industries have quite well defined limits, particularly when applied to young people, and there is general agreement with the suggested maxima of 25 kg (compact load) for youths and an arbitrary maximum of 58 kg overall.[97]

Because of the multiplicity of factors associated with the onset of back pain to which reference has already been made, the pragmatic attitude that the job has to be done as economically as possible tends to prevail, with a reluctance to spend money on expensive adaptations to job specifications. Indeed, recent attempts in the UK to draw up guidelines or even introduce regulations on weight-lifting in general have led to considerable resistance by employers on the grounds that the current evidence, though suggestive, does not yet have enough precision in respect of relative risk. It follows that specific regulations are open to challenge, while those of a more general nature are merely going to act as a pretext for litigation by the unscrupulous. Furthermore, there still appears to be a wide gap between the view that there should be restrictions in relation to manual lifting by imposing an arbitrarily determined maximum weight and the general acceptance that prolonged heavy lifting of lesser weights might hasten the onset of degenerative changes.[98]

Despite these difficulties some encouragement

can perhaps be gleaned from the increasing interest in the United States of actuarial assessment of claims for compensation in association with back pain.[99,100] This, as well as increasing social concern with the passage of time, may see a greater acceptance of the idea that men should be assessed for their strength capacity and that tasks should be assessed for their load demands.[67,68]

Until there is more widespread acceptance of the evidence which has been discussed in this chapter, it will be necessary to continue to practise prevention by education and encouragement. Physical effort, especially when it is sustained for long periods or is carried out in awkward stooping postures, does appear to result in significantly higher proportions of disc disease, but not with the less definitive forms of back pain. Furthermore, there is a high amount of sickness absence associated with both these conditions, particularly among those engaged in tasks which make heavy demands on the back. The demonstrable effects on the trunk of handling heavy loads in different postures[101] provide strong support for the view that special instruction should be given to those lifting and handling heavy and bulky loads so as to reduce injury from such causes.

A booklet circulated by the Industrial Welfare Society[102] is one convenient way of disseminating this information to all load-handlers. In addition, modification of loads (where this is possible) is probably advisable, but neither instructions nor modified loads alone or in combination provide the whole answer. Wherever the industrial concern is large enough, a specially-appointed instructor may be justified,[103] but this can hardly be regarded as a practical solution for smaller organizations. Limited evaluation has suggested that absence due to back pain can be reduced by systematic instruction,[104] but the experiment could bear repeating in a wider range of occupations before such instruction could be justified in terms of statutory requirements.

One of the difficulties about theoretical and even practical teaching is that there may be a failure to take account of the combination of awkward posture and weight distribution facing the individual in the working situation. Thus, instruction in lifting a compact 25 kg crate from an even surface has only limited application if the same weight is distributed in bulky form and has to be manhandled from the bottom of a ship's hold where the, docker finds himself obliged to stand with his legs apart and perhaps with one leg higher than the other. Similarly, the high prevalence rate of disc disease among coal miners engaged on work away from the coal face[7] may well be attributable to sudden (though not necessarily very great) demands for effort by unaccustomed lumbar muscles. It is possible that these problems may be resolved by further ergonomic research based on continuous monitoring to which reference has already been made.[71,83,93]

Wall posters[105] may be helpful in supplementing formal courses of instruction, and to a limited extent they may be useful on their own. Unfortunately, diagrams depicting the correct way to carry out procedures may lose credibility if they appear to be impractical to those performing the tasks on a day-to-day basis, and one such diagram may bring discredit on several others in a series which has overall potential usefulness.

Another method of primary prevention in relation to the onset of back pain in employees would be to modify conditions of work. Factors that have been given special consideration in this respect are those relating to climatic conditions. As already discussed (see page 24), there appears to be general agreement that the prevalence of back pain (as distinct from sickness absence) is affected little if at all by climatic conditions. There is thus insufficient evidence at present to support the view that low back pain could be prevented or even reduced mainly by encouraging more people to seek indoor employment. On the other hand, it is quite common for a worker engaged in a hot, sweaty job to blame an episode of low back pain on exposure to a draught or cold on his back while he was overheated.

Training in posture and advice in respect of daily living including housework, driving, recreational activities and relaxation, whether seated or in bed, by films[106] or booklets[107] can be used to add interest to these aspects of health education. Unfortunately, the ideas promolgated by these methods tend to follow well-established doctrines for preventing back problems, and many have little or no basis in terms of scientific observation and trials.

Pre-employment screening for predictive factors

Low back pain is an important cause of industrial compensation in the United States[108,109] because employers can be held responsible for allowing those with known defects to undertake potentially hazardous activities; one estimate[110] puts the cost of non-skeletal back injuries at nearly US$25 million in New York State in one year. However, one attempt to reduce this litigiously-induced hazard resulted in 1181 of a total of 4103 potential employees being rejected for production work.[100,111] Such rigid exclusions may be justified[112-115] if the aim is merely to reduce successful claims, but unless alternative employment can be found, these measures are not necessarily in the best interests of those trying to support a family. This is particularly true of those with minor deformities, since only a limited number can be expected to succumb to severe back pain.

If routine examinations of the back were to be made, it is possible (at least under existing statutory and voluntary insurance schemes in Britain and the United States) that early identification of changes could prove to be contrary to the interests of manual workers. This is because there may be an adverse effect on a claim where it can be shown that signs were demonstrable in advance of the event which is alleged to be responsible for the onset of symptoms.

Another possible predictive factor that has been studied is the range of movement of the spine, and in particular the lumbar segment — the modified Schober test[116,117] (see also Chapter 11). Indeed, Beiring-Sorensen[118] makes such a claim, but the known effects of age, race and length of the lumbar spine[119] suggest that caution should be used in relation to this predictor at the present time. The indications appear to be that, while the range of movement of the lumbar spine may be useful in assessing clinical progress in some patients with painful symptoms, the technique has a disappointingly low sensitivity and specificity as a predictor of future episodes in those who in other respects appear to be healthy.[118]

Claims have also been made that those with a narrowed lumen of the spinal canal are more likely to suffer from back pain than those with wider canals.[120] It has been suggested that this is particularly likely because a trefoil-shaped canal allows minimal additional intrusion before the nerve roots become compressed.[121] It has also been claimed that a higher proportion of those with back pain attending hospital have narrow canals, as gauged by ultrasonography, than a control population.[122] The

technique for measurement requires special training to ensure reproducibility, but if a cohort study in the mining industry which is currently being undertaken confirms the findings prospectively, then the method may have potential as a predictive factor.

More difficult to evaluate prospectively is the significance of spondylolisthesis in the onset of low back pain. There is general agreement that many cases of low back pain are associated with this condition[123] and that those involved in heavy manual work are likely to be at risk from such a development. However, there are few reliable clinical signs demonstrable in advance, while the, routine use of X-rays as part of a pre-employment examination schedule with the special requirements needed to detect the condition[124] would seem to be unjustified at the present time.

Early detection of progressive disease

An alternative to initial examination is to make routine checks at intervals on employees to discover disease early: the idea being to treat the disease successfully or modify activity so that the consequences are either reduced in severity or delayed in their progress. The value of this technique is generally unimpressive as far as low back pain is concerned.[125,126] However, there is an increasing body of opinion which takes the view that the discovery of spondylolisthesis in a heavy manual worker developing low back pain is an indication for suggesting a change of job.

When someone already in employment (or indeed an aspiring employee at an initial examination) is found to be developing the sitigmata associated with chronic back pain, there are two possible courses open, and neither is very effective. These are traditionally divided into therapy and rehabilitation, but in what is often a chronic and progressive condition such as low back pain the two tend to merge into a continuous process.

Therapy

Detailed aspects of treatment are considered elsewhere. However, it is axiomatic that selection of the right therapy may prove more practical than either primary or secondary measures in preventing chronic or recurring low back pain, particularly in the working population. As has been indicated (see Table 2.3),[12] many patients with low back pain are treated successfully by their general practitioners. This may be because many recover completely; one observer[127] claims this to be as high as 85%, but the more generally agreed figure is that some two-thirds recover within six to eight weeks of onset, and many of these, but by no means all, have no further problem. The difficulty is to identify which patients comprise the remaining third who will proceed to chronicity and which of those who appear to recover relapse when they return to work.

Since more serious and long-standing cases of low back pain tend to be referred to hospital, it would seem reasonable to look at the characteristics of such patients with a view to assessing the likelihood of relapse. The technique of cluster analysis based on data obtained systematically from such patients may be helpful in throwing light on this problem.[128] It is also important to ensure that occupational therapists combine their skills with doctors, physiotherapists and others, so that treatment such as muscle-strengthening exercises can be supplemented by occupational activities appropriate to the sort of tasks which the patient will have to do after returning to work.

Opinion is divided on whether physical activity programmes are of as much value as has been claimed.[128-130] Some observers[62] have noted that the strength of abdominal muscles in younger men was lower in patients with low back pain than in negative controls; this in turn led to the conclusion that muscular strength may have a bearing on the protection afforded to the spine both by the abdominal muscles themselves and their lumbar counterparts. However, in older patients there was little difference between those with back pain and controls as far as muscular strength was concerned, except where back pain had led to incapacity lasting for at least a month.

Patient selection

When patients are selected by physicians for a regime such as local injection complemented by hydrotherapy and active exercises,[131] then a remarkably high success rate can be achieved. However, selection of this kind inevitably means that others will be passed over for one reason or another,

and the hospital specialist has little chance of finding out how large a proportion of those in need are omitted in this way. The view held by many patients and their doctors is that 'nothing can be done', and this in turn means a reduction in referral rates: thus it may often be difficult or even impossible to determine accurately the size of the population from which a sample of hospital patients is drawn, or how many in that population may have symptoms comparable to those found in patients referred to hospital.

Occupational health

Perhaps one of the most contentious areas of therapy in relation to back pain is the interface between general practitioners and hospital care on the one hand and remedial services offered at the place of work on the other. In the minds of purists, occupational medicine is a preventive service aimed particularly at health education and environmental control. However, the chance of ensuring a graded return to full muscular effort at the place of work with supporting therapy has potential not only for reducing the duration of sickness absence but also for ensuring surveillance during the recovery period. Such work-based therapy would seem to be a natural extension of the back pain school[132] in the overall management of low back pain.

Heterodox therapy

Under the existing terms of the National Health Service in the UK, it is difficult to obtain treatment without payment from chiropractors, osteopaths and others who are not necessarily on the medical register. Furthermore, it is likely that this situation will prevail for the foreseeable future.[133] However, in the United States there is more widespread recognition of the use of such therapeutic procedures. What is perhaps more important from the occupational point of view is the concept that greater use of these facilities might be made available in the medical centres at workplaces, since this could go some way to overcoming the barrier between orthodox and heterodox therapies. Such a combination could also prove an excellent milieu for evaluative trials of different types of therapy. Furthermore, it is important to bear in mind that, even though it is desirable to aim for permanent relief of symptoms, this may not always be possible. Thus, when treatment has to be repeated from time to time, it is obviously less disruptive to working patterns if the necessary therapy can be given in a place adjacent to the site of work.

Rehabilitation

Apart from preventive measures and successful treatment, other measures may be taken to modify the effects of established disease in those wanting to continue work, and increasing attention is being paid to the important question of rehabilitating persistent back pain sufferers. Efficiency in this field can be achieved only if correct diagnosis and therapy have been established, since the long-term prognosis of the disease depends on these.[134,135] There is also a need for co-operation between industrial medical officers and personal physicians to prevent chronicity and ensure the best chance of return to productive employment. In such circumstances a useful contribution has been made by industries themselves through the establishment of special rehabilitation workshops within factory complexes.[136,137] Their greatest success appears to be in the reduction of absence time following fractures and other acute injuries, but men with disc disease have also had their periods of absence from work substantially reduced.

Other important aspects of successful rehabilitation include accurate job descriptions in placing men with disabilities, and having an industrial medical officer as a member of the supervising team. Workers in firms large enough to justify occupational physicians appear to be at a great advantage from the point of view of ultimate placement of those with residual handicaps. Although the number of people with back pain requiring such intensive rehabilitation may appear to be comparatively small, it is possible that reported cases may represent only the tip of the iceberg and that, if this quality of care were more widely available to assess the chances of preventing such people becoming chronically unemployed, then many more cases might come to light.

Industrial rehabilitation

Income. At present the sickness absence rates for those with low back pain, particularly disc disease, among those who are still regularly employed is fairly high.[6] However, people with poor work records are continually at risk of losing their jobs and, having done so, may find it difficult to regain employment. Often it is impracticable (e.g. on grounds of intellectual ability) to channel such people into work deemed more suitable on physical grounds. Furthermore, reduction in income from such a change may be unacceptable, particularly when general agreement is lacking about cause and effect in relation to chronic low back pain. Another difficulty associated with trying to persuade those disabled with low back pain to take up new occupations concerns membership of a trades union which may be denied those who are trying to transfer from one trade to another.[138]

Industrial injury. For those who cannot be rehabilitated to the stage of returning to work immediately, there is an added difficulty which has financial implications. Low back pain is not generally regarded as 'industrial' in the statutory sense, even though there is a growing amount of evidence, some of which has been discussed in this chapter, that many cases (especially those with disc disorders and degenerative changes of other joints in the spine) may be related to occupations imposing a prolonged physical strain on the back. However, there is still a long way to go before back pain as such can be considered an industrial disease. Thus it is possible for two men, each disabled with identical signs of low back pain, to receive financial payments at different rates. If the clinical findings can be related to a reported injury at work (even if the injury was trivial), then compensation may be claimed in some countries, either through statutory boards or through law courts. Other countries, including Britain, recognize the occupational component by paying Industrial Injury Benefit to those who can prove their case. By way of contrast, a man doing similar work with identical symptoms but who is unable to recall an 'injury' (or who failed to put it on record) will have to accept the standard payments of the basic sickness insurance or social security payments ('sickness benefit' in the UK), which is generally at a lower rate.

It is also possible that excessive effort or prolonged stooping may be more a feature of hobbies than work, and that resulting degenerative changes may set the stage for a comparatively trivial injury at work to cause prolonged disability. Accordingly, criteria will have to be a lot clearer before compensation can be paid out routinely to a man suffering from low back pain merely on the grounds that he was engaged in heavy manual work for a number of years. For some time to come, a clearcut history of injury or acute strain at the onset of symptoms will be *sine qua non* for those seeking to claim at the higher rate of benefit.

Rehabilitation centres. Rehabilitation is based on the principles of adequate treatment, assessment of residual disability and re-employment in a suitable job; it is implicit that the last-named may require the employee to undergo a process of retraining for alternative work within the constraints of the residual disability.

In Britain, Scandinavia and other countries where statutory health services and their social (welfare) counterpart are highly developed, there tends to be a pattern of industrial rehabilitation which is based on nationally determined standards. In Britain, for instance, this is vested in the Department of Employment and the Manpower Services Commission, with two divisions[139,142] responsible respectively for re-employment (Employment Service Division, including Employment Rehabilitation Centres and Disablement Resettlement Officers) and retraining (Training Services Division, including attachment to special centres or colleges for retraining purposes). In countries where such developments have not been introduced nationally it is left to hospitals, large employing firms and voluntary agencies to develop such rehabilitative services; if payment is required, this is met either by insurance, lawcourt claims or grants from the state or voluntary agencies, subject to the financial circumstances of the individual in need.

Registration of disabled persons. It was strongly believed at one time that the inclusion of names on a special register[140] might afford protection to those with chronic disability, including low back pain. Unfortunately the use of such a register to protect the interests of those with chronic back pain who were trying to continue work in a normal situation was found to be of limited value, because there was often lack of understanding of the purpose of such a register by doctors, managers and by the disabled people themselves.[141] However, registers are still available in some countries (including Britain) to help those with low back pain find employment.[142]

Fortunately, the number of people with disabilities limited to low back pain whose handicap is so severe that it is necessary to seek work in sheltered employment is very low, even though there are indications that there is a substantial number of so-called 'unemployables' with low back pain present in the community and receiving long-term supplementary benefit.[44]

Whether or not there is a register in operation, there is a public duty on society to identify those who are handicapped and in need of help. The responsibility for this identification is sometimes placed on local authorities, but even in Britain, where this is a statutory requirement, the successful compilation of such lists of handicapped persons is far from complete, and many of those who have mobility or dependency problems in respect of daily living activities remain unknown or are identified by chance encounters with medical services or other agencies.

One of the reasons for the difficulty is that it is not always clear what is meant by 'rehabilitation'. The tendency to overstress the importance of detecting impairments or abnormalities and the emphasis on establishing a firm diagnosis in general medical training tend to mask the importance of assessing disability — i.e. loss of activity.[143] Even less attention seems to be paid in general medical training to considering handicaps — i.e. the social impact of disability in relation to occupational and recreational aspirations of the individual and activities in relation to daily living (ADL).

Different people approach the problem from different standpoints, so psychometry, counselling, training and placement are essential features of any rehabilitation programme.[144] Both the Tonbridge and Mair reports,[145,146] though not devoting space specifically to back pain or disc disease, make similar points and emphasize that one important detriment to rehabilitation is the fragmentation of the caring services. Thus the health services (National Health Service in the UK and others elsewhere, whether in the private or public sector), welfare departments (Social Services Departments in the UK or local authorities and central government departments of employment supported by financial help from statutory benefits or insurance policies, as well as all the voluntary organizations, are all important. Each service may be relevant to the care of chronically handicapped persons, whatever their impairments. Those with back pain are no exception, even though the complaints from which they suffer, which are seldom life-threatening, may not have the dramatic appeal of some others.

CONCLUSIONS

Occupational aspects of low back pain are of growing interest, and research in this field is extending, but it is only fair to say that the interest and research have been concentrated in a comparatively recent period and that much still requires to be done. Low back pain is an important cause of sickness absence and to a lesser extent of prolonged handicap; it also makes substantial demands on health care services. Evidence that occupational hazards cause permanent changes in the discs, apophyseal joints or ligamentous structures around the vertebrae is difficult to assess, a problem which is not lessened by the lack of diagnostic clarity associated with many painful conditions of the lower back.

Effective primary prevention of all low back pain seems to be out of reach at the present time, and secondary prevention, either by initial or ongoing screening examinations, is ineffective because of inadequate knowledge of cause and effect in relation to impairment. Treatment, though often completely successful, still leaves many sufferers, so that the number of patients of working age who require ongoing care and rehabilitation for long-term low back pain is unlikely to diminish. In the immediate future there is also a feeling that a number of people with low back pain may be written off as being unemployable, without consideration for the requirements for sheltered employment that this implies. More energetic and multidisciplinary rehabilitative measures might encourage more of these unfortunates to re-enter the struggle to obtain fresh employment.

An increased awareness on the part of the medical profession as a whole could make a substantial contribution to help cope with low back pain in relation to occupation. It is too easy to dub a man who has no apparent physical abnormality as psychogenic or, worse still, a malingerer. Unfortunately, there are those who for one reason or another do overplay their symptoms, and this leads to unjust stigmatization for many other chronic sufferers.

Accurate information is still required about the cause of low back pain and what the characteristics are of some workers or their jobs that give them a better chance of returning to work; also opinion is divided about the best method of treating and rehabilitating affected individuals. Somehow these difficulties must be resolved. One possible way to unravel the problem might be for those engaged in the practice of occupational medicine, both in industry itself and in the more rarefied atmosphere of academic departments, to collaborate in multidisciplinary research with general practitioners, hospital specialists and those without orthodox medical qualifications who are actually engaged in treating this condition, with the aim of achieving occupational independence for the largest possible number of those affected.

REFERENCES

1   Bell A 1969 Challenges: guest editorial. Industr. Med. Surg. 38: 28–30
2   Lawrence J S 1969 Disc degeneration. Its frequency and relationship to symptoms. Ann. Rheum. Dis. 28: 121–138
3   Kellgren J H, Lawrence J S, Aitken-Swan J 1953 Rheumatic complaints in an urban population. Ann. Rheum. Dis. 12: 5–15
4   Arthritis and Rheumatism Council Field Unit 1969 Digest of morbidity and mortality data on rheumatic diseases. Ann. Rheum. Dis. 28: 443–446
5   Wood P H N, McLeish C L 1974 Digest of data on rheumatic diseases. Ann. Rheum. Dis. 33: 93–105
6   Benn R T, Wood P H N 1975 Pain in the back: an attempt to estimate the size of the problem. Rheum. Rehab. 14: 121–128
7   Anderson J A D, Duthie J J R, Moody B P 1962 Rheumatic complaints in a mining population. Ann. Rheum. Dis. 21: 342–352
8   Anderson J A D, Duthie J J R 1963 Rheumatic complaints in dockyard workers. Ann. Rheum. Dis. 22: 401–409

9   Partridge R E H, Anderson J A D, McCarthy M A, Duthie J J R 1965 Rheumatism in light industry. Ann. Rheum. Dis. 24: 332–340

10 Arthritis and Rheumatism Council Industrial Survey Unit 1969 Rheumatism in Industry (London)

11 Anderson J A D 1983 Occupational factors in arthritis and rheumatism. In: Hawkins C, Currey H L F (eds) Collected reports on rheumatic diseases 1959–1983 Arthritis and Rheumatism Council for Research, London, p 238–241

12 Anderson J A D 1971 Rheumatism in industry: a review. Br. J. Indust. Med. 28: 103–121

13 Sweetman B J 1978 Low back pain, sickness absence and work factors. PhD, University of London

14 Magora A 1970 Investigation of the relation between low back pain and occupation. I. Age, sex, community and other factors. Industr. Med. Surg. 39: 465–471

15 Wickstrom G 1978 Effect of work on degenerative back disease: a review. Scand. J. Work Env. Health 4 Suppl 1: 1–12

16 Timi P G, Wieser C, Zinn W M 1977 The transitional vertebra of the lumbosacral spine: its radiological classification, incidence, prevalence and clinical significance. Rheum. Rehab. 16: 180–187

17 Onishi N, Watanabe A, Shindo H, Tagaya S, Saito M 1983 Lower back load on workers handling heavy materials. J. Human Ergol. 12: 211 (abstr)

18 Lockshin M D, Higgins I T T, Higgins M W, Dodge H J, Canale N 1969 Rheumatism in mining communities in Marion County. Am. J. Epidem. 90: 17–29

19 Caplan P S, Freedman L M J, Connelly T P 1962 Degenerative joint disease of the lumbar spine in coal miners — a clinical and X-ray study. Arth. Rheum. 5: 288 (abstr)

20 Anderson J A D 1977 Problem of classification of back pain. Rheum. Rehab. 16: 34–36

21 World Health Organization 1977 International classification of diseases 9th revn, HMSO, London

22 Anderson J A D 1985 Arthrosis and its relation to work. Scand. J. Work Env. Health 10: 429–433

23 Bergquist-Ullman M, Larsson U 1977 A controlled prospective study with special reference to therapy and confounding factors. Acta Orth. Scand. 170: 1–177

24 Hirsh A 1886 Handbook of geographical and historical pathology 3. The New Sydenham Society, trans by Chrichton from 2nd German edn, ch XVIII 511–512

25 Glover J R 1960 Back pain and hyperaesthesia. Lancet 1: 1165–1169

26 Hirsch C 1966 Etiology and pathogenesis of low back pain. Israel J. Med. Sci. 2: 362–370

27 Hirsch C, Ingelmark B E, Miller M 1963 The anatomical basis for low back pain. Acta Orth. Scand. 33: 1–17

28 Kellgren J H 1939 On the distribution of pain arising from deep somatic structures with charts of segmented pain areas. Clin. Sci. 4: 35–46

29 Tichy H, Seidel K 1969 Beitraege zur Rheumatologie, vol 14. Volk und Gesundheit, Berlin

30 Heald C B 1952 Fibrositis in industry and the Laughton-Scott technique. Trans. Assoc. Indus. Offrs 2: 106–109

31 British Medical Association 1953 Report of annual meeting. Br. Med. J. 2: 205

32 Sweetman B J, Anderson J A D 1974 Proc. Soc. Back Pain Res. (unpublished)

33 Faculty of Community Medicine 1978 Evidence for Cochrane working group. Newsletter Fac. Comm. Med. Roy. Coll. Phys. 5: 72–79

34 Social Security Disability Application Statistics 1973 Unpublished data, US Government

35 National Center for Health Statistics 1977 Limitation of activity due to chronic condition series 10, No. 111. Department of Health Education and Welfare, United States

36 Kelsey J, White A, Pastides H, Bisbee G 1979 The impact of musculoskeletal disorders on the population of the United States. J. Bone Joint Surg. (Am.) 61: 959–964

37 Kertesz A, Kormos R 1976 Low back pain in the workmen of Canada. Canad. Med. Assoc. J. 115: 901–903

38 McCracken W J 1977 Low back pain in workmen. Canad. Med. Assoc. J. 116: 1343–1344

39 Chaffin D B 1966 Manual materials handling: the cause of overexertion injury and illness in industry. J. Environ. Pathol. Toxicol. 2: 31–66

40 Anderson J A D 1977 Sickness absence and back pain. Evidence to the Cochrane working party. (unpublished)

41 Partridge R E H, Duthie J J R 1968 Rheumatism in dockers and civil servants. Ann. Rheum. Dis. 27: 559–568

42 Yoke C, Ann T 1979 Study of lumbar disc pathology among a group of dockworkers. Ann. Acad. Med. Singapore 8: 81–85

43 White A W M 1966 Low back pain in men receiving workmen's compensation. Canad. Med. Assoc. J. 95: 50–56

44 Anderson J A D, Duthie J J R, Moody B P 1963 Rheumatic diseases affecting men registered as disabled. Ann. Rheum. Dis. 22: 188–193

45 Jefferys M, Millard J B, Hyman M, Warren M D 1969 A set of tests for measuring motor impairment in prevalence studies. J. Chron. Dis. 22: 303–319

46 Horal J 1969 The clinical appearance of low back disorders in Gothenburg, Sweden. Acta Orth. Scand. Suppl 118

47 Taylor P J 1967 Shift and day work: a comparison of sickness absence, lateness and other absence behaviour in an oil refinery from 1962 to 1965. Br. J. Industr. Med. 24: 93–102

48 Taylor P J 1967 Individual variations in sickness absence. Br. J. Industr. Med. 24: 169–177

49 Froggatt P 1970 Short-term absence from industry I, II, III. Br. J. Industr. Med. 27: 199–312

50 Stocks P 1949 Sickness in the population of England and Wales in 1944–47. General register office studies on medical and population subjects, No. 2, HMSO, London

51 Parsons T 1951 The social system. Free Press, Glencoe

52 Abrams N R 1960 In: Hollander J L (ed) Arthritis, 6th edn. p 811–829

53 Pommer G 1927 Uber die mikroskopischen Kennzeichen und die einstehungs Bedingungen der Arthritis deformans. Virchow's Arch. Path. Anat. 263: 434–514

54 Fenkill J 1969 Some considerations in the employment of arthritics in industry. Arch. Indust. Hlth 20: 359–364

55 Magora A 1973 Investigation of the relation between low back pain and occupation. VI: physiological requirements — bending, rotated, reaching and sudden maximal effort. Scand. J. Rehab. Med. 5: 186–190

56 Anderson J A D 1981 Low back pain — cause and prevention of long-term handicap (a critical review). Int. Rehab. Med. 3: 89–93

57 Rowe M L 1971 Low back disability in industry: updated position. J. Occup. Med. 13: 476–478

58 Bremner J M, Lawrence J S, Miall W E 1968 Degenerative joint disease in a Jamaican rural population. Ann. Rheum. Dis. 27: 326–332

59 Arnott A W, Grieve D W 1969 The relationship between torque and velocity of axial rotation of the human trunk during maximum effort. J. Physiol. (Lond.) 201: 87–88

60 Troup J D G, Roantree W B, Archibald R 1970 Industry and the low back problem. New Scientist 45: 65–67

61 Jayson M I V, Barks J S 1973 Structural changes in the intervertebral disc. Ann. Rheum. Dis. 32: 10–15

62 Nachemson A, Lindh M 1969 Measurement of abdominal and back muscle strength with and without low back pain. Scand. J. Rehab. Med. 1: 60–65

63 Movin A 1967 Myelographic appearances of disc protrusions in different positions. Acta Radiol. Diagn. 6: 524–528

64 Jacoby R K, Sims-Williams H, Jayson M I V, Baddeley H 1976 Radiographic stereoplotting. Ann. Rheum. Dis. 35: 168–170

65 Vernon-Roberts B, Pirie C J 1977 Degenerative changes in the intervertebral discs of the lumbar spine and the sequelae. Rheum. Rehab. 16: 13–21

66 Bosman A 1974 Personal communication

67 Chaffin D B, Park K S 1973 A longitudinal study of low back pain as association with weight-lifting factors. Amer. Industr. Hyg. Assoc. J.

68 Chaffin D B 1979 Manual materials handling: the cause of overexertion injury and illness in industry. J. Environ. Pathol. Toxicol. 2: 31–66

69 Keyserling W M, Herrin G D, Chaffin D B, Armstrong T J, Foss M L 1980 Am. Indust. Hyg. Assoc. J. 41: 730–736

70 Friewalds A, Chaffin D B, Garg A, Lee K S 1984 A dynamic biomechanical evaluation of lifting maximal acceptable loads. J. Biomech. 17: 251–262

71 Davis P R, Stubbs D A, Ridd J E 1977 Radio pills: their use in monitoring back stress. Med. Engin. and Tech. 1: 209–215

72 Andersson G B J, Ortengren R, Nachemson A 1977 Intradiskal pressure, intra-abdominal pressure and myoelectric back muscle activity related to posture and loading. Clin. Orthop. 129: 156–164

73 Andersson G B J, Ortengren R, Nachemson A, Elfstrom G 1974 Lumbar disc pressure and myoelectric back muscle activity during sitting. Scand. J. Rehab. Med. 6: 104–114

74 International Labour Organization 1966 Report of conference on maximum weight. Geneva

75 Panjabi M 1977 Effects of preload on load displacement curves of the lumbar spine. Orthop. Clin. North Am. 8: 169–192

76 Andersson G B J, Ortengren R, Herberts P 1977 Quantative electromyographic studies of back muscle activity. Orthop. Clin. North Am. 8: 85–96

77 Jayasinghe W J, Harding R H, Anderson J A D, Sweetman B J 1978 An electromyographic investigation of postural fatigue in low back pain — a preliminary study. Electromyogr. Clin. Neurophysiol. 18: 191–198

78 Griffin M J, Witham E M, Parsons K C 1982 Vibration and comfort I. Transitional seat vibration. Ergonomics 25: 142–162

79 Matthews J 1964 Ride comfort for tractor operators. I. Review of existing information. J. Agric. Engng. Res. 9: 3–31

80 Matthews J 1964 Ride comfort for tractor operators. II. Analysis of ride vibrations of pneumatic tyred tractors. J. Agric. Engng. Res. 9: 147–158

81 Sjoflot L 1982 The tractor as a place of work. Ergonomics 25: 11–18

82 Stayner R M, Collins T S, Lines J A 1984 Tractor ride vibration simulation as an aid to design. J. Agric. Engng. Res. 29: 345–355

83 Anderson J A D 1980 Occupational aspects of low back pain. Clin. Rheum. Dis. 6: 17–35

84 Maeda K, Okazaki F, Suemaga T, Sakurai T, Takamatsu M 1980 Low back pain related to bowing posture of greenhouse farmers. J. Human Ergol. 9: 117–123

85 Rosegger R, Rosegger S 1960 Health effects of tractor driving. J. Agric. Engng. Res. 5: 241–274

86 Bottoms D J, Barber T S, Chisholm C J 1979 Improving access to tractor cab: an experimental study

87 Bottoms D J, Barber T S 1978 A swivelling seat to improve tractor drivers posture. Applied Ergonomics 9: 77–84

88 Pheasant S T, Harris C M 1982 Human strength in the operation of tractor pedals. Ergonomics 25: 53–64

89 Allawi A 1978 Occupational factors in back pain. PhD thesis, University of London

90 Davis P R, Stubbs D A 1977 Safe levels of manual forces for young males. Applied Ergonomics 8: 141–150

91 Sweetman B J, Moore C S, Jayasinghe W J, Anderson J A D 1976 Monitoring work factors relating to back pain. Postgrad. Med. J. 52: (Suppl 7) 151–155

92 Otun E O, Henrich I, Anderson J A D, Crooks J 1984 'PADAS' An ambulatory electronic system to monitor and evaluate factors relating to back pain at work. Proceedings of the Ergonomics Society Conference (unpublished)

93 Sweetman B J, Edwards G S, Anderson J A D 1978 A measurement of limb activity in a back pain study in industry. In: Stott F D, Rafferty E B, Sleight P, Gould (eds) ISAM 1977 p 231–238

94 Bradshaw P 1957 Some aspects of cervical spondylosis. Quart. J. Med. 26: 177–208

95 Bull J, El Gammal T, Popham M 1969 A possible genetic factor in cervical spondylosis. Br. J. Radiol. 42: 9–16

96 Boasson M, Forestier J, Certonciny A, Forestier F, Auquier L 1969 Durée des manifestations douloureuses dans les arthroses vertébrales. Rev. Rhum. 36: 151–160

97 Troup J D G 1965 Relation of lumbar spine disorders to heavy manual work and lifting. Lancet 1: 857–861

98 United States Public Health Service 1973 DHEW Publication No. (HRA), p 74-1514

99 Snook S H 1982 Workloads. In: Nelson M (ed) Proceedings of the Colt Symposium on low back pain and industrial and social disablement. Back Pain Association, Teddington, Middlesex, p 30–35

100 Kosiak M, Aurelius J R, Hartfiel W F 1966 Backache in industry. J. Occup. Med. 8: 51–58
101 Berkson M, Schultz A, Nachemson A, Andersson G 1977 Voluntary strength of male adults with acute low back syndromes. Clin. Orthop. 129: 84–95
102 Anderson T McL 1960 Manual of lifting and handling. Industrial Welfare Society, London
103 Glover J R, Davies B T 1951 Manual handling and lifting. Its introduction to a 6000 employee works. J. Indust. Nurses 13: 1–12
104 Blow R J 1974 Proceedings of the Society of Back Pain Research (unpublished)
105 Back Pain Association Ltd 1978 Poster on lifting methods
106 I am Jo's spine 1976 Film distributed by Reader's Digest
107 Devlin D 1975 You and your back. Pan, London
108 Pillmore G U 1960 The occupational low back hazard. Industr. Med. Surg. 29: 28–32
109 Becker W F 1961 Prevention of low back disability. J. Occup. Med. 3: 329–335
110 Wilson P D 1962 Low back pain, a problem of industry. Arch. Env. Hlth 4: 505–510
111 Kosiak M, Aurelius J R, Hartfiel W F 1968 The low back problem. J. Occup. Med. 10: 588–593
112 Diveley R L, Kiene R H, Meyer P P W 1956 Low back pain. JAMA 160: 729–731
113 Diveley R L, Oglevie R R 1956 Pre-employment examination of the low back. JAMA 160: 856–858
114 Harte J D 1974 Is pre-employment medical examination of value? Proc. Roy. Soc. Med. 67: 177–180
115 Thomson D 1974 Civil service experience of pre-employment examinations. Proc. Roy. Soc. Med. 67: 182–184
116 Macrae I F, Wright V 1969 Measurement of back movement. Ann. Rheum. Dis. 28: 584–589
117 Anderson J A D, Sweetman B J 1975 A combined flexirule–hydrogoniometer for measurement of lumbar spine and its sagittal movement. Rheum. Rehab. 14: 173–179
118 Biering-Sorensen F 1984 Physical measurements as risk indicators for low-back from over a one year period. Spine 9: 106–119
119 Anderson J A D 1982 Measurement of movement of the thoraco-lumbar spine. Clin. Rheum. Dis. 8: 631–653
120 Porter R, Wicks M, Ottewell D 1978 Measurement of spinal canal by diagnostic ultrasound. J. Bone Joint Surg. (Br) 60: 481–484
121 Jayson M, Nelson D 1983 Spinal stenosis and low back pain. In: Hawkins C, Currey H L F (eds) Collected Rep. Rheum. Dis. 1959–1983 Arthritis and Rheumatism Council for Research, London p 106–109
122 Porter R, Hibbert C, Wicks M 1978 The spinal canal in symptomless lumbar disc lesions. J. Bone Joint Surg. (Br) 60: 485–487
123 Wiltse J J 1977 Surgery for intervertebral disk disease of the lumbar spine. Clin. Orth. 129: 22–45
124 Epstein B S, Epstein J A, Jones M D 1977 Degenerative spondylolisthesis with an intact neural arch. Radiol. Clin. N. Am. 15: 275–287
125 Rowe M L 1969 Low back pain in industry. J. Occup. Med. 11: 161–169
126 Magnuson H J 1969 A periodic examination program for occupational health. J. Occup. Med. 11: 349–354
127 Gordon E J 1968 Diagnosis and treatment of acute low back disorders. Industr. Med. Surg. 37: 756–761
128 Anderson J A D, Sweetman B S 1985 Clinical trials in low back pain. Recent Prog. Med. (in press)
129 Duggar B C, Swengros C V 1969 The design activity programs for industry. J. Occup. Med. 11: 322–329
130 Kraus H, Raab W 1961 Hypokinetic disease. Thomas, Springfield
131 Burry H C, Graham R 1970 Personal communication
132 Zachrisson M 1974 The low back school. Danderyd Hospital, Sweden
133 Department of Health and Social Security 1970 The future structure of the National Health Service. HMSO, London
134 Duthie J J R 1970 Rheumatology as a speciality in medicine: a personal appraisal. Scot. Med. J. 15: 165–168
135 Bianco A J 1968 Low back pain and sciatica: diagnosis and indications for treatment. J. Bone Jt. Surg. (Am) 50: 170–181
136 Stewart D 1954 Industrial rehabilitation. In: Mereweather E R A (ed) Industrial medicine and hygiene, vol I. Butterworth, London. ch 12, p 280–320
137 Plewes L W, Barron J N, Thompson A R,, Newell H H 1946 Rehabilitation in industry. Lancet 2: 699–702
138 Daniel J W 1969 Rehabilitation and resettlement of patients suffering from rheumatological disorders. J. Roy. Coll. Gen. Pract. 18: Suppl 3: 29–32
139 Manpower Services Commission 1982 Employing disabled people. HMSO, London
140 Townsend P 1973 The social minority. Allen Lane, London, p 108
141 Taylor P J, Fairrie A J 1968 Chronic disability in men of middle age. Br. J. Prev. Soc. Med. 22: 183–192
142 Manpower Services Commission, Employment Services Division 1979 The Disabled Persons (Employment) Acts 1944 and 1958: employees obligations. HMSO, London
143 World Health Organization 1980 International classification of impairments, disabilities and handicaps. WHO, Geneva
144 Notkin H 1951 Vocational training and public health. Am. J. Pub. Hlth 41: 1096–1100
145 Department of Health and Social Security 1972 Rehabilitation. Report of a sub-committee of the Standing Medical Advisory Committee (Tunbridge R, Chairman). HMSO, London
146 Scottish Home and Health Department 1972 Medical rehabilitation (Mair A, Chairman). HMSO, Edinburgh

Pathology of intervertebral discs and apophyseal joints

INTERVERTEBRAL DISC LESIONS

Terminology

The clinical condition 'degenerative spondylosis' is commonly signified radiologically by the presence of osteophytes (syndesmophytes) arising from the anterolateral margins of the vertebral bodies, and may sometimes be accompanied by a clinical history of back pain. The importance of pathological changes in the discs in the pathogenesis of these vertebral body osteophytes has been stressed by various workers, who have applied the terms 'spondylosis deformans' or 'spinal osteophytosis' to demarcate this state of affairs from true osteoarthrosis ('spondylosis') affecting the apophyseal (posterior intervertebral) synovial joints.

However, pathological changes in the intervertebral discs, osteophytes arising from the margins of the vertebral bodies and osteoarthrosis of the apophyseal joints co-exist in a majority of cases (Fig. 3.1) and are almost certainly pathogenetically interrelated.[1] Thus the term 'degenerative spondylosis' can be used with advantage to encompass the situation when one or more of these pathological changes are present. The questions that need to be answered in any consideration of lumbar spondylosis are:

1. What is the sequence of changes during which the 'normal' intervertebral disc seen in the young adult is transformed to a disc exhibiting advanced degenerative changes?
2. What is the role of disc prolapse in disc degeneration?
3. What is the role of disc degeneration and prolapse in the genesis of vertebral body osteophytes and osteoarthrosis of the apophyseal joints?
4. Which of the pathological features observed in lumbar spondylosis could be concerned in giving rise to low back pain?

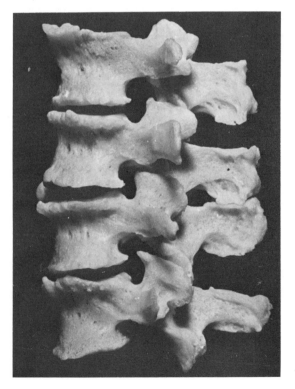

Fig. 3.1 Lateral view of part of macerated lumbar spine in advanced spondylosis, showing narrowing of intervertebral (disc) spaces, flange-like osteophytes arising from anterolateral borders of vertebral bodies, osteophytes arising from posterolateral borders of vertebral bodies, osteophytes arising from margins of apophyseal joints and projecting into intervertebral foramina, and pseudo-arthrosis between spines of vertebrae

Incidence

Autopsy studies report considerably higher percentages of the incidence of spondylosis than do clinical radiological studies. Thus the examination of 4253 spines obtained at autopsy by Schmorl[2,3] revealed evidence of the condition in 60% of women and 80% of men by the age of 49 years, and in 95% of both sexes by the age of 70 years. More recently, a very detailed pathological study of 100 lumbar spines has shown that degenerative changes (i.e. alterations from the young adult morphology) are present in the intervertebral discs of all subjects by middle age and, indeed, are present in many spines by the age of 30 years.[1]

The differences in the frequency of spondylosis in clinical radiological studies compared with pathological studies must be due to the inability of routine clinical radiographs to demonstrate the presence of small bony spurs and minor disc abnormalities which are easily seen in autopsy specimens on pathological examination. It remains to be seen if newer imaging techniques such as discography, CT scanning, ultrasound and stereoscopic radiography are capable of visualizing minor structural changes in spinal components.

The pathological findings could be interpreted as suggesting that, if all forms and degrees of severity of spondylosis are capable of giving rise to back pain, this could provide an adequate explanation for complaints of back pain in subjects over the age of 50 years even when radiological abnormalities of the spine may not be visible. However, in retrospective examination of the case histories of subjects in whom the lumbar spine has been carefully examined at autopsy[1] it is apparent that, in many instances, marked spondylotic changes do not appear to have given rise to back pain of such severity that it has been thought necessary by the patient to volunteer this information. Moreover, it is also known that some patients may have radiological and laboratory evidence of osteoporosis, Paget's disease, osteomyelitis, metastatic tumour and other diseases affecting the spine without any evidence of back pain being elicited. Thus structural deviations from the young normal spine observed in pathological studies must not be automatically interpreted as signifying definite causes of back pain, but must be regarded only as either potential causes in some individuals or as part of a combination of abnormalities which cumulatively can give rise to back pain.

Until better diagnostic techniques are capable of detecting minor abnormalities in spinal structure in life, the correlation of observed pathology in autopsy spines with the genesis of pain will remain largely speculative.

The normal disc

In childhood the opposing vertebral bodies are completely covered by thin plates of cartilage forming the epiphysis. After puberty, secondary centres of ossification appear in these epiphyses and fuse with the primary bone after the age of 21. However, they ossify only the periphery of the cartilaginous plates, the central part remaining cartilaginous. In advanced life this central portion may also become peripherally or wholly ossified. Thus, in the adult, the opposing vertebral bodies are covered centrally by thin laminae of hyaline cartilage. The cartilage end-plates, which are up to 1 mm thick, and the peripheral rims of bone, up to 10 mm wide, formed by ossification of the cartilage, are united by a peripheral ring of fibrous tissue and fibrocartilage, the annulus fibrosus.

The annulus fibrosus is largely composed of concentric layers of fibrous tissue (Figs 3.2, 3.3). The fibres of each layer are parallel and run spirally at an angle of 45° to the bodies of the vertebrae, and the fibres of alternate layers are at right angles to each other (Fig. 3.3). This arrangement results in great strength of union of the vertebral bodies, while at the same time the criss-cross arrangement of fibres resists torsional and flexional deformity and ensures resistance to rupture of the annulus. Enclosed by the annulus is the semi-gelatinous nucleus pulposus containing about 80% water, and ground substance consisting principally of collagen and protein-polysaccharide. Being an incompressible liquid, the nucleus distributes pressure evenly in a centrifugal manner on the annulus fibrosus and the cartilage end-plates. Under normal conditions, the annulus fibrosus and the cartilage end-plates (supported by the underlying bone) are strong enough to resist displacement of the nucleus.

The posterior longitudinal ligament runs down the posterior surfaces of the vertebral bodies inside

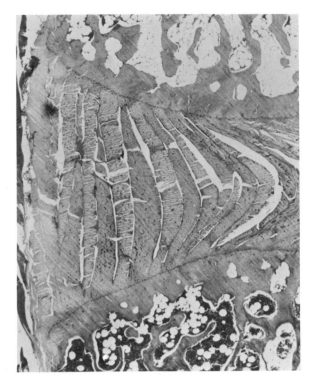

Fig. 3.2 Section through annulus fibrosus showing separate layers of fibrous tissue

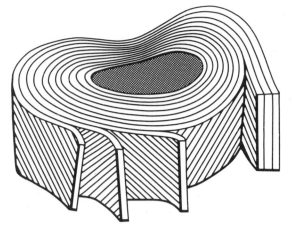

Fig. 3.3 Diagrammatic representation of intervertebral disc showing how collagen fibres of successive layers are arranged at right angles to each other and run spirally at an angle of 45°

the spinal canal and is firmly united to the intervertebral discs by lateral expansions which give it a serrated appearance. The anterior longitudinal ligament extends down the front of the spine but is not attached to the intervertebral discs.

There is a gradual decrease in the water content of the disc during life.[4] At birth, the water content of the annulus fibrosus is about 80% and of the nucleus pulposus about 90%. By the third decade, the annulus contains about 70% water and the nucleus about 75%. Thereafter, the annulus retains a relatively constant water content of about 70%, whereas the water content of the nucleus diminishes progressively to approach that of the annulus.

At birth, the discs consist almost entirely of nucleus, with a thin surrounding annulus. In childhood and adolescence the nuclei are gelatinous and turgid, so that the contents bulge spontaneously from the cut surface of the disc at autopsy. In childhood, the nuclei are composed predominantly of semigelatinous material traversed by a few delicate collagen fibrils and sometimes contain stellate chordal cells. Apart from the water content,

the collagen accounts for only about 15% of the dry solids of the young nucleus, and the remainder is protein-polysaccharide.[5] By the third decade the nuclei are semisolid and have lost much of their turgescence. Microscopy shows that this is associated with an apparent progressive centripetal encroachment of collagen into the nucleus from the inner layers of the annulus, a reduction in the number of healthy cells in the nucleus and a reduction in metachromatic staining indicating changes in the protein polysaccharides of the nucleus. After middle life, in the majority of the spines examined, the nuclei are solid, non-turgescent, dry and granular to the touch, and frequently they merge with the annulus so that it is not possible to ascertain where annulus ends and nucleus begins. There is a reduction or loss of metachromatic staining and a marked increase in collagen content which has been confirmed by biochemical analysis. A further decrease in the number of healthy nuclear cells also appears to take place during this period. These changes result in the progressive loss of resilience and turgescence of the disc as age advances, and are accompanied by a progressive reduction in the thickness of each disc.

Disc degeneration

In elderly subjects, the nuclei are not infrequently brown in colour (Fig. 3.4). This change is usually associated with a desiccated and friable consistency of the nucleus, and is frequently associated with the degenerative lesions described below. The brown pigment has not been identified, but there is no evidence to show that it arises from haemorrhage into the nucleus.

After middle age, splits and clefts are frequently found in the tissues of the disc. In the majority of cases, these clefts begin to appear about mid-way between the centre of the disc and the cartilage end-plates, and they are usually orientated parallel to the end-plates (Figs. 3.5–3.7). As the clefts become larger, they therefore tend to isolate progressively the central portion of the disc from the surrounding tissue. By the upper and lower clefts meeting peripherally, part of the central portion of the disc may become completely isolated to form a loose body

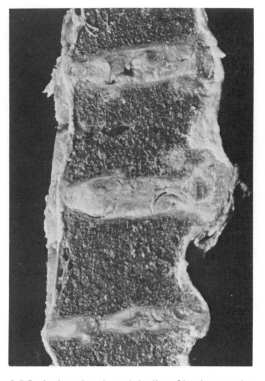

Fig. 3.5 Sagittal section through bodies of lumbar vertebrae, showing 'brown degeneration' of nuclei, fissuring of nuclei, collapse of discs with anterior protrusions and osteophytes which have formed at the margins of the bodies above and below each protrusion

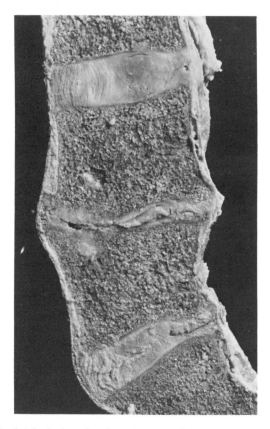

Fig. 3.4 Sagittal section through bodies of lumbar vertebrae, showing 'brown degeneration' of upper disc; degeneration, posterior thinning and cleft formation in lower disc; and collapse, fissuring and protrusion of middle disc which has resulted in osteophyte formation at the margins of the vertebral bodies on each side

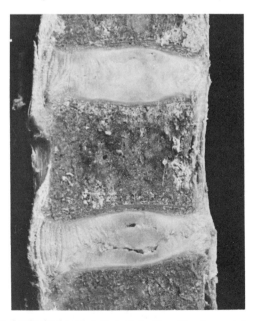

Fig. 3.6 Sagittal section through bodies of lumbar vertebrae. Lower disc has nuclear clefts extending towards the annulus posteriorly (right)

contained in a cavity, similar to a sequestrum of dead bone in osteomyelitis (Fig. 3.7). The clefts tend to extend more frequently in the posterior and posterolateral directions than anteriorly, and they often extend into the posterior part of the annulus. They sometimes pass through all layers of the annulus (Figs. 3.7, 3.8) and may even extend into the peridural space. The clefts passing into and through the annulus appear unlikely to have been formed as a result of disc herniation in the majority of cases, since microscopic examination has revealed that recognizable nuclear material is rarely present within the clefts. Where the clefts extend into the annulus, microscopy occasionally reveals vascular ingrowth around the margins of the cleft (Fig. 3.9) indicating a repair reaction; this suggests that the

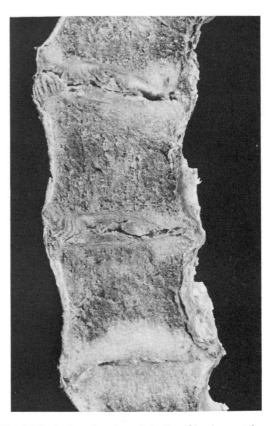

Fig. 3.8 Sagittal section through bodies of lumbar vertebrae, showing marked degenerative changes in discs with extensive fissures of nuclei and clefts extending through annuli. Collapse of discs has resulted in marked bone sclerosis in vertebral bodies on both sides of lower disc and, to a lesser extent, in relation to the posterior parts of the discs above

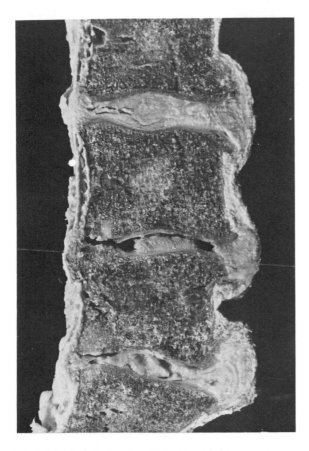

Fig. 3.7 Sagittal section through bodies of lumbar vertebrae. There has been marked degeneration of the discs with clefts extending posteriorly through the annulus (left). A portion of the lower disc has become isolated from the remainder of the disc substance. There has been disc collapse and anterior protrusion with marked osteophyte formation (right)

clefts could extend into the annulus by a tearing process rather than tissue breakdown by a degenerative process, at least in certain instances.

In some cases there are marked degenerative changes in the annulus which are often associated with the appearance of circumferential clefts between the layers of fibrous tissue. It would appear that these circumferential tears occur most frequently in the posterolateral part of the annulus,[6] and it has been postulated that repeated minor trauma may induce these tears to enlarge and coalesce to form one or more radial tears predisposing to disc herniations.[6]

Other clefts in the anterior annulus are visible by microscopy near the attachments of the annulus to the vertebral bodies,[3,1,7] and are directed at right angles to the directions of the collagen bundles of the

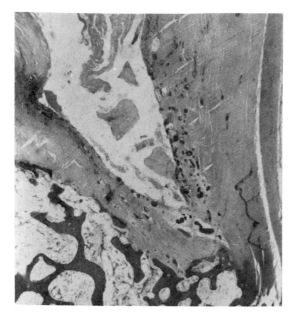

Fig. 3.9 Sagittal section through lumbar intervertebral disc, showing cleft extending deeply into posterior annulus with extensive vascular ingrowth around the margins of the cleft (reproduced with permission from Vernon-Roberts & Pirie[1])

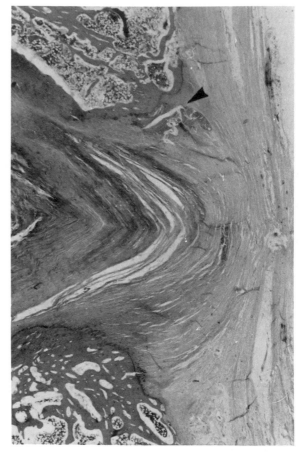

Fig. 3.10 Sagittal section through lumbar intervertebral disc, showing circumferential clefts in anterior annulus, and transverse cleft (arrow) separating annular fibres near their attachment to the upper vertebral body (reproduced with permission from Vernon-Roberts & Pirie[1])

annulus (Fig. 3.10). The fact that these clefts may contain fibrin and sometimes exhibit vascular ingrowth into the surrounding tissue again suggests that they are formed as the result of episodes of traumatic tearing rather than because of a purely degenerative process.

A recent pathological study[7] suggests that the majority of subjects aged over 50 years have at least one vertebral rim affected. The rim lesions were present more frequently in the upper than the lower rim and were more common anteriorly than posteriorly. They were associated radiographically with vertebral rim sclerosis, with or without a cup-shaped defect in the rim, and osteophytes confined to one side of the disc.

These internal derangements of the disc are more commonly present and are more severe when there is also evidence of true disc prolapse, either in the form of Schmorl's nodes, present in over 50% of spines, or posterior prolapse, present in over 10% of spines.[1] However, single or multiple Schmorl's nodes may be present in some adolescent or young adult spines with no associated evidence of disc degeneration or narrowing.

When there has been a breach in the cartilage end-plate, producing a microscopically or macroscopically visible Schmorl's node, there may be vascular invasion of the disc through this breach, which may be followed by calcification or ossification of the disc. Much less frequently, the disc may become vascularized from the periphery of the annulus.

Small 'islands' of bone may be present within the anterior and anterolateral margins of the annulus without any other strikingly abnormal findings.

Reduction of the disc height

To a limited extent narrowing of the disc height occurs progressively during adult life as the hydration of the nucleus diminishes. The narrowing process is accelerated and more marked when there is internal disruption of the disc by cleft formation or prolapse, and minor mechanical traumas probably play a part in this process. The disc narrowing is associated with bulging of the annulus right around the circumference of the disc.[6]

Some authors have used the term 'resorption' to describe the process of disc narrowing,[6,8] but it seems very unlikely that true 'resorption' leading to narrowing could occur in the absence of prior vascularization followed by fibrous tissue formation. This conclusion is based also upon the personal experience of this author of extensive material available for pathological examination after partial or total surgical removal of discs for 'discitis' and fusion and of autopsy material. It would appear, therefore, that the term 'resorption' may be usefully retained for radiological descriptive purposes[9] but is misleading in terms of the pathological sequence leading to disc narrowing.

The importance of a marked loss of disc height lies in the resulting posterior joint subluxation with facet overriding, facet intrusion into the nerve root canal and intervertebral foramen with narrowing of the lateral recess, and sclerosis of the vertebral end-plate. These changes may be associated with low lumbar pain with radiation into the leg[9] probably due to spinal nerve entrapment just medial to the intervertebral foramen.[6]

Herniation of the nucleus pulposus

It is clear that there is a constant tendency to displacement of the nucleus due to the forces acting on it. Normally the cartilage end-plates and the annulus are sufficiently strong to prevent displacement of the nucleus, even under conditions of great stress. In all discs, however, there are two potentially weak points:

1. the cartilage end-plate, which is supported by the very thin subchondral bone plate and the underlying trabecular bone; and
2. the posterior segment of the annulus which is not only thinner than the anterior and lateral segments but is also less firmly attached to the bone.

It is at these two points that herniation is liable to occur.

Lateral or anterior ruptures of the annulus are probably rare. By contrast, anterolateral bulging (without rupture) of the annulus is a frequent occurrence after extrusion of the nucleus in another direction (posteriorly or vertically) has caused the disc to collapse; it occurs anteriorly because of the forward tilting of the vertebral bodies pivoting on the apophyseal joints, and laterally because of the presence in the mid-line of the anterior longitudinal ligament.[10]

It seems likely that herniation is associated with an episode of trauma. It may be that congenital or acquired defects of the cartilage end-plates or posterior annulus are predisposing factors in some cases. It is clear that herniation of the nucleus is more likely to occur when it is still turgescent, and is less likely after middle age when the nucleus has become desiccated and collagenized.

Posterior prolapse

Much less common than vertical prolapse is posterior prolapse of disc tissue into the spinal canal or posterolateral prolapse into the intervertebral foramina. Posterior prolapse is, however, an important cause of acute and chronic back pain and neurological symptoms. Andrae[11] examined 368 spines at autopsy and found posterior displacements of disc tissue in 56 (15.2%). They were present in 11.5% of male and 18.7% of female spines. About one-half of the affected spines showed involvement at several sites, and it was not unusual to find two prolapses affecting a single disc. While in his series Andrae did not find any posterior disc prolapses in any subject less than 30 years, there have been numerous observations of posterior prolapses requiring surgical treatment in children, adolescents and adults below this age.[8-10] These findings suggest that disc prolapses in younger persons when the nucleus is still semigelatinous and turgescent are likely to be larger and produce more dramatic symptoms than they would in older persons when the nucleus has become collagenized and has lost its turgescence.

Although a history of preceding trauma may be elicited in many instances, the question remains open as to whether trauma can tear or displace a completely healthy disc, or whether trauma is only the final step in the posterior protrusion of a disc prolapse already in progress. There is no doubt that the discs of the lumbar spine are subjected to severe stresses in everyday life,[15] and it seems likely that fatigue damage, similar to fatigue fractures in bone, could take place in disc tissue when demands surpass functional ability. Schmorl & Junghanns[3] report that early fissure formation and disintegration may be found in discs at an age when the physiology of ageing does not explain the disc changes, and they are of the opinion that clefts extend in linear fashion posteriorly and posterolaterally to prepare the way for subsequent protrusion. This would be in keeping with the view that most prolapses probably occur before the discs lose their turgescence in middle age, and that discs exhibiting marked degenerative changes in elderly subjects rarely participate in posterior herniations.

Posterior herniations are rarely central in position, since the emerging tissue usually tracks around the lateral edge of the posterior longitudinal ligament (Fig. 3.11). Moreover, they are very often situated slightly above or below the central horizontal plane of the affected disc, since the emerging tissue also tracks above or below the lateral expansions of the posterior longitudinal ligament (Fig. 3.11) which are firmly attached to the outer layers of the annulus. This explains why sciatic pain and neurological symptoms are commonly unilateral.

Collins[10] expressed the opinion that there is seldom a gross breach of the annulus, and that the semifluid nuclear material appears to escape by dissecting its way between the fibres. He also stated that some of the inner fibres of the annulus may be fractured, but the outer ones may often be intact and separated rather than ruptured by the herniated nucleus. In contrast, Schmorl & Junghanns[3] state that the prolapsed tissue contains parts of the annulus and cartilage end-plate in addition to nuclear material. However, material removed surgically shortly after a well-documented acute prolapse may show only nuclear material with gelatinous matrix and chordoma-like cells, or mainly fibrocartilage; after a somewhat longer interval the protrusion may become vascularized, organised, chondrified or even ossified.

Occasionally, large posterior protrusions take the form of small sessile or nipple-shaped swellings covered by the loose extra-dural areolar tissue of the spinal canal (Fig. 3.11). Ultimately, the shape and size is determined by the bulk and consistency of the

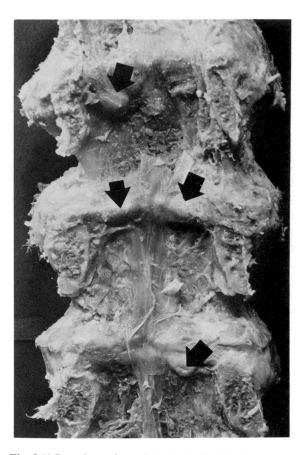

Fig. 3.11 Posterior surfaces of lumbar bodies following removal of neural arches. Multiple posterolateral disc protrusions (arrows) can be seen situated on each side of posterior longitudinal ligament and below its lateral expansions

extruded material. The presence and severity of pain, and the presence or absence of neurological symptoms, depend on the size and direction of the protrusion, but posterolateral prolapses extending into the intervertebral foramina are the type that usually produce the characteristic clinical picture of disc prolapse with sciatica.

Experiments on cadavers and examinations made during surgical exploration of disc prolapses have shown that some protrusions alternately project into the spinal canal and retreat into the disc substance during certain spinal movements, whereas other protrusions are fixed within the canal. Whatever the type of protrusion, its expansion is eventually halted at some stage by a combination of factors which include vascularization and fibrosis, loss of turgescence by the nucleus and a reduction in physical stresses on the disc by inhibition of movement for reasons of altered mechanics and the presence of pain. These factors produce the circumstances favourable for 'healing' and 'stabilization' of the prolapse to take place. Following vascularization and fibrosis, a reduction in the bulk of the prolapse may follow due to cicatrization; alternatively, the protrusion may become calcified or ossified and become visible radiographically. However, this 'healing' process is not necessarily accompanied by a relief of symptoms, because it is dependent upon the size and location of the prolapse, the degree of spinal rigidity achieved and other changes in adjacent structures. Moreover, it is not certain whether an 'arrested' prolapse may later enlarge by proliferation of the organizing connective tissues, or become the site for repeated episodes of prolapse punctuated by episodes of quiescence.

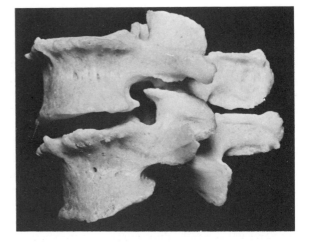

Fig. 3.12 Part of macerated lumbar spine showing a large osteophyte protruding anteriorly into intervertebral foramen from margin of apophyseal articular surface, and a smaller osteophyte extending posteriorly from upper vertebral body following posterior disc protrusion

Formation of osteophytes

Probably the most important factor concerned in stabilizing a disc prolapse is the formation of osteophytes encasing the prolapsed tissue as a result of periosteal elevation or some non-specific 'irritation'. These posterior vertebral body osteophytes occur much less frequently than those commonly seen on the anterolateral margins of the vertebral bodies. When osteophytes form as a result of posterior mid-line protrusions they are never large enough to narrow the spinal canal; however, when they form posterolaterally in relation to the intervertebral foramina, they may alone or together with the prolapsed disc tissue produce pressure effects on the spinal nerves and give rise to symptoms similar to those caused by disc prolapse alone. Pressure on the nerves may also be aggravated by osteophytes projecting into the intervertebral foramina from the margins of osteoarthritic apophyseal joints[1] (Fig. 3.12).

Vertical prolapse of disc into vertebral bodies

Schmorl's nodes are frequently found at autopsy when the vertebral bodies are bisected (Fig. 3.13). Schmorl himself found them in about 38% of all spines examined.[3] Men were involved more frequently (39.9%) than women (34.3%). Between the

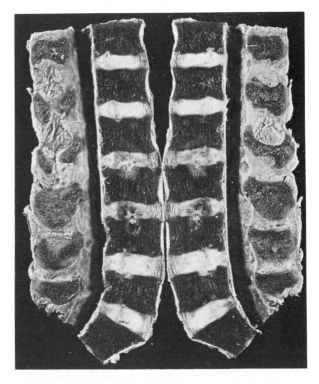

Fig. 3.13 Bisected lumbar spine showing numerous vertical disc protrusions (Schmorl's nodes)

ages of 18 and 59 they were twice as common in men as in women, but after the age of 60 they were twice as common in women as in men. Schmorl attributed the higher incidence in men in early life to their greater liability to accidental or occupational trauma, and the higher incidence in elderly women to greater physical activity at an age when degenerative processes in the disc may predispose to its rupture.

However, recent autopsy studies have found that not only are Schmorl's nodes present in 76% of spines but they are present with equal frequency in subjects above and below the age of 50 years.[16] The recent findings are consistent with the view that the majority of Schmorl's nodes are probably present from an early age and only a small percentage form in adult life. This supports the concept that herniation of nuclear material is more likely to occur at an age when the nucleus is in a semifluid state. Discs having Schmorl's nodes tend to exhibit advanced degenerative changes at an early age, and in some instances, at least, the earliest degenerative changes are in the region of the herniation.[1]

In marked contrast to the frequency of Schmorl's nodes demonstrable at autopsy, Schmorl's nodes are demonstrable by clinical radiography in only about 13.5% of cases.[3] The majority of Schmorl's nodes cannot be detected radiographically because the herniations are too small to produce visible changes, or the loss of tissue from the nucleus is not large enough to produce appreciable narrowing of the intervertebral (disc) space (Figs 3.13, 3.14). The demonstration of Schmorl's nodes radiographically may only be possible when the prolapse is large enough to produce visible loss of vertebral body bone, and tomography may be necessary to establish the true nature of the lesion. In fact, Schmorl's nodes are more easily diagnosed radiographically when they become surrounded, first by a reactive cartilaginous casing, and later by an osseous casing (Fig. 3.15). Moreover, in a proportion of cases, prolapse is eventually followed by vascularization (Fig. 3.16), fibrosis, calcification and ossification of the extruded material, and this process may extend into the disc itself.

The protrusion of nuclear material cranially or caudally into the adjacent vertebral body is only possible when there is a gap in the cartilage end-plate and subchondral bone plate. Normal cartilage end-plates do not have gaps. Congenital 'weaknesses' of

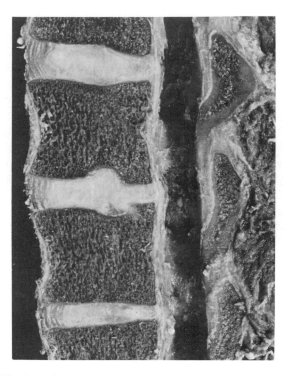

Fig. 3.14 Bisected lumbar spine showing large Schmorl's nodes arising from middle disc. Despite some posterior narrowing of the affected disc, there is little evidence of overall narrowing of the intervertebral space when compared with the normal disc above

the cartilage end-plates may predispose to gap formation; thus in some instances the cartilage opposite the nucleus is much thinner than normal, or a fibrous scar may be present where the end-plate

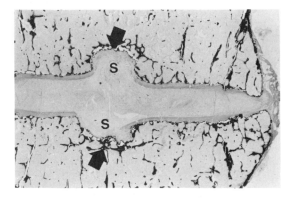

Fig. 3.15 Section through Schmorl's nodes (S) showing formation of increased trabecular bone (arrows) which limits further expansion of the nodes

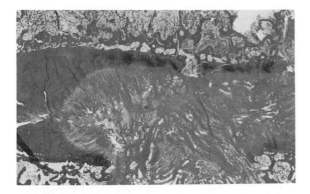

Fig. 3.16 Extensive vascularization of nucleus by vessels extending through defect in cartilage end-plate following organization of a Schmorl's node

was perforated by the axial vessels of the disc in embryonic life. However, apart from those rare conditions in young persons associated with the presence of multiple nodes (adolescent kyphosis, Scheuermann's disease), it seems likely that the majority of Schmorl's nodes are the result of acquired lesions of the cartilage end-plate. Schmorl described small necrotic areas of degenerate cartilage irregularly distributed in the end-plate[3] which could be the sites of herniation.

However, it is probable that most herniations occur as a direct result of single or repeated episodes of trauma causing the extrusion of nuclear tissue through tears in the cartilage of the end-plate and fractures in the subchondral bone. While the usual stress of everyday life may be sufficient to induce a tear in a previously damaged or abnormal end-plate, there is also no doubt that a single severe traumatic episode may be sufficient to rupture a previously normal healthy disc. In those few cases where it has been possible to carry out a pathological examination of a recently injured spine, it is occasionally possible to find tears in the cartilage end-plates associated with herniation of nuclear tissue into the adjoining bone, causing fractures of trabeculae and surrounding haemorrhage.

The majority of Schmorl's nodes are not more than 5 mm in diameter. Most are mushroom-shaped, since the nuclear material spreads out after passing through a relatively small defect in the cartilage end-plate. They are usually situated slightly posterior to the central axis of the vertebral body

(Fig. 3.13), although small nodes are not infrequently seen in other positions. After the extrusion of nuclear material, it is generally considered that the following pathological changes occur. At first, a cavity containing the extruded material is created by fracture of trabeculae and necrosis of marrow tissues in the immediate area of the prolapse. An inflammatory reaction is set up around the herniated material and there is resorption of necrotic bone and marrow. The enlargement of the prolapse may continue rapidly or slowly in this way until the forces causing further herniation disappear or are successfully opposed by reactive changes surrounding the prolapse. Thus the further progression and pressure changes that cause enlargement of the disc prolapse are arrested as soon as the nucleus loses its turgescence as a result of age changes, a decrease in water content or degenerative changes; further expansion is also halted by the formation of a cartilaginous or bony shell around the extruded tissue.

The cartilaginous 'cap' which forms around the extruded tissue is sometimes the result of metaplastic cartilage forming in the marrow at the periphery of the lesion. The extruded material may be surrounded by a zone of increased trabecular bone formation which produces the bony shell limiting further expansion into the vertebral body (Fig. 3.15). The trabeculae forming the walls of these bony shells may exhibit numerous healing trabecular microfractures,[17] indicating that repeated abnormally high stresses are placed on these trabeculae. Frequently there is little or no reactive cartilage or bone formation around the herniation, but the extruded material may be invaded by blood vessels which extend through the gap, in the end-plate into the original disc substance (Fig. 3.16); this vascularization of the node and disc may be followed by fibrosis, calcification or ossification, and will frequently result in radiographically visible changes.

The effect of degeneration and prolapse of the intervertebral discs is to narrow the intervertebral space. This has important consequences:

1. Spinal movements are greatly diminished in the affected segments
2. Forward tilting of the vertebral bodies occurs, and may lead to kyphosis if many discs are affected

3. Marginal osteophytes form anteriorly and laterally, and

4. Abnormal stresses are placed on the apophyseal (posterior intervertebral) joints and cause osteoarthritis, which may be severe.

End-plate changes

In association with advanced degenerative changes in the discs, there is frequently focal, and occasionally complete, disappearance of cartilage from the end-plate region. Fissures may also appear in the cartilage of the end-plates. The bone plate underlying the cartilage end-plates usually becomes irregular owing to focal ossification of the cartilage and indentation of thinned areas by disc substances; double bone plates are frequently formed, and the trabecular bone is usually increased. When disc degeneration is very advanced and the disc space markedly reduced in height, there may be dense bony sclerosis of the adjoining vertebral bodies (see Fig. 3.8).

Vertebral body osteophytes

Some degree of osteophyte formation at the peripheral margins of the vertebral bodies is seen in all cases where there are degenerative changes in the discs, i.e. in all persons after middle age has been reached. They are most frequently seen only on the anterolateral borders of the vertebral bodies and, while occasionally single, they are often multiple and form a row of nodular protruberances down one or both sides of the vertebral column (Figs 3.17, 3.18). The more severe the degenerative changes in the discs, then the more marked are the osteophytes that form in relation to the affected segment. Thus, one or more pairs of large 'beaked' or 'kissing' osteophytes are not infrequently seen in advanced degenerative disc disease, and are particularly prominent when some degree of scoliosis is also present.

Microscopic examination of sections taken through these anterolateral osteophytes reveals that: they form initially by advancing endochondral ossification of the annulus (Fig. 3.19); the spaces between them are occupied by forward extensions of disc tissue (Figs 3.20–3.22); they only rarely become united by bony ankylosis; the remainder of the

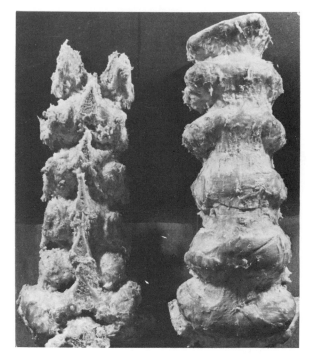

Fig. 3.17 Intact lumbar spine in advanced spondylosis. Anterior view (left) shows large anterolateral osteophytes arising from margins of vertebral bodies. Posterior view (right) shows apophyseal joints enlarged and misshapen due to severe osteoarthritis changes

affected disc shows advanced degenerative changes (Fig. 3.22); there is frequently evidence of Schmorl's node formation; and they increase in size largely by the formation of subperiosteal new bone. The osteophytic bone, at first coarsely trabeculated or compact, later becomes cancellous and the marrow cavities formed communicate freely with those of the vertebral body (Fig. 3.20).

Forming less frequently and reaching a smaller size than the anterolateral osteophytes are osteophytes arising at the posterior margins of the vertebral bodies (see Figs 3.12 and 3.23). They form when there has been wedge-shaped narrowing of the disc, clefts extending through the posterior annulus and true prolapse of the nucleus pulposus through the annulus. In the case of posterior mid-line protrusions, the osteophytes are seldom large enough to narrow the spinal canal. However, when they form posterolaterally in relation to the intervertebral foramina, they may alone or together with protruding disc tissue compress the emerging spinal nerves. Commonly, pressure on the nerves is

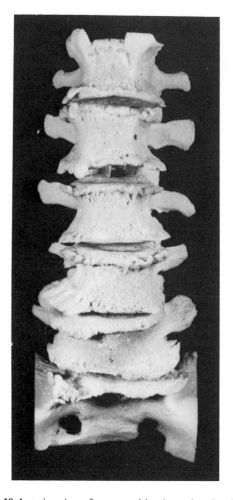

Fig. 3.18 Anterior view of macerated lumbar spine showing large osteophytes which have formed on the margins of the vertebral bodies following disc degeneration (reproduced with permission from Vernon-Roberts & Pirie[1])

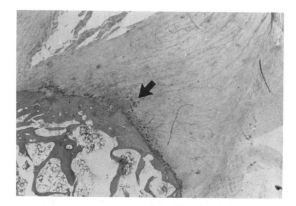

Fig. 3.19 Sagittal section through lumbar intervertebral disc showing a vertebral body osteophyte forming (arrow) by endochondral ossification of metaplastic cartilage in anterior annulus (reproduced with permission from Vernon-Roberts & Pirie[1])

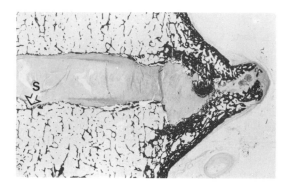

Fig. 3.20 Section through anterolateral disc protrusion. Large osteophytes (right) are composed of dense trabecular bone. A small Schmorl's node (S) is present where the cartilage end-plate is deficient

aggravated by osteophytes projecting into the intervertebral foramina from the margins of osteoarthritic apophyseal joints at the level of the affected disc (see Figs 3.12 and 3.23). A combination of posterior protrusion with osteophyte formation and large apophyseal joint osteophytes may produce a marked degree of narrowing of the spinal canal in relation to one or more affected discs (Fig. 3.23).

Schmorl[3] held the view that the formation of marginal osteophytes is initiated by tears in the region of the peripheral rim of the annulus, which allows the protrusion of disc tissue and stretching of the attachments of the anterior longitudinal ligament, with subsequent bony-spur formation. By contrast, Collins[10] proposed that the primary event in marginal osteophyte formation was the effective collapse of the disc due to degeneration or prolapse. He suggested that the marginal osteophytes were formed as a result of forward tilting of the vertebrae, which produced forward protrusion of the disc, the protruding disc material elevating the periosteum on each side of the anterior longitudinal ligament to

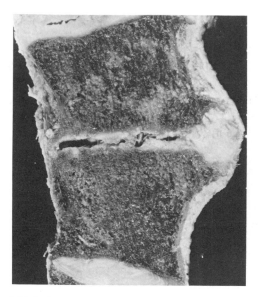

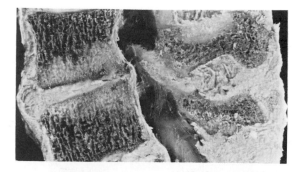

Fig. 3.23 Part of bisected lumbar spine. Anterior and posterior protrusion accompanied by marked collapse of intervertebral disc, with bone sclerosis in vertebral bodies on each side of affected disc. Slight narrowing of spinal canal by posterior disc protrusion and osteophyte formation has been markedly aggravated by the intrusion of apophyseal osteophytes and proliferation of adjoining soft tissues

Fig. 3.21 Sagittal section through vertebral bodies at lumbosacral junction. Large osteophytes are present on each side of the anterior disc protrusion (right), and the affected disc exhibits marked degenerative changes

produce subperiosteal new bone formation antero-laterally.

Recent findings[1] show that, although some marginal new bone formation is sometimes associated with the annular tears described by Schmorl, the size and extent of marginal osteophyte formation is directly related to the degree of degenerative narrowing of the intervertebral space and tilting of the vertebral bodies, as stated by Collins. However,

the findings also suggest that marginal osteophytes form, at least initially, by the endochondral ossification of metaplastic cartilage appearing near the attachments of the annulus to the bone, the role of periosteal elevation in the process of marginal osteophyte formation being unclear.

OSTEOARTHRITIS OF THE APOPHYSEAL (POSTERIOR INTERVERTEBRAL) JOINTS

Structural abnormalities in the disc are always accompanied by osteoarthritic changes in the associated apophyseal joints, while osteoarthritic changes in the apophyseal joints are absent or

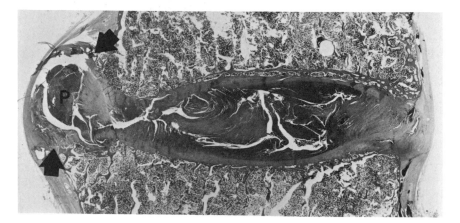

Fig. 3.22 Section through anterolateral disc protrusion showing fissuring of nucleus, and protrusion (P) enclosed by osteophytes (arrows)

minimal when the discs are relatively normal in structure or when there are only early degenerative changes. In the presence of marked degenerative changes in the disc there are always marked osteoarthritic degenerative changes in the apophyseal joints at the same level. Changes are also frequently seen at one or two levels above and below severely affected discs, i.e. they may involve levels at which the discs show minor changes only.

In the presence of conditions such as kyphosis, scoliosis, block vertebrae, spondylolisthesis, fractures, vertebral body collapse and hereditary disease affecting the spine, severe degrees of osteoarthritis of the apophyseal joints are commonly encountered. Apart from these circumstances, while mild degrees of kyphosis and scoliosis are commonly seen in spines at autopsy, in the majority of cases the severity of osteoarthritis appears to be inversely related to the preservation of disc structure.

The examination of apophyseal joints in macerated specimens of whole spines and in thin sections examined microscopically[1] has revealed that osteoarthritis of the apophyseal joints differs from that which is described in large weight-bearing joints such as the hip. An intact covering of hyaline cartilage is frequently retained by the articular surfaces even when large osteophytes have formed, and there is dense sclerosis of the subchondral bone (Fig. 3.24). Indeed, the retention of articular cartilage late in the course of the disease, combined with osteophyte formation and sclerosis of subchondral bone early in the course of the disease, may indicate that remodelling due to changing stresses consequent upon disc dysfunction is the main stimulus to the apophyseal joint changes.

However, in relation to advanced degenerative disc disease, particularly in the lower lumbar spine, the apophyseal joints may exhibit the classic changes of severe osteoarthritis, with areas of bone exposure and eburnation due to complete loss of articular cartilage, cysts, and pseudocysts in the bone, dense bone sclerosis and osteophytosis (Fig. 3.25). In such advanced cases it is not uncommon to find pseudoarthroses where the osteophytes impinge upon the dorsal surfaces of the laminae of the neural arches (Fig. 3.26).

The osteophytic outgrowths from the margins of the apophyseal joints commonly project into the intervertebral foramina, where they may compress the contents (see Figs 3.12 and 3.23). This may be particularly significant when osteoarthritis complicates or occurs as a sequel to a posterolateral disc

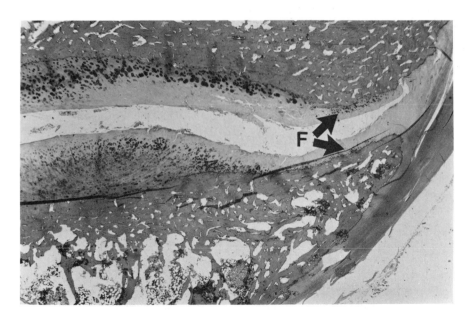

Fig. 3.24 Section through apophyseal joints showing large osteophytes (right) with articular surfaces covered by fibro-cartilage (F). Hyaline cartilage (left) shows moderate osteoarthritic changes and there is dense sclerosis of the subarticular bone

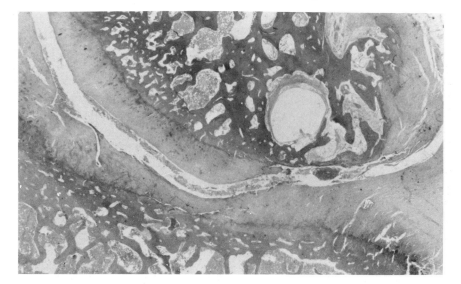

Fig. 3.25 Section through lumbar apophyseal joint showing advanced osteoarthritic changes of fibrillation of cartilage, bone exposure and cyst formation (reproduced with permission from Vernon-Roberts & Pirie[1])

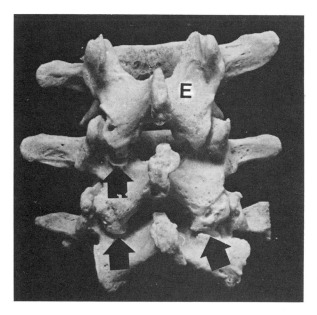

Fig. 3.26 Posterior view of portion of macerated lumbar spine showing osteophytes arising from margins of apophyseal joints, and pseudo-arthroses (arrows) between osteophytes and laminae

prolapse that already narrows part of the foramen. A further factor is the reactive proliferation of capsular and soft tissues, including the adjacent ligamentum flavum, overlying apophyseal osteophytes. This causes further narrowing of the intervertebral

foramina and sometimes bulges markedly into the spinal canal so as to cause some degree of spinal stenosis. In this way a marked degree of spinal stenosis may be produced when the spinal canal is already narrow or has a trefoil-shaped cross-section, or when it is already narrowed by posterior protrusion of the discs in the affected segment.

Bony ankylosis between pairs of apophyseal joints rarely takes place in the absence of ankylosing spondylitis or ankylosing hyperostosis.

An occasional finding in apophyseal joints is the presence of a breach in the subchondral bone plate, with protrusion of a portion of the articular cartilage into the subarticular bone (Fig. 3.27). This feature appears to be independent of disc degeneration or prolapse and of the degree of apophyseal joint osteoarthritis. The appearance of this lesion suggests that it represents traumatic herniation of the articular cartilage following fracture of the sub-chondral bone plates.

The apophyseal joints of spines displaying advanced osteophyte formation on the margins of the vertebral bodies usually exhibit marked osteoarthritic changes. Thus, marked changes in disc structure are always accompanied by significant osteoarthritic changes in the associated apophyseal joints. By contrast, marked osteoarthritic changes in the apophyseal joints are rarely seen when the discs are

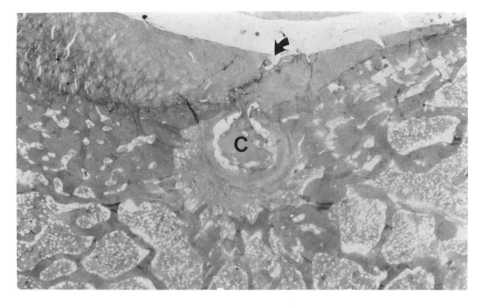

Fig. 3.27 Section through lumbar apophyseal joint showing fissure in articular cartilage (arrow) with defect in underlying bony end-plate, and portion of articular cartilage (C) impacted in subchondral bone (reproduced with permission from Vernon-Roberts & Pirie[1])

relatively normal in structure. Some authors[18,19,6] have stressed the concept of the two posterior joints and the disc forming the 'three-joint complex' such that lesions affecting the disc also affect the posterior joints and vice versa. They have also stressed the fact that the posterior joints are aligned obliquely and the discs are greater in height anteriorly than posteriorly at the two lower lumbar levels. They have suggested that these anatomical features place the two lower lumbar discs at risk.

Although pathological changes in some apophyseal joints similar to those of advanced osteoarthritis affecting the hip or knee may be found, bone exposure is relatively uncommon in the apophyseal joints and affects a small area of the articular surface, cysts are infrequent, marked sclerosis of subchondral bone accompanies early fibrillation of cartilage in the absence of bone exposure, and large osteophytes are frequently formed in the presence of minimal changes in the articular cartilage. The presence of marked bone sclerosis and osteophyte formation accompanying minimal changes in the cartilage could suggest that additional bone is formed in response to increased or altered mechanical stresses, possibly consequent upon primary disc degeneration, and that the majority of apophyseal joint changes are not pathogenetically related to

osteoarthritis of the synovial joints of the appendicular skeleton.

Additional support for this view that the apophyseal joints are subjected to abnormal mechanical stresses comes from the finding of protrusion of articular cartilage through the subchondral bone plate into the underlying trabecular bone in some cases,[1] a finding that has not been reported in osteoarthritic joints of the appendicular skeleton. This view is also supported by a recent report of small fractures of apophyseal facets identified by stereoscopic radiography.[20]

CONCLUSIONS

In conclusion, the sequence of events giving rise to the condition of 'degenerative spondylosis' as it affects the lumbar spine may be postulated on the basis of the pathological findings presented here (Fig. 3.28). The initial event is a structural derangement of the intervertebral disc arising from the normal ageing process, degeneration or prolapse. This is followed by a localized or generalized thinning of the disc with consequent forward tilting of the upper vertebral body about the axes of the apophyseal joints. The forward tilting of the upper

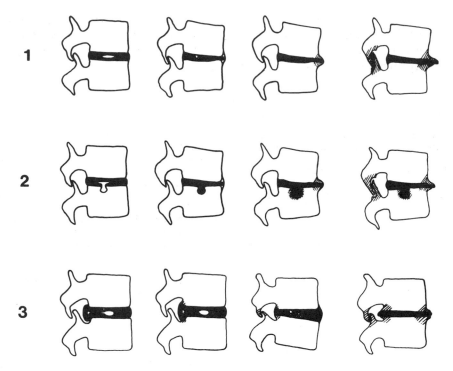

Fig. 3.28 Representation of postulated pathogenesis of lumbar spondylosis. The sequence of events runs from left to right on the diagram. The initial event may be (1) primary disc degeneration (due to ageing?), (2) vertical prolapse (Schmorl's nodes), or (3) posterior prolapse. In each case this results in disappearance of nuclear material, thinning of the disc, bulging of the annulus and osteophyte formation at the margins of the vertebral bodies. The ensuing changes in the mechanics of the spine result in osteophyte formation (shaded) on the apophyseal joints at the level of the affected disc

vertebral body results in anterolateral bulging of the annulus and stimulation of marginal osteophyte formation. The abnormal stresses placed upon the apophyseal joints lead to bone remodelling and, in some instances, true osteoarthritis. Finally, alone or together, each of these pathological changes contributes to changes in the mechanics of the spine at the level of the affected disc or discs.

The major question remaining to be answered is: 'Which of the pathological lesions present in the spine in lumbar spondylosis are concerned in giving rise to back pain?' In theory, pain could arise from the following sites:

1. From within the disc following the ingrowth of nerves accompanying vascularization of clefts and prolapses — it is probable that the nucleus pulposus frequently gains a nerve supply by this process
2. By pressure on pain-sensitive structures (outer annulus, ligaments, dura, nerve roots) by osteophytes arising from the margins of the vertebral bodies
3. By posteroslateral disc prolapses or osteophytes stabilizing such prolapses impinging on nerve roots in intervertebral foramina
4. From osteoarthritis of the apophyseal joints
5. From pseudoarthroses formed on the neural arches of the vertebrae following disc degeneration
6. From fractures of facets or facetal end-plates of the apophyseal joints
7. From narrowing of the spinal canal by posterior disc prolapses and apophyseal osteophytes, particularly when there is already a narrow spinal canal, and
8. From trabecular microfractures in vertebral bodies in association with osteoporosis and Schmorl's nodes.

While most of the above are still speculative possibilities, it may be a minor consolation to clinicians and others who have to deal with the problem of low back pain to know that even clinically and radiologically 'normal' spines can have pathological changes which, until proved otherwise, could be the cause of much stress to both doctor and patient.

REFERENCES

1   Vernon-Roberts B, Pirie C J 1977 Degenerative changes in the intervertebral discs and their sequelae. Rheumat. Rehab. 16: 13–00

2   Schmorl G, Junghanns H 1932 Die gesunde und kranke Wirbelsaule im Röntgenbild. Leipzig

3   Schmorl G, Junghanns H 1971 The human spine in health and disease (trans. E F Besemann). Grune & Stratton, New York

4   Puschel J 1930 Der Wassengelhalf normaler und degenerierter Zurachenwirbelscheiben. Beitr. Path. Anat. 84: 123–000

5   Eyring E J 1969 The biochemistry and physiology of the intervertebral disc. Clin. Orthop. 67: 16–00

6   Kirkcaldy-Willis W H, Wedge J T, Yong-Hing K, Rei K, Reilly J 1978 Pathology and pathogenesis of lumbar spondylosis and stenosis. Spine 3: 319–000

7   Hilton R C, Ball J 1984 Vertebral rim lesions in the dorsolumbar spine. Ann. Rheum Dis 43: 302–000

8   Crock H V 1970 A reappraisal of intervertebral disc lesions. Med. J. Aust. 1: 983–000

9   Venner R M, Crock H V 1981 Clinical studies of isolated disc resorption in the lumbar spine. J. Bone Jt Surg. 63-B: 491–000

10   Collins D H 1949 The pathology of articular and spinal diseases. Edward Arnold, London

11   Andrae R 1929 Uber Knorpelnotchen am hinteren Ende der Wirbelbandscheiben im Bereiche des Spinalkanals. Beitr. Path. Anat. 82: 464–000

12   Key I 1950 Intervertebral disc lesions in children and adolescents. J. Bone Jt Surg. 32A: 97–000

13   King A B 1950 Surgical removal of a ruptured intervertebral disc in early childhood. J. Pediat. 55: 57–00

14   Wahren H 1939 Hernie des Nucleus pulposus bei einem 12 jahrigen Kind. Acta Orth. Scand. 10: 286–000

15   Nachemson A 1966 The load on lumbar discs in different positions of the body. Clin. Orth. 45: 107–000

16   Hilton R C, Ball J, Benn R T 1976 Vertebral end-plate lesions (Schmorl's nodes) in the dorso-lumbar spine. Ann. Rheum. Dis. 35: 127–000

17   Vernon-Roberts B, Pirie C J 1973 Healing trabecular microfractures in the bodies of lumbar vertebrae. Ann. Rheum. Dis. 32: 406–000

18   Farfan H F 1969 Effects of torsion on the intervertebral joints. Canad. J. Surg. 12: 336–000

19   Farfan H F, Sullivan J B 1967 The relation of facet orientation to intervertebral disc failure. Canad. J. Surg. 10: 179–000

20   Sims-Williams H, Jayson M I V, Baddeley H 1978 Small spinal fractures in back pain patients. Ann. Rheum. Dis. 37: 262–000

The neurology of low back pain

I have assumed that no demonstration is required of how necessary the knowledge of human parts is for us who have enlisted under the banner of medicine, since the conscience of each and all will bear full testimony to the fact that in the cure of illness the knowledge of those parts lays rightful claim to first, second and third place; and this knowledge is to be sought primarily from the affected portion. . . .

Andreas Vesalius, *Epitome* (1543)*

INTRODUCTION

Pain is the commonest of all clinical symptoms encountered in medical and surgical practice, and no matter where it is felt in the body and no matter from what cause it is always an expression of a disturbance of neurological function. As such, its differential diagnosis and treatment should (ideally) be founded in every case upon precise understanding of the neurological mechanisms involved in its production, but unfortunately — because the necessary anatomical, physiological and pathological information is seldom available in sufficient detail — this is often not possible in practice, so that the clinician confronted by a patient in pain must perforce in many instances adopt a pragmatic approach in his or her attempts to relieve this distressing complaint.

This is particularly so with backache, the complexities of the understanding of which are compounded by the fact that as a clinical problem it engages (often by chance) the disparate specialized interests of neurologists and neurosurgeons, orthopaedic surgeons and physicians, rheumatologists,

gynaecologists and physiotherapists — to say nothing of general practitioners, osteopaths and chiropractors. These difficulties are especially regrettable in the case of low back pain, in view of the fact that it is the commonest cause of occupational and domestic disability in industrialized societies[1] and that, along with headache, it is the most frequent variety of pain with which general practitioners have to contend in their daily work.[2]

For these reasons, this chapter attempts to draw together the relevant threads of data from contemporary neuro-anatomical, neurophysiological and clinical studies into a systematized pattern that may serve as an operational basis for a more ordered approach to the multifaceted problems presented by patients suffering from low back pain, which, for the purposes of this discussion, is taken to refer to pain experienced in the lumbosacral region. To this end, attention is first directed to current understanding of the basic mechanisms involved in the production of pain in general, which understanding is fundamental to the clinical consideration of pain occurring anywhere in the body, and then to those mechanisms that are specifically relevant to low back pain; this is followed by an attempt to relate this information to the principal varieties of such pain that are encountered in clinical practice.

THE EXPERIENCE OF PAIN — GENERAL PRINCIPLES

Contrary to long-standing traditional views,[3] it is now clear that pain as a phenomenon of human experience is *not* a primary sensation in the sense that vision, hearing, smell, taste, touch, pressure, thermal sensibility and kinaesthesis are. On the contrary, it is

*From the introductory Letter in which Vesalius dedicated his Epitome to King Philip II of Spain (In *The Epitome of Andreas Vesalius*, transl. by L R Lind (1949). M I T Press, Cambridge, Mass.).

an abnormal affective state, i.e. an emotional disturbance, that is called into being by the development of mechanical and/or chemical changes in the tissues of the body of which the nature and magnitude are such that they give rise to activity in afferent systems within the neuraxis that are normally quiescent.[4] In other words, *pain is an unpleasant emotional state* that is aroused by unusual patterns of activity in specific (*nociceptive*) afferent systems, and one that is coloured by the variety of somatic and visceral reflex responses and by the hormonal changes that are simultaneously evoked by such activity.

Pain is not, as it has often been thought to be,[5] merely an unpleasant sensation evoked by particularly intense stimulation of any morphological variety of tissue receptor nerve ending.* Furthermore, and contrary to the empirical beliefs still held by many doctors, it is not so much the precise nature or absolute intensity of a tissue abnormality that determines whether or not it will be painful — or if it is, the intensity of the associated painful experience — as the extent to which the afferent activity that it evokes is channelled into and through those particular (nociceptive) central pathways whose intracerebral connections (q.v.) are such that they will evoke the experience of pain when activated to an appropriate degree. This discrepancy between the degree of tissue disturbance and the subjective intensity of the resulting pain — although empirically familiar to experienced physicians and surgeons — is nonetheless often dismissed, or attributed to some underlying psychiatric disorder in the patient, on the grounds that it is inexplicable in terms of the conventional view of pain as a primary sensation, but as will become apparent later in this chapter, it is a natural product of the fact that the centripetal flow of nociceptive afferent activity is subject to varying degrees of facilitatory and inhibitory modulation at many of the central synapses through which it must pass on its course from the peripheral tissues to the cerebral cortex to evoke therein the emotional disturbance that is pain. No matter how bizarre its clinical presentation may appear to be, then, a complaint of pain is always indicative of some variety or degree of tissue

dysfunction — unless the complainant is to be regarded as a malingerer.[6]

But although pain is an affective state, it differs uniquely from all other affective states of human experience in that it is always invested with a local habitation in the sufferer's body,[7] for unlike other affective states (such as elation or sorrow, for example), pain is always felt in some particular part of the body with varying degrees of precision.* This somatotopic attribution of pain may, however, sometimes be erroneous — as in patients with referred pain, or in those in whom the painful part of the body is in fact no longer present, as with the 'phantom pain' that may follow amputation of a limb or a breast.[8]

It is also essential to remind clinicians that although the emotional experience of pain is regarded by most individuals in contemporary civilized society as highly unpleasant and undesirable, and thus as something to be avoided or got rid of as soon as psossible, this is not always the case, even in apparently sophisticated societies. Thus, even today in some cultures and in certain religious sects (including some of the more extreme varieties of Christianity, and in the Hindu and Islamic faiths) pain is regarded as morally elevating, or as a means, especially when self-inflicted, of expiating feelings of guilt attached to some supposed transgression of ethical or social principles.[9] These attitudes were also earlier expressed in many of the initiation ceremonies practised in primitive tribal cultures, and in the activities of the flagellant orders of medieval European Christianity.

Such a penitential concept of pain is still extant in our own society, for it is implicit in the word itself, which has always carried the connotation in the English language of being an experience that is chastening, by virtue of its etymological origin.[10] The modern English word *pain* entered medieval English from the Latin root *poena* by way of the Norman French word *peine*, both of which signify a penalty or punishment (as does the modern French word *peine*), and this was the sole meaning of the English word 'pain' originally, bodily suffering then being described in early English by another word,

*This concept was first clearly appreciated by Erasmus Darwin (1731–1802) — the grandfather of Charles Darwin — and propounded by him in his book *Zoonomia* (1794), in which he emphasized that pain was *not* a sensation.

*It might be noted in passing that the seventeenth-century Dutch philosopher Benedictus de Spinoza (1632–1677) long ago — and with remarkable prescience — classified pain (in his *Ethics*) as 'a localized form of sorrow', and thus as one of the 'primary emotions'.

dolour (or dolor), also of Latin (and Norman French) origin, as is the modern French word douleur, the Spanish dolor and the Italian dolore. This differentiation, in turn, derives from Attic Greek usage, in which οδυνγ or λυπγ were used to designate bodily (or mental) suffering whereas ποινγ was the word for punishment or penalty. The linguistic distinction between 'pain' and 'dolour' was observed by all the early writers in English from Chaucer to Shakespeare, but gradually disappeared from the English language after the translators of the so-called Authorized Version of the Bible (1611) used the word 'pain' indiscriminately in both senses, so that the idea of pain as punishment became inevitably linked in popular usage with the description of bodily suffering.* This dual linguistic concept of the word 'pain' is still widespread among English-speaking people (to whom it is peculiar among speakers of the principal modern European languages†), and continues subconsciously to influence the attitude of many of them to painful experiences and their description of their suffering — which is the reason for this etymological digression in the present context.

It should also be noted that some psychiatrically disturbed individuals (e.g. hypochondriacs and masochists) may actually derive personal emotional satisfaction from the experience of pain,[11] sometimes to the point of deliberately resisting or attempting to circumvent therapeutic attempts to relieve them of it. Yet others may utilize it (consciously or subconsciously) as a protective device in the face of emotional, domestic or occupational stress, as may be the case with some of the complaints of backache encountered in psychiatric, medico-legal, industrial medical and gynaecological practice. On the other hand, there is a very small number of individuals, often otherwise apparently normal, who entirely lack the capacity to experience pain that is possessed by the rest of the human race.[12]

It has often been claimed that the apparent ubiquity of the experience of low back pain is an inevitable consequence of the evolutionary assumption of the erect posture by the human species. But such an assumption is extremely dubious,[13] not least

*Thanks are due to Miss Maria Wyke (of Somerville College, Oxford) for etymological assistance.
†Thus, in German, bodily suffering is specifically designated by the word Schmerz, whereas the word for penalty or punishment is Strafe.

in the light of the much greater incidence of this complaint in industrialized as compared with hunter–gatherer societies, which rather suggests that it is individual lifestyle rather than bipedal evolution that is primarily at fault. At the outset of this account, then, it is asserted that low back pain is not biologically inevitable but, on the contrary, is preventable — and should it occur, treatable — provided that adequately detailed information regarding its various modes of production be forthcoming. To this end, this chapter attempts to provide some of the relevant neurological data that are now available, based on the thesis that a clinician confronted with a patient with this complaint should regard the patient as someone with a pain that happens to be in the lower back, rather than as someone with a back that happens to be painful.

PERIPHERAL NOCICEPTIVE SYSTEMS IN THE BACK

With the foregoing general considerations as background, the structural and functional features of the neurological systems innervating the tissues of the lower back of which the abnormal activity may give rise to the experience of lumbosacral pain are now reviewed.

Nociceptive receptor systems in the lumbosacral tissues

In spite of prolonged argument for over a century, there is now no doubt that most (albeit not all) tissues of the body, including those in the lower back, are provided with a morphologically distinct system of receptor nerve endings that are sensitive to mechanical and chemical tissue dysfunction, and which are therefore categorized as nociceptive receptors. As with other regions of the back,[14] this system is represented in the lumbosacral region[15] by plexiform and freely-ending unmyelinated nerve fibres that are distributed tridimensionally (see below) throughout the skin, subcutaneous and adipose tissue; the fasciae, aponeuroses and ligaments; the vertebral periosteum and marrow; the adventitial sheaths of blood vessels (both arteries and veins); and the fibrous capsules (although not the articular cartilage or synovial tissue) of the lumbar apophyseal (facet) and sacroiliac joints (see Table 4.1). In normal circumstances, this nociceptive receptor system remains largely inactive, but it becomes active when its constituent unmyelinated nerve fibres are depolarized[16] by the application of mechanical forces to the containing tissue that sufficiently stress, deform or damage it (as with pressure, distraction, distension, abrasion, contusion, laceration or tearing), or by their exposure to sufficient concentrations in the surrounding tissue fluid of irritating chemical substances (such as lactic acid, potassium ions, polypeptide kinins, 5-hydroxytryptamine, prostaglandins and histamine[17] that are released from traumatized, inflamed, necrosing or metabolically abnormal (and especially ischaemic) tissues.

The clinically relevant details of the distribution of the lumbosacral tissue nociceptive receptor system (Table 4.1) are as follows:

1. In the skin and subcutaneous (including the adipose) tissues of the back. As with the similar tissues elsewhere in the body,[18] the receptor system here consists of a dense network of unmyelinated nerve fibres that weaves tridimensionally throughout the tissue, and from which still finer nerve terminals pass superficially towards the skin surface between the epidermal cells.

2. Throughout the fibrous capsules of the synovial joints between the articular processes of contiguous lumbar vertebrae, and of the sacroiliac joints.[19] In these joint systems, the tridimensional plexus of unmyelinated nerve fibres is morphologically identical with that present in the fibrous capsules of all the other synovial joints in the body,[20] including those of the joints in other regions of the vertebral column.[21]

Table 4.1 Distribution of lumbosacral nociceptive receptor systems

---

1. Skin, subcutaneous and adipose tissue
2. Fibrous capsules of apophyseal (facet) and sacroiliac joints
3. Longitudinal spinal, interspinous, flaval and sacroiliac ligaments
4. Periosteum covering vertebral bodies and arches (and attached fasciae, tendons and aponeuroses)
5. Dura mater and epidural fibro-adipose tissue
6. Walls of blood vessels supplying the spinal and sacroiliac joints, and in vertebral cancellous bone
7. Walls of epidural and paravertebral veins
8. Walls of intramuscular arteries within lumbosacral muscles

---

3. In the longitudinal spinal, interspinous, flaval and sacroiliac ligaments.[22] In these ligaments, as with ligaments elsewhere in the body,[23] the nociceptive receptor system is not plexiform but instead consists of unmyelinated free nerve endings that weave between the bundles of ligamentous fibres. Furthermore, it should be noted that there are significant differences in the density of the nociceptive innervation of the individual spinal ligaments,[24] this being greatest in the posterior longitudinal ligament, less in the other, longitudinal and sacroiliac ligaments, and least in the interspinous and flaval ligaments.

4. In the periosteum covering the vertebral bodies and arches,[25] and in the fasciae, aponeuroses and tendons attached thereto.[26] In these tissues, the nociceptive receptor system consists of a plexus of unmyelinated nerve fibres of varying density that is similar to, but less dense than, that in the apophyseal joint capsules, and the plexus system in the vertebral periosteum (and joint capsules) is continuous with that in the tendons, fasciae and aponeuroses that are attached to the vertebral bodies and arches and to the joint capsules.

5. In the dura mater and epidural fibro-adipose tissue within the lower end of (as elsewhere within) the vertebral column.[27] In the spinal dura mater, and extending into the dural sleeves that surround the nerve roots, the nociceptive receptor system is again represented by a plexiform array of unmyelinated nerve fibres, but this system is largely confined to the anterior aspect of the dural tube (a fact evidenced, inter alia, by the experience of lumbar puncture), and its density is less than that of the similar plexiform system in the joint capsules and vertebral periosteum. Also in the fibro-adipose tissue that occupies the space between the dural tube and the bony walls of the spinal canal, i.e. the epidural tissue, there is an identical nociceptive plexus system, but its density in this tissue is less in the lower than in the upper regions of the vertebral column.

6. In the walls of the arteries and arterioles supplying the intervertebral apophyseal and sacroiliac joints, and of the blood vessels in the cancellous interior of the vertebral bodies and arches and of the sacrum and ilium.[28] This peri-arterial nociceptive system consists of a dense plexus of unmyelinated nerve fibres, embedded in the adventitial sheaths of the blood vessels, that may be irritated in a variety of

ways (to be described later). It should be emphasized at this point, however, that the bony tissues of the lumbosacral region (apart from their cancellous interior) contain no receptor nerve endings of any description, and hence can never be the direct source of low back pain.[29]

7. In the adventitial sheaths of the paravertebral and epidural veins.[30] A dense plexus of veins extends along the entire length of the vertebral column, both external to the vertebral bodies and within the epidural space,[31] and the whole of this continuous vertebral venous system is enmeshed by a nociceptive plexus of unmyelinated nerve fibres,[32] the clinical significance of which will be considered later in this account. This perivenular plexus thus constitutes a second spinal perivascular nociceptive system additional to that represented by the periarterial system described above.

8. In the adventitial sheaths of the arteries and arterioles that ramify through and supply the paravertebral and other muscles of the lower back. This intramuscular perivascular nociceptive system is identical to that in all the other striated muscles of the body,[33] and its irritation is a frequent and potent cause of low back pain, as will be described later.

It will be remarked that thus far no mention has been made of a nociceptive innervation of the intervertebral discs in the lower spine, in spite of the fact that low back pain has often been attributed to disease of these structures giving rise to irritation of nerve endings that are assumed to be present therein.[34] This omission arises from the fact that, once a child assumes the erect posture, the unmyelinated nerve terminals, which are certainly present in the immature intervertebral discs of the fetus and neonate,[35] rapidly degenerate and disappear, so that in the mature human spine no nerve endings of any description remain in the nucleus pulposus or annulus fibrosus of the intervertebral discs in any region of the vertebral column.[36] Clinicians should note that the only place where a nociceptive receptor system is directly related to the intervertebral discs is in the fibro-elastic tissue that binds the posterior surface of each annulus fibrosus to the related portion of the posterior longitudinal ligament,[37] where it may be directly irritated by (the relatively rare) central disc protrusion or nuclear herniation. The much more common posterolateral herniation of the nucleus pulposus impinges on and irritates the nociceptive plexus embedded in the anterior aspect of the dural sleeves surrounding the related spine nerve roots that has been described previously.

Nociceptive afferent pathways from the lower back

The afferent pathways through which nerve impulses evoked from the lumbosacral nociceptive receptor systems just described are delivered into the spinal cord are represented[38] by small myelinated and unmyelinated nerve fibres 5 μm or less in diameter — and which therefore belong to the Group III category[39] of human peripheral nerve fibres — whose cell bodies are all located in the dorsal root ganglia of the lumbar and sacral spinal nerves. The very small diameter of these nociceptive afferents from the lumbosacral tissues determines[40] their slow conduction velocity, their relative insensitivity to transcutaneous electrical stimulation of the nerve trunks containing them (q.v.) and, above all, their extreme sensitivity to blockade produced by subarachnoid or epidural injection of local anaesthetic drugs.

The nociceptive afferents from all the tissues of the lower back that lie posterior to the vertical plane through the intervertebral foramina traverse individual branches of the posterior primary rami of the spinal nerves to reach the dorsal spinal roots, whereas the more anteriorly located tissues are innervated through specific anterior branches of the same spinal nerves, including the recurrent sinuvertebral nerve.[41] The clinically relevant details of this afferent innervation are as follows:

1. Afferents from the dermatomes (and related subcutaneous tissues) of the lower back[42] are conveyed through the *lateral* branches of the posterior primary rami of the lumbar dorsal nerve roots and the upper two sacral nerve roots. But it should be noted, especially in relation to some clinical matters to be considered later, that the nociceptive afferent innervation of individual dermatomes is not unisegmental but is, instead, plurisegmental, with considerable variation from person to person, and that there is a good deal of overlap between adjacent dermatomes in this respect.[43] Thus, individual lumbosacral dermatomes may receive their nociceptive afferent innervation from a minimum of three and a maximum of five

contiguous dorsal nerve roots in different subjects.

2. Afferents from the lumbar apophyseal and sacroiliac joints, the vertebral arches and sacral cancellous bone and periosteum (and the tendons, fasciae and aponeuroses attached thereto), and from the flaval and interspinous ligaments (together with those from the perivascular receptor system in the related back muscles) enter the *medial* branches of the posterior primary rami of the lumbar and sacral nerves,[44] and this innervation is again plurisegmental.

3. The nociceptive receptor system in the capsule of each apophyseal joint is innervated from both *primary* and *secondary* articular nerves, the former being independent and variable nerve filaments that run directly to the joints from the spinal nerves as they emerge from the intervertebral foramina, and the latter arising as intramuscular branches of the muscle nerves supplying some of the back muscles and reaching the joints by running through the substance of the muscles and their joint capsule attachments.[45] It should also be emphasized (because of its clinical relevance to matters of diagnosis, and to the surgical and manipulative treatment of low back pain) that nowhere in the vertebral column, including its lumbar region, does an individual apophyseal joint receive its nociceptive innervation exclusively from the segmentally related dorsal nerve root. Certainly each joint does receive such a segmental innervation, but in addition it is innervated by articular nerves that descend to it from rostrally located dorsal nerve roots and ascend to it from more caudal nerve roots.[46] For the above reason, claims that lumbar apophyseal joints can be denervated by blind percutaneous surgical procedures purporting to divide segmentally related articular nerves or dorsal nerve roots are clearly unfounded.

4. Afferents from the nociceptive receptor systems in the posterior and anterior longitudinal spinal ligaments, the anterior dura mater and dural sleeves, the walls of the epidural veins and the epidural fibro-adipose tissue, the periosteum covering the vertebral bodies (and the walls of the blood vessels in their cancellous interior) traverse various branches of the recurrent sinuvertebral nerves (of von Luschka) to reach the dorsal nerve roots.[47] These nerves arise from each spinal nerve just distal to the dorsal root ganglion as the nerve root emerges from the intervertebral foramen and immediately turn me-

dially (applied to the posterior surface of the annulus fibrosus of the related intervertebral disc) to re-enter the spinal canal, within which they are distributed intersegmentally (through ascending and descending collateral branches that run along the edges of the posterior longitudinal ligament) to the tissues mentioned above. Because of its application to the posterior surface of the annulus fibrosus as the sinuvertebral nerve re-enters the spinal canal, it will be clear that this nerve is readily impinged upon as posterolateral herniation of the nucleus pulposus develops, and in this connection it is relevant to point out that the sinuvertebral branch of the second lumbar nerve regularly gives off a long descending collateral branch that extends caudally (alongside the posterior longitudinal ligament) as far as the fifth lumbar vertebra, so that afferent inputs may be fed into the second lumbar nerve root as a result of lesions expanding posteriorly into the spinal canal from vertebral bodies or intervertebral discs lying well below this level, and thus give rise to pain experienced in regions of the back that may mislead the clinician unaware of this anatomical fact.

5. In addition to the above pathways, further nociceptive inputs are delivered into the dorsal nerve roots by afferent fibres from the perivascular plexus in the walls of the paravertebral system of veins.[48] These afferents not only convey activity from the nociceptive receptor system already described as being embedded in the adventitial sheaths of these veins, but also from receptor systems located in some other spinal tissues; for a proportion of the nociceptive afferents from the vertebral periosteum, the cancellous bone within the vertebrae, the anterior longitudinal ligament and the apophyseal joint capsules join and run through the perivenular plexus system (sometimes after traversing the lower sympathetic ganglia and trunk) before finally entering the dorsal spinal nerve roots.

Intraspinal distribution of lumbosacral nociceptive afferents

As the preganglionic portion of each lumbar and sacral dorsal nerve root approaches the spinal cord within the spinal canal it divides[49] into two rami — anterior and posterior, and all the afferent fibres that are 5 μm or less in diameter entering the root from the periphery are diverted into the anterior ramus, while the other larger fibres are aggregated into the posterior ramus. Thus, the nociceptive afferents from the tissues of the lumbosacral region are delivered into the spinal cord by way of the anterior ramus, while the larger-diameter afferents from the same tissues (including those innervating the corpuscular mechanoreceptors in the skin and in the capsules of the apophyseal and sacroiliac joints, and the muscle spindles and tendon organs in the back muscles) enter by way of the posterior ramus.

On entering the spinal cord, the anteriorly located nociceptive afferents give off[50] short ascending and descending branches that for one or two segments run up and down in the spinal white matter (in the dorsolateral tract of Lissauer), together with direct medially-orientated branches. All of these branches then penetrate into the dorsal horn of the spinal grey matter, where they terminate by synapsing on various groups of relay neurones located therein. Many of them run anteriorly through the dorsal horns to synapse on neurones located[51] at the base thereof (in the *basal spinal nucleus*), the axons of which then cross the spinal cord in the anterior grey commissure to turn upwards in the contralateral anterolateral tracts to reach the brain (see below); while others project polysynaptically through interneurones[52] located in the *apical* and *intermediate* nuclei of the dorsal horn ultimately to reach the anteriorly located motoneurone pools of the back, thigh, and abdominal muscles. Transmission of nociceptive afferent activity through the former ascending projection system underlies (as will be described later) the evocation of the experience of pain in the lumbosacral region, while the simultaneous transmission of activity through the latter intraspinal polysynaptic system of reflexogenic pathways contributes to the changes in motor unit activity in the back, abdominal and lower limb musculature[53] that are associated with nociceptive irritation in the lumbosacral tissues and which result in the clinically apparent disorders of posture and gait that are associated therewith.

CENTRAL LUMBOSACRAL NOCICEPTIVE PROJECTION SYSTEMS

Ascending spinal projections

Should nociceptive afferent activity of peripheral lumbosacral origin result in trans-synaptic activation of the neurones located in the basal spinal nucleus,* the efferent discharges thereby evoked therefrom are propagated rostrally into the brain in the *anterolateral spinal tracts*.[54] In the lumbosacral region of the spinal cord the majority of the axons of the nociceptive relay neurones in the basal spinal nucleus cross the cord obliquely (in the anterior grey commissure) to turn upwards into the contralateral tract, and very few (unlike the situation in more rostral regions of the spinal cord) ascend ipsilaterally. Furthermore, within each anterolateral tract the ascending fibres are disposed in somatotopically organized groups in oblique laminae like the segments of a fan, such that the fibres transmitting activity of lumbosacral tissue origin lie, in the supralumbar regions of the spinal cord, dorsal and lateral to those conveying activity from more rostrally located tissues.[55] These neuro-anatomical details are not merely of academic interest, and are mentioned here because they are of vital concern to the neurosurgeon contemplating the performance of the operation of anterolateral spinal tractotomy[56] for the relief of severe, persistent pain in the lower part of the body.

It should be noted that the spinal tract system designated herein as the 'anterolateral tract' is the one traditionally (but, as it turns out, erroneously) known as the 'spinothalamic tract'. The latter designation was based on the earlier assumption that all of its constituent fibres ascend without synaptic interruption to the thalamus. More recent clinical surgical experience[57] and experimental study,[58] however, indicate that this is not so. On the contrary, less than 30% of the fibres (namely, those of relatively larger diameter and, hence, of faster conduction velocity) in this tract system actually terminate in the thalamus: most of the remainder are of finer diameter and slower conduction velocity (50–60% of them being unmyelinated) and do not reach the thalamus but terminate on neurones in the brain-stem reticular system (see below) and other brain-stem nuclei,[59] while still others re-enter the spinal grey matter to synapse on internuncial neurones located therein after ascending for varying distances within the anterolateral tracts.[60] Thus, in

---

*This is not an inevitable process, and some of the clinically significant mechanisms that may modulate it are considered later in this chapter.

terms of their operation as a cerebral nociceptive input system, the anterolateral tracts constitute a double-barrelled system, one barrel firing, through a small proportion of relatively fast-conducting, paucisynaptic pathways, into the thalamic nuclei, and the other, larger, barrel firing, through a multitude of more slowly conducting, multisynaptic pathways, ultimately into the brain-stem reticular system. The clinical significance of each of these components of the central lumbosacral nociceptive input system is further considered below.

Nociceptive relays in the brain stem

The fibres in the spinal anterolateral tract system that do not terminate on internuncial neurones within the spinal grey matter continue their ascent into the medulla oblongata (wherein they lie ventrolaterally near the surface of the brain stem) and mesencephalon (wherein they lie dorsolaterally).[61]

As the ascending tract traverses the lower brain stem just dorsal to the inferior olivary nuclei, most of its smaller diameter fibres leave it to enter (as described above) the adjacent longitudinal column of neurones that is the *reticular system*,[62] while more rostrally others deviate dorsally into the tectum of the midbrain.[63] Activity conveyed in the former (reticulopetal) group of fibres is then propagated further rostrally (and slowly) through a large series of intermediate synaptic relays within the mesencephalic portion of the reticular system, ultimately to the centre-median and intralaminar nuclear complexes of the thalamus,[64] while activity in the latter (tectopetal) projection is delivered to neurones located in the tectal nuclei.[65]

The remaining small proportion of larger-diameter fibres ascends still further through the mesencephalon to the diencephalon, finally to enter the *thalamus*, wherein they terminate (in the case of the fibres conveying impulses of lumbosacral origin) on neurones in the lateral portion of the posteroventral nucleus,[66] in the intralaminar nuclear system[67] and pulvinar,[68] and in the magnocellular portion of the lateral geniculate body.[69]

These anatomical and physiological observations on the various modes of termination of the fibres in the anterolateral spinal tracts reinforce the suggestion, made above, that afferent activity, originating in the nociceptive receptor systems located in the lumbosacral tissues is propagated into the brain to evoke the experience of low back pain through two parallel pathways — one being a relatively rapidly-conducting, paucisynaptic system that feeds mainly into the posterolateral ventral nucleus of the thalamus, and the other a very slowly-conducting, multisynaptic system whose activity is eventually delivered to the intralaminar and centre-median thalamic nuclear complexes. Furthermore, it is much more likely[70] that the familiar dual nature of the experience of pain that follows transient peripheral nociceptive receptor stimulation — the so-called 'fast' and 'slow' varieties of pain — arises from the difference in the time course of transmission of the resulting afferent activity through these two central pathways finally to the cerebral cortex (see below), rather than that it is due, as the traditional explanation would have it, to differences in the conduction velocity of afferent impulses in two distinct groups of peripheral afferent nerve fibres supposedly different in diameter from one another, especially since no such dichotomy of peripheral nociceptive nerve fibre diameters exists, there being instead (as pointed out earlier) a continuous spectrum of such fibre diameters from 5 μm down to less than 1 μm. Additionally, it might be noted in this context that direct electrical stimulation of the anterolateral spinal tract system with appropriately selected stimulus parameters in patients undergoing spinal surgery with local anaesthesia[71] can separately evoke either of these two varieties of painful experience, as a result of selective activation of differing fibre diameter populations within the tract (the few large-diameter fibres therein having a lower threshold than the many small-diameter fibres).

It should also be emphasized that in none of the thalamic nuclear relay sites mentioned above (with the possible exception of the intralaminar nuclei) are there neurones that respond uniquely to peripheral noxious stimulation. Instead, all of them are individually capable of activation as a result either of noxious or of innocuous, i.e. mechanoreceptor, peripheral stimulation,[72] and this intrathalamic synaptic convergence of nociceptive receptor and mechanoreceptor inputs on the cells of the posteroventral thalamus nucleus especially may exert a significant influence on the perceptual capacity to localize the peripheral source of pain,[73] as well as contributing to the modulation of its subjectively apparent intensity (see below). Furthermore, neurosurgical experience[74] has shown that in spite of the relatively wide diversity of thalamic nuclei upon which ascending nociceptive inputs terminate, localized surgical lesions placed stereotactically in certain of them (especially the intralaminar and centremedian nuclei) may sometimes result in relief of persistent pain for varying periods of time; and, on the other hand, direct electrical stimulation of the same nuclei in unanaesthetized human subjects and animals produces, in the former, pain felt in specific regions of the body, including the lumbosacral area, and in the latter behavioural responses indicative of the experience of pain.[75]

While much still remains to be determined regarding the relative rôles of the different thalamic synaptic relays in generating and modulating the experience of pain, the experimental and clinical data currently available leave little doubt that evocation of this experience depends upon the development of a critical degree of activity in several of the thalamic nuclear systems in response to discharges delivered to them (both directly and indirectly) by way of the central nociceptive afferent pathways projecting thereto — which, in the case of low back pain, means the relevant fibres of the anterolateral spinal tracts. But as already indicated, and as will be discussed in more detail later, generation of this critical degree of activity in the thalamic nuclei depends not only upon the intensity and duration of peripheral nociceptive receptor stimulation but also upon the extent to which centripetal trans-synaptic flow of the afferent discharges resulting therefrom is modulated (in the spinal grey matter and in the thalamic nuclei themselves) by coincident inputs from peripheral tissue mechanoreceptors and by the on-going activity of central projection systems to these same synaptic sites (see below). Nevertheless, once such a degree of activity has been generated in the neurones of the thalamic nuclei it is inevitably dispersed intracerebrally therefrom in four directions simultaneously, and each component of this quadruple extrathalamic projection system makes a specific contribution to the patient's global experience of pain,[76] as follows.

Thalamic nociceptive dispersal systems

Perceptual component

In the case of pain in the lower back, impulses reaching the lateral portion of the posteroventral nucleus of the thalamus are relayed therefrom — in fibres of the thalamocortical radiation that ascend through the posterior limb of the internal capsule — mainly to neurones in the superior paracentral, both pre-and post-central,[77] regions of the cerebral cortex.[78] Because of the predominantly contralateral input of lumbosacral tissue receptors into the spinal anterolateral tract system (see above), each half of the lumbosacral region projects largely to the superior paracentral region of the opposite cerebral hemisphere (somatic sensory area I), and there is only a meagre input from this region of the body to the inferior parietal lobe (somatic sensory area II) of the ipsilateral hemisphere.

Within the paracentral cortical projection area, the receptor systems in the lumbosacral tissues transmit their activity to vertically disposed columns of neurones that are somatotopically organized within a small region of cortex that is located around the point where the central fissure (of Rolando) cuts across the superior margin of the cerebral hemisphere.[79] Furthermore, within this small cortical area afferent activity from cutaneous (and subcutaneous) receptors is projected to cortical neurones that lie closer to the central fissure than do those that receive inputs from more deeply located tissues[80] such as the spinal joints and ligaments, while intramuscular receptors project to neurones lying in, or anterior to, the central fissure[81] as well as to others located in the superior postcentral and parietal cortical regions.[82]

Activation of this somatotopically organized thalamocortical projection system underlies the patient's capacity to recognize (with varying degrees of precision) the peripheral anatomical location of the source of pain and its qualitative nature, i.e. whether pressing, pricking, bursting, stabbing, throbbing or burning, but it does not provoke the experience of pain as such.[83] Thus, experimental peripheral nociceptive stimulation, in the absence of coincident mechanoreceptor stimulation (a situation, however, that is rare in clinical practice except in respect of pain that is the result of the chemical abnormalities in tissues that have been described earlier) results in little or no activation of cortical neurones in sensory area I,[84] while direct electrical stimulation of cortical sensory area I (or II) in unanaesthetized patients never evokes pain, although it gives rise to a galaxy of non-painful somatic sensory experiences in the related parts of the body.[85] Furthermore, localized traumatic, infarctive or neoplastic lesions involving cortical sensory area I do not impair patient's awareness of the painful nature of peripheral nociceptive stimulation, although they seriously interfere with his or her ability to identify its anatomical location,[86] and the same applies with surgical or pathological lesions confined to the posteroventral nucleus of the thalamus from which the paracentral cortical projection system arises.[87]

Taken together, the above observations indicate[88] that the thalamic projections to the paracentral region of the cerebral cortex contribute what may be called the *perceptual component* of painful experiences — that is to say, the sufferer's awareness of whereabouts in his or her body the source of pain is located and his or her capacity to apply qualitative discriminations to its nature — but nothing 'hurts' as a result of activation of this thalamocortical projection system. Furthermore, this perceptual information appears to be related not so much to the activity derived from irritated peripheral nociceptive receptor systems as to the degree of activity being coincidentally evoked from related tissue mechanoreceptors by the pain-provoking stimulus, which latter activity is transmitted through the posterior spinal column-lemniscal system to the same posteroventral thalamic nuclear neurones and thence to the same cortical neurones as receive the nociceptive input from the identical part of the body. This proposal receives support from the clinically obvious fact that the precision of the description of their experience given by patients with pain of mechanical origin (see above) is much greater than when their pain is of purely chemical origin, for the majority of adjectives used by patients in qualifying the nature of their pain are descriptive of mechanical (e.g. pressing, pricking, bursting, stabbing, throbbing) rather than of chemical (e.g. burning) experience, and the long-familiar clinical observation[89] that lesions of the dorsal spinal columns seriously impair a patient's capacity to identify the location and nature of a painful stimulus in the lower part of the body, even though the intensity of his or her now diffused pain is then considerably enhanced (see below).

Affective component

As indicated at the beginning of this account, pain is an affective disorder, and evocation of this emotional disturbance is contingent upon activation of a second set of thalamocortical projections, namely, those that pass from the medial and anterior thalamic nuclei to neurones in the frontal cortex by way of the anterior limb of the internal capsule. Within this massive thalamocortical radiation system, it is its inferior portion, which passes from the dorsomedial nuclei of the thalamus to the orbital surface of the frontal lobes,[90] and its medial portion, which projects from the anterior thalamic nuclei to the cingulate cortex,[91] that are of special significance in relation to the evocation of pain, for it is in the synaptic systems of these two regions of the cerebral cortex that things 'hurt' when nociceptive afferent activity arrives therein.[92]

Within the thalamus, secondary intrathalamic connexions[93] link the relay nuclei within which the spinothalamic components of the anterolateral tract system terminate (principally, the posteroventral nucleus) to the dorsomedial and anterior nuclei, from which axons ascend to synapse (inter alia) with neurones in the orbitofrontal and cingulate regions of the cerebral cortex, which cortical regions form part of the so-called 'limbic system' that is concerned with emotional behaviour.[94] Nociceptive afferent impulses reaching the thalamus from the lumbosacral tissues are thus propagated to the orbitofrontal and cingulate regions of the cerebral cortex coincidentally with their delivery to the superior paracentral regions of the cortex, and clinical evidence (see below) clearly indicates that it is the arrival of such activity in the former regions of cortex that specifically underlies the evocation of the unpleasant emotional experience that is pain; in the present context, then, it might be said that it is in these regions of the brain that a backache 'aches'.

Clinical study of the effects of selective neurosurgical interruption of the above-mentioned orbitofrontal thalamic projection system in patients with persistent pain, either at its distal end in the operation of orbitofrontal leucotomy[95] or at its origin in the thalamus by the performance of stereotatic thalamotomy,[96] confirms the above proposals; for in either instance the procedure, when successful, relieves the distress of which the patient complains and his or her need for powerful analgesic drugs — in other words, it relieves the pain — but does not remove his or her perceptual awareness of a bodily abnormality. Thus, after such operations the patient remains aware that something is still wrong with a particular part of his body but no longer complains that it hurts him,[97] the reason being that the surgical procedure has interrupted the thalamic projection into the limbic sectors of cortex where the emotional experience of pain is evoked, but has left the perceptual projection system (see above) to the paracentral cortex intact. Finally, further emphasis is lent to the validity of the distinction being made here between the emotional disturbance that *is* pain and the perceptual component *of* this experience, by the observation[98] that, in unanaesthetized patients, direct electrical stimulation of the intralaminar thalamic nuclei, which project to the orbitofrontal and cingulate, but not to the paracentral regions of the cerebral cortex, results in intense unlocalized pain felt in the entire contralateral half of the body.

Memory component

A third (but much smaller) thalamocortical projection system links some of the medial thalamic nuclei (and pulvinar) on each side of the brain to the cortex of the related temporal lobe,[99] in the synaptic circuits of the ventromedial parts of which (with their associated structures) are located the recent and long-term memory storage systems of the brain,[100] and these regions of the temporal lobe also receive secondary inputs from the cortical sectors mentioned earlier through many corticocortical association fibres.[101] Thus it is that nociceptive (and mechanoreceptor) afferent activity reaching the thalamus and the limbic and paracentral cortical sectors to which the thalamic relay nuclei project (see above) is transferred into the memory-storage system; and it is by this means that a subject builds up his or her memory of past painful experiences such as backache.

Clinical experience and specific neuropsychological study indicate, however, that the efficacy of the transfer of such input information from the short-term to the long-term memory storage system is not simply a function of the intensity of individual episodes of painful experience.[102] Instead, the vividness and duration with which the memory of pain is preserved appear to relate much more to the length of time a painful experience lasts (as with chronic painful disorders) or to the frequency with which it is repeated (as with recurrent episodes of acute pain.)

Visceral-hormonal reflex component

A fourth (non-cortical) projection system passes from some of the secondary, and especially the medial, thalamic nuclei to the subjacent hypothalamic nuclei located in the ventral diencephalon, which nuclei also receive inputs from (inter alia) neurones in the adjacent portions of the brain-stem reticular system and in the limbic sectors of the cerebral cortex.[103] As the discharges from certain of the nuclear subgroups within the hypothalamus continuously control the global efferent activity in the sympathetic and parasympathetic outflows from the neuraxis,[104] and as neurones within these same hypothalamic nuclei are also the source[105] of the hypophysoportal hormones that regulate the secretory activity of the adenohypophysis as well as of the antidiuretic and oxytocic hormones, it will be apparent that the above-mentioned thalamo-hypothalamic projection system provides the means whereby nociceptive afferent activity entering the brain evokes the complex of visceral reflex effects such as those involving the cardiovascular and gastro-intestinal systems, and the hormonal changes that are inevitably associated with the experience of pain.[106]

Arising out of the above observations, it should be emphasized here — because of the frequent attempts that have been, and continue to be, made to find measurable parameters of physiological function that might serve as so-called 'objective' indices of the intensity of painful experiences[107] — especially in patients with persistent low back pain — that the thalamo-hypothalamic mechanisms just described operate reflexly, and hence the magnitude of the changes in visceral nervous activity and in hormonal status thereby produced in patients in pain *do not correlate* with the intensity of the emotional experience (simultaneously evoked in the synaptic circuits of the orbitofrontal and cingulate regions of the cerebral cortex) that is pain. In short, the visceral and hormonal changes and the experience of pain are epiphenomena that are evoked in parallel by the arrival of nociceptive afferent activity in the thalamus, and (for reasons that will become apparent later) are not directly related quantitatively. Hence, clinical attempts to use measurements of changes in pupillary diameter, in heart rate and arterial blood pressure, in electrical skin resistance or skin temperature, or in plasma catecholamine concentration as indices of the intensity of painful experiences are entirely fallacious, for they are based on the false assumption of an equation between the hypothalamic reflex effects of peripheral nociceptive receptor stimulation and the affective response thereto. Since a complaint of pain is a description of a subjective emotional change whose intensity is independent of the concurrent reflex changes in the sufferer's body, attempts to assess its severity should be based on the use of self-rating scales based on established psychological principles,[108] and this applies as much to lumbosacral pain as to pain anywhere else in the body.

MODULATION OF THE AWARENESS OF LOW BACK PAIN

The quadripartite dispersal within the brain of activity of nociceptive receptor origin that has just been described indicates that each of the thalamic projection systems contributes its own specific component to the global experience of pain. But nowhere within this fourfold intracerebral projection system is there any neurological mechanism that can explain the vagaries of the experience of pain that are so apparent to the sufferer in his or her everyday life. Thus, personal introspective experience reveals all too clearly that the intensity of a pain with which one happens to be afflicted varies widely with one's prevailing emotional mood, with the extent to which one's attention may be engaged by concentration on one's daily tasks, and in response to suggestion by others.[109] Furthermore, experienced clinicians are well aware of the fact that individual patients vary in the intensity of their experience of pain from day to day and from time to time in the course of the day,[110] and that different patients with apparently comparable pathological lesions giving rise to pain may report widely differing degrees of suffering.[111]

Nevertheless, these familiar everyday aspects of the experience of pain have always been ignored or dismissed by those wedded to the traditional view of pain as a 'sensory modality' whose intensity is directly determined by the activity inevitably provoked in a direct on-line projection system from peripheral 'pain receptors' to a supposed 'pain centre' located somewhere within the brain.[112] Fortunately, however, in recent years a series of neuro-anatomical, neurophysiological and neuropharmacological studies has shed considerable light on these clinically important matters (which are especially significant in relation to backache) by revealing that the experience of pain may be modulated up or down in its intensity by concurrent activity in a number of peripheral and central neurological systems that play upon the nociceptive afferent system at various synaptic stages in its course within the neuraxis.

Peripheral modulation of pain

The large-diameter afferents derived from the various mechanoreceptors (including the apophyseal articular mechanoreceptors and the muscle spindles) that are distributed through the lumbosacral tissues enter the spinal cord through the posterior rami of the dorsal nerve roots (see above), and immediately divide into many ascending, intersegmental and segmental collateral branches.[113] Among these branches, however, are some that penetrate into the adjacent dorsal horns of spinal grey matter to synapse therein on neurones located in the apical spinal nucleus (containing the substantia gelatinosa Rolandi, and including lamina II of Rexed,[114] on which are also subtended collaterals from the much finer nociceptive afferent fibres traversing the dorsolateral tract of Lissauer,[115] as described earlier. The axons of the apical spinal interneurones then turn laterally out of the dorsal horn to join the dorsolateral tract, within which they ascend and descend for varying distances[116] and from which they re-enter the spinal grey matter to reach[114] the basal spinal nucleus (or lamina V of Rexed). Therein they terminate (in axo-axonic synapses) on the presynaptic terminals of the nociceptive afferents that directly reach, as described previously, the relay neurones located in the basal spinal nucleus — and the influence of the apical spinal neurones, exerted through their presynaptic axo-axonic synapses on the terminations of the peripheral nociceptive afferent fibres, is inhibitory.[117] Thus it is that the probability that nociceptive afferent discharges originating in the lumbosacral tissues will effect trans-synaptic activation of the relay neurones in the basal spinal nucleus, and thus be propagated up into the brain to evoke the experience of pain, is inversely related to the on-going frequency of discharge from mechanoreceptors located in these same (or related) tissues — which discharge through the presynaptic inhibitory effect that it exerts through the apical spinal interneurones on the trans-synaptic propagation of nociceptive afferent activity through the basal spinal nuclear relays into the anterolateral spinal tracts (see above), depresses the centripetal flow of such activity.

These seemingly arcane matters are not merely of academic neurological interest, but have considerable practical significance for the understanding of the clinical phenomena of pain in general and of low back pain in particular, for they indicate that the centripetal projection into the central nervous system of afferent activity from the nociceptive receptor systems located in the lumbosacral tissues is not a directly inevitable on-line process (which, as pointed out previously, is often assumed to be the case), but instead is continuously modulated at its synaptic portal of entry into the neuraxis (i.e. in the basal spinal nucleus) by the concurrent activity emanating from the mechanoreceptors located in these same or related tissues. This mechanism provides one of the several reasons (others will be described later) why the intensity of the experience of low back pain is not simply a direct function of the intensity of mechanical or chemical irritation of the lumbosacral tissue nociceptive receptor systems, but is related (inter alia) inversely to the prevailing activity of the tissue mechanoreceptors.

In this connexion, it is relevant to point out that all human beings, as well as many animals, are instinctively aware that rubbing or pressing on painful regions of the body may temporarily abort the pain being experienced therein. Again, midwives have long known from their empirical experience that one of the most effective ways of alleviating the low back pain associated with the first and second stages of labour is to carry out prolonged, deep massage of the mother's lumbosacral tissues. In actual fact massage, compression and vibration of tissues, which procedures may be usefully employed

for the relief of pain,[118] including that in the lumbosacral region, as physiotherapists well know, are all techniques that stimulate the slowly adapting and rapidly adapting mechanoreceptors located therein, and thereby generate central presynaptic inhibitory blockade of nociceptive afferent activity through the mechanisms described above. The same mechanisms may also be operated for therapeutic purposes by selective transcutaneous electrical stimulation of the large-diameter (and hence low threshold) mechanoreceptor afferent nerve fibres in appropriate peripheral nerves,[119] but the most effective means of producing massive peripheral mechanoreceptor stimulation in patients with low back pain, and thus prolonged and effective relief of their discomfort, is to persuade them to spend their sitting time in rocking chairs (q.v.) instead of in static chairs.[120]

These observations may also explain why the minor traumata to which many tissues in the body, including those in the lumbosacral region, are continuously exposed in everyday life do not, in the majority of people, give rise to significant degrees of pain, for such daily traumatic stimuli are usually mechanical in nature, and hence activate mechanoreceptors at the same time as they irritate the nociceptive receptors in the affected tissues. Furthermore, the operation of this peripheral modulating system, in conjunction with the central modulating mechanisms to be described below, may provide the reason why the many attempts made over the past 35 years to measure so-called 'pain thresholds' in human subjects[121] have largely proved irrelevant to the practical problems associated with the assessment of pain in clinical practice,[122] including lumbosacral pain, for most of the techniques used for this purpose take no account of the possible effects of, or do not evoke, afferent discharges from the mechanoreceptors located in the tissue (usually the skin but sometimes the muscles) being tested, although activation of these latter receptors is very frequently involved in clinical pain-producing situations. In this same context, it is perhaps worth reminding clinicians that the majority of people do not seek therapeutic assistance because their pain 'threshold' has been exceeded — for this happens almost every day in most individuals — but because the limits of their pain 'tolerance' have been reached, from which it follows (as will be mentioned again later) that it is measurement of the *pain tolerance* of individual patients that is the clinically relevant parameter worth determining, not their pain threshold.

While much still remains to be done in developing the applications of the experimental data that are now available in the field of pain research to the specific clinical problems that are presented by the different varieties of low back pain (see below), there can be no doubt that recognition of the modulating influence of peripheral tissue mechanoreceptor activity upon the centripetal trans-synaptic propagation of nociceptive afferent activity has already proved helpful in a number of circumstances. Thus, it seems[123] that the extreme cutaneous hyperalgesia that afflicts patients with post-herpetic neuralgia is the result, of selective destruction of the parent dorsal root ganglion cells of the large-diameter mechanoreceptor afferents in the affected peripheral nerves, with consequent loss of their normal presynaptic inhibitory effects on centripetal synaptic nociceptive afferent transmission until (and if) these mechanoreceptor afferent neurones regenerate. A comparable mechanism may underlie the production of the zones of hyperaesthesia that have been observed in the skin of the lower back[124] of some patients with lumbosacral pain, for it may be that in such patients the mechanoreceptors located in the apophyseal joints of the lumbar spine[125] are destroyed (as the result of trauma, or of degenerative or inflammatory diseases involving this region of the vertebral column) and as a result their normal inhibitory effects on nociceptive afferent transmission are lost, although no direct neuropathological evidence of this proposal is yet available. Furthermore, as increasing age in adult life is associated with progressive, selective degeneration of peripheral tissue mechanoreceptors and their large-diameter afferent fibres in peripheral nerves throughout the body,[126] the resulting gradual loss of their central inhibitory effects on centripetal nociceptive afferent transmission may contribute to the diminishing pain tolerance that characterizes middle aged and elderly patients,[127] and thus to the greater incidence and severity of non-traumatic backache in older than in younger subjects.[128] In the present context, it is also relevant to point out that chronic degenerative neurological diseases (for example, tabes dorsalis) that involve selective degeneration of

the dorsal root ganglion cells of the peripheral spinal mechanoreceptor afferent nerve fibres are associated with cutaneous hyperalgesia and episodes of 'spontaneous' pain felt in various regions, including the lumbosacral area, of the lower part of the body,[129] and that direct electrical stimulation of the dorsal spinal columns with implanted electrodes — and thus antidromic activation of the ascending collaterals therein derived from peripheral mechanoreceptor afferents — has been found[130] to produce relief in patients suffering from persistent pain by retrograde (i.e. antidromic) activation of the inhibitory interneurones in the apical spinal nucleus that have already been described.

Finally, it must be emphasised here that one of the most effective, and non-intrusive, methods of producing sustained relief of persistent lumbosacral pain is to install the patient in a rocking chair for as many hours of the day as is possible. The effectiveness of this simple mode of therapy arises from the fact that the rhythmic oscillations of the body thereby engendered generate fluctuating discharges from the various mechanoreceptors located in the moving joints and muscles of the lower part of the body (including those in the lumbosacral region) that maintain prolonged presynaptic inhibitory blockade (through the mechanisms described previously) of peripheral nociceptive inputs. Clinical experience with the use of rocking chairs by patients with persistent low back pain, as well as by those with chronic pain in the joints and muscles of the lower limbs, has already shown[131] that it has a significant effect in ameliorating the severity of their discomfort, a fact reflected, inter alia, in a marked reduction in the patients' daily intake of analgesic drugs. In addition, since low back pain in older subjects is often associated with co-incident chronic respiratory disease such as bronchitis, emphysema or asthma, or with cardiovascular dysfunction as in arteriosclerosis, it is worth pointing out here that the use of rocking chairs not only produces useful degrees of pain relief but also assists impaired pulmonary ventilation and defective haemodynamics, in the latter case, particularly, by augmenting venous return from the lower limbs.

Central modulation of pain

In addition to the modulating influence of peripheral tissue mechanoreceptor inputs that has just been described, awareness of pain is further modulated by at least three central projection systems within the neuraxis that influence the sequential centripetal propagation of afferent activity of lumbosacral nociceptive receptor origin through its synaptic relays in the spinal grey matter, in the thalamus, and in the cerebral cortex itself.

In the spinal cord

The centripetal flow of nociceptive impulses through the synapses in the basal nuclei of the dorsal horns of the spinal grey matter up to the brain is modified through descending projection systems derived from neurones located in the caudal region of the brain stem reticular system, and in the paracentral regions of the cerebral cortex.

Reticulofugal system

Axons descend in the reticulospinal tracts from large neurones located medially in the caudal (pontomedullary) part of the reticular system to synapse[132] with the interneurones in the apical nucleus of the spinal grey matter that exert presynaptic inhibitory effects, which probably involve 5-hydroxytryptamine as a transmitter agent,[133] on the nociceptive afferent terminals subtended on the projection neurones in the basal spinal nucleus, upon which inter-neurones the reticular projections exert a facilitatory influence. As this reticulofugal projection system is discharging continuously at varying frequencies throughout life, it will be clear that its activity normally restricts (to varying degrees) the onward flow into the spinal cord and brain of impulses of peripheral nociceptive receptor origin[134] — including those from the tissues of the lower back — thereby reinforcing the similar effect of inputs from mechanoreceptors located in the same (and related) tissues in depressing awareness of the effects of nociceptive irritation in the lumbosacral tissues.

The normal inhibitory effect of the activity of this reticulofugal cascade system on noticeptive afferent transmission is *augmented*[135] when one's attention is diverted away from a painful site in the body by stimulation elsewhere, or by concentration of atten-

tion on some particular task; when sleep supervenes; when hypnosis is induced; when hysterical anaesthesia develops; and when the blood concentration of catecholamines becomes very high, as in states of great emotional tension. These facts (inter alia) may explain why distraction of attention or counter-irritation elsewhere in the body diminishes awareness of lumbosacral pain, why hypnotic suggestion may be effective in alleviating backache in some patients, and why soldiers in battle (with consequent high blood concentrations of catecholamines) may sustain severe injuries without complaining of pain.[136] It is also relevant for the clinician to note that numbers of drugs, if administered in individually appropriate doses, may selectively increase the activity of the reticular neurones that operate this inhibitory system,[137] and thereby reduce a patient's awareness of pain without diminishing his or her general state of alertness. Examples of such drugs are methylamphetamine, chlorpromazine (Largactil), diazepam (Valium), and morphine and its analogues.

Conversely, a *reduction* in the centrifugal inhibitory effect of the caudal reticulospinal projection system on spinal nociceptive afferent transmission enhances the intensity of on-going painful experiences, and also increases the probability that a particular peripheral tissue stimulus (whether mechanical or chemical) will evoke an attack of pain.[138] Such a situation may arise[139] with exposure to sudden, intense painful stimuli that canalize attention on the lumbosacral tissues; with specific direction of the patient's attention to those tissues in the absence of distracting stimuli; and following the administration of small doses of ethyl ether or barbiturates.[140] Clinicians should note particularly that it is for this latter reason that patients suffering from chronic backache, or repeated attacks of episodic lumbosacral pain, should never be given small doses of barbiturates of any type,[141] including quinalbarbitone (Seconal), pentobarbitone (Nembutal) and phenobarbitone (Luminal) for soporific or sedative purposes, for then the pain will be intensified to the point where it becomes excruciating agony. Indeed, one of the worst things that can happen to a patient with backache is for some well-meaning doctor to prescribe a barbiturate for her 'to help her get a good night's sleep', for the exact reverse will often be the case.

Corticofugal system

The modulating influence of this descending reticular projection system on spinal synaptic transmission is, in turn, regulated from the cerebral cortex by way of projections from several cortical sectors (especially the frontal and paracentral regions) to neurones located in the caudal portion of the reticular system.[142] Some of these corticoreticular fibres exert a facilitatory influence[143] upon the reticulospinal neurones to which they project, and thus (when increasingly excited) enhance reticular blockade of spinal synaptic transmission of nociceptive activity, while others have the reverse effect, and several studies[144] in the past decade suggest that variations in the activity of this system, and especially that part of it derived from the superior frontal and anterior parietal regions, may underlie the changes in awareness of peripheral, nociceptive stimuli that are associated with alterations in the direction of attention and with induction of hypnosis, to which reference has already been made.

In addition to these direct corticoreticular projections, there is an indirect (multisynaptic) projection system that influences the caudal reticular neurones through facilitatory relays on interneurones located in the midbrain, particularly in the periaqueductal grey matter. The synaptic transmitter agents that excite these interneurones are amines with a molecular structure closely resembling that of morphine, and hence are designated as *endorphins*,[145] and it now appears that the enhanced activity of the pain-suppressive reticular neurones that is produced by morphine and its analogues (see above) results from activation by these drugs of the endorphin-sensitive interneurones in the midbrain[146] that project to the caudal reticular neurones. Thus, it seems that there are two parallel pathways by which corticoreticular modulation of pain may be achieved — one direct, and the other indirect through the endorphin relays in the midbrain — but the precise clinical circumstances in which one or other of these systems may operate to influence lumbosacral pain are still uncertain.

There is also evidence[147] of still more direct corticofugal modulation of nociceptive afferent transmission through spinal synaptic relays, operated through fibres that arise from neurones in the paracentral regions of the cerebral cortex and descend (mainly contralaterally) in the corticospinal tract system to terminate in several of the internuncial synaptic relay systems in the dorsal horns of the spinal cord, transmission through which they may facilitate or inhibit.[148] Some of these corticospinal fibres may terminate in facilitatory synapses on neurones in the apical spinal nucleus, excitation of which leads secondarily to presynaptic inhibition of nociceptive afferent transmission,[149] but others appear to end in presynaptic inhibitory axo-axonic synapses on the larger diameter mechanoreceptor afferent collaterals[150] subtended on these same spinal interneurones, and their activity would then result eventually in enhancement of centripetal transmission of nociceptive afferent activity. Nevertheless, whatever the precise functional details of these terminations may be, it is now clear that the regions of cerebral cortex to which the 'perceptual' projections (see above) of the lumbosacral afferent systems are delivered exert both negative and positive feedback influences on the centripetal transmission of activity within these systems at the spinal level, which processes may assist in 'sharpening' the subjective localization of the evocative stimulus within the lumbosacral tissues. It may also be noted here that pathological destruction of the cells and nerve fibre terminals in the dorsal horns of the spinal cord, as occurs in some patients with syringomyelia,[151] leads to the development of intense burning pain in the related tissues, presumably because of the resulting loss of the inhibitory effects normally exerted on nociceptive afferent transmission by the cells of the apical spinal nuclei and the peripheral mechanoreceptor, reticulofugal, and corticofugal projection systems related thereto.

In the thalamus

Additional modulation of the centripetal propagation of nociceptive spinothalamic tract activity is provided more rostrally through projections to the thalamic relay nuclei from the cerebral cortex. These corticothalamic projections,[152] like those entering the corticospinal tracts described above, arise from neurones located (inter alia) in the para-central regions of the cerebral cortex and descend through the internal capsule to synapse with the thalamic neurones on which the spinothalamic fibres relay, on which neurones they exert long-lasting postsynaptic inhibitory effects.[153] Supplementary post-synaptic (as well as presynaptic) inhibitory effects on thalamic synaptic transmission of nociceptive afferent activity may also be exerted from more widely dispersed cortical neurones located in the frontal, parietal and temporal regions[154] and in other parts of the cortical limbic system,[155] either through direct cortico-thalamic projections, or indirectly through sub-cortical relays in the caudate nucleus.[156]

It therefore seems that neurones located in each of the cortical regions to which centripetal spino-thalamic activity is dispersed to evoke the perceptual, emotional and memory aspects of painful experiences, exert a retrograde inhibitory (i.e. negative feedback) influence on the thalamic sites through which such nociceptive activity is relayed to the cerebral cortex, and thereby 'damp down' awareness of pain. The precise circumstances in which these corticofugal inhibitory projections to the primary and secondary thalamic relay nuclei operate is still unknown, especially in relation to backache, although loss of their normal inhibitory influence on account of interruption of their pathways by destructive internal capsular or parathalamic lesions (such as may occur in patients with cerebral vascular disease, or following intracerebral stereotactic surgery) may have something to do with the production of the syndrome of so-called 'thalamic pain'.[157]

In the cerebral cortex

The excitability of the neurones in each of the cortical sectors within which the thalamocortical projections terminate is continuously modulated by ascending activity that reaches them (mainly through relays in some of the 'non-specific' thalamic nuclei) from neurones located in the rostral (and particularly the mesencephalic) portions of the brain stem reticular system, via the reticulocortical projection system.[158] The influence of this continuously active system on cortical neurones is generally facilitatory, so that their excitability at any moment is a function of the prevailing frequency of reti-culocortical discharge, and for this reason, this system was originally designated as the 'reticular activating system'.[159] More recent study has led to some modifications of the original anatomical implications of this latter term, but the functional concept of cortical activation provided from neuro-nes located in the rostral brain stem has been thoroughly validated, both in experimental and clinical contexts.[160]

It now seems[161] that this cortical activating system is operated from rostral reticular and 'non-specific' thalamic (for example, midline and intralaminar) neurones, and functions as a driving (or 'alerting') mechanism for the synaptic systems within most of the cortical mantle, to which it contributes an unceasing but fluctuating stream of facilitatory impulses. Thus, an individual's prevailing global awareness of the environment (that is, his or her 'state of consciousness'), and the intensity of all his or her sensory and emotional experiences (including pain), is continuously modulated by the degree of activity prevailing in this system.[162] As nociceptive afferent activity originating in the lumbosacral tissues is channelled into the brain stem reticular and intralaminar thalamic neuronal systems from the spinothalamic tracts, and thereby influences cortical activation through the pathways outlined above, it will be clear that the state of excitability obtaining in the cells of the reticular system and intralaminar thalamic nuclei at the time when nociceptive impulses are delivered thereto will, from moment to moment, determine the magnitude of the responses of these cells to such an input and thus, through their corticopetal projections, influence the intensity of a patient's experience of backache.[163] In this con-nection, it is relevant to note that peripheral nociceptive stimulation has been shown[164] to be a particularly potent means of evoking augmented activity in the reticular system and in the cortical activating system.

Experimental and clinical studies extending over the past 15 years have shown that many afferent, metabolic, hormonal and pharmacological influen-ces too numerous to describe in detail here[165] may produce moment-to-moment fluctuations in the excitability of reticular and other cortical-activating neurones, and thus in the intensity of the awareness of pain. For example, cortical activation is *enhanced*, and pain is thereby intensified, in states of persisting anxiety: by a moderate increase in the blood concentration of catecholamines; by moderate degrees of hypercarbia, such as obtain in chronic respiratory disease; by the taking of drugs such as dextro-amphetamine (Benzedrine), cannabis indica (marijuana) and lysergic acid diethylamide (LSD-50); and by the intake of small amounts of alcohol or caffeine. For this reason, therefore, small amounts of alcohol in the form of brandy or whisky, or caffeine in cups of tea or coffee, should *never* be given to patients in pain,[166] as these socially conventional gestures merely intensify the pain. Conversely, cortical activation is *reduced* and pain is thereby diminished: by emotional tranquillity (induced by suggestion, for instance); by the onset of sleep; by hypocarbia (induced by hyperventilation, for instance*); by the intake of large amounts of alcohol (which may, in fact, be used as an anaesthetic agent); and by the administration of drugs such as meperidine (Pethidine) and the volatile and non-volatile general anaesthetic agents.

As the cortical activating system projects (inter alia) to the orbitofrontal, paracentral (and inferior parietal) and temporal sectors of the cerebral cortex, it follows that should afferent impulses from lumbosacral nociceptive receptors be delivered into the brain at a time when reticulocortical excitability is augmented for any of the reasons mentioned above, the backache will be felt to be intense, it will be relatively well localized within the lumbosacral tissues, and it is likely to be remembered relatively vividly, whereas, should the same afferent input enter the brain at a time when reticulocortical excitability is diminished (again for any of the reasons already mentioned), the pain will be felt to be less severe, it will be poorly localized, and memory of the experience is likely to be imprecise and short-lived. In this way, then, the intensity of the emotional experience of backache, the precision of its perceptual localization within the lumbosacral tissues and the vividness with which it is likely to be remembered are all conditioned by the degree of activity prevailing in the rostral activating projections to the orbitofrontal, paracentral and parietal, and temporal sectors of the cerebral cortex, and thus — as well as for the reasons already mentioned — are not solely determined by the physical or

chemical intensity of the peripheral nociceptive stimulus. When these observations are added to the other reasons already mentioned, it is hardly surprising that an individual's *pain tolerance* is a widely varying parameter of his or her experience and that it bears little relation to his or her relatively constant *pain threshold*.[167]

CLINICAL CATEGORIES OF LOW BACK PAIN

Having outlined the nature and distribution of the nociceptive receptor systems located within the various tissues of the lumbosacral region, the pathways by which afferent fibres from these receptors transmit activity therefrom into and through the spinal cord and brain, and the mechanisms by which such transmission of nociceptive afferent activity may be modulated from peripheral and central sources, an attempt can now be made to relate these data to some of the varieties of low back pain that are encountered in clinical practice, general accounts of which may be found in other parts of this book and in representative reviews published elsewhere.[168] To this end, it is operationally convenient, and apposite for diagnostic and therapeutic purposes, to classify low back pain into four principal categories[169] in terms of the neurological mechanisms whose disordered activity may give rise to pain experienced in the lumbosacral region. These groups are summarized for convenience in Table 4.2 and will now be discussed in order.

Primary backache

When low back pain is the result of direct mechanical or chemical irritation of the nociceptive receptor nerve endings embedded in the various lumbosacral tissues, it may be designated as *primary backache*. In this situation, then, the pain is experienced by the patient, with varying degrees of precision, in those tissues within which the pathological disturbance, whether mechanical or chemical, or both, is operating, and within this category further subdivision is possible in terms of the particular tissues containing the irritated nociceptive nerve endings, as follows.

*In this connection, it may be noted here that hyperventilation (produced by excitation of respiratory neurones in the caudal reticular system (see Wyke, 1974c) is one of the reflex consequences of painful stimulation; and that many primitive tribal and religious rituals that are utilised to produce analgesia in the participants (see Sargant, 1957) involve procedures that induce hyperventilation in them.

Table 4.2 Classification of spinal pain syndromes

1. *Primary backache*
   a. Cutaneous and subcutaneous
   b. Myofascial (muscles and fasciae):
      (i)   Trauma
      (ii) Spasm
      (iii) Fatigue
      (iv) Inflammation
   c. Articular and ligamentous:
      (i) Apophyseal and sacroiliac joints
      (ii) Spinal ligaments
   d. Osseous (vertebral and sacral):
      (i) Intravertebral
      (ii) Periosteal
   e. Vascular (venous)
   f. Dural

2. *Secondary backache*
   a. Compressive lesions
   b. Degenerative lesions

3. *Referred backache*
   a. Gynaecological
   b. Urinary tract
   c. Prostate
   d. Appendix

4. *Psychosomatic backache*
   a. Depression and anxiety
   b. Hysteria
   c. Malingering

Cutaneous pain

The nociceptive receptor system distributed through the skin and subcutaneous (including the adipose) tissues of the back may be irritated by a wide variety of cutaneous lesions of which the diagnostic recognition usually presents little difficulty to the experienced clinician and which, therefore, do not require detailed enumeration here. Suffice it to say that direct involvement of the superficial tissues of the back by trauma (involving contusion, laceration or burning), by ulceration (as in a number of dermatological diseases, and in tabes dorsalis), by neoplasms (especially those extending superficially from more deeply located tissues) or by infective lesions (as with abscesses and cellulitis) are the major causes of superficial primary low back pain, and to these may be added the superficial burning pain that is experienced when some portion of the lumbosacral skin is involved in the acute (erythematous and vesicular) stage of herpes zoster infection.

Myofascial pain

One of the commonest causes of low back pain is provided by irritation of the nociceptive receptor system that is distributed through the muscle masses of the lower back, their fascial sheaths and intramuscular septa and the tendons that attach them to the vertebral column and pelvis. Such irritation usually arises as a result of mechanical trauma to these tissues or of the reflex spasm or fatigue of the muscles, and less often because of inflammatory changes therein. Its existence is indicated by the patient with backache stating that the pain is felt in the deep tissues of the back lateral to the lumbar spine, that it restricts (and is made worse by) movements of the spine in particular directions, and that it is relieved by the local application of heat and by lying flat in the supine position; and by the fact that when asked to indicate the site of maximum pain with his fingertips, he or she places them over some part of the laterally located paravertebral muscle masses or their spinal attachments.

Trauma. The rapid development of high tensions in the muscles of the lower back, as when attempting to lift heavy weights while in a stooping position,[170] may lead to avulsion of some of the tendinous attachments of these muscles to the pelvic or lumbosacral skeleton, or, less often, and usually when the muscles are initially relaxed, as they are in the fully flexed position,[171] to rupture of muscle fibres and tearing of their fascial sheaths. The pain experienced is more intense in the former than in the latter case,[172] but in either instance it consists of a sharp stab at the moment of injury, followed by an incrementing dull ache that may persist thereafter for many days or even weeks, together with intense, relatively localized deep tenderness and reflex spasm of the affected muscles. The initial stabbing pain results from disruption of the unmyelinated nerve terminals that ramify through the tendons and fascial sheaths of the muscles, or which surround the intramuscular blood vessels, while the prolonged aching pain is due to irritation of the same nerve endings located in the vicinity of the injury by the chemical changes that develop and persist in the interstitial fluid of the damaged tissue.

Muscle spasm. Everyday experience provides clear testimony of the fact that when excessive motor unit activity is maintained for prolonged periods in any muscle, a dull aching pain develops in that muscle, which also becomes tender to pressure. This pain arises because of irritation of the plexus of un-myelinated nerve fibres distributed through the adventitial sheaths of the intramuscular blood vessels by the chemical changes that develop in the interstitial fluid of the muscles, especially the increase therein in lactic acid and K^+ ion concentration that results from the abnormal metabolic activity of the hyperactive muscle fibres. These changes occur more rapidly in the muscles of untrained (i.e. sedentary) than of trained (i.e. active or athletic) subjects, and their development is influenced by muscle temperature and blood flow rate, being, for example, more readily provoked in cold than in warm, and in elderly than in young subjects.[173]

These considerations apply to the muscles of the lower back as much as to striated muscles elsewhere in the body, for persisting reflex hyperactivity may develop in these muscles in response to abnormal activity of the receptors located in the joints of the vertebral column[174] as a result of postural abnormalities (such as those associated with certain occupations, with the later stages of pregnancy and with prolonged wearing of high-heeled shoes,[175] for example), of pathological changes in the vertebral column (as with degenerative disc diseases, rheumatoid arthritis, osteoarthritis, osteoporosis and osteomalacia), or of irritative lesions involving segmentally related viscera (especially the genito-urinary system). In the investigation of patients with low back pain, then, it is essential to examine the individual components of the lumbosacral musculature for evidence of spasm, and to obtain reliable information this may require the use of static and dynamic multichannel electromyography.[176] If such spasm be present, further investigations are necessary to determine whether it is the reflex result, of mechanical, structural or inflammatory abnormalities in the skeletal and articular tissues of the lumbosacral spine, or whether it is reflexly provoked from a lesion located elsewhere in segmentally related visceral tissues. In the latter case, backache due to reflex muscle spasm should not be confused with referred backache (see below).

Muscle fatigue. Everyday experience also demonstrates all too clearly that muscles subjected to prolonged work become fatigued, and as a result become locally painful and tender, and this applies to the back muscles, as when they are kept hyperactive by the assumption of persistently distorted standing or sitting postures, or by the demands of occupation or athletic activity.[177] Although the mechanisms involved in the production of muscular fatigue are complex and still not clearly understood,[178] there is no doubt that the muscular discomfort with which the process is associated, and which becomes increasingly evident on cessation of the excessive muscular activity, depends on an inadequate muscle blood flow[179] and results from biochemical changes in the muscles[180] similar to those already described (see above) for the pain due to reflex muscle spasm, and it may be relevant that experimental studies have shown[181] that increased activity occurs in the small-diameter nociceptive afferent fibres in muscle nerves as a result of reduction in muscle blood flow and following the cessation of periods of severe muscular activity. Despite this, however, the electromyographic appearances presented by fatigued muscles[182] are different from those of muscles involved in reflex spasm, which is a matter of practical importance in the clinical differential diagnosis of muscular low back pain. Finally, it should be noted that not all the backache associated with postural or occupational fatigue is derived from the nociceptive receptor system within the back muscles, for part of it, and in some instances, most of it, is provided by coincident mechanical irritation of the nerve endings in the lumbar spinal ligaments and apophyseal joints, and in the capsules of the sacroiliac joints. However, to the extent that backache is the product of muscular fatigue, and is therefore a reflection of inadequate muscle blood floow, it may be relieved by resting the affected muscles[183] and by adopting measures that promote muscle blood flow (and lymphatic drainage), such as massage and the local application of heat (externally with hot-water bottles, or, preferably, internally with diathermy).

Inflammation. In popular usage (and often, even by doctors) non-traumatic backache is still frequently ascribed to 'rheumatism' or 'fibrositis', the implication being that the symptom of backache reflects some inflammatory change in the connective tissues of the back. In the context of this chapter, it is worth noting that the term *fibrositis* was originally coined by a distinguished neurological physician[184] to indicate a hypothetical inflammation of fibrous tissue as a cause of pain, and this concept was later taken up by rheumatologists,[185] one of whom once stated[186] that fibrositis 'is the most common form of rheumatic disease'. Despite the eminence of some of the protagonists of this view, however, it has to be emphasized here that inflammatory changes in the connective tissues related to the back muscles (if this is what is meant by 'fibrositis', or 'fasciitis') have never been shown, even by biopsy studies, to be a cause of backache;[187] for this reason, then, clinicians should cease using the term 'fibrositis' (or 'fasciitis') in this sense in relation to backache unless and until such time as evidence for its occurrence is available.

The term *myositis* refers to non-suppurative inflammation of the muscles,[188] and while this, unlike fibrositis, is a specific pathological entity, it rarely involves the muscles of the lower back as a cause of pain, except as a complication or aftermath of some acute pyrexial conditions such as meningitis, influenza, rheumatic fever, typhus and dengue fever, and malaria.[189] Occasionally, backache may also arise because of the involvement of the blood vessels in the lumbosacral musculature in the syndrome of polymyalgia rheumatica.[190]

From this discussion it will be apparent that, contrary to the traditional opinions of many doctors, inflammatory disorders of the back muscles and their related connective tissues are seldom the cause of low back pain except as a complication of some acute febrile illnesses. Far more often, backache of myofascial origin is the result of muscular fatigue, reflex muscle spasm or trauma, which factors should therefore receive more prominent consideration in differential diagnosis than vague and unsubstantiated entities such as 'rheumatism' or 'fibrositis'.

Articular and ligamentous pain

Apart from myofascial pain, the only other common cause of primary low back pain is provided by mechanical or, less often, chemical irritation of the nociceptive receptor system that is distributed through the fibrous capsules of the lumbar apophyseal and sacroiliac joints, and through the ligaments related to the vertebral column.[191] When asked to indicate the location of their backache, patients with this variety of pain usually point to the lumbar spine (in or close to the midline) or to the sacroiliac joint region, but local tenderness on pressure over the designated area is usually less evident than in the case of myofascial pain, or may even be absent, although tapping of the spinous processes of the lumbar vertebrae with a percussion hammer may elicit localised pain. Furthermore, because irritation of the receptor system in the lumbar apophyseal joint capsules may give rise to reflex spasm of the paravertebral musculature, such patients may also complain of pain (and indicate tenderness) in the deep soft tissues lateral to the lumbar spine. In such cases, zones of cutaneous hyperaesthesia may also be found on examination extending laterally across the lumbar region,[192] and the patient may additionally indicate zones of (referred) pain in the buttock, inguinal region or thigh.

Articular pain. Mechanical stresses of sufficient magnitude to excite the nociceptive receptor system in the capsules of the lumbar apophyseal joints (and of the sacroiliac joints) may be created by postural abnormalities involving this region of the spine,[193] or by the development therein of abnormal forces during movement.[194] Examples of the former static situation are the more frequently encountered, and are represented in the backache engendered by prolonged standing or sitting in inappropriate postures (as in women in late pregnancy or wearing high-heeled shoes, in workers at factory benches or at office desks, or in drivers sitting for long periods in motor vehicle seats); by persistently sleeping in beds with sagging mattresses; by the development of weakness or atrophy of the back muscles (as a result of old age, or confinement to bed for long periods); or on account of a reduction in the vertical height of the lumbar spine (for example, as a result of senile or post-menopausal osteoporosis, of vertebral body collapse following trauma or metastatic neoplastic involvement, or following intervertebral disc degeneration); or as a result of malformations of the lower vertebral column.[195]

Apart from the special dynamic forces that may be engendered in athletics, gymnastics, ballet-dancing and ice-skating, the latter situation is usually associated with occupations that involve frequent and prolonged stooping, such as gardening, and in the building trade. It should also be borne in mind that the manipulation of anaesthetized (and especially, curarized) patients into special postures — such as the lithotomy and Trendelenburg positions

— for prolonged periods gives rise to abnormal stresses in the lumbar apophyseal joints that may result in backache that long outlasts the immediate post-operative period, and that similar considerations apply, especially in women, to some of the more extreme postures that may be adopted during sexual intercourse. It is also pertinent here to point out that the development of oedema in the capsular tissues of the lumbar apophyseal and sacroiliac joints (as a result of trauma or inflammation — see below) may, as in other joints, generate sufficient mechanical distortion of those tissues to stimulate the nociceptive receptor system contained therein, and thus augment the pain being experienced as a result of its direct chemical irritation.[196]

Inflammatory processes[197] involving the joint tissues in the lower back irritate their contained receptor systems as a result of the associated chemical changes that occur in the tissue fluid of the affected joint capsules. Examples of such varieties of backache are provided by the lumbosacral arthritis that may be associated with diseases such as tuberculosis, typhoid fever, dengue fever, syphilis, brucellosis, gonorrhoea and non-specific urethritis (Reiter's syndrome), and more often by rheumatoid arthritis (including ankylosing spondylitis) and by osteoarthritis. In this connexion it must be emphasized, however, that backache of articular origin is determined in these circumstances exclusively by the extent of inflammatory involvement of the fibrous capsules of the apophyseal joints, and bears no relation to the severity of pathological change in the articular cartilages, intra-articular menisci or synovial tissue therein, for, as pointed out previously, these latter tissues contain no nerve endings of any description.[198] It is hardly surprising, therefore, that in many of the circumstances mentioned the severity of backache may bear little relation to the magnitude of the structural changes, if any, revealed by radiological studies of the lumbosacral region.

Ligamentous pain. Irritation of the receptor system distributed through the complex of ligaments and aponeuroses attached to the bones of the lumbosacral region is often additionally associated with irritation of the nerve endings, located in the joint capsules in the circumstances that have been described, but not always.

Thus, although the fact has been demonstrated repeatedly over the past 30 years,[199] it is still not sufficiently appreciated by the generality of doctors that much of the static postural support for the lower spine in the erect, sitting and fully flexed positions of the body is provided by the passive elastic tension of the ligaments and aponeuroses attached thereto, rather than by neurologically engendered motor unit activity in the paravertebral musculature. As these connective tissues, like the capsules of the related apophyseal and sacroiliac joints, are richly innervated by nociceptive nerve endings, it will be clear that backache is readily produced from these tissues when they are subjected to abnormal mechanical stresses (as by prolonged standing, especially while wearing high-heeled shoes; by persistently distorted postures in occupational circumstances, or as a result of structural abnormalities of the vertebral column; or by attempts to lift or support heavy weights), or when their elasticity is decreased, as it inevitably is with advancing age, or as a result of the hormonal changes associated with ingestion of oestrogen-containing oral contraceptive agents or with developing pregnancy. It is highly probable, therefore, that a good deal of the so-called 'fatigue backache' that is encountered in everyday life arises from this ligamentous source, although additional irritation of the nociceptive receptor system in the back muscles or in the joint capsules may reinforce the pain in the circumstances already described.

Much less often, direct mechanical irritation of the nerve endings in the posterior longitudinal ligament and in the fibro-adipose tissue that binds it to the annulus fibrosus may be produced by central posterior protrusion of the nucleus pulposus of an intervertebral disc, to produce severe midline backache, to which bilateral paravertebral pain may be added by associated reflex muscle spasm. The midline pain may be further intensified if the pressure of the herniated nucleus be transmitted through a degenerate ligament[200] to the anterior surface of the lumbar dural tube.

It will also be clear that should these ligamentous connective tissues become involved in inflammatory processes, as may be the case in some of the 'rheumatic' affections,[201] then the resulting chemical irritation of their contained nociceptive receptor endings will give rise to pain in the back. It is probable, however, that such disorders are usually accompanied by comparable inflammatory changes in the lumbar apophyseal and/or sacroiliac joints and therefore reinforce the pain being experienced in the back, rather than represent its exclusive source, although some rheumatologists might not accept this view. Furthermore, in view of what has been said previously concerning 'fibrositis', it should be noted here that this term is sometimes also used by physicians to embrace the inflammatory changes in ligaments to which reference has just been made, but although such changes do occur, the word 'fibrositis' should be eliminated from the professional medical vocabulary because of its vagueness and should not be used, especially as a pseudo-diagnosis, to designate ligamentous inflammation. In scientific, as opposed to folk, medicine, it is essential to call a spade a spade and not to invent pseudo-pathological states (as 'fibrositis') in the absence of evidence of their occurrence, nor to cloak aetiological ignorance in Galenic or Greek etymology (as by use of the term 'idiopathic'); and nowhere is this more essential than in the study of backache.

Finally, before leaving this matter of spinal ligamentous pain, reference must be made to some 40-year-old clinical experiments[202] involving the injection of hypertonic saline solutions into the vertebral connective tissues, because these studies continue to be cited in rheumatological literature as evidence for a segmental nociceptive innervation of these tissues. Although such saline solutions provide a very effective chemical irritant for connective tissue nociceptive receptors, it must be emphasized here that because of the diffuse distribution of this receptor system through the vertebral connective tissues, and because of the widespread intersegmental linkages between their afferent nerve fibres, attempts to use such a procedure as a means of delineating a supposed segmental nociceptive innervation of the spinal tissues are clearly fallacious,[203] especially as it is impossible (even with the introduction of radio-opaque material into the injected solution) to be certain just how much of the diffuse nociceptive afferent system is being stimulated by any given volume of hypertonic saline.

Osseous pain

Backache may be produced by irritation of the perivascular receptor system that is distributed through the cancellous bone of the vertebral bodies

and arches, and of the sacrum.[204] This may arise on account of the mechanical irritation of this system occasioned by trauma to the lower back (especially in the case of crush fractures of the lumbar vertebrae, or fractures of the sacrum), or by collapse of the vertebral bodies as a result of their involvement in osteomalacia, senile or postmenopausal osteoporosis,[205] or by metastatic neoplasms (derived especially from the prostate, uterus, breast, colon and bladder,[206] or by the lesions of myelomatosis.[207] Much less often, low back pain may indicate the presence of a primary neoplasm in the bones of the lower spine, of which chordomata (occurring usually in the sacrum) and angiomata are the only significantly frequent examples in practice,[207] or it may be the result of vertebral erosion by an abdominal aortic aneurysm.

If osseous lesions of the lower spine and sacrum involve the enclosing periosteum and the nociceptive receptor system located therein, the resulting pain is much more intense than otherwise. Thus, if the traumatic or neoplastic lesions already mentioned result respectively in tearing or invasion of the lumbar vertebral or sacral periosteum the associated pain is often extreme, while severe pain is also produced by involvement of the vertebral and sacral periosteum in the inflammatory processes of osteitis, especially if subperiosteal abscess development occurs, as with pyogenic or tuberculous osteitis[208] and osteomyelitis. Similar remarks apply in respect of the pain produced by the hypertrophic vertebral changes associated with Paget's disease, osteitis deformans,[209] in which the lumbar vertebrae are involved in 75% of cases, and which, in its milder forms, provides an important though often overlooked cause of low back pain in patients over the age of 40 years.

Vascular pain

Backache of vascular origin may arise in two ways: one, the primary variety, being far more common than the other, the secondary variety. Primary vascular backache arises from mechanical irritation of the nerve endings located in the walls of the vertebral venous plexus as a result of excessive distension of these vessels by the development of abnormally high venous pressures therein,[210] and although still seldom recognized as a cause of low back pain, this mechanism should receive serious consideration from clinicians working in this field.

Because the vertebral venous system is in free communication with the mass of veins in the chest, abdomen and pelvis,[211] elevations of pressure in the thoracic and abdominal cavities are transmitted directly to and provoke distension of the vertebral veins,[212] and if the walls of these veins be sufficiently stretched thereby, their contained nerve endings are stimulated mechanically to provoke diffuse pain felt deeply in the back. Such elevations of venous pressure may be extreme during the process of lifting or supporting heavy weights, as the abdominal and thoracic muscles then contract — after an initial deep inspiration — against a closed glottis,[213] while similar, and even more marked phasic elevations of pressure occur during prolonged bouts of coughing,[214] during vomiting, during parturition, during straining at stool by constipated patients, and during obstructed micturition, as in men with prostatic enlargement.[215] On the other hand, persisting elevations of vertebral venous pressure are associated with the later stages of pregnancy, with chronic emphysema, and with congestive heart failure.[216] From a diagnostic viewpoint, it is worth noting that the backache that may occur in all these situations is frequently associated with diffuse headache due to accompanying distension of the intracranial veins and sinuses, with which the vertebral venous plexus is in communication at its rostral end.[217]

It may also be pointed out that should there be a pre-existing irritative lesion of the dural nerve root sleeves — as with posterolateral prolapse of the nucleus pulposus of an intervertebral disc, or because of a displacement fracture of a vertebra or the pressure of an intraspinal tumour — quite moderate distension of the epidural veins (to degrees less than that required to excite their own contained nerve endings) as a result of coughing, laughing, sneezing or straining may provoke or intensify pain in the back and/or leg by increasing the pressure on the affected nerve root sleeves.

Dural pain

Mention was made previously of the fact that the spinal dural tube has little or no nociceptive innervation on its posterior aspect (which is why posterior dural penetration with a lumbar puncture needle is painless) but is densely innervated on its anterior aspect. Compressive lesions that impinge on the anterior portion of the dura mater, or on its sleeve-like extensions into the intervertebral foramina, may therefore give rise to pain experienced in or close to the midline of the lower back. This situation is encountered with fractures of the lumbar or upper sacral vertebrae in which fragments of bone are displaced posteriorly or posterolaterally, or when posterior dislocation of a lumbar vertebra occurs as a result of trauma. It also develops when the herniated nucleus pulposus of a lumbar intervertebral disc impinges on the anterior aspect of the dura mater or, more often, on a dural sleeve, and this latter state of affairs will be compounded should posterolateral osteophytes develop from the edges of the vertebrae related to the affected intervertebral disc.[218] It is probably these mechanisms that determine (in part) the extent to which backache occurs in the presence of a prolapsed nucleus pulposus, in addition to, or even in lieu of, sciatica.

In the interests of completeness, it should also be mentioned that seepage into the dura mater (and epidural adipose tissue) of solutions of irritant materials introduced into the lumbar subarachnoid fluid may produce chemical irritation of the nerve endings located therein.[219] This used to be a frequent cause of iatrogenic backache when relatively high concentrations of penicillin were injected into the subarachnoid fluid in the treatment of meningitis, but seldom occurs nowadays.

Secondary backache

Secondary low back pain is defined[220] as pain experienced in the lumbosacral region as a result of some disturbance of function in the afferent nerve fibres that link the receptor systems located peripherally in the vertebral and paravertebral tissues with the spinal cord. In such cases, then, the pathological change giving rise to backache is not to be sought in the tissues of the body in which the patient feels the pain to be, but somewhere along the course, from periphery to dorsal nerve roots, of the afferent nerve fibres that innervate those tissues. Such pathological changes may be subdivided into two categories, involving either interruption of the normal centripetal flow of nociceptive inhibitory activity in the large diameter mechanoreceptor afferent fibres in the lumbosacral nerves (see above) or enhancement of activity as a result of their irritation somewhere along their course in the small-diameter nociceptive afferents in the same nerves, or a combination of the two. Furthermore, such changes may affect the afferent fibres in either the posterior primary or sinuvertebral branches of the dorsal nerve roots, or in the dorsal nerve roots themselves.

Compressive lesions

Because of the correlation between the diameter of nerve fibres and their metabolic activity,[221] conduction in the larger-diameter mechanoreceptor afferent fibres in the spinal nerves is interfered with earlier and more severely by any disturbance of the blood flow through the vasa nervorum than is conduction through the smaller-diameter nociceptive afferent fibres in the same nerves,[222] with consequent selective loss of the inhibitory effects of the former upon central centripetal trans-synaptic propagation of activity in the latter system. Such changes occur in the early stages of compressive lesions of nerves or nerve roots, or as result of vascular pathological changes involving the vasa nervorum,[223] as in arteriosclerosis, for instance.

In the present context, the most obvious example of such a compressive lesion is represented by posterolateral herniation of the nucleus pulposus of a lumbar intervertebral disc, more frequently, that between the fourth and fifth lumbar and less often that between the fifth lumbar and first sacral vertebrae. As such a protrusion develops it impinges initially on the sinuvertebral nerve, in which it not only interrupts mechanoreceptor afferent activity but may also irritate the contained nociceptive afferent fibres and thereby, because of the terminal distribution of the sinuvertebral nerve fibres, give rise to pain in the lower back in the absence of sciatica, although it should be emphasized, contrary to popular impression, that less than 5% of patients with backache have prolapsed intervertebral discs, whereas 70% of patients with such a lesion have backache as the initial symptom.[224] Should the nuclear protrusion develop further, it begins to impinge on the related dorsal nerve roots (and their containing dural sleeves) as a result of which the

backache becomes more severe and more widely distributed, being reinforced by concomitant reflex muscle spasm, and to it are added sensory changes (paraesthesiae and numbness) and pain experienced in the distribution of the sciatic nerve,[225] which symptoms are discussed elsewhere in this volume. It should also be noted that because of the considerable obliquity of the dorsal nerve roots within the lower end of the adult spinal canal, an expanding posterolateral protrusion from the disc between the fourth and fifth lumbar vertebrae impinges not only on the fifth lumbar dorsal root but also involves the first sacral root,[226] and it is relevant to reiterate at this point that irritative compression of the descending branch of the second lumbar nerve within the posterior longitudinal ligament by posterior herniation of the nuclei of one or other of the more rostral lumbar intervertebral discs may give rise to pain experienced in the fifth lumbar dermatomal region of the back, which may mislead the clinician who is unaware of this neuro-anatomical peculiarity. It may also be useful here to dispose of a widespread misconception regarding the production or enhancement of the pain associated with prolapse of lumbar intervertebral disc nuclei by forward flexion of the trunk (or neck) or by straight-leg raising (the so-called Lasègue's sign), which assumes that the effect is due to traction on the affected nerve roots by the spinal cord riding up in the vertebral canal, in the former case, or by peripheral stretching forces, in the latter. Neither of these views is tenable, in view of the fact that during flexion and extension movements of the trunk or neck the spinal cord does not move vertically within the vertebral canal,[227] and because the nerve roots are firmly anchored within their dural sleeves to the walls of the intervertebral foramina.[228] On the contrary, in both sets of circumstances the intraspinal pressure is increased (and nerve root irritation is thereby increased) because of the changes in the transverse diameter of the spinal cord and in the volume of blood in the epidural veins that then occur.

From the above account, it should be apparent that progressing compressive lesions of the lumbosacral intraspinal nerve roots, whether they be due to disc herniations, displacement fractures, or the development of extramedullary neoplasms, exert a specific sequence of effects on the nerve fibres contained therein that are reflected in the changing clinical phenomena presented as the lesion expands within the spinal canal, additional to any effects that may arise from direct compression of the lower end of the spinal cord itself above the level of the second lumbar vertebra. Considering these effects solely in terms of low back pain — and ignoring all the other somatic and visceral sensory and reflex effects that may occur but which are outside the terms of reference of this chapter — the initial change is an increase in the pain sensitivity (especially in response to static and dynamic mechanical forces) of the articular, ligamentous and muscular tissues of the back as the mechanoreceptor activity normally derived therefrom is interfered with. As the nerve root compression develops, this is followed by intermittent or continuous irritation of the smaller diameter nociceptive afferent fibres in the same nerve roots and their dural sleeves, so that the backache becomes more severe and is less readily relieved by changes of posture or activity. Similar remarks may also apply to the production of the backache that may be associated with caudal spinal stenosis,[229] and with spondylolisthesis.[230]

Degenerative lesions

Should compression of the intraspinal nerve roots persist to the extent that the resulting chronic ischaemia results in degeneration of the mechanoreceptor, but not the nociceptive, afferent fibres contained therein,[231] the backache becomes almost continuous and the patient finds that rest in bed, or the assumption of postures that previously ameliorated his symptoms, now give him little or no relief from his distress. In severe cases the patient may be unable to sit or lie down for more than brief periods, and spends most of his time walking about in order to produce maximum stimulation of his surviving mechanoreceptor afferent systems and thus inhibit his pain.

Similar selective degeneration of mechanoreceptor afferents in the lumbosacral nerves is encountered in patients in whom the vasa nervorum are the site of occlusive vascular disease. This occurs uniformly, as already indicated, in elderly patients as arteriosclerotic changes develop in their small blood vessels, and may account in part for the increasing incidence of postural backache in older subjects. Ischaemic inactivation of mechanoreceptor afferents

combined with ischaemic irritation of nociceptive afferents, due to arteriosclerotic changes in the blood vessels supplying the lumbosacral nerve roots, may also account for the clinical phenomenon of 'spinal claudication', in which patients develop increasing backache, with or without accompanying pain in the distribution of the sciatic nerves, on walking.[232] Any idea that this latter pain is generated by irritation of receptor systems within the lumbosacral musculature (in a manner similar to the production of calf pain in the intermittent claudication associated with Buerger's disease) is untenable, in view of the evanescent activity of the low back musculature associated with walking.[233] Occlusive disease of the vasa nervorum, resulting in degeneration of the myelinated mechanoreceptor afferent fibres in the spinal nerves, also occurs in diabetes mellitus and in rheumatoid arthritis,[234] and this may reinforce the backache experienced in the latter disease as a result of the primary inflammatory changes that occur in the capsules of the lumbar apophyseal and sacroiliac joints.

Finally, it should be noted that selective degeneration of the dorsal root ganglion cells of mechanoreceptor afferent fibres in the lumbosacral nerves may occur in tabes dorsalis, and as a late result of herpes zoster infection, contributing to the intense backache that may be experienced in the former condition and to the production of post-herpetic neuralgia in the latter.

Referred backache

Pain may be experienced in the lower back, although the causative lesion lies neither in the tissues in which the pain is felt nor along the course of the afferent fibres that innervate these tissues, but instead involves some tissue or organ whose innervation is segmentally related to that of the superficial tissues of the lumbosacral region, and this variety constitutes *referred backache*.[235] In such circumstances, the development of the primary visceral (or peritoneal) disorder is accompanied by pain, and often hyperaesthesia, in one or more sectors of the skin in the lumbosacral area, in which reflex vasomotor changes may also occur, and this is frequently associated with reflex spasm in segmentally related portions of the lumbosacral musculature, in which more deeply felt backache may be experienced in addition to the superficial localised cutaneous pain. Such referred pain generally does not occur until the initiating disorder has been present for some time — thus its presence is more often indicative of chronic rather than of acute visceral or peritoneal lesions — but it may outlast the disappearance of the directly causative visceral pain, as after treatment of a visceral lesion, for instance.

In the past, there have been many theories purporting to explain the phenomenon of referred pain,[236] but most of them have been found wanting in relation to the observed facts of clinical experience with the problem. Fortunately, however, the recent studies of the central connexions of spinal dorsal root afferents already described have thrown considerable light on the matter, especially in view of the demonstration that nociceptive afferents from visceral tissues project onto the same relay cells in lamina V of the basal spinal nucleus as do the afferents from segmentally related areas of skin.[237] Because of this convergence of visceral and cutaneous nociceptive input systems on the relay cells in lamina V, whose excitation is the essential prerequisite for centripetal transmission of nociceptive activity into the brain and thus for the evocation of the experience of pain, it will be apparent that normally trivial stimuli applied to the related area of skin may induce these relay cells to fire should their excitability be sufficiently increased by pre-existing afferent activity emanating from visceral nociceptive nerve endings; the resulting pain is then perceived to reside in the skin.

Gynaecological

In clinical practice, referred low backache is encountered most frequently in a gynaecological context, the common example being dysmenorrhoea, in which low back pain may occur with or, less often, without accompanying suprapubic pain immediately before and on the first one or two days of each menstrual period. As the nociceptive innervation of the uterus is largely confined to the lining of the cervix, the referred backache is generated by distension of this structure, a fact illustrated also by the backache produced by surgical dilatation of the cervix in unanaesthetized patients and by the initial cervical dilatation at the onset (i.e., the 'first stage') of labour. Pain may also be referred to the back in women with lesions of the ovaries or fallopian tubes, as in salpingitis and ectopic pregnancy, with uterine prolapse or retroversion, especially when associated with myomatosis, or with carcinoma of the uterine cervix, for which reasons a detailed gynaecological history and investigation is an essential part of the examination of any woman with non-traumatic low back pain. In connexion with the periodicity that is so often observed in referred backache of gynaecological origin, even with continuously present lesions, it is worth noting that a monthly cyclical variation in pain sensitivity has been demonstrated in normal premenopausal women,[238] and that this cyclical fluctuation is suppressed by the intake of oestrogen-containing oral contraceptive agents.[239] although, as already mentioned, the latter may sometimes produce low back pain often accompanied, incidentally, by temporomandibular articular pain,[240] as one of the complications of their use.

Urinary tract

In either sex, patients with lesions of the upper urinary tract frequently present with referred backache as one of their symptomatic features. This is particularly the case with pyelitis and pyelonephritis, and in patients with renal calculi, but low back pain may also be associated with hydronephrosis or neoplastic lesions that involve the renal pelvis, which is where the nociceptive innervation of the kidney is mainly concentrated.

Prostate

Apart from urinary tract disorders, in men the various forms of prostatitis, especially if chronic, provide the principal cause of referred low back pain, but it may also occur in a small proportion of patients with prostatic carcinoma. However, pain referred from the prostate is usually experienced in the sacral rather than in the lumbar region, the latter being the usual site of reference of pain of renal origin.

Appendix

Occasionally also, right-sided low back pain may be associated with the presence of an inflamed retrocaecal appendix.

Psychosomatic backache

It is often said that many cases of backache are 'psychogenic', the implication being that the complaint of pain in the back is entirely of psychological origin and is unrelated to any structural or functional change in the tissues of the back, and therefore is 'imaginary' or 'unreal', and many patients with persistent backache regard the final seal as having been set on disbelief in the 'reality' of their complaint when, as a last desperate resort, they are referred to a psychiatrist after having been seen by a succession of specialists, usually including orthopaedic surgeons, rheumatologists, neurologists or neurosurgeons and — in the case of women — gynaecologists. On the other hand, as already indicated early in this account, there is no doubt that a variety of psychological disturbances may be associated with backache,[241] either as aggravating factors, or as a result of its development for any of the reasons discussed previously. For this reason, the term *psychosomatic backache* is preferred here to categorize those cases in which such psychological disturbances, especially anxiety and depression, constitute the dominating feature of the overall clinical picture, and in which, therefore, psychological investigation and treatment is an essential part of their management. In this connection, it should also be pointed out, again contrary to a widespread 'clinical impression' among general practitioners especially, that specific studies of the matter[242] have failed to reveal any significant correlation between the occurrence of backache and specific personality characteristics of the sufferer therefrom.

Anxious depression

The commonest variety of psychosomatic backache is that associated with states of anxiety and depression, that is, with so-called 'agitated' or 'reactive' depression, for in this psychiatric syndrome backache is the most frequent 'somatic' complaint after headache.[243] Patients with this variety of psychosomatic backache form an identifiable diagnostic subgroup among the generality of sufferers from low back pain,[244] and their backache shows little response to purely physical methods of treatment. As patients with reactive depression are characteristically agitated, restless and tense, and as they show persisting hyperactivity of motor units in various muscle groups even when apparently at rest,[245] perhaps as a consequence of overactivity in the reticulospinal projection system that controls fusimotor neurone excitability,[246] it may be that the development of backache in these circumstances results from excessive motor unit activity in the back muscles. This view should be regarded as hypothetical at the moment, as no electromyographic studies have yet been carried out (as they should be) on the back muscles of such patients, but it receives some support from empirical clinical experience that administration of drugs that depress reticulospinal excitation of fusimotor neurones[247] may produce a significant improvement in the backache of which these patients complain, whereas antidepressive agents have little or no such effect.

Hysteria

A second, and less common, variety of psychosomatic backache is represented by those patients in whom the complaint of low back pain is a symptomatic manifestation of hysteria. Psychological tests have indicated[248] that some patients with persisting backache show higher than normal hysteria ratings, although whether this is cause or effect in relation to the backache remains undetermined. Nevertheless, most clinicians experienced in this field are familiar with the type of patient whose complaint of backache represents an hysterical reaction to a relatively trivial traumatic or mechanical disorder of the muscular, ligamentous or articular tissues of the back, especially when this has occurred in circumstances that may have medico-legal consequences as with accidents at work, or with road accidents.[249] A comparable psychoneurotic situation may also arise in women in consequence of the emotional stresses engendered by their domestic obligations, or as a protective conversion symptom related to their unwillingness to accept the sexual advances of a husband they no longer find attractive. All these patients, however, have certainly experienced some degree of disturbance in the tissues of the lumbosacral region, but the dominating feature of the clinical picture is the intensity of their emotional reaction to it, and its linkage, sometimes not at first sight obvious, with some personal emotional or financial advantage to the sufferer.

Malingering

The final variety of backache that requires mention in this category is that presented by malingerers, that is, the patients who are lying when they complain of low back pain, in that they are not experiencing, or have not experienced, such pain although they say that they are, or have. This situation is encountered relatively frequently in medico-legal circumstances in which a claim for compensation for injuries alleged to have been sustained at work or in a traffic accident is in question, and is very difficult to deal with, in view of the fact that pain is a subjective emotional disorder. For this latter reason, it must be said at once that there is no way in which a doctor can disprove a patient's claim that he or she is, or has been, in pain, but an experienced clinician, from detailed interrogation and examination of the patient, will be alerted to the possibility of malingering by the discrepancy between the patient's account of the distribution and severity of his or her alleged pain and the circumstances of the injury, and by the nature of the activities, especially recreational and sexual, in which the patient is currently able to indulge. It must be emphasized, however, that the absence of the conventional 'physical signs' of low back dysfunction, and even less of radiological evidence of structural lesions of the lumbosacral region, does not entitle the clinician to leap to the conclusion that the patient is a malingerer; furthermore, it should be realized that malingering is in itself a manifestation of psychoneurotic disorder, the cause of which requires clinical psychological investigation and treatment.

ACKNOWLEDGEMENTS

The personal research cited in this account was assisted by grants from the British Postgraduate Medical Federation of the University of London, the Camilla Samuel Fund, the National Fund for Research into Crippling Diseases and the Back Pain Association.

REFERENCES TO BIBLIOGRAPHY

1   Hirsch & Schajowicz, 1953; Rowe, 1969, 1971; Horal, 1969; Lawrence, 1969; Westrin, 1970; Wood, 1970; Simons and Mirabile, 1972.
2   Devine and Mersky, 1965; Rudd and Margolin, 1966; Dillane et al., 1966; Ward et al., 1968; Horal, 1969; Fisk, 1970; Westrin, 1970; Gilchrist, 1976.
3   For example, see Dallenbach, 1939; Wolff and Hardy, 1947; Wyke, 1947; Wolff and Wolf, 1948; Keele, 1957; Sweet, 1959.
4   Wyke, 1947, 1968, 1974a, 1979a; Noordenbos, 1959; Wolstenholme and O'Connor, 1959; Merskey and Spear, 1967; Merskey, 1968; Melzack and Casey, 1968; Sternbach, 1968; 1974; Melzack, 1973; Bonica, 1974; Bonica and Albe-Fessard, 1976.
5   See also Zotterman, 1939, 1959, 1972; Sweet, 1959; Iggo, 1959, 1963, 1972; Melzack and Wall, 1962, 1965; Wyke, 1968.
6   See Hardy et al., 1943, 1952; Kolb, 1952; Merskey, 1965, 1968; Devine and Mersky, 1965; Wyke, 1974; Bonica, 1974; Bonica and Albe-Fessard, 1976.
7   Wyke, 1958b, 1968, 1974a.
8   Henderson and Smyth, 1948; Kolb, 1954; Bressler et al., 1955; Simmel, 1959; Gillis, 1964; White and Sweet, 1969.
9   See Engel, 1951; Keele, 1957; Sargant, 1957; Wyke, 1958b, 1974a; Merskey and Spear, 1967; Sternbach, 1974.
10 Wyke, 1958.
11 Ellis, 1898; Merskey and Spear, 1967; Merskey, 1968; Sternbach et al., 1973b; Sternbach, 1974; Gilchrist, 1976.
12 Kunkle and Chapman, 1943; Jewsbury, 1951; Critchley, 1956; Sternbach, 1963, 1968; Bourland and Winkelmann, 1966; Merskey and Spear, 1967; Osuntokun et al., 1968.
13 For discussion of this matter, see Akerblom, 1948; Steindler, 1955; Davis, 1961, 1972; Asmussen and Klausen, 1962; Basmajian, 1974.
14 Wyke, 1967, 1970, 1972a, 1975, 1977, 1979a, b; Wyke and Molina, 1972; Wyke and Poláček, 1973, 1975; Vrettos and Wyke, 1974; Molina et al., 1976.
15 Wyke, 1967, 1977; Nade et al., 1978.
16 Iggo, 1959, 1963, 1966a, 1972; Bessou and Perl, 1969; Van Hees and Gybels, 1972; Bonica, 1974; Wyke, 1974a, 1979a; Bonica and Albe-Fessard, 1976.
17 Keele and Armstrong, 1964, 1968; Sicuteri et al., 1965; Lim, 1968; Benjamin, 1968; Bessou and Perl, 1969; Ferreira, 1972; Werle, 1972; Bonica, 1974; Bonica and Albe-Fessard, 1976.
18 Weddell, 1941; Wolstenholme and O'Connor, 1959; Montagna, 1960; Sinclair, 1967; Kenshalo, 1968; Wyke, 1979a.
19 Jung and Brunschwig, 1932; Ikari, 1954; Pedersen et al., 1956; Stilwell, 1956; Lewin et al., 1961; Hirsch et al., 1963; Jackson et al., 1966; Wyke, 1967, 1970, 1977; Nade et al., 1977.
20 For example, see Wyke, 1967, 1972a; Freeman and Wyke, 1967a, b; Dee, 1969; Wyke and Poláček, 1973, 1975.
21 Wyke, 1970, 1975, 1977, 1979b; Wyke and Molina, 1972; Vrettos and Wyke, 1974; Molina et al., 1976.
22 Rüdinger, 1857; Hovelacque, 1925; Jung and

Brunschwig, 1932; Roofe, 1940; Ehrenhaft, 1943;
Sinclair et al., 1948; Wiberg, 1949; Hirsch and
Schajowicz, 1953; Pedersen et al., 1956; Stilwell, 1956,
1957a, b; Mulligan, 1957; Malinský, 1959; Scapinelli,
1960; Hirsch et al., 1963; Jackson et al., 1966; Wyke,
1970, 1977; Nade et al., 1978.

23 For example, see Ralston et al., 1960; Wyke, 1967,
1972a; Freeman and Wyke, 1967a, b; Dee, 1969; Wyke
and Poláček, 1973, 1975.
24 Jackson et al., 1966; Wyke, 1970, 1977.
25 Purkyně, 1845; von Luschka, 1850; Ikari, 1954;
Pedersen et al., 1956; Stilwell, 1956, 1957a, b; Jackson
et al., 1966; Wyke, 1970, 1977.
26 Stilwell, 1957a, b; Ralston et al., 1960; Hirsch et al.,
1963; Wyke, 1977.
27 Hovelacque, 1925; Pedersen et al., 1956; Stilwell, 1956;
Bridge, 1959; Jackson et al., 1966; Edgar and Nundy,
1966; Wyke, 1970, 1977.
28 von Luschka, 1850; Hovelacque, 1925; Roofe, 1940;
Stilwell, 1956; Hirsch et al., 1963; Jackson et al., 1966;
Wyke, 1970, 1977.
29 Wyke, 1970, 1977.
30 Wyke, 1970, 1977.
31 Batson, 1940; Herlihy, 1947, 1948; Henriques, 1962;
Wyke, 1969, 1970, 1977.
32 Gardner, 1943; Pedersen et al., 1956; Stilwell, 1956;
Mulligan, 1957; Bridge, 1959; Wyke, 1970, 1977.
33 For example, see Feindel et al., 1948; Fernand and
Young, 1951; Polley, 1955; Bessou and Laporte, 1958;
Lim et al., 1962; Iggo, 1962, 1966b.
34 See Bradford and Spurling, 1945; Barr, 1951; Friberg,
1954; Cailliet, 1962; Armstrong, 1965; Lawrence, 1969;
Chamberlain, 1971.
35 Tsukada, 1938, 1939; Ehrenhaft, 1943; Malinský, 1959.
36 Jung and Brunschwig, 1932; Roofe, 1940; Wiberg,
1949; Stilwell, 1956; Malinský, 1959; Hirsch et al.,
1963; Jackson et al., 1966; Wyke, 1970, 1977.
37 Wyke, 1970, 1977.
38 Wyke, 1967, 1969, 1970, 1977, 1979a; Bonica, 1974;
Bonica and Albe-Fessard, 1976.
39 See Wyke, 1969.
40 See Wyke, 1969.
41 von Luschka, 1850; Rüdinger, 1857; Pederson et al.,
1956; Stilwell, 1956; Wyke, 1970, 1977.
42 See Head, 1920; Foerster, 1933; Judovich and Bates,
1944; Keegan, 1944; Keegan and Garrett, 1948; Hansen
and Schlick, 1962; Brodal, 1969.
43 See Brodal, 1969.
44 Wyke, 1977; Nade et al., 1978.
45 Wyke, 1970, 1977; Nade et al., 1978.
46 Roofe, 1940; Wiberg, 1949; Pedersen et al., 1956;
Mulligan, 1957; Pallie, 1959; Wyke, 1970, 1977, 1979b;
Nade et al., 1978.
47 von Luschka, 1850; Hovelacque, 1925; Roofe, 1940;
Kaplan, 1947; Wiberg, 1949; Stilwell, 1956; Pedersen et
al., 1956; Bridge, 1959; Wyke, 1970, 1977.
48 Purkyně, 1845; Stilwell, 1956; Mulligan, 1957; Bridge,
1959; Wyke, 1970, 1977.
49 Ranson and Clark, 1932; Rexed, 1944; Ranson and Clark,
1959; Brodal, 1969; Wyke, 1979a.
50 Ranson and Clark, 1959; Sprague and Ha, 1964;
Carpenter et al., 1968; Brodal, 1969.
51 Rexed, 1954; Wall and Cronly-Dillon, 1960; Wall,
1960, 1967; Sprague and Ha, 1964; Melzack and Wall,
1965; Scheibel and Scheibel, 1968; Brodal, 1969;

Christensen and Perl, 1970; Bonica, 1974; Price and
Meyer, 1974; Kerr, 1975; Meyer et al., 1975; Bonica
and Albe-Fessard, 1976; Nathan, 1976; Price and
Dubner, 1977; Wyke, 1977, 1979a.
52 Scheibel and Scheibel, 1966a; Brodal, 1969; Brazier,
1970.
53 Pedersen et al., 1956; Nade et al., 1978.
54 Wyke, 1947, 1979a; Ranson and Clark, 1959; Brodal,
1969; Handwerker and Zimmermann, 1972; Lippman
and Kerr, 1972; Trevino et al., 1972; Bonica, 1974;
Kerr, 1975; Bonica and Albe-Fessard, 1976.
55 Walker, 1940; Weaver and Walker, 1941; Gardner and
Cuneo, 1945; Morin et al., 1951; White and Sweet,
1969; Brodal, 1969.
56 See Nathan, 1963; White and Sweet, 1969.
57 Nathan, 1963; White and Sweet 1969; Noordenbos,
1972; Bonica, 1974; Bonica and Albe-Fessard, 1976.
58 Glees, 1953; Bowsher, 1957, 1962, 1976; Nauta, 1958;
Brodal, 1969; Wyke, 1979a.
59 Hàggqvist, 1936; Verhaart, 1954; Bowsher, 1962, 1976;
Mehler, 1962; Brodal, 1969; Lippman and Kerr, 1972;
Wyke, 1979a.
60 Bowsher, 1962; Mehler, 1962; White and Sweet, 1969;
Noordenbos, 1972.
61 Walker, 1940, 1942a, b; Wyke, 1947; Drake and
McKenzie, 1953; Ranson and Clark, 1959; Bowsher,
1962; Brodal, 1969.
62 Morin et al., 1951, 1966; Bowsher, 1957, 1961b, 1962,
1976; Brodal, 1957, 1969; Mehler et al., 1960; Mehler,
1962; Benjamin, 1970; Hassler, 1972; Curry and
Gordon, 1972; Rosén and Scheid, 1972; Bonica, 1974;
Bonica and Albe-Fessard, 1976; Wyke, 1979a.
63 Brodal, 1969.
64 Bowsher, 1957, 1976; Scheibel and Scheibel, 1966b;
Lund and Webster, 1967; Bowsher et al., 1968; Brodal,
1969; Mancia et al., 1971; Hassler, 1972; Curry and
Gordon, 1972; Bonica, 1974; Bonica and Albe-Fessard,
1976.
65 Brodal, 1969; Stein and Arigbeda, 1972.
66 Le Gros Clark, 1936; Walker, 1938, 1943; Wyke, 1947,
1979a; Bowsher, 1957, 1961a; Mehler et al., 1960;
Whitlock and Perl, 1961; Scheibel and Scheibel, 1966b;
Brodal, 1969; Dewulf, 1971; Hassler, 1972; Curry and
Gordon, 1972; Jabbur et al., 1972; Bonica, 1974; Bonica
and Albe-Fessard, 1976.
67 Poggio and Mountcastle, 1960; Albe-Fessard and
Bowsher, 1965; Scheibel and Scheibel, 1966b; Dewulf,
1971; Hassler, 1972; Curry and Gordon, 1972.
68 Majorossy and Kiss, 1969.
69 Mehler et al., 1960; Poggio and Mountcastle, 1960;
Bowsher, 1961a; Whitlock and Perl, 1961; Hassler, 1972.
70 See Bowsher, 1957, 1961a; Morse and Towe, 1964;
Hassler, 1972; Wyke, 1974a.
71 Sweet et al., 1950.
72 Hassler and Reichert, 1959; Poggio and Mountcastle,
1960; Hassler, 1960, 1972; Bowsher, 1961a;
Mountcastle et al., 1963; Calma, 1965; Casey, 1966;
Curry and Gordon, 1972; Curry, 1972; Jabbur et al.,
1972; Bonica, 1974.
73 See Mountcastle and Powell, 1959b; Poggio and
Mountcastle, 1960.
74 Hassler and Reichert, 1959; Mark et al., 1962, 1963;
Speigel and Wycis, 1962; Speigel et al., 1966; Kruger,
1966; Uemura and Watkins, 1968; Cassinari and Pagni,
1969; Hassler, 1972.

75   Monnier, 1953; Delgado, 1955; Hassler and Reichert, 1959; Hassler, 1961; Roberts, 1962.

76   Wyke, 1958b, 1968, 1974a, 1979a.

77   Walker, 1938; Chow and Pribram, 1956; Woolsey, 1964; Walker and Johnson, 1965; Albe-Fessard and Liebeskind, 1966; Purpura and Yahr, 1966; Pubols, 1968; Hand and Morrison, 1970.

78   Walker, 1938; Wyke, 1947, 1979a; Penfield and Rasmussen, 1950; Monnier, 1953; Penfield and Jasper, 1954; Wolsey, 1964; Purpura and Yahr, 1966; Brodal, 1969; Jones and Powell, 1969, 1970; Hand and Morrison, 1970; Dewulf, 1971.

79   See Penfield and Rasmussen, 1950; Penfield and Jasper, 1954; Brodal, 1969.

80   Powell and Mountcastle, 1959a, b; Mountcastle and Powell, 1959a; Rose and Mountcastle, 1959; Kelly et al., 1965; Whitsel et al., 1972.

81   Oscarsson and Rosén, 1963, 1966; Albe-Fessard and Liebeskind, 1966; Goldring et al., 1970; Phillips et al., 1971.

82   See Matthews, 1972.

83   Wyke, 1968, 1974a, 1979a; Nashold et al., 1972.

84   Mountcastle and Powell, 1959a.

85   Penfield and Rasmussen, 1950; Penfield and Jasper, 1954; Penfield and Faulk, 1955; Albe-Fessard, 1968.

86   Michelsen, 1943; Marshall, 1951; Sweet, 1959; White and Sweet, 1959.

87   Mark et al., 1963; Cooper, 1965; Cassinari and Pagni, 1969.

88   See Wyke, 1968, 1974a, 1979a.

89   For example, see Foerster, 1936.

90   Le Gros Clark and Boggon, 1935; Walker, 1938; Le Gros Clark, 1948; Purpura and Yahr, 1966; Brodal, 1969; Wyke, 1979a.

91   Le Gros Clark and Boggon, 1933; Walker, 1938; Purpura and Yahr, 1966; Brodal, 1969.

92   See Wyke, 1958b, 1968, 1974a, 1979a; White and Sweet, 1969.

93   Walker, 1938; Nauta and Whitlock, 1954; Scheibel and Scheibel, 1966b; Purpura and Yahr, 1966; Brodal, 1969; Desiraju and Purpura, 1970.

94   Walker, 1938; Le Gros Clark, 1948; Kaada, 1960; Purpura and Yahr, 1966; Brodal, 1969; Wyke, 1969, 1979a.

95   Freeman and Watts, 1950; Sweet, 1959; White and Sweet, 1969; Heppner, 1972.

96   Speigel and Wycis, 1962; Urabe and Tsubokawa, 1965; Speigel et al., 1966; White and Sweet, 1969; Cassinari and Pagni, 1969; Schürmann, 1972; Hassler, 1972; Forster et al., 1972.

97   Elithorn et al., 1955, 1958; Nemiah, 1962; Wyke, 1968, 1974a, 1979a.

98   Hassler, 1972.

99   Le Gros Clark, 1936; Walker, 1938; Purpura and Yahr, 1966; Brodal, 1969; Wyke, 1979a.

100   Penfield and Jasper, 1954; Penfield, 1958; Wyke, 1958a, 1979a; Barbizet, 1963; Kimble, 1965; Pribram and Broadbent, 1970; Newcombe, 1972.

101   See Ranson and Clark, 1959; Brodal, 1969.

102   Melzack and Scott, 1957; Nathan, 1962; Barbizet, 1963; Merskey and Spear, 1967; Wyke, 1974a.

103   Le Gros Clark et al., 1938; Fulton et al., 1940; Clara, 1953; Bernhaut et al., 1953; Ranson and Clark, 1959; Skultety, 1963; Haymaker et al., 1969; Brodal, 1969; Wyke, 1969, 1979a; Raisman, 1970; Martini et al., 1971.

104   Fulton et al., 1940; Miller, 1942; Haymaker et al., 1969; Brodal, 1969; Martini et al., 1971.

105   Harris, 1955; Harris et al., 1966; McCann et al., 1968; Haymaker et al., 1969; Brodal, 1969; McCann and Porter, 1969; Martini et al., 1971.

106   See Engel, 1959; Black, 1970; Wyke, 1979a.

107   See Beecher, 1956a, 1959, 1968; Janzen et al., 1972; Bonica, 1974; Bonica and Albe-Fessard, 1976 for details.

108   Melzack, 1973, 1975a; Bonica, 1974; Bonica and Albe-Fessard, 1976; Scott and Huskisson, 1976; Bailey and Davidson, 1976; Crockett et al., 1977.

109   Wolff and Goodell, 1943; West et al., 1952; Beecher, 1956a, 1959; Wyke, 1960, 1974, 1979a; Merskey and Spear, 1967; Melzack and Casey, 1968; Sternbach, 1968, 1974; Langen and Spoerri, 1968; Langen, 1972; Finer, 1972; Melzack, 1973; Glynn and Lloyd, 1976.

110   Wolff and Jarvik, 1963; Petrie, 1967; Beecher, 1968; Procacci, 1972; Glynn and Lloyd, 1976.

111   Wolff and Goodell, 1943; Beecher, 1956a, 1968; Sweet, 1959; Merskey and Spear, 1967; Petrie, 1967; Wyke, 1967, 1974a; Bond, 1972; Melzack, 1973.

112   See Wyke, 1947, 1979a; Keele, 1957; Melzack and Wall, 1965; Merskey and Spear, 1967; Melzack, 1972, 1973.

113   Ranson and Clark, 1959; Petit and Burgess, 1968; Brodal, 1969; Wall, 1970; Handwerker et al., 1975; Kerr, 1975; Wyke, 1979a.

114   Rexed, 1954; Ralston, 1965; Wall, 1967; Brodal, 1969; Price and Meyer, 1974.

115   Szentágothai, 1964; Mendell and Wall, 1965; Melzack and Wall, 1965, 1968; Mendell, 1966; Heimer and Wall, 1968; Wagman and Price, 1969; Wall, 1970; Gregor and Zimmermann, 1972; Handwerker et al., 1975; Kerr, 1975.

116   Earle, 1952; Nathan and Smith, 1959; Szentágothai, 1964; Brodal, 1969.

117   Melzack and Wall, 1965, 1968; Ralston, 1965; Mendell, 1966; Wall, 1969; Wagman and Price, 1969; Wyke, 1969, 1977, 1979a; Melzack, 1972; Janzen et al., 1972; Hassler, 1972; Gregor and Zimmermann, 1972; Bonica, 1974; Handwerker et al., 1975; Kerr, 1975; Bonica and Albe-Fessard, 1976; Nathan, 1976.

118   Russell and Spalding, 1950; Keidel, 1972; Wyke, 1974a, 1977, 1979a.

119   Bonica, 1974; Cauthen and Renner, 1975; Ray and Maurer, 1975; Long and Hagfors, 1975; Melzack, 1975b; Fox and Melzack, 1976; Bonica and Albe-Fessard, 1976; Wyke, 1979a.

120   Wyke, 1977, 1979a.

121   See Wolff and Goodell, 1943; Hardy et al., 1943; Chapman, 1944; Wolff and Wolf, 1948; Beecher, 1953, 1957, 1959, 1968; Wolff and Jarvik, 1963; Janzen et al., 1972; Bonica, 1974; Bonica and Albe-Fessard, 1976.

122   Beecher, 1959; Noordenbos, 1959; Woodrow et al., 1972; Wyke, 1979a.

123   Noordenbos, 1959.

124   Judovich and Bates, 1944; Glover, 1960.

125   Wyke, 1960, 1970, 1972, 1977, 1979a; Nade et al., 1978.

126   Rexed, 1944; Brodal, 1969; Ochoa and Mair, 1969; Arnold and Harriman, 1970.

127   Woodrow et al., 1972.

128   Katz et al., 1963; Rudd and Margolin, 1966; Ward et al., 1968.

129   For example, see Brodal, 1969.

130   Shealy et al., 1970; Nashold and Friedman, 1972; Goloskov and Le Roy, 1974; Fox, 1974; Long and Hagfors, 1975; Ray and Maurer, 1975.

131   Wyke, 1974b, 1977.

132   Olszewski and Baxter, 1954; Hagbarth and Kerr, 1954; Brodal, 1957, 1969; Scheibel and Scheibel, 1958, 1968; Hagbarth and Fex, 1959; Wolstencroft, 1964; Nyberg-Hansen, 1965; Ralston, 1965; Wall, 1967; Fox, 1970; Handwerker et al., 1975; Bonica, 1976; Mayer and Price, 1976; Wyke, 1979a.

133   Hillman and Wall, 1969; Hassler and Bak, 1970; Hassler, 1972; Akil and Mayer, 1972.

134   Hagbarth and Kerr, 1954; Wall, 1967; Hillman and Wall, 1969; Wyke, 1969, 1974a, 1979a.

135   Wyke, 1960, 1969, 1974a, 1979a; Taub, 1964; Sternbach, 1968, 1974; Langen and Spoerri, 1968; Hernández-Peón, 1969; Finer, 1972; Hilgard, 1975; Hilgard and Hilgard, 1975.

136   See Gammon and Starr, 1941; Beecher, 1956a, b, 1959; Wyke, 1960; Barber, 1963; Merskey and Spear, 1967; Lassner, 1967; Langen and Spoerri, 1968; Delius, 1972; Langen, 1972.

137   See Wyke, 1969; Janzen et al., 1972; Chapman and Feather, 1973 for details.

138   Melzack et al., 1958; Wyke, 1969, 1974a.

139   See Wyke, 1960, 1969; Melzack and Eisenberg, 1968; Melzack and Casey, 1968.

140   Wyke, 1968, 1969, 1974a.

141   Wyke, 1968, 1969, 1974a, b, 1977.

142   Hernández-Peón and Hagbarth, 1955; French et al., 1955; Brodal, 1957, 1969; Kuypers, 1958a, b, 1960; Magni and Willis, 1964; Bruckmoser et al., 1970; Wyke, 1979a.

143   Magni and Willis, 1964; Bruckmoser et al., 1970; Mayer and Price, 1976; Wyke, 1979a.

144   See Wyke, 1960, 1979a; Melzack and Wall, 1965, 1968; Melzack and Casey, 1968; Evans and Mulholland, 1969 for reviews.

145   Kosterlitz, 1976; Mayer and Price, 1976; Bonica and Albe-Fessard, 1976; Wyke, 1979a.

146   Satoh and Takagi, 1971; Kosterlitz, 1976.

147   Hagbarth and Fex, 1959; Kuypers, 1960; Nyberg-Hansen and Brodal, 1963; Carpenter et al., 1966; Hongo and Jankowska, 1967; Wall, 1967; Kawana, 1969; Brodal, 1969; Wiesendanger, 1969; Kuypers and Brinkman, 1970; Handwerker et al., 1975; Kerr, 1975; Sessle et al., 1976; Bonica and Albe-Fessard, 1976.

148   Carpenter et al., 1963; Fetz, 1968; Kasprzak et al., 1970; Handwerker et al., 1975; Kerr, 1975.

149   Hagbarth and Kerr, 1954; Fetz, 1968; Kasprzak et al., 1970.

150   Lindblom and Ottosson, 1957; Carpenter et al., 1963, 1966; Andersen et al., 1964c; Handwerker et al., 1975; Sessle et al., 1976.

151   Hassler, 1972.

152   Walker, 1938; Shimazu et al., 1965; Purpura and Yahr, 1966; Kusama et al., 1966; Jones and Powell, 1968, 1970; Kawana, 1969; Nümi and Inoshita, 1971.

153   Iwama and Yamamoto, 1961; Andersen et al., 1964a, b; Matano et al., 1972.

154   Purpura and Yahr, 1966; Sessle and Dubner, 1971.

155   See Delgado, 1955; Melzack and Casey, 1968.

156   Albe-Fessard and Krauthamer, 1964; Yamaguchi and Krauthamer, 1966.

157   See Déjerine and Roussy, 1906; Waltz and Ehni, 1966; Cassinari and Pagni, 1969;; Hassler, 1972.

158   Delafresnaye, 1954; Brodal, 1957, 1969; Jasper et al., 1958; Wyke, 1958b, 1960, 1968, 1969, 1974a, 1979a.

159   Moruzzi and Magoun, 1949; French et al., 1952; Delafresnaye, 1954; Rossi and Zanchetti, 1957; Magoun, 1963; Wyke, 1969.

160   For detailed discussion of these matters, see Scheibel and Scheibel, 1958, 1966b; Brodal, 1969; Wyke, 1969.

161   Bowsher, 1961b; Brodal, 1969; Wyke, 1969, 1974a, 1979a; Skinner, 1970.

162   French et al., 1952; French, 1952; Delafresnaye, 1954; Jasper et al., 1958; Wyke, 1960, 1968, 1969, 1974a, 1979a; Magoun, 1963.

163   See Scheibel and Scheibel, 1965; Wyke, 1968, 1969, 1974a, 1979a; Melzack and Casey, 1968; Bonica, 1974; Bonica and Albe-Fessard, 1976.

164   Hernández-Peón and Hagbarth, 1955; Roger et al., 1956; Pompeiano and Swett, 1962, 1963; Magni and Willis, 1964; Wolstencroft, 1964; Keidel, 1972.

165   See, for example, Magoun, 1963; Wyke, 1963, 1969, 1979a; Brodal, 1969 for discussion of these matters.

166   Wyke, 1972b.

167   Hardy et al., 1943, 1952; Wolff and Wolf, 1948; Beecher, 1956a, 1959, 1968; Wolff and Jarvik, 1963; Gelfand, 1964; Merskey and Spear, 1967; Wolf, 1968; Sternbach, 1968; Woodrow et al., 1972; Wyke, 1974a, 1979a; Bonica, 1974.

168   For example, Albee et al., 1945; Steindler, 1959; Cailliet, 1962; Hirsch, 1966; Kester, 1969; Chamberlain, 1971; Sternbach et al., 1973a; Leavitt et al., 1978.

169   See also Wyke, 1970.

170   Floyd and Silver, 1955; Davis, 1959; Pauly, 1966; Tichauer, 1971; Basmajian, 1974.

171   Floyd and Silver, 1951, 1955; Basmajian, 1974.

172   Steindler, 1959.

173   Merton, 1956; Edholm, 1960; Simons, 1976.

174   Pedersen et al., 1956; Eble, 1961; Wyke, 1970, 1977; Waters and Morris, 1970; Shealy, 1974; Basmajian, 1974; Mooney and Robertson, 1976; Nade et al., 1978.

175   Appleton, 1939; Joseph, 1960; Miyazaki, 1968.

176   See Morris et al., 1962; Pauly, 1966; Yamaji, 1968; Yamaji and Misu, 1968; Miyazaki, 1968; Wyke, 1970, 1977; Jonsson, 1970; Tichauer, 1971; Basmajian, 1974.

177   Lundervold, 1951; Steindler, 1959; Carlsöö, 1961; Davis, 1972; Simons, 1976.

178   See Merton, 1956; Scherrer and Monod, 1960; Basmajian, 1974.

179   Merton, 1954, 1956; Myers and Sullivan, 1968; Kuroda et al., 1970.

180   Edholm, 1960. Christensen, 1962; Kuroda et al., 1970.

181   Hnik et al., 1964; Hnik, 1966.

182   Merton, 1956; Scherrer et al., 1957; Scherrer and Monod, 1960; Lenman, 1969; Basmajian, 1974.

183   See also Waters and Morris, 1970.

184   Gowers, 1904.

185   Stockman, 1920; Copeman, 1951, 1964; Cyriax, 1970.

186   Copeman, 1951.

187   For example, see Steindler, 1959; Adams, 1969.

188   Pearson and Rose, 1961; Gardner-Medwin and Walton, 1969; Person, 1969; Simons, 1976.

189   Copeman, 1943; Gardner-Medwin and Walton, 1969.

190   Barber, 1957; Dixon et al., 1966; Pearson, 1969.

191   Wyke, 1970, 1977; Shealy, 1974; Mooney and Robertson, 1976.
192   Sinclair et al., 1948; Glover, 1960.
193   Floyd and Silver, 1950; Lundervold, 1951; Morton, 1952; Keegan, 1953; Steindler, 1959; Joseph, 1960; Wyke, 1977.
194   Davis, 1959, 1972; Davis et al., 1965; MacConaill and Basmajian, 1969; Wyke, 1977.
195   See Harris, 1959.
196   Wyke, 1970, 1977.
197   See Nassim and Burrows, 1959; Lawrence et al., 1964; Wyke, 1970.
198   Wyke, 1967, 1970, 1972a, 1977; Wyke and Poláček, 1973, 1975.
199   Floyd and Silver, 1951, 1955; Lundervold, 1951; Joseph, 1960; Carlsöö, 1961; Asmussen and Klausen, 1962; Rasch and Burke, 1963; MacConaill and Basmajian, 1969; Basmajian, 1974.
200   Beatty et al., 1968.
201   Stockman, 1920; Copeman, 1951, 1964; Hart, 1959; Cyriax, 1970.
202   Kellgren, 1939; Kellgren and Lewis, 1939; Inman and Saunders, 1944; Hirsch et al., 1963; Hockaday and Whitty, 1967.
203   Sinclair et al., 1948; Wyke, 1970, 1977.
204   Wyke, 1970, 1977; Hall, 1970.
205   Collins, 1959; Nassim, 1959; Nordin, 1973.
206   Sissons, 1959; Hall, 1970.
207   Sissons, 1959.
208   Cholmeley, 1959; Mantle, 1959; Wyke, 1970.
209   Collins, 1959; Wyke, 1970.
210   Wyke, 1970, 1977.
211   Batson, 1940; Herlihy, 1947; Henriques, 1962.
212   Herlihy, 1948; Wyke, 1969, 1970, 1977.
213   Bartelink, 1957; Bearn, 1961; Campbell et al., 1970; Wyke, 1974c.
214   Agostoni et al., 1960; Wyke, 1969; Campbell et al., 1970.
215   Wyke, 1969, 1970; Basmajian, 1974.
216   Wyke, 1969, 1970.
217   See Wyke, 1969, 1970.
218   Collins, 1959; Nathan, 1962.
219   Wyke, 1969, 1970.
220   See Wyke, 1970.
221   See Wyke, 1969.
222   Wyke, 1969, 1974d.
223   Wyke, 1969, 1974d.
224   Bradford and Spurling, 1945; Barr, 1951; Friberg,

1954; Rabinovitch, 1961; Hirsch, 1965; DePalma and Rothman, 1970.
225   Keegan, 1944; Bradford and Spurling, 1946; Keegan and Garrett, 1948; Friberg, 1954; Brieg, 1960; Rabinovitch, 1961; De Palma and Rothman, 1970; Edgar and Park, 1974.
226   Spurling and Grantham, 1940; Keegan, 1944; Bradford and Spurling, 1945; Keegan and Garrett, 1948; Brodal, 1969.
227   Brieg, 1960; Louis et al., 1967.
228   Brodal, 1969.
229   Joffe et al., 1966; Jones and Thomson, 1968; Schatzker and Pennal, 1968; Ehni et al., 1969; Nelson, 1973; Brodsky, 1975.
230   See Harris, 1959.
231   Wyke, 1969, 1974d.
232   Blau and Logue, 1961; Joffe et al., 1966; Ehni et al., 1969; Zulch, 1970; Nelson, 1973.
233   Battye and Joseph, 1966; Waters and Morris, 1972.
234   Weller et al., 1970.
235   See Wyke, 1970, 1977.
236   See, for example, Lewis, 1942; Wolff and Hardy, 1947; Nathan, 1956; Keele, 1957; Noordenbos, 1959; White and Sweet, 1969 for reviews and discussion.
237   Melzack and Wall, 1965; Pomeranz et al., 1968; Selzer and Spencer, 1969a, b; Bonica, 1974; Kerr, 1975; Bonica and Albe-Fessard, 1976.
238   Buzzelli et al., 1968; Procacci, 1972.
239   Procacci, 1972.
240   Wyke, 1974a.
241   Merskey, 1965; Devine and Merskey, 1965; Merskey and Spear, 1967; Minc, 1968; Westrin, 1970; Sternbach et al., 1973a, b; Sternbach, 1974; Forrest and Walkind, 1974; Bonica, 1974; Bonica and Albe-Fessard, 1976; Maruta et al., 1976; Gilchrist, 1976; Leavitt et al., 1978.
242   Partridge et al., 1968; Collette and Ludwig, 1968.
243   Devine and Merskey, 1965; Merskey, 1965; Merskey and Spear, 1967.
244   Westrin, 1970; Wolkind and Forrest, 1972; Sternbach et al., 1973a, b; Forrest and Wolkind, 1974; Gilchrist, 1976; Maruta et al., 1976.
245   Goldstein, 1965; Basmajian, 1974.
246   See Wyke, 1969.
247   Wyke, 1969.
248   Wolkind and Forrest, 1972; Sternbach et al., 1973a; Sternbach, 1974.
249   Devine and Merskey, 1965; White, 1966; Rowe, 1969, 1971; Westrin, 1970.

BIBLIOGRAPHY

Adams R D 1969 Pathological reactions of the skeletal muscle fibre in man. In: Walton J N (ed) Disorders of voluntary muscle, 2nd edn. Churchill, London p 143

Agostoni E, Sant'Ambrogio G, Carrasco H del P 1960 Elettromiografia del diaframma e pressione transdiaframmatica durante la tosse, lo sternuto ed il riso, Atti Accad. Nazion, Lincei, 28, 493

Åkerbom B 1948 Standing and sitting posture (trans. Ann Syngel). Nordiska Bokhandeln, Stockholm

Akil H, Mayer D J 1972 Antagonism of stimulation-produced analgesia by p-CPA, a serotonin synthesis inhibitor. Brain Res. 44: 692

Albee, F H, Powers E J, McDowell H C 1945 Surgery of the Spinal Column. Davis, Philadelphia

Albe-Fessard D 1968 Central nervous mechanisms involved in pain and analgesia. In: Lim R K S, Armstrong D, Pardo E G (eds) Pharmacology of Pain. Pergamon Press, Oxford, p 131

Albe-Fessard D, Bowsher D 1965 Responses of monkey thalamus to somatic stimuli under chloralose anaesthesia. Electroenceph. Clin. Neuro-physiol, 19: 1

Albe-Fessard D, Krauthamer G 1964 Inhibition of units of the non-specific afferent system by stimulation of the basal ganglia. J. Physiol. Lond. 175: 54

Albe-Fessard D, Liebeskind J 1966 Origine des messages somatosensitifs activant les cellules du cortex moteur chez le singe. Exper. Brain Res. 1: 127

Andersen P, Brooks C McC, Eccles J C, Sears T A 1964 The ventrobasal nucleus of the thalamus: potential fields, synaptic transmission and excitability of both presynaptic and postsynaptic components. J. Physiol. Lond. 174: 348

Andersen P, Eccles J C, Sears J C 1964a The ventrobasal complex of the thalamus: types of cells, their responses and their functional organisation. J. Physiol. Lond. 174: 370

Andersen P, Eccles J C, Sears J C 1964b Cortically evoked depolarisation of primary afferent fibres in the spinal cord. J. Neurophysiol. 27: 63

Appleton A B 1939 The effects of high-heeled shoes on posture. J. Chart. Soc. Massage Med. Gym. November, p 134

Armstrong J R 1965 Lumbar Disc Lesions, 3rd edn. Livingstone, Edinburgh and London

Arnold N, Harriman D G F 1970 The incidence of abnormality in control human peripheral nerves studied by single axon dissection. J. Neurol. Neurosurg. Psychiat. 33: 55

Bailey C A, Davidson P O 1976 The language of pain: intensity. Pain, 2: 319

Barber H S 1957 Myalgic syndrome with constitutional effects: polymyalgia rheumatica. Ann. Rheumat. Dis. 16: 230

Barber T X 1963 The effects of 'hypnosis' on pain. Psychosomat. Med. 25: 303

Barbizet J 1963 Defect of memorising of hippocampal-mammillary origin: a review. J. Neurol. Neurosurg. Psychiat. 26: 127

Barr J S 1951 Protruded discs and painful backs. J. Bone Jt. Surg. 33B: 3

Bartelink D L 1957 The role of abdominal pressure in relieving the pressure on the lumbar intervertebral discs. J. Bone Jt. Surg. 39B: 718

Basmajian J V 1974 Muscles alive. Their functions revealed by electromyography, 3rd edn. Williams and Wilkins, Baltimore

Batson O V 1940 The function of the vertebral veins and their role in the spread of metastases. Ann. Surg. 112: 138

Battye C K, Joseph J 1966 An investigation by telemetering of the activity of some muscles in walking. Med. Biol. Eng. 4: 125

Bearn J G 1961 The significance of the activity of the abdominal muscles in weight lifting. Acta Anat. Basel 45: 83

Beatty R A, Sugar O, Fox T A 1968 Protrusion of the posterior longitudinal ligament simulating herniated lumbar intervertebral disc. J. Neurol. Neurosurg. Psychiat. 31: 61

Becker D P, Gluck H, Nulsen F E, Jane J A 1969 An inquiry into the neurophysiological basis for pain. J. Neurosurg. 30: 1

Beecher H K 1953 A method for quantifying the intensity of pain. Science 118: 322

Beecher H K 1956a The subjective response and the reaction to sensation. Amer. J. Med. 20: 107

Beecher H K 1956b Relationship of significance of wound to the pain experienced. J. Amer. Med. Assoc. 161: 1609

Beecher H K 1957 The measurement of pain. Pharmacol. Rev. 9: 59

Beecher H K 1959 The measurement of subjective responses: quantitative effects of drugs. Oxford University Press, New York

Beecher H K 1968 The measurement of pain in man. In: Soulairac A, Cahn J, Charpentier N (eds) Pain. Academic Press, New York, p 207

Benjamin F B 1968 Release of intracellular potassium as a factor in pain production. In: Kenshalo D R (ed) The skin senses. Thomas, Springfield, Illinois, p 466

Benjamin R M 1970 Single neurons in the rat medulla responsive to nociceptive stimulation. Brain Res. 24: 525

Bernhaut M, Gellhorn E, Rasmussen A T 1953 Experimental contributions to the problem of consciousness. J. Neurophysiol. 16: 21

Bessou P, Laporte Y 1958 Activation des fibres afférentes amyéliniques d'origine musculaire. Compt. Rend. Soc. Biol. Paris 152: 1587

Bessou P, Perl E R 1969 Response of cutaneous sensory units with unmyelinated fibres to noxious stimuli. J. Neurophysiol. 32: 1025

Bishops G H 1966 Fiber size and myelinisation in afferent systems. In: Knighton R S, Dumke P R (eds) Pain: an international symposium. Little Brown, Boston, p 83

Black P 1970 Physiological correlates of emotion. Academic Press, New York

Blau J N, Logue V 1961 Intermittent claudication of the cauda equina. Lancet 1: 1018

Bond M R 1972 Psychological aspects of pain. In: Critchley M, O'Leary J L, Jennett B (eds) Scientific foundations of neurology. Heinemann, London, p 165

Bonica J J (ed) 1974 International symposium on pain. Raven Press, New York

Bonica J J, Albe-Fessard D (eds) 1976 Advances in pain research and therapy. Raven Press, New York

Bourland A, Winkelmann R K 1966 Study of cutaneous innervation in congenital anaesthesia. Archiv. Neurol. Chicago 14: 223

Bowsher D 1957 Termination of the central pain pathway in man: the conscious appreciation of pain. Brain 80: 606

Bowsher D 1961a The termination of secondary somatosensory neurons within the thalamus of Macaca mulatta: an experimental degeneration study. J. Comp. Neurol. 117: 213

Bowsher D 1961b The reticular formation and ascending reticular system: anatomical considerations. Brit. J. Anaesth. 33: 174

Bowsher D 1962 The topographic projection of fibres from the anterolateral quadrant of the spinal cord to the subdiencephalic brain stem in man. Psychiat. Neurol. Basel 143: 75

Bowsher D 1976 Role of the reticular system in response to noxious stimulation. Pain 2: 361

Bowsher D, Mallart A, Petit D, Albe-Fessard D 1968 A bulbar relay to the center median. J. Neurophysiol. 31: 288

Bradford F K, Spurling R G 1945 The intervertebral disc, 2nd edn. Thomas, Springfield, Illinois

Brazier Mary A B (ed) 1970 The interneuron. University of California Press, Berkeley

Bressler B, Cohen S I, Magmussen F 1955 Bilateral breast phantom and breast phantom pain. J. Nerv. Ment. Dis. 122: 315

Bridge C J 1959 Innervation of spinal meninges and epidural structures. Anat. Rec. 133: 553

Brieg A 1960 Biomechanics of the central nervous system. Some basic normal and pathologic phenomena. Year Book Publishers, Chicago

Brodal A 1957 The reticular formation of the brain stem. Anatomical aspects and functional correlations. Oliver & Boyd, Edinburgh

Brodal A 1969 Neurological anatomy in relation to clinical medicine, 2nd edn. Oxford University Press, London

Brodsky A E 1975 Low back pain syndromes due to spinal stenosis and posterior cauda equina compression. Bull. Hosp. Joint Dis. 36: 66

Bruckmoser P, Hepp-Raymond M C, Wiesendanger M 1970 Cortical influence on single neurons of the lateral reticular nucleus of the cat. Exper. Neurol. 26: 239

Burgess P R, Perl E R 1967 Myelinated afferent fibres responding specifically to noxious stimulation of the skin. J. Physiol. Lond. 190: 541

Buzzelli G, Voegelin M R, Procacci P, Bozza G 1968 Modificazioni della soglia del dolore cutaneo durante il ciclo mestruale. Bull. Soc. Ital. Biol. Sper. 44: 235

Cailliet R 1962 Low back pain syndrome. Davis, Philadelphia

Calma I 1965 The activity of the posterior group of thalamic nuclei in the cat. J. Physiol. Lond. 180: 350

Campbell E J M, Agostoni E, Newsom Davis J 1970 The respiratory muscles: mechanics and neural control, 2nd edn. Lloyd-Luke, London

Carlsöö S 1961 The static muscle load in different work positions: an electromyographic study. Ergonomics 4: 193

Carpenter D, Engberg L, Lundberg A 1966 Primary afferent depolarisation evoked from the brainstem and the cerebellum. Archiv. Ital. Biol. 104: 73

Carpenter D, Lundberg A, Norrsell U 1963 Primary afferent depolarisation evoked from the sensorimotor cortex. Acta Physiol. Scand. 59: 126

Carpenter M B, Stein B M, Shriver J E 1968 Central projections of spinal dorsal roots in the monkey. II. Lower thoracic, lumbosacral and coccygeal dorsal roots. Amer. J. Anat. 123: 75

Casey K L 1966 Unit analysis of nociceptive mechanisms in the thalamus of the awake squirrel monkey. J. Neurophysiol. 29: 727

Cassinari V, Pagni C A 1969 Central pain. A neurosurgical survey. Harvard University Press, Cambridge, Massachusetts

Cauthen J C, Renner E J 1975 Transcutaneous and peripheral nerve stimulation for chronic pain states. Surg. Neurol. 4: 102

Chamberlain G V P 1971 Backache I and II. Brit. Med. J. 99: 159

Chapman C R, Feather B W 1973 Effects of diazepam on human pain tolerance and pain sensitivity. Psychosom. Med. 35: 330

Chapman W P 1944 Measurements of pain sensitivity in normal control subjects and in psychoneurotic patients. Psychosomat. Med. 6: 252

Cholmeley J A 1959 Tuberculous disease of the spine. In: Nassim R, Burrows H J (eds) Modern trends in diseases of the vertebral column. Butterworths, London, p 137

Chow K L, Pribram K H 1956 Cortical projection of the thalamic ventrolateral nuclear group in monkeys. J. Comp. Neurol. 104: 57

Christensen B N, Perl E R 1970 Spinal neurons specifically excited by noxious or thermal stimuli: marginal zone, of the dorsal horn. J. Neurophysiol. 33: 293

Christensen E H 1962 Muscular work and fatigue. In: Rodhal K, Horvath S M (eds) Muscle as a tissue. McGraw-Hill, New York, p 176

Clara M 1953 Die Anatomie der Sensibilität unter besonderer Berücksichtigung der vegetativen Leitungsbahnen. Acta Neuroveg. Wien, 7: 4

Clark W E Le Gros 1936 The thalamic connections of the temporal lobe of the brain in the monkey. J. Anat. London 70: 447

Clark W E Le Gros 1948 The connections of the frontal lobes of the brain. Lancet 254: 353

Clark W E Le Gros, Beattie J, Riddoch G, Dott N M 1938 The hypothalamus. Morphological, functional, clinical and surgical aspects. Oliver & Boyd, Edinburgh

Clark W E Le Gros, Boggon R H 1933 On the connections of the anterior nucleus of the thalamus. J. Anat. Lond. 67: 215

Clark W E Le Gros, Boggon R H 1935 The thalamic connections of the parietal and frontal lobes of the brain in the monkey. Phil. Trans. Roy. Soc. Lond. 224B: 313

Collette J, Ludwig E G 1968 Low back disorders: an examination of the stereotype. Indust. Med. Surg. 37: 685

Collins D H 1959 Degenerative diseases. In: Nassim R, Burrows H J (eds) Modern trends in diseases of the vertebral column. Butterworths, London, p 101

Cooper I S 1965 Clinical and physiologic implications of thalamic surgery for disorders of sensory communication: I. Thalamic surgery for intractable pain. J. Neurol. Sci. 2: 493

Copeman W S C 1943 Aetiology of the fibrositic nodule: a clinical contribution. Brit. Med. J. 2: 263

Copeman W S C 1951 Fibrositis. In: Lord Horder (ed) The British Encyclopaedia of Medical Practice, 2nd edn. vol. 5. Butterworths, London, p 431

Copeman W S C (ed) 1964 Textbook of the rheumatic diseases, 3rd edn. Livingstone, Edinburgh

Critchley M 1956 Congenital indifference to pain. Ann. Inter. Med. 45: 737

Crockett D J, Prkachin K M, Craig K D 1977 Factors of the language of pain in patient and volunteer groups. Pain 4: 175

Curry M J 1972 The exteroceptive properties of neurones in the somatic part of the posterior group (PO). Brain Res. 44: 439

Curry M J, Gordon G 1972 The spinal input to the posterior group in the cat: an electrophysiological investigation. Brain Res. 44: 417

Cyriax J 1970 Textbook of orthopaedic medicine, 5th edn. Baillière, Tindall, London

Dallenbach K M 1939 Pain: history and present status. Amer. J. Psychol. 52: 331

Davis P R 1959 Posture of the trunk during the lifting of weights. Brit. Med. J. 1: 87

Davis P R 1961 Human lower lumbar vertebrae: some mechanical and osteological considerations. J. Anat. Lond. 95: 337

Davis P R 1972 The physical causation of disease. Roy. Soc. Health J. 92: 63

Davis P R, Troup J D G, Burnard J H 1965 Movements of the thoracic and lumbar spine when lifting: a chronocyclophotographic study. J. Anat. Lond. 99: 13

Dee R 1969 Structure and function of hip joint innervation. Ann. Roy. Coll. Surg. Engl. 45: 357

Déjerine J, Roussy G 1906 Le syndrome thalamique. Rev. Neurol. Paris 14: 521

Delafresnaye J F (ed) 1954 Brain mechanisms and consciousness. Blackwell, Oxford

Delgado J M R 1955 Cerebral structures involved in transmission and elaboration of noxious stimulation. J. Neurophysiol. 18: 261

Delius L 1972 Psychosomatic aspects of treating pain: the internist's viewpoint. In: Janzen R, Keidel W D, Herz A,

Steichele C (eds) Pain: basic principles, pharmacology, therapy. Thième, Stuttgart, p 161

DePalma A F, Rothman R H 1970 The intervertebral disc. Saunders, Philadelphia

Desiraju T, Purpura D P 1970 Organisation of specific-nonspecific thalamic inter-nuclear synaptic pathways. Brain Res. 21: 169

Devine R, Merskey H 1965 The description of pain in psychiatric and general medical patients. J. Psychosomat. Res. 9: 311

Dewulf A 1971 Anatomy of normal human thalamus. Elsevier, New York

Dillane J B, Fry J, Kalton G 1966 Acute back syndrome: a study from general practice. Brit. Med. J. 2: 82

Dixon A St J, Beardwell C, Kay A, Wanka J, Wong Y T 1966 Polymyalgia rheumatica and temporal arteritis. Ann. Rheumat. Dis. 25: 203

Drake C G, McKenzie K G 1953 Mesencephalic tractotomy for pain. J. Neurosurg. 10: 457

Earle K M 1952 The tract of Lissauer and its possible relation to the pain pathway. J. Comp. Neurol. 96: 93

Eble J N 1961 Reflex relationships of paravertebral muscles. Amer. J. Physiol. 200: 939

Edgar M A, Nundy S 1966 Innervation of the spinal dura mater. J. Neurol. Neurosurg. Psychiat. 29: 530

Edgar M A, Park W M 1974 Induced pain patterns on passive straight-leg raising in lower disc protrusion. J. Bone Jt. Surg. 56B: 658

Edholm O G 1960 Some effects of fatigue, temperature and training on muscular contraction in man. In: Bourne G H (ed) Structure and function of muscle, vol 2. Academic Press, New York, p 440

Ehni G, Clark K, Wilson C B, Alexander E 1969 Significance of the small lumbar spinal canal: a symposium. J. Neurosurg. 31: 490

Ehrenhaft J L 1943 Development of the vertebral column as related to certain congenital and pathological changes. Surg. Gynec. Obstet. 76: 282

Elithorn A, Glithero E, Slater E 1958 Leucotomy for pain. J. Neurol. Neurosurg. Psychiat. 21: 249

Elithorn A, Piercy M F, Crosskey M A 1955 Prefrontal leucotomy and the anticipation of pain. J. Neurol. Neurosurg. Psychiat. 18: 34

Ellis H Havelock 1898 Studies in the Psychology of Sex, Part I. Random House, New York

Engel B T 1959 Some physiological correlates of hunger and pain. J. Exper. Psychol. 57: 389

Evans C R, Mulholland T B (eds) 1969 Attention in neurophysiology. Butterworths, London

Feindel W H, Weddell G, Sinclair D C 1948 Pain sensibility in deep somatic structures. J. Neurol. Neurosurg. Psychiat. 11: 113

Fernand V S V, Young J Z 1961 The sizes of the nerve fibres of muscle nerves. Proc. Roy. Soc. Lond. 139B: 38

Ferreira S H 1972 Prostaglandins, aspirin-like drugs and analgesia. Nature New Biol. 240: 200

Fetz E E 1968 Pyramidal tract effects on interneurons in the cat lumbar dorsal horn. J. Neurophysiol. 31: 69

Finer B 1972 The use of hypnosis in the clinical management of pain. In: Janzen W D, Keidel Q D, Herz A, Steichele C (eds) Pain: basic principles, pharmacology, therapy. Thième, Stuttgart, p 168

Fisk J W 1970 Backache in general practice. J. Roy. Coll. Gen. Pract. 119: 92

Floyd W F, Silver P H S 1950 Electromyographic study of patterns of activity of the anterior abdominal wall muscles in man. J. Anat. Lond. 84: 132

Floyd W F, Silver P H S 1951 Function of erector spinae in flexion of the trunk. Lancet 1: 133

Floyd W F, Silver P H S 1955 The functions of the erectores spinae muscles in certain movements and postures in man. J. Physiol. Lond. 129: 184

Foerster O 1933 The dermatomes in man. Brain. 56: 11

Foerster O 1936 Symptomatologie der Erkrankungen des Rückenmarks und seiner Wurzein. In: Bumke F, Foerster O (eds) Handbuch der neurologie, vol 5. Springer, Berlin, p 1

Foltz E L, White L E 1962 Pain relief by frontal cingulumotomy. J. Neurosurg. 19: 89

Forrest A J, Wolkind S N 1974 Masked depression in men with low back pain. Rheumatol. Rehab. 13: 148

Forster D M C, Leksell L, Meyerson B A, Steiner L 1972 Gammathalamotomy in intractable pain. In: Janzen R, Keidel W D, Herz A, Steichele C (eds) Pain: basic principles, pharmacology, therapy. Thième, Stuttgart, p 194

Fox E J, Melzack R 1976 Transcutaneous electrical stimulation and acupuncture: comparison of treatment for low back pain. Pain 2: 141

Fox J E 1970 Reticulo-spinal neurons in the rat. Brain Res. 23: 35

Fox J L 1974 Dorsal column stimulation for relief of intractable pain: problems encountered with neuro-pacemakers. Surg. Neurol. 2: 59

Freeman M A R, Wyke B D 1967a The innervation of the knee joint: an anatomical and histological study in the cat. J. Anat. Lond. 101: 505

Freeman M A R, Wyke B D 1967b The innervation of the ankle joint: an anatomical and histological study in the cat. Acta Anat. Basel 68: 321

Freeman W, Watts J 1950 Psychosurgery in the treatment of mental disorders and intractable pain, 2nd edn. Thomas, Springfield, Illinois

French J D 1952 Brain lesions associated with prolonged unconsciousness. Archiv. Neurol. Psychiat. Chicago 68: 722

French J D, von Amerongen F K, Magoun H W 1952 An activating system in brain stem of monkey. Archiv. Neurol. Psychiat. Chicago 68: 577

French J D, Hernández-Peón R, Livingston R B 1955 Projections from cortex to cephalic brain stem (reticular formation) in monkey. J. Neurophysiol. 18: 74

Friberg S 1954 Lumbar disc degeneration in the problem of lumbago sciatica. Bull. Hosp. Joint. Dis. 15: 1

Fulton J F, Ranson S W, Frantz A M (eds) 1940 The hypothalamus and central levels of autonomic function. Williams & Wilkins, Baltimore

Gammon G D, Staff I 1941 Studies on relief of pain by counter-irritation. J. Clin. Invest. 20: 13

Gardner E D 1943 Surgical anatomy of the external carotid plexus. Archiv. Surg. 46: 238

Gardner E D, Cuneo H M 1945 Lateral spinothalamic tract and associated tracts in man. Archiv. Neurol. Psychiat. Chicago 53: 423

Gardner-Medwin D, Walton J N 1969 A classification of the neuromuscular disorders and a note on the clinical examination of the voluntary muscles. In: Walton J N (ed) Disorders of voluntary muscle, 2nd edn. Churchill, London, p 411

Gelfand S 1964 The relationship of experimental pain tolerance to pain threshold. Canad. J. Psychol. 18: 36

Gilchrist I C 1976 Psychiatric and social factors related to low-back pain in general practice. Rheumatol. Rehab. 15: 101

Gillis L 1964 The management of the painful amputation stump and a new theory for the phantom phenomena. Brit. J. Surg. 51: 87

Glees P 1953 The central pain tract. Acta Neuroveg. Wien 7: 160

Glover J R 1960 Back pain and hyperaesthesia. Lancet 1: 1165

Glynn C J, Lloyd J W 1976 The diurnal variation in perception of pain. Proc. Roy. Soc. 69B: 369

Goldring S, Aras E, Weber P C 1970 Comparative study of sensory input to motor cortex in animals and man. Electroenceph. Clin. Neurophysiol. 29: 537

Goldstein I B 1965 The relationship of muscle tension and autonomic activity to psychiatric disorders. Psychosomat. Med. 27: 39

Goloskov J, LeRoy P 1974 Pain and suffering: use of the dorsal column stimulator. Amer. J. Nursing 74: 506

Gowers W R 1904 Lumbago: its lesions and analogues. Brit. Med. J. 1: 117

Gregor M, Zimmermann M 1972 Characteristics of spinal neurons responding to cutaneous myelinated and unmyelinated fibres. J. Physiol. Lond. 221: 555

Hagbarth K E, Fex J 1959 Centrifugal influences on single unit activity in spinal sensory paths. J. Neurophysiol. 22: 321

Hagbarth K E, Kerr D I B 1954 Central influences on spinal afferent conduction. J. Neurophysiol. 17: 295

Häggqvist G 1936 Analyse der Faserverteilung in einem Rückenmarkquerschnitt (Th. 3). Zeit. Mikr.-Anat. Forsch. 39: 1

Hall J H 1970 The 'lumbar disc syndrome' produced by sacral metastases. Canad. J. Surg. 13: 149

Hand P J, Morrison A R 1970 Thalamocortical projections from the ventrobasal complex to somatic sensory area I and II. Exper. Neurol. 27: 291

Handwerker H O, Iggo A, Zimmermann M 1975 Segmental and supraspinal actions on dorsal horn neurones responding to noxious and non-noxious skin stimulation. Pain 1: 147

Handwerker H O, Zimmermann M 1972 Cortical evoked responses upon selective stimulation of cutaneous Group III fibers and the mediating spinal pathways. Brain Res. 36: 437

Hansen K, Schliack H 1962 Segmentale innervation: ihre Bedeutung für Klinik und Praxis. Thième, Stuttgart

Hardy J D, Wolff H G, Goodell H 1943 The pain threshold in man. Res. Pub. Assoc. Nerv. Ment. Dis. 23: 1

Hardy J D, Wolff H G, Goodell H 1952 Pain sensations and reactions. Williams & Wilkins, Baltimore

Harris G W 1955 Neural control of the pituitary gland. Arnold, London

Harris G W, Reed M, Fawcett C P 1966 Hypothalamic releasing factors and the control of anterior pituitary function. Brit. Med. Bull. 22: 266

Harris R I 1959 Congenital anomalies. In: Nassim R, Burrows H J (eds) Modern trends in diseases of the vertebral column. Butterworths, London, p 29

Hart F D 1959 Ankylosing spondylitis. In: Nassim R, Burrows H J (eds) Modern trends in diseases of the vertebral column. Butterworths, London, p 155

Hassler R 1960 Die zentrale Systeme des Schmerzes. Acta Neurochir. Wien 8: 353

Hassler R 1961 Motorische und sensible Effekte umschriebener Reizungen und Ausschaltungen in menschlichen Zwischenhirn. Nervenheilk, Deutsche Zeit 183: 148

Hassler R 1972 Afferent systems: the division of pain conduction into systems of pain sensation and pain awareness. In: Janzen R, Keidel W D, Herz A, Steichele C (eds) Pain: basic principles pharmacology, therapy. Thième, Stuttgart, p 98

Hassler R, Bak I J 1970 The fine structure of different types of synapses and their circuit arrangement in the substantia gelatinosa trigemini. In: Hassler R, Walker A E (eds) Trigeminal neuralgia: pathogenesis and pathophysiology. Saunders, Philadelphia, p 50

Hassler R, Riechert T 1959 Klinische und anatomische Befunde bei thalamischen Schmerzoperationen am Menschen. Archiv. Psychiat. Nervenkr. 200: 93

Haymaker W, Anderson E, Nauta W J H (eds) The hypothalamus. Thomas, Springfield, Illinois

Head H 1920 Studies in neurology. Frowde, Hodder & Stoughton, London

Heimer L, Wall P D 1968 The dorsal root distribution to the substantia gelatinosa of the rat with a note on the distribution in the cat. Exper. Brain Res. 6: 89

Henderson W R, Smyth G E 1948 Phantom limbs. J. Neurol. Neurosurg. Psychiat. 11: 88

Henriques C Q 1962 The veins of the vertebral column and their role in the spread of cancer. Ann. Roy. Coll. Surg. Engl. 31: 1

Heppner F 1972 Studies with rostral leucotomy. In: Janzen R, Keidel W D, Herz A, Steichele C (eds) Pain: basic principles, pharmacology, therapy. Thième, Stuttgart, p 217

Herlihy W F 1947 Revision of the venous system: the role of the vertebral veins. Med. J. Austral. 1: 661

Herlihy W F 1948 Experimental studies on the internal vertebral venous plexus. In: Phillips G, Wyke B D, Herlihy W F (eds) Essays in biology. Australasian Medical Publishing Company, Sydney, p 151

Hernández-Peón R 1969 A neurophysiological and evolutionary model of attention. In: Evans C R, Mulholland T B (eds) Attention in neurophysiology. Butterworths, London, p 417

Hernández-Peón R, Hagbarth K-E 1955 Interaction between afferent and cortically induced reticular responses. J. Neurophysiol. 18: 44

Hilgard E R 1975 The alleviation of pain by hypnosis. Pain 1: 213

Hilgard E R, Hilgard J R 1975 Hypnosis in the relief of pain. Kaufmann, Los Altos, California

Hillman P, Wall P D 1969 Inhibitory and excitatory factors influencing the receptive fields of lamina 5 spinal cord cells. Exper. Brain Res. 9: 284

Hirsch C 1965 Efficiency of surgery in low-back disorders: pathoanatomical experimental and clinical studies. J. Bone Jt. Surg. 47A: 991

Hirsch C 1966 Etiology and pathogenesis of low back pain. Israel J. Med. Sci. 2: 362

Hirsch C, Inglemark B-E, Miller M 1963 The anatomical basis for low back pain: studies on the presence of sensory nerve endings in ligamentous, capsular and intervertebral disc structures in the human lumbar spine. Acta Orthopaed. Scand. 33: 1

Hirsch C, Schajowicz F 1953 Studies on structural changes in the lumbar annulus fibrosus. Acta Orthopaed. Scand. 22: 184

Hnik P 1966 Increased sensory outflows from atrophying muscles and muscles after functional activity. In: Granit R (ed) Muscular afferents and motor control. Wiley, New York, p 445

Hnik P, Hudlická O, Stulcová B 1964 Activité afférente du muscle strié en rapport avec des changements circulatoires intramusculaires. J. Physiol. Paris 56: 569

Hockaday J M, Whitty C W M 1967 Patterns of referred pain in the normal subject. Brain 90: 481

Hongo T, Janowska E 1967 Effects from the sensorimotor cortex on the spinal cord in cats with transected pyramids. Exper. Brain Res. 3: 117

Horal J 1969 The clinical appearance of low back disorders in the city of Gothenburg, Sweden. Acta Orthopaed. Scand. Suppl 118: 1

Hovelacque A 1925 Le nerf sinu-vertébral. Ann. d'Anat. Pathol. Méd-chir. 2: 435

Iggo A 1959 A single unit analysis of cutaneous receptors with C afferent fibres. In: Wolstenholme G E W, O'Connor M (eds) Pain and itch. Churchill, London, p 41

Iggo A 1962 Non-myelinated visceral, muscular and cutaneous afferent fibres and pain. In: Keele C A, Smith R (eds) U F A W Symposium on assessment of pain in man and animals. Livingstone, London, p 74

Iggo A 1963 An electrophysiological analysis of afferent fibres in primate skin. Acta Neuroveg. Wien 24: 225

Iggo A 1966a Cutaneous receptors with a high sensitivity to mechanical displacement. In: de Reuck A V S, Knight J (eds) Touch, heat, pain. Churchill, London, p 237

Iggo A 1966b Muscle nociceptors with C. fibres. In: de Reuck A V S, Knight J (eds) Touch, heat, pain. Churchill, London, p 364

Iggo A 1972 The case for 'pain' receptors. In: Janzen R, Keidel W D, Herz A, Steichele C (eds) Pain: basic principles pharmacology, therapy. Thième, Stuttgart, p 60

Ikari C 1954 A study of the mechanism of low-back pain: the neurohistological examination of the disease. J. Bone Jt. Surg. 36A: 195

Inman V T, Saunders J B D 1944 Referred pain from skeletal structures. J. Nerv. Ment. Dis. 99: 660

Iwama K, Yamamoto C 1961 Impulse transmission of thalamic somatosensory relay nuclei as modified by electrical stimulation of the cerebral cortex. Jap. J. Physiol. 11: 169

Jabbur S J, Baker M A, Towe A L 1972 Wide-field neurons in thalamic nucleus ventralis posterolateralis of the cat. Exper. Neurol. 36: 213

Jackson H C, Winkelmann R K, Bickel W H 1966 Nerve endings in the human lumbar spinal column and related structures. J. Bone Jt. Surg. 48A: 1272

Janzen R, Keidel W D, Herz A, Steichele C (eds) 1972 Pain: basic principles, pharmacology, therapy. Thième, Stuttgart

Jasper H H, Proctor L D, Knighton R S, Noshay W C, Costello R T (eds) 1958 The reticular formation of the brain. Little, Brown, Boston

Jewsbury E C O 1951 Insensitivity to pain. Brain 74: 336

Joffe R, Appleby A, Arjona V 1966 Intermittent ischaemia of the cauda equina due to stenosis of the lumbar canal. J. Neurol. Neurosurg. Psychiat. 29: 315

Jones E G, Powell T P S 1968 The projection of the somatic sensory cortex upon the thalamus in the cat. Brain Res. 10: 369

Jones E G, Powell T P S 1969 The cortical projection of the ventroposterior nucleus of the thalamus in the cat. Brain Res. 13: 298

Jones E G, Powell T P S 1970 Connexions of the somatic sensory cortex of the rhesus monkey. III. Thalamic connexions. Brain 93: 37

Jones R A C, Thomson J L G 1968 The narrow lumbar canal. J. Bone Jt. Surg. 50B: 595

Jonsson B 1970 The functions of individual muscles in the lumbar part of the erector spinae muscle. Electromyography 10: 5

Joseph J 1960 Man's posture: electromyographic studies. Thomas, Springfield, Illinois

Judovich B, Bates W 1944 Segmental neuralgia in painful syndromes. Davis, Philadelphia

Jung A, Brunschwig A 1932 Recherches histologiques sur l'innervation des articulations des corps vertébraux. Presse Méd 40: 316

Kaada B 1960 Cingulate, posterior orbital, anterior insular and temporal pole cortex. In: Field J, Magoun H W, Hall V E (eds) Handbook of physiology, vol 2 section 1: Neurophysiology. American Physiological Society, Washington, p 1345

Kaplan E B 1947 Recurrent meningeal branch of the spinal nerves. Bull. Hosp. Joint Dis. 8: 108

Kasprzak H, Mann M D, Tapper D N 1970 Pyramidal modulation of responses of spinal neurons to natural stimulation of cutaneous receptors. Brain Res. 24: 121

Katz S, Ford A B, Moskowitz R W, Jackson B A, Jaffe M W 1963 Studies of illness in the aged. J. Amer. Med. Assoc. 185: 914

Kawana E 1969 Projections of the anterior ectosylvian gyrus to the thalamus, the dorsal column nuclei, the trigeminal nuclei and the spinal cord in cats. Brain Res. 14: 117

Keegan J J 1944 Neurosurgical interpretation of dermatome hypalgesia with herniation of the lumbar intervertebral disc. J. Bone Jt. Surg. 26A: 238

Keegan J J 1953 Alterations of the lumbar curve related to posture and seating. J. Bone Jt. Surg. 35A: 589

Keegan J J, Garrett F D 1948 The segmental distribution of the cutaneous nerves in the limbs of man. Anat. Rec. 102: 409

Keele C A, Armstrong D 1964 Substances producing pain and itch. Arnold, London

Keele C A, Armstrong D 1968 Mediators of pain. In: Lim R K S, Armstrong D, Pardo E G (eds) Pharmacology of pain. Pergamon Press, Oxford, p 3

Keele K D 1957 Anatomies of pain. Blackwell, Oxford

Keidel W D 1972 The problem of 'subjective' and 'objective' quantification of pain. In: Janzen R, Keidel W D, Herz A, Steichele C (eds) Pain: basic principles, pharmacology, therapy. Thième, Stuttgart, p 16

Kellgren J H 1939 On the distribution of pain arising from deep somatic structures with charts of segmental pain areas. Clin. Sci. 4: 35

Kellgren J H, Lewis T 1939 Observations relating to referred pain, viscero-motor reflexes and other associated phenomena. Clin. Sci. 4: 46

Kelly D L, Goldring S, O'Leary J L 1965 Average evoked somatosensory responses from exposed cortex of man. Archiv. Neurol. Chicago 13: 1

Kenshalo D R (ed) 1968 The skin senses. Thomas, Springfield, Illinois

Kerr F W L 1975 Neuroanatomical substrates of nociception in the spinal cord. Pain 1: 325

Kester N C 1969 Evaluation and medical management of low back pain. Med. Clin. Nth. Amer. 53: 525

Kimble D P (ed) 1965 Anatomy of memory. Science and Behavior Books, Palo Alto, California

Kolb L C 1952 Pain as a psychiatric problem. Lancet 72: 50

Kolb L C 1954 The painful phantom: psychology, physiology and treatment. Thomas, Springfield, Illinois

Kosterlitz H W (ed) 1976 Opiates and endogenous opioid peptides. North-Holland Press, Amsterdam

Kruger L 1966 The thalamic projection of pain. In: Knighton R S, Dumke P R (eds) Pain: an international symposium. Little, Brown, Boston, p 67

Kunkle E C, Chapman W P 1943 Insensitivity to pain in man. Res. Pub. Assoc. Nerv. Ment. Dis. 23: 100

Kuroda E, Klissouras V, Mulsum J H 1970 Electrical and metabolic activities and fatigue in human isometric contraction. J. Appl. Physiol. 29: 358

Kusama T, Otani T, Kawana E 1966 Projections of the motor, somatic sensory, auditory and visual cortices in cats. Prog. Brain Res. 21A: 292

Kuypers H G J M 1958a An anatomical analysis of corticobulbar connexions to the pons and lower brainstem in the cat. J. Anat. Lond. 92: 198

Kuypers H G J M 1958b Corticobulbar connexions to the pons and lower brainstem in man: an anatomical study. Brain 81: 364

Kuypers H G J M 1960 Central cortical projections to motor and somatosensory cell groups. Brain 83: 161

Kuypers H G J M, Brinkman J 1970 Precentral projections to different parts of the spinal intermediate zone in the rhesus monkey. Brain Res. 24: 29

Langen D 1972 Psychosomatic aspects in the treatment of pain. In: Janzen R, Keidel W D, Herz A, Steichele C (eds) Pain: basic principles, pharmacology, therapy. Thième, Stuttgart, p 164

Langen D, Spoerri T (eds) 1968 Hypnose und Schmerz. Karger, Basel

Lassner J (ed) 1967 Hypnosis and psychosomatic medicine. Springer, Berlin

Lawrence J S 1969 Disc degeneration: its frequency and relationship to symptoms. Ann. Rheumat. Dis. 28: 121

Lawrence J S, Sharp J, Ball J, Bier F 1964 Rheumatoid arthritis of the lumbar spine. Ann. Rheumat. Dis. 23: 205

Leavitt F, Garron D C, Whisler W W, Sheinkop M B 1978 Affective and sensory dimensions of back pain. Pain 4: 273

Lenman J A R 1969 Integration and analysis of the electromyogram and related techniques. In: Walton J N (ed) Disorders of voluntary muscle, 2nd edn. Churchill, London, p 843

Lewin T, Moffett R, Vüdik A 1961 The morphology of the lumbar synovial intervertebral joints. Acta Morph. Neerl-Scand. 4: 299

Lewis T 1942 Pain. Macmillan, New York

Lim R K S 1960 Visceral receptors and visceral pain. Ann. N.Y. Acad. Sci. 86: 73

Lim R K S 1968 Cutaneous and visceral pain, and somesthetic chemoreceptors. In: Kenshalo D R (ed) The skin senses. Thomas, Springfield, Illinois, p 458

Lim R K S, Guzman F, Rodgers D W 1962 Note on the muscle receptors concerned with pain. In: Barker D (ed) Symposium on muscle receptors. Hong Kong University Press, Hong Kong, p 215

Lindblom U F, Ottosson J L 1957 Influence of pyramidal stimulation upon the relay of coarse cutaneous afferents in the dorsal horn. Acta Physiol. Scand. 38: 309

Lippman H H, Kerr F W L 1972 Light and electron microscopic study of crossed ascending pathways in the anterolateral funiculus in monkey. Brain Res. 40: 496

Long D M, Hagfors N 1975 Electrical stimulation in the nervous system: the current status of electrical stimulation of the nervous system for the relief of pain. Pain 1: 109

Louis R, Laffont J, Conty C-R, Argème M 1967 Mobilité de la moelle épinière.Compt. Rend. Assoc. Anat. Paris 138: 817

Lund R D, Webster K E 1967 Thalamic afferents from the spinal cord and trigeminal nuclei: an experimental anatomical study in the rat. J. Comp. Neurol. 130: 313

Lundervold A J S 1951 Electromyographic investigations of position and manner of working in typewriting. Brøggers, Oslo

von Luschka H 1850 Die Nerven des menschlichen Wirbelkanales. Laupp & Siebeck, Tübingen

McCann S M, Dhariwal A P S, Porter J C 1968 Regulation of the adenohypophysis. Ann. Rev. Physiol. 30: 589

McCann S M, Porter J C 1969 Hypothalamic pituitary stimulating and inhibiting hormones. Physiol. Rev. 49: 240

MacConaill M A, Basmajian J V 1969 Muscles and movements. A basis for human kinesiology. Williams & Wilkins, Baltimore

Magni F, Willis W D 1964 Afferent connections to reticulospinal neurons. Prog. Brain Res. 12: 246

Magoun H W 1963 The waking brain, 2nd edn. Thomas, Springfield, Illinois

Majorossy K., Kiss A 1969 Cortical and subcortical connections of the pulvinar thalami. Acta Morph. Acad. Sci. Hung. 17: 342

Malinský J 1959 The ontogenetic development of nerve terminations in the intervertebral discs of man. Acta Anat. Basel 38: 96

Mancia M, Broggi G, Margnelli M 1971 Brain stem reticular effects on intralaminar thalamic neurons in the cat. Brain Res. 25: 638

Mantle J A 1959 Non-tuberculous infections of the spine. In: Nassim R, Burrows H J (eds) Modern trends in diseases of the vertebral column. Butterworths, London, p 142

Mark V H, Ervin F R, Yakovlev O I 1962 The treatment of pain by stereotaxic methods. Confinia Neurol. 22: 238

Mark V H, Ervin F R, Yakovlev P I 1963 Stereotactic thalamotomy. III. The verification of anatomical lesion sites in the human thalamus. Archiv. Neurol. Chicago 8: 528

Marshall J 1951 Sensory disturbances in cortical wounds with special reference to pain. J. Neurol. Neurosurg. Psychiat. 14: 187

Martini L, Motta M, Fraschini F (eds) 1971 The hypothalamus. Academic Press, New York

Matano S, Shigenaga Y, Hura T, Sakai A 1972 the cortico-thalamic and bulbar projections from the somatic sensory face area in the rat. Okajimas Folia Anat. Jap. 49: 249

Mayer D J, Price D 1976 Central nervous system mechanisms of analgesia. Pain 2: 379

Mayer D J, Price D D, Becker D P 1975 Neurophysiological characterization of the anterolateral spinal cord neurons contributing to pain perception in man. Pain 1: 51

Mehler W R 1962 The anatomy of the so-called 'pain tract' in man: an analysis of the course and distribution of the ascending fibers of the fasciculus anterolateralis. In: French J D, Porter R W (eds) Basic research in paraplegia. Thomas, Springfield, Illinois, p 26

Mehler W R, Feferman M E, Nauta W J H 1969 Ascending axon degeneration followigng anterolateral cordotomy: an experimental study in the monkey. Brain 83: 718

Melzack R 1972 Mechanisms of pathological pain. In: Critchley M, O'Leary J L, Jennett B (eds) Scientific foundations of neurology. Heinemann, London, p 153

Melzack R 1973 The puzzle of pain. Basic Books, New York

Melzack R 1975a The McGill pain questionnaire: major properties and scoring methods. Pain 1: 277

Melzack R 1975b Prolonged relief of pain by brief, intense transcutaneous somatic stimulation. Pain 1: 357

Melzack R, Casey K L 1968 Sensory, motivational and central control determinants of pain: a new conceptual model. In: Kenshalo D R (ed) The skin senses. Thomas, Springfield, Illinois, p 423

Melzack R, Eisenberg H 1968 Skin sensory afterglows. Science 159: 445

Melzack R, Scott T H 1957 The effect of early experience on the response to pain. J. Comp. Physiol. Psychol. 50: 155

Melzack R, Stotler W A, Livingston W K 1958 Effects of discrete brainstem lesions in cats on perception of noxious stimulation. J. Neurophysiol. 21: 353

Melzack R, Wall P D 1962 On the nature of cutaneous sensory mechanisms. Brain 85: 331

Melzack R, Wall P D 1965 Pain mechanisms: a new theory. Science 150: 971

Melzack R, Wall P D 1968 Gate control theory of pain. In: Soulairac A, Cahn J, Charpentier J (eds) Pain. Academic Press, New York

Mendell L M 1966 Physiological properties of unmyelinated fiber projection to the spinal cord. Exper. Neurol. 16: 316

Mendell L M, Wall P D 1965 Responses of single dorsal cord cells to peripheral cutaneous unmyelinated fibres. Nature 206: 97

Merskey H 1965 The characteristics of persistent pain in psychological illness. J. Psychosomat. Res. 9: 291

Merskey H 1968 Psychological aspects of pain. Postgrad. Med. J. 44: 297

Merskey H, Spear F G 1967 Pain: psychological and psychiatric aspects. Baillière, Tindall & Cassell, London

Merton P A 1954 Voluntary strength and fatigue. J. Physiol. Lond. 123: 553

Merton P A 1956 Problems of muscular fatigue. Brit. Med. Bull. 12: 219

Meruta T, Swanson D W, Swanson W M 1976 Pain as a psychiatric symptom: comparison between low back pain and depression. Psychosomatics 17: 123

Michelsen J J 1943 Subjective disturbances of the sense of pain from lesions of the cerebral cortex. Res. Pub. Assoc. Nerv. Ment. Dis. 23: 86

Miller H R 1942 Central autonomic regulations in health and disease. Grune & Stratton, New York

Minc S 1968 Psychological aspects of backache. Med. J. Austral. 1: 964

Miyazaki A 1968 Posture and low back pain: electromyographic evaluation. Electromyography 8: 191

Molina F, Ramcharan J E, Wyke B D 1976 Structure and function of articular receptor systems in the cervical spine. J. Bone Jt. Surg. 58B: 255

Monnier M 1953 Le rôle du thalamus dans l'organisation de la douleur. Acta Neuroveg. Wien 7: 85

Montagna W (ed) 1960 Cutaneous innervation. Pergamon Press, Oxford

Mooney V, Robertson J 1976 The facet syndrome. Clin. Orthoped. 115: 149

Morin F, Kennedy D T, Gardner E D 1966 Spinal afferents to the lateral reticular nucleus. I. An histological study. J. Comp. Neurol. 126: 511

Morin F, Schwartz H G, O'Leary J L 1951 Experimental study of the spinothalamic and related tracts. Acta Psychiat. Neurol. Scand. 26: 371

Morris J M, Benner G, Lucas D B 1962 An electromyographic study of the intrinsic muscles of the back in man. J. Anat. Lond. 96: 509

Morse R W, Towe A L 1964 The dual nature of the lemnisco-cortical afferent system in the cat. J. Physiol. Lond. 171: 231

Morton D J 1952 Human locomotion and body form. A study of gravity and man. Williams & Wilkins, Baltimore

Moruzzi G, Magoun H W 1949 Brain stem reticular formation and activation of the EEG. Electroenceph. Clin. Neurophysiol. 1: 455

Mountcastle V B, Covian M R, Harrison C R 1950 The relation of thalamic representation of some forms of deep sensibility. Res. Pub. Assoc. Nerv. Ment. Dis. 30: 339

Mountcastle V B, Poggio G F, Werner G 1963 The central cell response to peripheral stimuli varied over an intensity continuum J. Neurophysiol. 26: 507

Mountcastle V B, Powell T P S 1959a Central nervous mechanisms subserving position sense and kinesthesis. Bull. Johns Hopkins Hosp. 105: 173

Mountcastle V B, Powell T P S 1959b Neural mechanisms subserving cutaneous sensibility, with special reference to the role of afferent inhibition in sensory perception and discrimination. Bull. Johns Hopkins Hosp. 105: 201

Mulligan J H 1957 The innervation of the ligaments attached to the bodies of the vertebrae. J. Anat. Lond. 91: 455

Myers S J, Sullivan W P 1968 Effect of circulatory occlusion on time of muscular fatigue. J. Appl. Physiol. 24: 54

Nade S, Bell E, Wyke B D 1978 Articular neurology of the feline lumbar spine. Proc. Aust. N.Z. Orthop. Assoc. (Oct. 1977), p 6

Nashold B S, Friedman H 1972 Dorsal column stimulation for the relief of pain: preliminary report on 30 patients. J. Neurosurg. 36: 590

Nashold B S, Somjen G, Friedman H 1972 Parathesias and EEG potentials evoked by stimulation of the dorsal funiculi in man. Exper. Neurol. 36: 273

Nassim R 1959 Osteoporosis. In: Nassim R, Burrows H J (eds) Modern trends in diseases of the vertebral column. Butterworths, London, p 125

Nassim R, Burrows H J (eds) 1959 Modern trends in diseases of the vertebral column. Butterworths, London

Nathan H 1962 Osteophytes of the vertebral column: an anatomical study of their development according to age, race and sex, with considerations as to their etiology and significance. J. Bone Jt. Surg. 44A: 243

Nathan P W 1956 Reference of sensation at the spinal level. J. Neurol. Neurosurg. Psychiat. 19: 88

Nathan P W 1962 Pain traces left in the central nervous system. In: Keele C A, Smith R (eds) U F A W symposium on assessment of pain in man and animals. Livingstone, Edinburgh, p 129

Nathan P W 1963 Results of antero-lateral cordotomy for pain in cancer. J. Neurol. Neurosurg. Psychiat. 26: 353

Nathan P W 1976 The gate-control theory of pain: a critical review. Brain 99: 123

Nathan P W, Smith, Marion C 1959 Fasciculi proprii of the spinal cord: a review of present knowledge. Brain 82: 610

Nauta W J H 1958 Hippocampal projections and related neural pathways to the mid-brain in the cat. Brain 81: 319

Nauta W J H, Whitlock D G 1954 An anatomical analysis of the non-specific thalamic projection system. In: Delafresnaye J F (ed) Brain mechanisms and consciousness. Blackwell, Oxford, p 81

Nelson M A 1973 Lumbar spinal stenosis. J. Bone Jt. Surg. 55B: 506

Nemiah J C 1962 The effect of leukotomy on pain. Psychosomat. Med. 24: 75

Newcombe Freda 1972 Memory. In: Critchley M, O'Leary J L, Jennett B (eds) Scientific foundations of neurology. Heinemann, London, p 205

Noordenbos W 1959 Pain. Problems pertaining to the transmission of nerve impulses which give rise to pain. Elsevier, Amsterdam and London

Noordenbos W 1972 Remarks on afferent systems in the antero-lateral quadrant. In: Janzen R, Keidel W D, Herz A, Steichele C (eds) Pain: basic principles, pharmacology, therapy. Thième, Stuttgart, p 112

Nordin B E C 1973 Metabolic bone and stone disease. Churchill Livingstone, Edinburgh and London

Nümi K, Inoshita H 1971 Cortical projections of the lateral thalamic nuclei in the cat. Proc. Jap. Acad. 47: 664

Nyberg-Hansen R 1965 Sites and mode of termination of reticulo-spinal fibers in the cat: an experimental study with silver impregnation methods. J. Comp. Neurol. 124: 71

Nyberg-Hansen R, Brodal A 1963 Sites of termination of corticospinal fibers in the cat: an experimental study with silver impregnation methods. J. Comp. Neurol. 120: 369

Ochoa J, Mair W G P 1969 The normal sural nerve in man. II. Changes in the axons and Schwann cells due to aging. Acta Neuropathol. Berlin 13: 217

Olzewski J, Baxter D 1954 Cytoarchitecture of the human brain stem. Karger, Basel

Oscarsson O, Rosén I 1963 Cerebral projection of Group I afferents in fore-limb muscle nerves of cat. Experientia, Basel 19: 206

Oscarsson O, Rosén I 1966 Short-latency projections to the cat's cerebral cortex from skin and muscle afferents in the contralateral forelimb. J. Physiol. Lond. 182: 164

Osuntokun B O, Okeku E L, Luzzato L 1968 Congenital pain asymbolia and auditory imperception. J. Neurol. Neurosurg. Psychiat. 31: 291

Pallie W 1959 The intersegmental anastomoses of posterior spinal rootlets and their significance. J. Neurosurg. 16: 188

Partridge R E H, Anderson J A D, McCarthy M A, Duthie J J R 1968 Rheumatic complaints among workers in iron foundries. Ann. Rheumat. Dis. 27: 441

Pauly J E 1966 An electromyographic analysis of certain movements and exercises. I. Some deep muscles of the back. Anat. Rec. 155: 223

Pearson C M 1969 Polymyositis and related disorders. In: Walton J N (ed) Disorders of voluntary muscle, 2nd edn. Churchill, London, p 501

Pearson C M, Rose A S 1961 Myositis: the inflammatory disorders of muscle. Res. Pub. Assoc. Nerv. Ment. Dis. 38: 422

Pedersen H S, Blunck C F J, Gardner E D 1956 The anatomy of the lumbosacral posterior rami and meningeal branches of spinal nerves (sinu-vertebral nerves): with an experimental study of their functions. J. Bone Jt. Surg. 38A: 377

Penfield W 1958 The rôle of the temporal cortex in recall of past experience and interpretation of the present. In: Wolstenholme G E W, O'Connor C M (eds) The neurological basis of behaviour. Churchill, London, p 149

Penfield W, Faulk M E 1955 The insula: further observations on its function. Brain 78: 445

Penfield W, Jasper H 1954 Epilepsy and the functional anatomy of the human brain. Churchill, London

Penfield W, Rasmussen T 1950 The cerebral cortex of man. Macmillan, New York

Petit D, Burgess P R 1968 Dorsal column projections of receptors in cat hairy skin supplied by myelinated fibers. J. Neurophysiol. 31: 849

Petrie A 1967 Individuality in pain and suffering. University of Chicago Press

Phillips C G, Powell T P S, Wiesendanger M 1971 Projection from low-threshold muscle afferents of hand and forearm to area 3a of baboon's cortex. J. Physiol. Lond. 217: 419

Poggio G F, Mountcastle V B 1960 A study of the functional contributions of the lemniscal and spinothalamic systems to somatic sensibility. Bull. Johns Hopkins Hosp. 106: 266

Polley E H 1955 Innervation of blood vessels in striated muscle and skin. J. Comp. Neurol. 103: 253

Pomeranz B, Wall P D, Weber W V 1968 Cord cells responding to fine myelinated afferents from viscera, skin and muscle. J. Physiol. Lond. 199: 511

Pompeiano O, Swett J E 1962 Identification of cutaneous and muscular afferent fibers producing EEG synchronisation or arousal in normal cats. Archiv. Ital. Biol. 100: 343

Pompeiano O, Swett J E 1963 Actions of graded cutaneous and muscular afferent volleys on brain stem units in the decerebrate, cerebellectomised cat. Archiv. Ital. Biol. 101: 552

Powell T P S, Mountcastle V B 1959a Some aspects of the functional organisation of the postcentral gyrus of the monkey: a correlation of findings obtained in a single unit analysis with cyto-architecture. Bull. Johns Hopkins Hosp. 105: 133

Powell T P S, Mountcastle V bB 1959b The cyto-architecture of the postcentral gyrus of the monkey Macaca mulatta. Bull. Johns Hopkins Hosp. 106: 108

Pribram K H, Broadbent D E 1970 Biology of memory. Academic Press, New York

Price D D, Dubner R 1977 Neurons that subserve the sensory-discriminative aspects of pain. Pain 3: 307

Price D D, Meyer D J 1974 Physiological laminar organisation of the dorsal horn of M. mulatta. Brain Res. 79: 321

Procacci P 1972 Circadian and circatrigintan changes in the cutaneous pricking pain threshold. In: Janzen R, Keidel W D, Herz A, Steichele C (eds) Pain: basic principles, pharmacology, therapy. Thième, Stuttgart, p 45

Pubols B H 1968 Retrograde degeneration study of somatic sensory thalamocortical connections in brain of Virginia opossum. Brain Res. 7: 232

Purkyně J E 1845 Mikroskopisch-neurologische Beobachtungn. Archiv. Anat. Physiol. Wiss. Med. 281

Purpura D P, Yahr M D (eds) The thalamus. Columbia University Press, New York

Rabinovitch R 1961 Diseases of the intervertebral disc and its surrounding tissues. Thomas, Springfield, Illinois

Raisman G 1970 An evaluation of the basic pattern of connections between the limbic system and the hypothalamus. Amer. J. Anat. 129: 197

Ralston H J 1965 The organisation of the substantia gelatinosa Rolandi in the cat lumbosacral cord. Zeit Zellforsch 67: 1

Ralston H J, Miller M R, Kasahara M 1960 Nerve endings in human fasciae, tendons, ligaments, periosteum and joint synovial membrane. Anat. Rec. 136: 137

Ranson S W, Clark S L 1959 The anatomy of the nervous system, 10th edn. Saunders, Philadelphia

Rasch P J, Burke R K 1962 Kinesiology and applied anatomy. The science of human movement, 2nd edn. Lea & Febiger, Philadelphia

Ray C D, Mauer D D 1975 Electrical neurological stimulation systems: a review of contemporary methodology. Surg. Neurol. 4: 82

de Reuck A V S, Knight J (eds) 1966 Touch, heat and pain. Churchill, London

Rexed B 1944 Contributions to the knowledge of the post-natal development of the peripheral nervous system in man. Acta Psychiat. Kbh. Suppl 33: 1

Rexed B 1954 A cytoarchitectonic atlas of the spinal cord in the cat. J. Comp. Neurol. 100: 297

Robezrts W W 1962 Fearlike behaviour elicited from dorsomedial thalamus of cat. J. Comp. Physiol. Psychol. 55: 191

Roger A, Rossi G F, Zirondoli A 1956 Le rôle des afférences des nerfs craniens dans le maintien de l'état vigile de la préparation 'encéphale isolé'. Electroenceph. Clin. Neurophysiol. 8: 1

Roofe P G 1940 Innervation of annulus fibrosus and posterior longitudinal ligament. Archiv. Neurol. Psychiat. Chicago 44: 100

Ross J E, Mountcastle V B 1959 Touch and kinesthesia. In: Field J, Magoun H W, Hall V E (eds) Handbook of physiology, Section 1. Neurophysiology, vol 1. American Physiological Society, Washington, p 387

Rosén I, Scheid P 1972 Cutaneous afferent responses in neurones of the lateral reticular nucleus. Brain Res. 43: 259

Rossi G F, Zanchetti A 1957 The brain stem reticular formation. Archiv. Ital. Biol. 95: 199

Rowe M L 1969 Low back pain in industry: a position paper. J. Occup. Med. 11: 161

Rowe M L 1971 Low back disability in industry: updated position. J. Occup. Med. 13: 476

Rudd J L, Margolin R J 1966 A study of back cases in an outpatient clinic. J. Assoc. Phys. Ment. Rehab. 20: 20

Rüdinger N 1857 Die Gelenknerven des menschlichen Körpers. Ferdinand Enke, Erlangen

Russell W R, Spalding J M K 1950 Treatment of painful amputation stumps. Brit. Med. J. 2: 68

Sargant W 1957 Battle for the mind. Heinemann, London

Satoh M, Takagi H 1971 Enhancement by morphine of the central descending inhibitory influence on spinal sensory transmission. Europ. J. Pharmacol. 14: 60

Scapinelli R 1960 I ligamenti interspinosi dell'uomo ed i strutturali in rapporto all'età. Archiv. Ital. Anat. Embriol. 65: 364

Schatzker J, Pennal G F 1968 Spinal stenosis, a cause of cauda equina compression. J. Bone Jt. Surg. 50B: 606

Scheibel M E, Scheibel A B 1958 Structural substrates for integrative patterns in the brain stem reticular core. In: Jasper H H, Proctor L D, Knighton R S, Noshay W C (eds) Reticular formation of the brain. Little, Brown, Boston, p 31

Scheibel M E, Scheibel A B 1965 Periodic sensory nonresponsiveness in reticular neurons. Archiv. Ital. Biol. 103: 300

Scheibel M E, Scheibel A B 1966a Spinal motoneurons, interneurons and Renshaw cells: a Golgi study. Archiv. Ital. Biol. 104: 328

Scheibel M E, Scheibel A B 1966b Patterns of organisation in specific and nonspecific thalamic fields. In: Purpura D P, Yahr M D (eds) The thalamus. Columbia University Press, New York, p 13

Scheibel M E, Scheibel A B 1967 Structural organisation of non-specific thalamic nuclei and their projection toward cortex. Brain Res. 6: 60

Scheibel M E, Scheibel A B 1968 Terminal axonal patterns in cat spinal cord. II. The dorsal horn. Brain Res. 9: 32

Scherrer J, Lefebvre J, Bourguignon A 1957 Activité électrique du muscle strié squeletique et fatigue. Proc. 4th Int. Congr. Electroenceph. Clin. Neurophysiol. Brussels, p 99

Scherrer J, Monod H 1960 Le travail musculaire local et la fatigue chez l'homme. J. Physiol., Paris 52: 419

Schumann K 1972 Fundamental principles of the surgical treatment of pain. In: Janzen R, Keidel W D, Herz A, Steichele C (eds) Pain: basic principles, pharmacology, therapy. Thième, Stuttgart, p 181

Scott J, Huskisson E C 1976 Graphic representation of pain. Pain 2: 175

Selzer M, Spencer W A 1969a Convergence of visceral and cutaneous afferent pathways in the lumbar spinal cord. Brain Res. 14: 331

Selzer M, Spencer W A 1969b Interactions between visceral and cutaneous afferents in the spinal cord: reciprocal primary afferent fiber depolarisation. Brain Res. 14: 349

Sessle B J, Dubner R 1971 Presynaptic depolarisation and hyperpolarisation of trigeminal primary and thalamic afferents. In: Dubner R, Kawamura Y (eds) Oral-facial sensory and motor mechanisms. Appleton-Century-Crofts, New York, p 279

Shealy C N 1974 The role of the spinal facets in back and sciatic pain. Headache 14: 101

Shealy C N, Mortimer J T, Hagfors N R 1970 Dorsal column electroanalgesia. J. Neurosurg. 32: 560

Shimazu H, Yanagisawa N, Garoutte B 1965 Cortico-pyramidal influences on thalamic somatosensory transmission in the cat. Jap. J. Physiol. 15: 101

Sicuteri F, Fanciullaci M, Franchi G, del Biancho P L 1965 Serotonin-bradykinin potentiation of the pain receptors in man. Life Sci. 4: 309

Simmel N L 1959 Phantoms, phantom pain and 'denial'. Amer. J. Psychotherap. 13: 603

Simons D G 1976 Muscle pain syndromes. Part II. Amer. J. Phys. Med. 55: 15

Simons G R, Mirabile M P 1972 An analysis and interpretation of industrial medical data, with concentration on back problems. J. Occup. Med. 14: 227

Sinclair D C 1967 Cutaneous sensation. Oxford University Press, London

Sinclair D C, Feindel W H, Weddell G, Falconer M A 1948 The intervertebral ligaments as a source of segmental pain. J.b Bone Jt. Surg. 30B: 515

Sissons H A 1959 Tumours of the vertebral column. In: Nassim R, Burrows H H (eds) Modern trends in diseases of the vertebral column. Butterworths, London, p 192

Skinner J E 1970 Electrocortical desynchronisation during functional blockade of the mesencephalic reticular formation. Brain Res. 22: 254

Skultety F M 1963 Stimulation of periaqueductal gray and hypothalamus. Archiv. Neurol. Chicago 8: 608

Speigel E A, Wycis H T 1962 Stereoencephalotomy. II. Clinical and physiological applications. Grune & Stratton, New York

Speigel E A, Wycis H T, Szekely E G, Gildenberg P L 1966 Medial and basal thalamotomy in so-called intractable pain. In: Knighton R S, Dumke P R (eds) Pain: an international symposium. Little, Brown, Boston, p 503

Sprague J M, Ha H 1964 The terminal fields of dorsal root fibers in the lumbosacral cord of the cat, and the dendritic organisation of the motor nuclei. In: Eccles J C, Schadé

J P (eds) Organisation of the spinal cord. Elsevier, Amsterdam, p 120

Stein B E, Arigbede M O 1972 Unimodal and multimodal response properties of neurons in the cat's superior colliculus. Exper. Neurol. 26: 179

Steindler A 1955 Kinesiology of the human body under normal and pathological conditions. Thomas, Springfield, Illinois

Steindler A 1959 Lectures on the interpretation of pain in orthopedic practice. Thomas, Springfield, Illinois

Sternbach R A 1963 Congenital insensitivity to pain: a critique. Psychol. Bull. 60: 252

Sternbach R A 1968 Pain: a psychophysiological analysis. Academic Press, New York

Sternbach R A 1974 Pain patients: traits and treatment. Academic Press, New York

Sternbach R A, Wolf S R, Murphy R W, Akeson W H 1973a Aspects of chronic low back pain. Psychosomatics 14: 52

Sternbach R A, Wolf S R, Murphy R W, Akeson W H 1973b Traits of pain patients: the low-back 'loser'. Psychosomatics 14: 226

Stilwell D L 1956 The nerve supply of the vertebral column and its associated structures in the monkey. Anat. Rec. 125: 139

Stilwell D L 1957a Regional variations in the innervation of deep fasciae and aponeuroses. Anat. Rec. 127: 635

Stilwell D L 1957b The innervation of tendons and aponeuroses. Amer. J. Anat. 100: 289

Stockman R 1920 Rheumatism and arthritis. Green, Edinburgh

Sweet W H 1959 Pain. In: Field J, Magoun H W, Hall V E (eds) Handbook of physiology. Section 1. Neurophysiology. American Physiological Society, Washington, vol. 1, p 459

Sweet W H, White J C, Selverstone B, Nilges R 1950 Sensory responses from anterior roots and from surface and interior of spinal cord in man. Trans. Amer. Neurol. Assoc. 75: 165

Szentágothai J 1964 Neuronal and synaptic arrangement in the substantia gelatinosa Rolandi. J. Comp. Neurol. 122: 219

Taub A 1964 Local, segmental and supraspinal interaction with a dorsolateral spinal cutaneous afferent system. Exper. Neurol. 10: 357

Tichauer E R 1971 A pilot study of the biomechanics of lifting in simulated industrial work situations. J. Safety Res. 3: 98

Trevino D L, Maunz R A, Bryan R N, Willis W D 1972 Location of cells of origin of the spinothalamic tract in the lumbar enlargement of cat. Exper. Neurol. 34: 64

Tsukada K 1938 Histologische studien über die zwischenwirbelscheibe des menschen: histologische befunde des foetus. Mitt. Med. Akad. Kioto 24:(1057), 1172

Tsukada K 1939 Histologische studien über die zwischenwirbelscheibe des menschen: Alters-veränderungen. Mitt. Med. Akad. Kioto 25:(1), 79

Uemura K, Watkins E S 1968 Stereotaxic thalamotomy for intractable pain: study of clinico-pathological correlation for the best target point. Neurol. Med.-chir. 10: 325

Urabe M, Tsubokawa T 1965 Stereotaxic thalamotomy for the relief of intractable pain. Tohoku J. Exper. Med. 85: 286

Van Hees J, Gybels J M 1972 Pain related to single afferent C fibers from human skin. Brain Res. 48: 397

Verhaart W J C 1954 Fiber tracts and fiber patterns in the anterior and the lateral funiculus of the cord in Macaca ira. Acta Anat., Basel 20: 330

Vrettos X C, Wyke B D 1974 Articular reflexogenic systems in the costovertebral joints. J. Bone Jt. Surg. 56B: 382

Wagman I H, Price D D 1969 Responses of dorsal horn cells of M. mulatta to cutaneous and sural nerve A and C fiber stimuli. J. Neurophysiol. 32: 803

Walker A E 1938 The primate thalamus. University of Chicago Press, Chicago

Walker A E 1940 The spinothalamic tract in man. Archiv. Neurol. Psychiat., Chicago 43: 284

Walker A E 1942a Relief of pain by mesencephalic tractotomy. Archiv. Neurol. Psychiat., Chicago 48: 865

Walker A E 1942b Somatotopic localisation of spinothalamic and secondary trigeminal tracts in mesencephalon. Archiv. Neurol. Psychiat., Chicago 48: 884

Walker A E 1943 Central representation of pain. Res. Pub. Assoc. Nerv. Ment. Dis. 23: 63

Wall P D 1960 Cord cells responding to touch, damage and temperature of skin. J. Neurophysiol. 23: 197

Wall P D 1967 The laminar organisation of dorsal horn and effects of descending impulses. J. Physiol. Lond. 188: 403

Wall P D 1970 The sensory and motor role of impulses travelling in the dorsal columns towards the cerebral cortex. Brain 93: 505

Wall P D, Cronly-Dillon J R 1960 Pain, itch and vibration. Archiv. Neurol., Chicago 2: 365

Waltz T A, Ehni G 1966 The thalamic syndrome and its mechanism. J. Neurosurg. 24: 735

Ward T, Knowelden J, Sharrad W J W 1968 Low back pain: an epidemiological survey of low back pain in a rural practice. J. Coll. Gen. Pract. 15: 128

Waters R L, Morris J M 1970 Effect of spinal supports on the electrical activity of muscles of the trunk. J. Bone Jt. Surg. 52A: 51

Waters R L, Morris J M 1972 Electrical activity of muscles of the trunk during walking. J. Anat. Lond. 111: 191

Weaver T A, Walker A E 1941 Topical arrangement within the spinothalamic tract of the monkey. Archiv. Neurol. Psychiat., Chicago 46: 877

Weller R O, Bruckner F E, Chamberlain M A 1970 Rheumatoid neuropathy: a histological and electrophysiological study. J. Neurol. Neurosurg. Psychiat. 33: 592

Werle E 1972 On endogenous pain-producing substances, with particular reference to plasmakinins. In: Janzen R, Keidel W D, Herz A, Steichele C (eds) Pain: basic principles, pharmacology, therapy. Thième, Stuttgart, p 86

West L J, Niell K C, Hardy J D 1952 Effects of hypnotic suggestion on pain perception and galvanic skin response. Archiv. Neurol. Psychiat., Chicago 68: 549

Westrin C-G 1970 Low back sick-listing: a nosological and medical insurance investigation. Acta Socio-med. Scand. 2-3: 127

White A W M 1966 Low back pain in men receiving workman's compensation. Canad. Med. Assoc. J. 95: 50

White J C, Sweet W H 1969 Pain and the neurosurgeon: a forty years' experience. Thomas, Springfield, Illinois

Whitlock D G, Perl E R 1961 Thalamic projections of spinothalamic pathways in monkey. Exper. Neurol. 3: 240

Whitsel B L, Roppolo J R, Werner G 1972 Cortical information processing of stimulus motion on primate skin. J. Neurophysiol. 35: 691

Wiberg G 1949 Back pain in relation to the nerve supply of the intervertebral disc. Acta Orthopaed. Scand. 19: 211

Wiesendanger M 1969 The pyramidal tract: recent investigations on its morphology and function. Ergeb. Physiol. 61: 72

Wolf S 1968 Pain perception and reaction. In: Schwartz L,

Chayes C M (eds) Facial pain and mandibular dysfunction. Saunders, Philadelphia, p 7

Wolff B B, Jarvik M E 1963 Variations in cutaneous and deep somatic pain sensitivity. Canad. J. Psychol. 17: 37

Wolff H G, Goodell H 1943 The relation of attitudes and suggestion to the perception of and reaction to pain. Res. Pub. Assoc. Nerv. Ment. Dis. 23: 434

Wolff H G, Hardy J D 1947 On the nature of pain. Physiol. Rev. 27: 167

Wolff H G, Wolf S 1948 Pain. Thomas, Springfield, Illinois

Wolkind S N, Forrest A J 1972 Low back pain: a psychiatric investigation. Postgrad. Med. J. 48: 76

Wolstencroft J H 1964 Reticulospinal neurones. J. Physiol. Lond. 174: 91

Wolstenholme G E W, O'Connor M (eds) 1959 Pain and itch: nervous mechanisms. Churchill, London

Wood P H N. Statistical appendix — digest of data on the rheumatic diseases. 2. Recent trends in sickness absence and mortality. Ann. Rheumat. Dis. 29: 324

Woodrow K M, Friedman G D, Siegelaub A B, Collen M F 1972 Pain tolerance: differences according to age, sex and race. Psychosomat. Med. 34: 548

Woolsey C N 1964 Cortical localisation as defined by evoked potential and electrical stimulation studies. In: Schaltenbrand G, Woolsey C N (eds) Cerebral localisation and organisation. University of Wisconsin Press, Madison, p 17

Wyke B D 1947 The pain pathway. Bull. N.S.W. Postgrad. Comm. Med. Univ. Syd. 3: 1

Wyke B D 1958a Surgical considerations of the temporal lobes. Ann. Roy. Coll. Surg. Engl. 22: 117

Wyke B D 1958b The surgical physiology of facial pain. Brit. Dent. J. 104: 153

Wyke B D 1960 Neurological aspects of hypnosis. Dental and Medical Society for the Study of Hypnosis, London

Wyke B D 1963 Brain function and metabolic disorders. Butterworths, London

Wyke B D 1967 The neurology of joints. Ann. Roy. Coll. Surg. Engl. 41: 25

Wyke B D 1968 The neurology of facial pain. Brit. J. Hosp. Med. 1: 46

Wyke B D 1969 Principles of general neurology. Elsevier, Amsterdam and London

Wyke B D 1970 The neurological basis of thoracic spinal pain. Rheumatol. Phys. Med. 10: 356

Wyke B D 1972a Articular neurology: a review. Physiotherapy 58: 94

Wyke B D 1972b Pain and hypnosis. New Scientist 56: 585

Wyke B D 1974a Neurological aspects of the diagnosis and treatment of facial pain. In: Cohen B, Kramer I (eds) Scientific foundations of dentistry. Heinemann, London, p 278

Wyke B D 1974b Neurological mechanisms of pain in relation to rheumatology. Communication to Royal Society of Medicine (Section of Rheumatology), London, 9 January 1974

Wyke B D (ed) 1974c Ventilatory and phonatory control systems: an international symposium. Oxford University Press, London

Wyke B D 1974d Clinical physiology of peripheral nerve injuries. In: Wells C, Kyle J, Dunphy J E (eds) Scientific foundations of surgery, 2nd edn. Heinemann, London, p 242

Wyke B D 1975 Morphological and functional features of the innervation of the costovertebral joints. Folia Morphol., Prague 23: 296

Wyke B D 1977 Neurological mechanisms of spinal pain. In: Hernández Conesa S, Seiquer J (eds) Patología de la Columna Vertebral. Ferrer Internacional, Murcia, Spain, p 45

Wyke B D 1979a Neurological mechanisms in the experience of pain. Acupuncture Electrotherap. Res. J. 4: 27

Wyke B D 1979b Neurology of the cervical spinal joints. Physiotherapy 65: 72

Wyke B D, Molina F 1972 Articular reflexology of the cervical spine. Proc. 6th Int. Congr. Phys. Med., Barcelona, p 4

Wyke B D, Poláček P 1973 Strukturálni a funkcni charakteristika kloubniho receptorvého aparátu. Acta Chir. Orthop. Traum. Česk 40: 489

Wyke B D, Poláček P 1975 Articular neurology: the present position. J. Bone Jt. Surg. 57B: 401

Yamaguchi I, Krauthamer G 1966 Inhibitions d'activités corticales associatives par la stimulation de l'écorce cérébrale. Compt. Rend. Acad. Sci., Paris 262: 1013

Yamaji K, Misu A 1968 Kinesiologic study with electromyography of low back pain. Electromyography 8: 189

Zulch K J 1970 The pathogenesis of 'intermittent spinovascular insufficiency' ('spinal claudication of Déjerline') and other vascular syndromes of the spinal cord. Vasc. Surg. 4: 116

Biochemistry of the intervertebral disc

INTRODUCTION

Although cartilage and intervertebral disc show some degree of similarity in the types of collagens and proteoglycans present in their matrices, it is becoming evident that there are as many differences as similarities between the two tissues and that the disc should be considered as a tissue in its own right. Essentially the disc represents three distinct types of extracellular matrix: the nucleus, annulus and end-plates, the latter being essentially cartilage. Age changes are more evident in the nucleus than in the annulus and these are deleterious, leading to generalized loss of function. A particular feature of the adult intervertebral disc is that it is the largest avascular tissue in the body, and this presents nutritional problems for the sparse population of cells within its matrix.

In this chapter we will describe the embryonic development of the disc and its structural components as well as age and degenerative changes. Where possible, we will concentrate on human material, but inevitably a considerable proportion of research into the biochemistry of the disc has been on animal material.

EMBRYONIC DEVELOPMENT

During the early stages of embryogenesis, the mesoderm which forms around the notochordal process differentiates to mesenchyme from whence derive the cells of the intervertebral disc.[1] The annulus fibrosus and nucleus pulposus both develop from the dense tissue of the perichordal disc, which itself arises through a series of differentiations from the ventromedial cells of the somites (sclerotome)

into which the mesoderm divides early in embryogenesis (21 days).[2] The loose connective tissue of the vertebral body derives from the same source.[3-6] It should be noted that the notochord is not the progenitor of the nucleus pulposus, though this is sometimes stated to be the case. The notochord derives from the endoderm, and its role is strictly an organizational one, inducing the migration of the sclerotome cells which subsequently undergo differentiation into chondrocytes.

Chondrogenesis

The biochemical and ultrastructural changes which occur in the sclerotome and notochord prior, during and subsequent to chondrification have been studied extensively in the chick embryo,[7-9] but not in humans, although similar, if not identical, changes probably occur. Bancroft & Bellairs[10] suggested that the chick notochord and its secretion products are chemotactic for sclerotome cells, ensuring their correct anatomical position for the development of the intervertebral disc. The cells of the sclerotome do not possess a prominent endoplasmic reticulum, Golgi apparatus or the characteristic crenated surface of differentiated chondrocytes until they are 'in position' and in contact with the 'inducer' macromolecules produced by the notochord. These macromolecules, which are both polyanionic and fibrillar but have not been characterized, are synthesized prior to sclerotome migration. Once the sclerotome and notochord are close to, but not in direct contact with, each other[1] the notochordal cells synthesize increasing amounts of chondroitin-sulphate-rich proteoglycans[11] and type II collagen.[12] In vitro studies in chicks have shown that both chondroitin-sulphate proteoglycans[13] and type II collagen[14] stimulate sclerotome cells to undergo chondrogenesis, indicating that the notochord per se is not a prerequisite. However, these sclerotome cells could have been 'programmed' by the notochord in vivo prior to the in vitro experiments. Kosher & Lash[11] have also suggested that the sclerotome cells must possess an inherent chondrogenic 'bias' (i.e. the appropriate enzymic pathways characteristic of chondrocytes) before they can interact with, and respond to, the extracellular matrix 'inducer' macromolecules of the notochord. It has also been suggested[7] that proteoglycans and collagen stabilize chondrogenesis, rather than induce it.

The mechanism of interaction between the extracellular matrix and sclerotome cells involves specific receptors on the cell surface.[13] During chondrogenesis the sclerotome cells became polygonal with a well-developed endoplasmic reticulum, Golgi apparatus and the characteristic crenated cell membrane of differentiated chondrocytes. Subsequently they synthesize the characteristic cartilage-specific macromolecules. Kosher & Savage[15] suggest that these events are triggered by collagen binding to cell receptors and lowering the cyclic AMP levels inside the cells. The influence of matrix on differentiated adult cells may be by a similar mechanism. The mature chondrocyte certainly conditions its own environment, possibly by receptor-mediated feedback of information from extracellular macromolecules with which it is in direct contact.[16]

ANATOMY OF THE INTERVERTEBRAL DISC

The human spine contains 23 intervertebral discs which have the same general anatomy, although the lumbar discs are much larger than cervical and thoracic discs. Each disc consists of three major elements: the cartilaginous end-plates, the annulus fibrosus and the nucleus pulposus, which together form the partially mobile articulating joints (amphiarthroses) between the individual vertebral bodies.

The end-plates

The end-plates consist of hyaline cartilage which is approximately 1 mm thick at the periphery and slightly thinner centrally. They overlay the perforated bone of the vertebral bodies and are linked directly to the annulus fibrosus by a series of dense collagenous fibres.

Annulus fibrosus

The annulus fibrosus consists of concentric lamellae of highly-oriented collagen fibres which encapsulate the nucleus pulposus. The fibres are parallel to each other but diagonally oriented at an angle to the spinal axis and lie in opposite directions in adjacent lamellae, the fibres of alternating lamellae being approximately in register. This 'criss-cross' arrangement is essential for the biomechanical properties of the fibres and function of the intervertebral disc (see Chapter 6).

The adjacent lamellae are separated by a proteoglycan-rich gel which transmits the applied pressure from the nucleus pulposus, itself a gel, to the lamellar fibres and is analogous to the brake fluid in a car.[17]

Nucleus pulposus

The nucleus pulposus is essentially a highly hydrated gel of proteoglycans enveloped by collagen fibrils which are randomly distributed. The young nucleus is a gelatinous fluid and transmits the pressure from applied loads equally in all directions to the annulus. With increasing age it becomes more fibrous due to an increase in both collagens and non-collagenous proteins, decrease in the quantity of proteoglycans and an accompanying loss of water resulting in impaired hydrostatic function.

CELLS OF THE INTERVERTEBRAL DISC

Cellularity

Maroudas et al[18] have compared the mean cell density in the three regions of the human intervertebral disc (Table 5.1). The number of cells decreases dramatically across the intervertebral disc from the end-plate to the nucleus, and this has important connotations with regard to the nutritional status of the disc.

Cell types

The intervertebral disc and vertebral body develop from the same sclerotome cells, implying that these

Table 5.1 Biochemical composition of the human intervertebral disc*

Zone of intervertebral disc	Age (yrs)	Water content (%)	Major extracellular matrix macromolecules (% dry weight)			Minor components	Mean cell density (cells × 10^3 per mm^3 tissue)
			Collagen	Proteoglycan	Non-collagenous proteins		
	Birth	90	—	—	—		—
Nucleus pulposus	5–25	80	15–20	65	20–45	Cells	3.8
	60	70		30			4.7
						Intra- and extracellular enzymes	
Annulus fibrosus	5–25	60–70	50–60	20	5–25		7.7
	60			10		Age pigment	11.6
Cartilage end-plate†	15–20	72	66	18			14
	60						17
[Vertebral aspect]	Birth	[81]	[37]	[15]			

*compiled from references cited in text.
†figures quoted are for the end plate as a whole and for its vertebral aspect and are assumed to be similar in composition to articular and epiphysial cartilage respectively.

are the only type of cells present in the early embryonic vertebral skeleton.

Cartilage end-plate

The cells of the cartilaginous end-plate are typically chondrocytic and rounded and are embedded in a homogeneous matrix typical of hyaline cartilage.[18] An ossification layer of columnar cells, responsible for the endochondral growth of the vertebral body, is present at the end-plate/vertebral body margin in the neonate. During maturation the end-plate thins and fuses anteriorly and posteriorly to the epiphysial ring, and by the third decade no columnar cells remain.

Nucleus pulposus

Although the cells of the nucleus of young spines have been classified as fibrocytes,[19] most workers agree that they are in fact chondrocytes.[20-22] These cells lie in pericellular lacunae which are rich in proteoglycans and surrounded by an outer fibrillar ring of collagen, features identical to those of healthy cartilage cells.[23,8] Other types of chondrocytes have also been observed which resemble those in the deep zones of degenerating articular cartilage and pre-

sumably result from either normal ageing or pathological changes. These include: (a) groups of cells surrounded by a common halo consisting of an outer fibrillar ring and inner broader region containing proteoglycans, and (b) single (or two) cells surrounded by a poorly defined fibrillar ring which are 'necrotic'[22] Matrix vesicles similar to those found in the deep calcifying layers of articular cartilage are also seen near the necrotic cells.

Annulus fibrosus

The cells in the human annulus have been variously defined as fibrocytes,[19] chondrocytes[22] and as a mixed population of both types of cell.[24] Most workers agree that the morphology of the cells in the outer annulus is different from those of the inner annulus, the cells of the outer annulus being spindle-shaped, whereas those of the inner annulus are typically chondrocytic and rounded.[25,18,22] This is also true for the cat annulus, where the outermost cells have been likened to tendon cells.[26]

The heterogeneity, particularly with respect to collagen types, in the extracellular matrix of the annulus implies the presence of multiple cell types or of an alteration of the phenotypic expression of the same cell type due to environmental or humoral factors. Chondrocytes in particular can easily de-differentiate in vitro and lose their characteristic morphology and phenotypic expression, becoming fibroblast-like and synthesizing types I and III collagens rather than type II collagen.[7,27,9] However, morphological and phenotypic changes are not necessarily synchronized: polygonal cells can synthesize type I collagen and fibroblast-like cells can synthesize type II collagen.[28,29] De-differentiated chondrocytes deposit an extracellular meshwork of fibronectin rather than proteoglycan,[30,28,31] type V collagen rather than $[1\alpha\ 2\alpha\ 3\alpha]$ collagen.[32] It is quite conceivable that the same chondrocytic cells could be modulated in vivo to produce all the types of extracellular matrix macromolecules found in the human annulus, nucleus and cartilage end-plate.

It must not be forgotten that, distinct from the synthesis of macromolecules, the cells of the intervertebral disc also synthesize specific enzymes, some of which are important in the turnover of the extracellular matrix.

NUTRITION OF THE INTERVERTEBRAL DISC

Source and transport of nutrients

At birth, small blood vessels penetrate the disc from the vertebral bone and lateral margins of the annulus, but the adult disc is totally avascular. The lumbar discs are in fact the largest avascular tissues in the body (5 cm wide and 1.25 cm thick). The cells of the discs must therefore derive their nutrients and dispose of their waste metabolic products by diffusion from and to blood vessels at the disc margins. It has been suggested that inadequate nutrition of the disc (particularly the nucleus pulposus) may be a major factor in disc degeneration.[33,34]

Early studies, using a dye injected into rabbits, indicated that exchange of solutes occurred at both the annular edge and the vertebral bodies.[35] Subsequent studies on the human disc in vitro, using either a dye[34] or ^{14}C-glucose,[18] confirmed that nutrients entered the disc at these specific sites and that the mode of transport was by passive diffusion. The centre of the cartilage end-plate was more permeable than the peripheral parts, due to a greater number of vascular contacts between the marrow spaces in the vertebral bone and the central region of the end-plate.

More precise quantitative data on the rates of penetration and utilization of various solutes were obtained by in vivo studies using large dogs.[36] The in vivo studies eliminated errors which could arise in vitro due to (a) tissue swelling and loss of proteoglycans, and (b) blockage of blood vessels in the absence of any circulation. Similar amounts of uncharged solutes, such as glucose or oxygen, entered the disc at the periphery of the annulus and centre of the end-plate. Negatively-charged sulphate, however, was partially excluded from entering via the end-plate due to electrostatic repulsion by the glycosaminoglycans of the nucleus. Thus only one-third of the total sulphate entered by this route, the remainder diffusing via the periphery of the annulus.

Metabolism of nutrients

Respiration and glycolysis

Chondrocytes thrive in an avascular environment yet form an extremely organized extracellular matrix. It has long been known that chondrocytes of articular cartilage derive their energy from anaerobic glycolysis at very low oxygen tensions and display the Pasteur effect, i.e. an increase in rate of glycolysis with decrease in oxygen tension.[37,38] Recent studies by Holm et al[39] have confirmed previous assumptions[18] that the intervertebral disc also metabolizes glucose by anaerobic glycolysis. Their studies showed that only 1.5% of the glucose taken up was converted to carbon dioxide, even at high oxygen tensions. The concentration profiles of oxygen and lactic acid within the inner annulus and nucleus, were measured in the dog and extrapolated to the human disc. This led to the conclusion that the human nucleus could be at risk on two accounts: (a) the lactic acid concentration was sufficient to decrease the pH by one or two units, which could enhance (or perhaps inhibit) the activity of degradative enzymes; (b) the oxygen tension was very low and there may not be sufficient glucose diffusing from the outer disc to meet the corresponding increase in glycolytic rate, resulting in an inadequate amount of ATP which would be needed to meet the energy requirements of the cell. Eventually this must lead to cell death.

The variation in oxygen utilization at different sites in the intervertebral disc is consistent not only with the oxygen available by diffusion but also with the cell density at these sites: there are more cells in the outer annulus, where the oxygen tension is higher, than in the nucleus. There may be either a single population of near-facultative anaerobes present, or a mixed population of obligatory anaerobes and aerobes, as was suggested for articular cartilage.[38] The different populations may be distributed at specific sites in relation to their oxygen requirements. The latter hypothesis would be more consistent with the varying amounts and specific distribution of the extracellular macromolecules throughout the disc, as well as with the changing morphology of the cells themselves.

Sulphate metabolism

Early autoradiographic studies showed that the uptake of ^{35}S-sulphate varied across the intervertebral disc in guinea pigs[40] and rabbits.[41] The most actively labelled cells, and therefore those most actively synthesizing proteoglycan, were found at the inner annulus/nucleus junction or transition zone.[41]

In the case of the canine disc, the fastest turnover of sulphated glycosaminoglycans occurred in the outer annulus, where the concentration was low and the slowest turnover was in the nucleus.[36] Both turnover rates were in the order of years rather than months.

THE EXTRACELLULAR MATRIX

Ultrastructural morphology

Several studies have investigated the ultrastructure of the matrix of the cartilage end-plate, annulus fibrosus and nucleus pulposus.

The cartilage end-plate consists of typical chondrocytic cells[18] embedded in a matrix which shows a histochemical staining pattern characteristic of hyaline articular cartilage.[42] The arrangement of cells in the end-plate is also analogous to that in articular cartilage, the cells of the deep zone near the vertebral bone forming columns perpendicular to the bone surface.[42] Early in development, during endochondral bone formation, the vertebral aspect of the end-plate is comparable to the epiphysial cartilage of long bones.

The lamellae of the annulus fibrosus are essentially fibrocartilaginous, consisting of highly-oriented collagen fibrils which form sheets of collagen with increasing age.[43–45] The fibrils also appear to stream off from the ends of the cells and align parallel to existing fibres, suggesting a functional relationship between the cells and fibrillogenesis.[46,25] Electron-dense material has also been observed sheathing the collagen fibrils[47] and may represent proteoglycan and/or protein, since a strong association between collagen, proteoglycan and non-collagenous proteins is indicated by biochemical studies. The fine filaments of electron-dense alcianophilic material (staining with alcian blue) are also thought to represent proteoglycans.[48] The collagenous lamellae and interlamellar proteoglycans/glycoproteins form a looser network in the inner annulus and transition zone than in the outer annulus.

Except for the spindle-shaped cells in the dense fibrillar tissue of the outer annulus, the cells of both the annulus and nucleus have a highly specialized pericellular matrix, consisting of fine filamentous material separated from the major collagen fibres by a fibrillar ring or capsule.[26,20–22]

Ultrastructural studies on the nucleus pulposus indicate a delicate meshwork of collagen fibrils within a 'watery' matrix of proteoglycans.[20,21,49,22] The collagen fibrils are smaller in diameter, more randomly distributed and less oriented than those of the annulus.[25,20,21] Several studies have also demonstrated the presence of unusual banded structures in the human and rabbit nucleus pulposus but not in the annulus fibrosus.[50,51,21,22] These are predominantly located within or near the edge of the lacunae, often forming a complete corona round the cell[51] and consist of alternating light and dark bands approximately 40 and 45 nm wide respectively. The dark bands are composed of a closely-spaced electron-dense doublet separated by a lucent strip through which course fine filaments.[50] Although their chemical composition is unknown, their morphology is identical to the fibrillar form of type VI collagen which is located around the chondrocytes and which has been extracted from the disc (see pp. 103, 109, Fig. 5.1).

Biochemical composition

The gross anatomical structure of the three regions of the intervertebral disc which determines their respective functions depends ultimately on (a) the different proportions and types of the major macromolecules — collagen, proteoglycan, non-collagenous protein, elastin — and (b) the specific interactions between these macromolecules and between the macromolecules and smaller molecules, notably water (Table 5.1).

Water content

The water content of the nucleus pulposus decreases from about 90% at birth to approximately 80% at 20 years and 70% above 60 years.[52-55] The annulus fibrosus contains less water (60–70%), and this does not change significantly with age.[52] A water content of approximately 72% would be expected for the end-plate cartilage if similar to that of human articular cartilage[56] with a possibly higher content (81%) in the vertebral aspect analogous to epiphysial cartilage.[57]

Collagen

The nucleus and annulus contain 15–20% and 50–60% collagen per dry weight respectively (Table 5.1), and these quantities show little change with age.[58,59,53] Human articular and epiphysial cartilage contain 66% and 37% collagen respectively,[57,56] and similar values are expected for the analogous regions of the end-plate. These figures are at best approximations. All the calculations for the collagen content are based on the hydroxyproline content of type I collagen reported in old literature. It is now known that the hydroxyproline content varies with collagen type and tissue source.

Proteoglycans

One of the major functions of proteoglycans is to retain water within a tissue, and hence the amount of proteoglycans in the nucleus (65%) is much greater (particularly in early life) than in the annulus (20%).[58,52] In contrast to collagen, the proteoglycan content decreases with age, being particularly marked in the nucleus, and probably accounts for the observed decrease in water content (see Table 5.1).

The proteoglycan content of articular cartilage (18% per dry weight) is similar to that of the annulus, and a similar value is expected for the end-plate cartilage.

Non-collagenous proteins and elastin

In contrast to proteoglycan, the amount of non-collagenous protein increases with age, varying in the range 5–25% in the annulus and 20–45% in the nucleus.[59] Elastin and its associated microfibrils are also present in both the annulus and nucleus, but in very small amounts (Table 5.1).

Minor components

The remaining components making up the dry weight of the disc include the extracellular enzymes, age pigment, as well as the cells themselves.

The collagens

Collagen is not a single species, as was originally thought. The name collagen is now used collectively to describe a family (possibly families) of glyco-proteins (collagen types) which have a similar basic structure but which also exhibit a considerable variation in fine structure required for their specific functions (Table 5.2).

Basic collagen structure

Common to all collagen types is the 'triple helix' in which three left-handed helices (α-chains) twist together to form a right-handed superhelix. In the primary structure of the helical regions of all collagens glycine occurs at every third residue leading to the repeat sequence (Gly-X-Y), and the cyclic amino-acids proline and hydroxyproline together account for approximately a third of the remaining amino-acids.[63-65] The hydroxyproline is nearly always present in the Y position and is essential for the stability of the triple helix, the hydroxyl group forming hydrogen bonds (probably via water bridges) between the three chains.[66,67] The remaining residues are grouped together in clusters of polar and non-polar residues and influence the assembly of the individual collagen molecules into a quaternary structure, which is fibrillar in the case of most of the major collagen types, but may exhibit

Table 5.2 Molecular configuration, physico-chemical properties and tissue distribution of collagen types (references as cited in text, unless stated)

Collagen type	Molecular configuration	Physico-chemical properties	$M_r \times 10^3$ pro α- or α-chains	Tissue source
I	[α1(I)]₂α2(I)	Low glycosylation, forms thick fibrils, no S-S bonds		Annulus fibrosus, skin, bone, tendon placental tissue, cornea lung, liver
I trimer	[α1(I)]₃	—		skin, tumours, tendon, liver[60]
II	[α1(II)]₃	Moderately glycosylated, forms narrow fibrils, no S-S bonds	95	Annulus fibrosus, nucleus pulposus cartilage, vitreous body
III	[α1(III)]₃	Low glycosylation, forms thin fibrils, S-S bonds present		Fetal skin, aorta, uterus, placental tissue, synovia, liver, lung
IV	[proα1(IV)]₂proα2(IV)	Highly glycosylated, does not form fibrils, S-S bonds present, interrupted helix	170–180	Lens capsule, renal glomerulus placental tissue, tumour, aorta Descemet's membrane
V	[α1(V)]₂α2(V) [α1(V), α2(V), α3(V)] [α1(V)]₃	Highly glycosylated, forms fine fibrils, no S-S bonds	105–120	Annulus fibrosus, placental tissues skin, bone, tendon, synovia, cornea, aorta, lung, liver, uterus
VI	[α1(VI), α2(VI), α3(VI)] pro-form	Highly glycosylated, forms long filaments, highly S-S bonded	140	Placental tissue, uterus, skin, liver, aorta, lung, nuchal ligament
VII	[α1(VII)]₃	S-S bonded, forms anchoring fibrils, single interruption in helix	170	Amniotic membrane, skin, oesophagus[61]
VIII	[α1(VIII)]₃?	No S-S bonds, interrupted helix	177	Culture fluids from endothelial, astrocytoma and other cell types from normal and malignant tissues[62]
IX	[α1(IX), α2(IX), α3(IX)] pro-form?	Highly glycosylated, does not form fibrils, S-S bonded, interrupted helix	84	Annulus fibrosus, nucleus pulposus cartilage, vitreous body
X	[α1(X)]₃	Glycosylated, no S-S bonds, fibril form unknown	49	Calcifying cartilage
1α2α3α (XI?)	[1α2α3α]	Glycosylated, no S-S bonds, forms fine fibrils similar to type V?	100–120	Annulus fibrosus, nucleus pulposus cartilage, vitreous body

different forms in the case of other collagens. Of particular significance is the genetically determined position of certain lysine and hydroxylysine residues which undergo a series of specific reactions leading to the formation of covalent intermolecular cross-links once the molecules have assembled into their specific quaternary arrangements. The hydroxyly-sine residues are also the potential sites for glycosy-lation, which is one of the major factors responsible for the 'fine tuning' of collagen structure to suit the specific individual requirements of different tissues.

Collagen types

There are at least 15 genetically distinct collagens which exist singly or together in different propor-tions in the various connective tissues (Table 5.2), and ten of these (types I–X) have been classified (for reviews on type I–V collagens.[68–71]).

Interstitial collagens — types I, II and III

It was perhaps fortuitous that all the early structural studies were carried out on a soluble form of collagen now known to consist only of one type (type I),[71] and it was not until the late 1960s and early 1970s that the concept of genetically distinct collagen types became evident with the demonstration of a different collagen type in cartilage (type II)[72,73] and skin (type III).[73]

Types I, II and III collagens are the three most abundant collagens in the body which form fibrils with different anatomical arrangements in the various connective tissues.[68,74,75]

In the main, the intervertebral disc with its end-plates contains only types I and II and type II collagen. However, recent work has shown the presence of one of the three or four probable types of type V collagen and type VI collagen, as well as a so far unclassified collagen [$1\alpha2\alpha3\alpha$] and the two newest collagens described types IX and X. Un-fortunately the complexity does not end there, as type III collagen has also been shown to be a component of the degenerated disc. The three main types of collagen not yet identified in disc (!) are types IV, VII and VIII and, of these, only type IV will be described here, since this collagen has structural features which are similar to type IX collagen and which may be relevant to the function of this collagen in the disc.

Type I collagen is the major collagen of tendon, bone and adult skin and consists of two identical α-chains [$\alpha1(I)$] and one dissimilar chain [$\alpha2(I)$], the molecule designated [$\alpha1(I)$]$_2\alpha2$. Type II collagen is the predominant species in avascular tissues such as cartilage, intervertebral disc and vitreous humour, and contains three identical α-chains with a different amino-acid composition from both the $\alpha1$ and $\alpha2$ chains of type I collagen. The α-chains are designated $\alpha1(II)$ and the molecule [$\alpha1(II)$]$_3$. Type II collagen has a higher hydroxylysine content and is more glycosylated than types I and III collagens. Type III collagen is a major component of the more disten-sible connective tissues such as uterus, placental membranes, skin and blood vessels, and also provides a loose reticular network in parenchymal tissues such as liver and lung. The three α-chains of type III collagen, like type II, are also identical [$\alpha1(III)$] but differ in amino-acid composition from those of types I and II collagens; the molecule is designated [$\alpha1(III)$]$_3$. Unlike types I and II col-lagens, type III contains cysteine residues, these being present at the carboxy terminus of the helix, forming two stable disulphide bonds between the three chains.[76] Single $\alpha1(III)$ chains are therefore observed only after reduction of these bonds.

Types I, II and III collagens have a molecular mass of approximately 285 000 (each α-chain being approximately 95 000 M_r and consisting of just over 1000 amino-acid residues). Short non-helical sequences are present at both the amino and carboxy terminal ends of each α-chain and contain the specific lysine and hydroxylysine residues which participate in cross-linking. The helical molecules, together with their non-helical terminal peptides, formerly known as telopeptides, form the basic tropocollagen units necessary for fibril formation and are approximately 285 nm long and 1.4 nm in diameter.[74]

Biosynthesis, secretion and extracellular processing of types I, II and III collagens

The biosynthesis of collagen involves a large number of post-translational modifications which occur both intracellularly and extracellularly. The collagen molecules are also synthesized and secreted in a much larger precursor (procollagen) form, large extension (pro)peptides being present at both the amino and carboxy terminal ends.

The initial translation product of the procollagen mRNA has an additional hydrophobic amino-terminal 'pre', 'signal' or 'leader' sequence which binds to the rough endoplasmic reticulum membrane and leads the nascent polypeptide chain into the membrane.[77] This 'pre' sequence is cleaved early in translation.

The major intracellular modifications are the hydroxylation of peptide-bound proline and lysine to form predominantly 4-hydroxyproline and occasionally 3-hydroxyproline isomers and hydroxylysine.[78] The hydroxylation reactions are catalysed by specific enzymes (hydroxylases) which require Fe^{2+}, 2-oxoglutarate, O_2 and ascorbic acid. As stated above, the hydroxyl group of hydroxyproline is important for helical stability. The hydroxyl group of hydroxylysine enhances the stability of the intermolecular cross-links formed between modified lysine and hydroxylysine residues. Hydroxylysine also serves as the site for a further post-translational modification — glycosylation. Either galactose or the disaccharide glucosylgalactose is attached to the hydroxyl group in a reaction catalysed by specific sugar transferases.[79,78] The hydroxylation and glycosylation reactions occur prior to the formation of the triple helix.

The propeptides of the procollagen α-chains contain oligosaccharides of mannose and N-acetyl glucosamine, sugars which are not present in the triple helical domain. The propeptides are distinct for each procollagen type. However, all the amino terminal propeptides (pN peptides) of the $\alpha 1$ chains of types I, II and III collagens have non-collagenous and collagenous domains linked to the telopeptide regions, but only the pN peptides of type III procollagen are cross-linked by interchain disulphide bonds.[80–83] In contrast, the carboxyterminal propeptides (pC peptides) of all three procollagens are non-collagenous and cross-linked by interchain disulphide bonds. The formation of these bonds directs the folding of the three α-chains into a triple helix and dictates the correct combination of α-chains for a particular collagen type.[84]

The procollagens are secreted from cells in the form of structured but non-fibrillar aggregates which are more stable at body temperature than the unaggregated molecules.[85,86] The propeptides are believed to prevent normal fibrillogenesis occurring intracellularly.[84]

Specific extracellular post-translational modifications occur once the procollagens have been secreted. The pN and pC propeptides are cleaved by specific pN and pC proteases, the order and rate of cleavage varying for the different collagen types.[78] This results in the formation of the basic tropocollagen molecules, which then spontaneously aggregate into fibrils. The pN propeptides, after cleavage, regulate collagen biosynthesis by a feedback mechanism.[87]

The aggregation of tropocollagen monomers into fibrils is highly specific: the monomers are staggered by exactly 234 amino-acids (D-period) which allow maximum electrostatic and hydrophobic interaction and the interchain alignment of lysine and/or hydroxylysine residues for cross-link formation.[84] The amino groups of specific lysines/hydroxylysines in the amino and carboxy telopeptides are first oxidized to aldelyde groups by the enzyme lysyl oxidase which only acts on the assembled fibrils.[88,89] The aldehyde derivatives then condense spontaneously with the ϵ-amino group of lysine/hydroxylysine on an adjacent molecule to form the cross-links. Cross-links involving hydroxylysine-derived aldehydes are more stable than those arising from lysine-derived aldehydes, but both types of cross-link probably react further to form the more complex stable trifunctional cross-links (hydroxypyridinium) which are observed on ageing.[90]

The fibrils of type I, II and III collagens exhibit the same characteristic 234 amino-acid D-periodicity (67nm), when examined by electron microscopy, which results from the specific overlap of molecules.[74] However, the ultimate diameter and arrangement of the different types of collagen fibrils varies widely in different tissues and appears to depend on several factors. These include the extent of hydroxylysine glycosylation,[91,78] the interaction of the collagen molecules with other extracellular matrix macromolecules, particularly proteoglycans,[92,93] and possibly the presence of procollagen molecules in which the amino propeptide has not been cleaved.[94,95]

Basement membrane (type IV) collagen

Basement membranes are specialized condensations of the extracellular matrix which are elaborated by specific epithelial and endothelial cells and contain type IV collagen. Type IV collagen is not itself present in the intervertebral disc, but another collagen (type IX) with similar characteristics is present.

Type IV collagen is synthesized as a procollagen but, unlike types I, II and III collagens, is incorporated directly into the extracellular matrix without *apparent* processing.[96-98] It therefore does not form the 67 nm periodic fibrils but aggregates into either filamentous, network or hexagonal structures, depending on its specific function in a particular tissue.[99,100] However, some processing (however limited) or perhaps conformational change must take place extracellularly in order to prevent aggregation occurring within the cells.

The aggregation of type IV (pro) collagen involves the interaction between the globular C-terminal propeptides of two molecules and between specialized triple-helical N-terminal domains of four molecules.[100,101] The tetrameric arrangement connecting the four triple helices is further stabilized by disulphide bonds and lysine/hydroxylysine-derived cross-links[102,103] and is known as the 7S domain. The major triple helical region of type IV collagen is longer than that of the fibrillar collagens and contains several non-helical interruptions[104] which, together with the non-helical regions linking the C-terminal propeptides and 7S domain to the main helical body, make type IV collagen extremely flexible (an important property for many of its functions).[105] There are two genetically distinct chains which are highly glycosylated and probably exist in the molecular form of $[(pro)\alpha1(IV)]_2$ $(pro)\alpha2(IV)$.[106,107]

Minor collagens

A large proportion of the insoluble cross-linked collagen which in the early days had resisted extraction can be solubilized by pepsin digestion[108] which cleaves the non-helical regions and releases the individual intact triple helical molecules into solution. This procedure also facilitated the isolation of types II and III collagens and, together with improved fractionation techniques, has resulted in the isolation of several important minor collagens. In general, minor collagens can be divided into two groups: those which are mainly found in tissues containing type I or more usually types I and III collagens and those which occur predominantly in type II collagen-rich tissues. Several minor collagens are present in the intervertebral disc, since this tissue contains both types I and II collagens.

Type V collagen

Type V collagen is an interstitial collagen and is *not* present in basement membranes as was originally believed.[70,71] Neither is it a constituent of hyaline cartilage[109,110] as has been so often quoted on the basis of two earlier reports.[111,112] Immunolocalization studies indicate that it occurs mainly in an area adjacent to the cell membrane[113,114] and in biosynthetic studies it is virtually restricted to the cell layer.[115,116] It is therefore often referred to as a pericellular collagen,[117] although it is also found between the major collagen fibrils of the interstitium.[118]

Type V collagen is highly glycosylated and exists in more than one molecular form.[69] Three genetically distinct α-chains have been described, $\alpha1(V)$, $\alpha2(V)$[119,120] and $\alpha3(V)$;[121-124] the molecular form — $[\alpha1(V)]_2\alpha2(V)$ — is the most common species.[122,125,126] Many tissues, however, contain two molecular forms, $[\alpha1(V)]_2\alpha2(V)$ and $[\alpha1(V), \alpha2(V), \alpha3(V)]$ — and in these tissues there appears to be a positive relationship between the second form and type VI collagen.[122] The length of the type V collagen helix is comparable to that of types I, II and III collagens,[125] although the procollagen forms of type V are much larger and are processed more slowly than those of the interstitial collagens. A considerable portion of the propeptides is retained unprocessed in the extracellular matrix.[127-129]

Immuno-electronmicroscopy has shown that type V collagen exists in vivo as fine filaments of approximately 9 nm diameter,[118] but whether these filaments exhibit the characteristic 67 nm periodicity observed for type V fibrils formed in vitro[130,131] is not known.

Type VI collagen

This collagen, which was first isolated from pepsin digests of aortic intima,[120] is a highly disulphide-bonded triple helical aggregate which on reduction gives rise to three major collagenous chains of molecular mass 35–55 000. It is now known to exist in a wide variety of tissues.[122,132–139] The earlier extremely varied nomenclature for this collagen (HMW aggregate, intima collagen and SC collagen) has now been replaced by the classification type VI collagen.[140,135] It has been suggested that the three major pepsin-derived chains are distinct: $\alpha 1(VI)$, $\alpha 2(VI)$ and $\alpha 3(VI)$,[135] although other workers have observed only two chains occurring in a 2:1 ratio.[138]

Several research groups have recently identified the in vivo form of type VI collagen using either non-enzymic methods to extract whole tissue or biosynthetic studies and specific type VI collagen antibodies.[141–147] The individual chains of this in vivo form have a molecular mass of approximately 140 000, indicating that large non-collagenous portions are present. Electron microscopy indicates that these are at the ends of the short collagenous domains, but whether there are three genetically distinct chains of M_r 140 000 and these represent procollagen forms that have not been processed extracellularly has not been established. Type VI collagen forms filamentous structures in vitro and may be a component of microfibrillar structures in vivo.[141,140] This collagen and type V collagen have been identified in the fetal bovine intervertebral disc.

[$1\alpha 2\alpha 3\alpha$] collagen

Three α-chains designated 1α, 2α, 3α, were first isolated from human cartilage, the 1α, 2α chains exhibiting type V collagen-like properties, while the 3α chain was similar to the $\alpha 1(II)$ chain but was more glycosylated.[148] However, although the 1α and 2α chains are genetically distinct from the $\alpha 1(V)$ and $\alpha 2(V)$ chains,[149] there has been a reluctance to classify this collagen. Recent observations, however, certainly suggest that the three chains occur within the same triple helix-[$1\alpha 2\alpha 3\alpha$].[150,151] [$1\alpha 2\alpha 3\alpha$] collagen represents approximately 8–10% of total collagen present in hyaline cartilage, and immunolocalization studies have shown that it is present in the territorial matrix region around the chondrocytes.[152] The function of the [$1\alpha 2\alpha 3\alpha$] collagen in cartilaginous tissues is probably analogous to that of type V collagen present in other tissues.

The [$1\alpha 2\alpha 3\alpha$] collagen has a helical length comparable to types I, II, III and V collagens,[153] but the nature of its procollagen forms is not known.

Type IX collagen

A number of short-chain disulphide-bonded triple helical fragments have been characterized, the nomenclature for which is somewhat diverse.[154–162] Those from pepsin digests of mammalian cartilaginous tissues were approximately one-third and one-seventh the length of type II collagen and were designated cartilage-phosphate-soluble (C-PS) 1 and 2 collagens respectively because of their preferential solubility in phosphate buffers.[154,155]

C-PS1 consisted of three disulphide-bonded apparently identical chains of molecular mass 33 000, whereas C-PS2 contained three dissimilar chains with molecular masses of 10 000, 12 000 and 16 000 linked by disulphide bonds. It was subsequently suggested that C-PS1 and C-PS2 collagens were linked together in vivo in one larger molecule.[150] An additional non-disulphide-bonded triple helical fragment (C-PS3) containing chains of molecular mass 10 000, 13 000 and 15 000 and with similar solubility properties to C-PS1 and C-PS2 has also been isolated from mammalian tissues.[163] In the case of chick cartilage, C-PS3 is linked to C-PS1 by a region which is largely pepsin-resistant.[157,162] Recent biosynthetic studies have indicated that the fragments are indeed linked together to form a larger molecule.[164–166] However, the definitive proof has arisen from the isolation of a cDNA encoding one of the three chains of the chick collagen which is made up of three collagenous domains (COL1, COL2, COL3) and four non-collagenous domains.[167] The size and amino-acid sequence of the various domains indicates that COL1, COL2, COL3 correspond closely to single chains of the C-PS2, C-PS1 and C-PS3 mammalian fragments respectively. Since the three chains are dissimilar and distinct from other known collagens, it is designated type IX collagen — [$\alpha 1(IX)$, $\alpha 2(IX)$, $\alpha 3(IX)$].[168,169]

Immunolocalization studies using antibodies to the pepsin-derived fragments have shown that type IX collagen is present in the territorial/pericellular regions in the cartilage matrix.[170,152,158] Since the distribution of this collagen increases from the superficial zone to the deeper zone of articular cartilage[171] and parallels that of the pericellular capsules observed surrounding the chondrocytes,[23] it is tempting to suggest that the capsules are made up of type IX collagen and act as a protective barrier around the cells analogous to basement membranes in other tissues. Indeed the phosphate solubility property is only shown by one other known collagen — basement membrane type IV collagen,[71] which in addition contains similar interruptions within the helix as well as similar compositional features.[155] Very recently the genes for type IX collagen and also for type IV collagen have been shown to differ from those of the interstitial collagens which have very specific base pairing characteristics. However, it is not certain whether the genes for types IV and IX collagens have similar characteristics to each other.[172,173]

Type X collagen

Type X collagen is the new nomenclature for a short non-disulphide-bonded collagen previously called G collagen[174,165,175,176] or short-chain cartilage collagen[177-179] which is synthesized by chondrocytes involved in endochondral calcification, as well as those derived from the presumptive calcification region of chick sterna.[180] Each procollagen chain has a molecular mass of 59 000 which is cleaved by pepsin to give a species of molecular mass 45 000. Recent studies have shown that limited processing of the procollagen chains to chains of M_r 49 000 occurs prior to deposition in the extracellular matrix, and the molecular configuration of this collagen is designated $[\alpha 1(X)]_3$.[181]

Collagens of the intervertebral disc

Cartilage end-plates

The end-plate is similar ultrastructurally to articular cartilage, which suggests that the collagens in the two tissues would be similar, if not identical. It is therefore more than likely that types II, IX and $[1\alpha 2\alpha 3\alpha]$ collagens are present. Type X collagen is probably specifically located in its vertebral aspect, this region being responsible for endochondral bone formation.

Nucleus pulposus

Early studies indicated that the collagen of the whole human disc had a similar hydroxylysine content to that of cartilage[182,183] Pearson et al[184] deduced from

the high content of hydroxylysine and its glycosides in human nucleus pulposus that cartilage and nucleus pulposus contained the same collagen, which by 1972 had been established as type II collagen.[72] These studies were subsequently confirmed by Eyre and Muir, who digested the nucleus pulposus of both the pig and human intervertebral disc with cyanogen bromide (CNBr).[185-187] This reagent cleaves polypeptide chains specifically at methionine residues and, since all collagens have few methionine residues, cleavage results in the formation of several large CNBr peptides which act as a 'fingerprint' for the collagen type. All other proteins (except elastin, which contains no methionine) are completely digested. When the CNBr peptide profile of the nucleus pulposus was examined by ion-exchange chromatography or SDS/polyacrylamide-gel electrophoresis, it was found to be characteristic of type II collagen. Type II collagen was also the only collagen observed in the human nucleus after pepsin digestion and purification of the solubilized collagen.[188]

The fraction of hydroxylysine residues which was substituted with either glucosylgalactose or galactose was 66–68% for the type II collagen of both nucleus pulposus and articular cartilage. However, the ratio of glucosylgalactose to galactose in the collagen of nucleus was 1.36:1 compared to 0.61:1 for the cartilage collagen.[189,187] The nucleus pulposus collagen will therefore be more hydrated than that of cartilage and thus may augment the role of proteoglycans. This difference may reflect the different degrees to which the two tissues resist compressive forces.

The type II collagen fibrils of the human nucleus pulposus are stabilized by the same types of intermolecular cross-links found in cartilage.[188] These 'reducible' cross-links predominate in young tissue but decrease on ageing and are replaced by more stable cross-links which have recently been shown to be identical to the hydroxypyridinium cross-links observed in mature cartilage.[190,191]

Recent studies, using pepsin digestion followed by rigorous fractionation techniques, have shown that human nucleus pulposus like cartilage contains the $[1\alpha 2\alpha 3\alpha]$ collagen and the short-chain disulphide-bonded collagens C-PS1 and C-PS2,[154,155] the latter now known to be part of the same larger collagen molecule designated type IX collagen. Gel electrophoresis of these collagens indicates that they do not differ significantly in the degree of glycosylation from those of cartilage (Fig. 5.1[154,155]) but differences in the *type* of glycosides as in the case of type II collagen cannot be excluded.

Annulus fibrosus

CNBr peptide analysis of pig and human annulus fibrosus indicated the presence of both types I and II collagens, and the amount of each collagen in the two species was quantified by estimating the relative amounts of two CNBr peptides which were specific for types I and II collagens respectively.[189,185-187] Pig annulus contained 80% type I and 20% type II collagen, whereas the human annulus contained 40% type I and 60% type II collagen, and it was suggested that the higher content of type II collagen reflected an evolutionary adaptation to an upright position and hence different spinal loading.[187]

The hydroxylysine content of the human annulus collagen as a whole was not significantly different from that of the nucleus and indicated that the type I collagen was similar to that of the fibrocartilaginous semilunar meniscus.[187] The percentage of hydroxylysine residues glycosylated was 51%, intermediate between that of the nucleus (66–68%) and semilunar meniscus (35%), but the glucosylgalactose to galactose ratio (1.36:1) was analogous to both

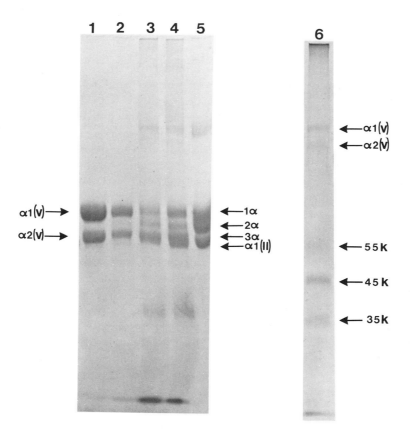

Fig. 5.1 Sodium dodecyl sulphate/polyacrylamide gel electrophoresis of intervertebral disc collagens. The different collagen types were separated from pepsin digests of human and bovine intervertebral discs according to Ayad et al[154,155] and analysed on 5% gels (lanes 1–5) or 8% gels (lane 6).
Lane 1:   type V collagen standard (fetal calf skin)
Lane 2:   fetal bovine disc (types V and [1α2α3α] collagens)
Lane 3:   human (16 yrs) nucleus pulposus ([1α2α3α] and traces of type II collagen)
Lane 4:   human (16 yrs) annulus fibrosus (types V, [1α2α3α] and traces of type II collagen)
Lane 5:   [1α2α3α] collagen standard (bovine nasal cartilage)
Lane 6:   fetal bovine disc (35K, 45K, 55K pepsin-derived fragments of type VI collagen plus type V collagen)

nucleus (1.37:1) and meniscus (1.33:1).[189,187] The more highly glycosylated type I collagen of the annulus compared with that of skin, tendon or bone probably dictates the specific fibrillar arrangement of this collagen in the lamellae of the annulus.

Analysis of the human annulus collagen solubilized by pepsin digestion at 4°C failed to detect any type I collagen[187,192] perhaps because it was not solubilized or was complexed with glycosaminoglycans in the digest.[187,193] Pepsin digestion at 15°C, however, did release some soluble type I collagen.[188]

The development of improved fractionation techniques has resulted in the isolation of several minor collagens from pepsin digests of the annulus fibrosus. These include the $[1\alpha2\alpha3\alpha]$ and C-PS1/C-PS2 (type IX) collagens, the same collagens as those seen in the nucleus pulposus.[154,155] However, gel electrophoresis of the $[1\alpha2\alpha3\alpha]$ collagen fraction from the annulus (Fig. 5.1) indicated a greater proportion of the 1α and 3α chains relative to the 2α chain, and this was shown to be due to the presence of the $\alpha1$ and $\alpha2$ chains of type V collagen which have similar electrophoretic mobilities to the 1α and 3α chains respectively. An even greater proportion of type V collagen relative to the $[1\alpha2\alpha3\alpha]$ collagen was found when the whole fetal bovine disc was examined (Fig. 5.1). The presence of type V is consistent with the fibrocartilaginous nature of the annulus and analogous to the presence of type V in the bovine semilunar meniscus.[194] The increased proportion of the $[1\alpha2\alpha3\alpha]$ collagen relative to type V collagen in human compared to bovine tissues is also consistent with the higher proportion of type II collagen relative to type I collagen in human tissue, and again probably reflects an evolutionary adaptation to the upright position. It is almost certain that types I and V collagens are synthesized by the same fibroblastic-like cells and the type II and $[1\alpha2\alpha3\alpha]$ collagens by the chondrocytic cells. The above observations also support the recent finding that a switch from type II to type I collagen by chick chondrocytes is paralleled by a switch from the synthesis of $[1\alpha2\alpha3\alpha]$ collagen to type V collagen.[32]

Pepsin digests of fetal bovine disc also contained collagenous peptides characteristic of the pepsinized form of type VI collagen (Fig. 5.1) which has not been isolated previously from cartilaginous tissues, although it has been demonstrated in bovine cartilage by immunofluorescence techniques.[109]

Spatial distribution of collagen types in the intervertebral disc

CNBr peptide analysis of serial sections across the annulus indicated a specific distribution for the types I and II collagens: the outer annulus contained virtually all type I collagen, the transition zone virtually all type II collagen and the intermediate regions had increasing amounts of type II relative to type I collagen from outer annulus to the transition zone.[186] This is consistent with the morphology of the cells in the various regions, those of the outer annulus resembling fibroblasts and the remaining cells being typically chondrocytic.

Immunofluorescent localization studies using antibodies to types I and II collagens confirmed the CNBr peptide analyses in both the pig[195,196] and human[197,198] annulus and nucleus.

The $[1\alpha2\alpha3\alpha]$ and type IX collagens have not been localized in the intervertebral disc, but by analogy with cartilage[152,171] they would be expected to locate (and form a protective barrier) around the chondrocytes in all three regions of the disc, since the pericellular environment is identical to that found in hyaline cartilage.

PROTEOGLYCANS

Proteoglycans are polyanionic macromolecules consisting of mixtures of acidic polysaccharides, known collectively as glycosaminoglycans (GAGS) in association with a small quantity of protein. The individual glycosaminoglycans all consist of repeating disaccharide units of an N-acetylated hexosamine (glucosamine or galactosamine) and either uronic acid (glucuronic or iduronic) or galactose (Table 5.3).

With one exception (hyaluronic acid) all are O-sulphated (on the hexosamine residue) and covalently linked to a central protein core. The resulting macromolecules are called proteoglycans, a term introduced in 1967[199] to replace the old nomenclature of protein polysaccharides. At the same time the term GAG replaced the former term mucopolysaccharide. Early methods of preparation involving high-speed homogenization produced shearing forces which split the protein polysaccharides (PP) which were therefore extremely heterogeneous. They were, however, fractionated into two main classes of light

Table 5.3 Composition of glycosaminoglycans in the mammalian intervertebral disc

Glycosaminoglycan	Repeat disaccharide unit -[hexuronic acid or hexose with hexosamine]-	Linkage to protein core
Hyaluronic acid	-[D-glucuronic acid D-N-acetylglucosamine]-	?

Chondroitin-4-sulphate	-[D-glucuronic acid D-N-acetylgalactosamine]-
	                                         |
	                                4 sulphate
		–Gal-Gal-Xyl-Ser
		                      |

Chondroitin-6-sulphate	-[D-glucuronic acid D-N-acetylgalactosamine]-
	                                         |
	                                6 sulphate
		-Gal-Gal-Xyl-Ser
		                      |

Keratan sulphate	-[D-galactose D-N-acetylglucosamine]-
	        | |
	   6 sulphate 6 sulphate
		-Gal-N-acetyl-Ser
		            (Thr)
		        |
		        Gal
		        |
		        N-acetylneuraminic
		        acid

Dermatan sulphate*	-[L-iduronic acid D-N-acetylgalactosamine]-
	      or
	-[D-glucuronic acid 4 or 6 sulphate]-
		-Gal-Gal-Xyl-Ser
		                      |

*Not detected in human intervertebral disc

fraction (PPL), which could be further fractionated in the ultracentrifuge, and a heavy high molecular weight fraction (PPH) which also contained collagen. The relationship between PPL, PPH and the proteoglycans produced by the dissociative extraction procedure is discussed by Hamerman et al.[200] The proteoglycans of different tissues contain different proportions and types of glycosaminoglycans. Proteoglycans of the hyaline cartilage are the most well-characterized.[201,202] A brief account of their structure and function will be presented here, since (a) identical proteoglycans are presumed to occur in the cartilaginous end-plates of the disc, and (b) similar but not identical proteoglycans occur in both the annulus fibrosus and nucleus pulposus.

Hyaline cartilage end-plate proteoglycans

Composition and structure of PG subunit

The glycosaminoglycans of the end-plate proteoglycan are predominantly chondroitin 4- and 6-sulphates with small proportions of keratan sulphate attached to the same protein core (Table 5.3).[203] The widely accepted 'bottle-brush structure' (see below) was evident as early as 1958[204] but it was not until efficient non-degradative methods of preparing proteoglycans were developed[205,206] that the structure of proteoglycans could be fully elucidated. These methods (involving the use of dissociative solvents such as 4M-guanidinium chloride follwed by CsCl

density gradient centrifugation) established that the proteoglycan subunit consisted of 87% chondroitin sulphate, 6% keratan sulphate and 7% protein, and that the polydispersity of proteoglycans was due to variable amounts of chondroitin sulphate.[203]

Specific enzymic degradation studies established that the molecular weight of the individual glycosaminoglycan side chains was similar, the average molecular mass for chondroitin and keratan sulphate being 15–20 000 and 5–8000 respectively.[207] Subsequent studies established the order of the side chains on the protein core as well as the hyaluronate-binding site.[208,209]

The protein core has a molecular mass 2.3×10^5 and is divided into three main parts: (1) a globular domain of 60–80 000 molecular mass which contains interchain disulphide bonds and is specific for binding to hyaluronic acid and to link protein; (2) a region of 200–250 amino-acids to which most of the keratan sulphate is attached; and (3) a region of approximately 1000 amino-acids for the attachment of chondroitin sulphate. The chondroitin sulphate chains are attached to the protein core by a xylosyl serine linkage between a neutral trisaccharide: galactosyl-galactosyl-xylose and a serine residue on the protein core,[210] xylose forming an O-glycosidic link with the hydroxyl group of the serine residue. Keratan sulphate is linked by two different bonds, one between N-acetyl galactosamine, a minor component sugar at one end of the carbohydrate molecule and serine or threonine on the protein core,[211] and another involving glutamic acid.[212] In addition, small (1200–2000 M_r) oligosaccharides are found along the protein core, some linked to serine or threonine, others to aspartic acid, the latter mainly in the hyaluronate-binding region.[213,214] There are approximately 100 chondroitin sulphate chains,[215] which are grouped together in clusters of (on average) four,[207] 50 keratan sulphate chains and 50 oligosaccharides per protein core, probably consisting of a single polypeptide chain.[201] This leads to an average molecular mass for the proteoglycan subunit (monomer) of $0.5–4 \times 10^6$ and the characteristic 'bottle-brush' structure, confirmed by electron microscopy using the Kleineschmidt technique.[216,217]

Aggregation of proteoglycan subunits (Monomers)

In cartilaginous tissues proteoglycan subunits are organized as huge multimolecular aggregates by specific interaction with hyaluronic acid. Approximately 200 subunits bind per hyaluronic acid molecule, resulting in a molecular mass of 350×10^6.[201] The binding to hyaluronic acid is specific and is a function of the protein core, requiring intact arginine, lysine and tryptophan residues as well as disulphide bonds.[218] In the formation of these aggregates, a decasaccharide is the minimum length of the hyaluronic acid required.[219,220] The N-acetyl *glucosamine* residues of hyaluronic acid are also essential, since de-sulphated chondroitin sulphate containing N-acetyl *galactosamine* will not form aggregates.[221]

Despite its importance in the aggregation of proteoglycans, hyaluronic acid in cartilage accounts for only 1% of the total glycosaminoglycans, and most of this participates in aggregate formation.

Proteoglycans, once aggregated, are further stabilized by interaction with a specific globular protein known as link protein, of which there are two structurally related molecular forms, both of which are glycoproteins.[222,223] The link glycoprotein locks the proteoglycan subunits on to the hyaluronic acid chain.

A small proportion of proteoglycans do not interact with hyaluronic acid: these are smaller, having lower protein and keratan sulphate content and a different protein core.[220] Only 75% of the total

cartilage proteoglycans are extractable from the tissue by dissociative solvents. However, chemical modification of the non-extractable proteoglycans indicates that they are similar to the extractable type, their insolubility being due to non-specific entanglement within the collagen fibrillar meshwork.[224]

Biosynthesis of proteoglycans

The biosynthesis and secretion of proteoglycans, link-proteins and hyaluronic acid by chondrocytes has been reviewed by Kleine.[225] Proteoglycans are formed by a stepwise addition of activated single monosaccharides from their respective nucleotide sugar on to the growing protein core. Sulphation occurs at a later stage in synthesis by transfer of 'active' sulphate. Recent subcellular localization studies[226] indicate that the N-linked oligosaccharides are added in the rough endoplasmic reticulum, whereas glycosaminoglycans are added predominantly in the smooth membranes. Link protein is formed by the normal synthetic pathway for glycoproteins. Since the formation of link-stable aggregates is an extracellular event and does not take place instantaneously,[227] the pathways leading to the biosynthesis and secretion of proteoglycan subunit, link protein and hyaluronate must be separate and there must be some delaying mechanism preventing aggregation and stabilization outside the cell.

Functions of proteoglycans

Cartilaginous tissues have the highest known concentration of proteoglycans. The major function of proteoglycans lies in the ability of the negatively-charged side chains to repel one another and occupy large volumes in free solution, i.e. their space-filling function.[202] In the cartilage end-plate matrix they are under compression and act as molecular springs resisting external forces by increasing their internal charge density and filling more space when the external force is removed. The swelling pressure created by proteoglycans is resisted by the collagen fibrils which are under tension. The formation of aggregates ensures that the molecules do not move away but are trapped more easily within the collagen network, and it is possible that the delay in extracellular aggregate formation allows their diffusion away from the cells and their entrapment at specific sites where their resistance to compressive forces is required most.[202]

Proteoglycans of the intervertebral disc

Most studies on the structure of cartilage proteoglycans have been carried out using bovine or porcine tissues, but in the case of disc proteoglycans human tissue has been studied extensively. This should be remembered when comparing cartilage and disc. Unless otherwise stated, only human intervertebral disc will be described.

Disc proteoglycans are more easily extracted than those of cartilage, a high percentage being extractable by non-dissociative solvents.[228,229] The ease of extractability decreases across the disc: 92% of the uronic acid is extracted from the nucleus as compared to 75% for the annulus.[230] This may be due to the increasing collagen content from the nucleus to annulus leading to physical entrapment of the proteoglycan.[228]

Chondroitin sulphate and keratan sulphate are the major glycosaminoglycans, but chondroitin-6-sulphate predominates in the young disc and is the only isomer after middle age.[231,232] The two glycosaminoglycans are also linked to the same polypeptide of the protein core[233] by similar linkages to those found in cartilage.[234,212] However, disc proteoglycans have a much higher keratan sulphate to chondroitin sulphate ratio[228,231] and a higher protein content.[233,230]

Fibrocartilaginous tissues such as the semilunar meniscus contain dermatan sulphate (Table 5.3).[235] Although the annulus fibrosus is a fibrocartilaginous tissue, no dermatan sulphate has been found in the human annulus, whereas its presence has been reported in the cat annulus.[236] Dermatan sulphate interacts strongly with type I collagen,[93,237] and although less of this collagen is present in human annulus than in that from quadruped animals, there is still sufficient (40%) to have supposed that, if dermatan sulphate were present, it could have been detected.

Estimations of chain length for keratan sulphate and chondroitin sulphate in the disc vary widely with species, age and method of preparation. However, values reported for human tissue are similar to those of bovine cartilage: 20 000 for chondroitin sulphate and 10 000 for keratan sulphate.[231,230]

It is generally agreed that the proteoglycans *extracted* from disc are smaller and more polydispersed than those *extracted* from cartilage, the average mass of the disc macromolecules being approximately half (1×10^6) that of the cartilage macromolecules.[58,229] The size and polydispersity of proteoglycans extracted from the nucleus and annulus are similar.[228,58]

A detailed investigation of disc proteoglycan structure was carried out using non-degradative extraction procedures.[230] A model was proposed to explain the differences in chemical composition and molecular mass between the proteoglycans of disc and those of cartilage. This model envisages a molecule in which the keratan-sulphate-rich and hyaluronate binding regions of the protein core are similar to the cartilage molecule but in which the chondroitin-sulphate-binding region is drastically shortened.

Disc proteoglycans are capable, like those of cartilage, of forming aggregates with hyaluronic acid, but the aggregates are much smaller, presumably due to the smaller size of the proteoglycan subunits[228,230] although there may also be fewer of them. Possibly the most significant difference between the proteoglycans of the two tissues lies in the *proportion* of proteoglycan subunits *capable* of forming aggregates. Only 5–10% of the proteoglycans extracted from whole human disc were capable of forming aggregates, compared to 40–60% for human cartilage proteoglycans.[229] When the annulus and nucleus were analysed separately, most of the non-aggregating proteoglycans were concentrated in the nucleus. Values for the quantities of proteoglycans capable of aggregating range from 15–20% in the nucleus to 40–65% in the annulus, depending on age.[58,238,230]

It would seem that the hyaluronic acid binding site on the proteoglycan subunit in disc is either absent or altered in some way so that it is unable to aggregate. The concentration of hyaluronic acid in disc is greater than that found in cartilage: nucleus 1.8%, annulus 12% and cartilage 1%,[240] suggesting that lack of aggregated macromolecules is an intrinsic property of the proteoglycan subunits or link glycoprotein. An abnormality of link glycoprotein has been suggested by Tengblad et al,[239,241] who were the first people to have identified link protein in disc. Using antibodies to these proteins,

Tengblad and his colleagues showed that the link protein of both the human annulus and nucleus reacts with antibodies to that of human articular cartilage link protein. The disc link protein also binds to hyaluronic acid and proteoglycans, has a similar molecular weight to cartilage link protein, but is less effective in stabilizing the proteoglycan aggregates. Thus aggregation may be normal, as is suggested from the biosynthetic studies, but the aggregates formed may be less stable than those in cartilage.

It is obviously important to know whether the significant difference in hydrodynamic size and aggregating ability observed between the proteoglycans of the annulus, nucleus and cartilage are (a) inherent and reflect the different functions of these tissues in response to external forces or (b) due to other factors relating to their degradation by endogenous enzymes. It is equally possible that both suggestions are correct. In other words, the metabolism of the aggregates is different from cartilage, but this is because the disc will function more effectively with shorter proteoglycan aggregates.

Artefactual results arising from degradation during the extraction procedure have been effectively ruled out by the work of Stevens et al,[242] who added labelled newly synthesized porcine cartilage proteoglycans to extracts of human disc. No change in either amount or size of the labelled cartilage material was demonstrated. The biosynthetic studies of Oegema et al[243] have indicated that the proteoglycans of human nucleus pulposus are synthesized initially as large molecular mass aggregates. The newly synthesized molecules have a larger core protein and a greater potential for aggregation than those extracted under associative conditions in the presence of proteinase inhibitors. They suggested that the avascular nature of the nucleus pulposus may be responsible for the inability of the tissue to dispose of partially-metabolized aggregates. In other words, the thickness of the disc would make diffusion of degraded proteoglycan considerably slower than in the thinner hyaline cartilage of articular surfaces and end-plates.

It is reasonable to conclude that the proteoglycans of nucleus, annulus and cartilage are synthesized as a similar, if somewhat heterogeneous, population of macromolecules and are also probably metabolized in the same manner in all tissues. The resultant products may, however, diffuse into bone or synovial fluid in the case of end-plate or cartilage but be retained in thicker avascular tissues such as the nucleus pulposus or deeper layers of the annulus. The question remains as to whether the retention of these smaller aggregates is necessary for the specific function of the disc or whether it is responsible for the nucleus losing its hydrostatic function with age and becoming fibrous.

Proteoglycan distribution

Biochemical analyses of proteoglycans in the human disc have indicated an increase in their concentration from the outer annulus to the nucleus[58,240,42] (Table 5.1). This radial distribution was confirmed by immunolocalization studies using antiproteoglycan antibodies on both pig[196] and human[197] discs. Intense staining was observed in the nucleus and inner annulus of both species. However, in the case of the outer annulus, a reticular pattern was observed in the pig, but staining was largely negative in the human.

Minor proteoglycans

There may be minor proteoglycan species with specific functions present in the disc which have yet to be isolated. In this respect two unusual proteoglycans have been extracted from chick cartilage which are quite distinct from the major characteristic cartilage proteoglycans. One has a very small core protein and large glycosaminoglycan side chains and is synthesized in a higher-molecular-weight precursor form containing glycoprotein oligosaccharides.[244] The other consists of a disulphide-bonded collagenous core and only two large side chains of the non-cartilage type glycosaminoglycan dermatan sulphate and has been implicated in cell–cell and cell–matrix interactions.[245] The collagenous core is apparently identical to type IX collagen,[246] and hence a similar macromolecule probably occurs in the human intervertebral disc. It is becoming increasingly apparent that there is a wide distribution of macromolecules with properties intermediate between the extreme forms of proteoglycans, collagens and glycoproteins which may have a unique functional significance.

Proteoglycan–collagen interactions

Several studies have indicated that proteoglycans and glycosaminoglycans influence type I collagen fibrillodgenesis in vitro.[247-249] However, these studies do not explain the interactions, or lack of them in vivo between specific types of proteoglycans and collagens which have unique anatomical arrangements within a particular tissue. These associations have been demonstrated largely by electron microscopy, but unfortunately ultrastructural studies often give artefactual results due to poor staining procedures and 'drying out' effects. Recent electron microscopical studies by Scott and co-workers,[93,250,251] using a specific cationic dye at physiological pH, have overcome these problems and have shown that dermatan sulphate proteoglycan interacts strongly with type I collagen molecules on the outer surface of developing fibrils in tendon. The proteodermatan sulphate binds specifically at the 'gap' region between non-overlapping collagen molecules, the amount bound being inversely proportional to fibril diameter. The authors suggest that this is a probable mechanism for controlling the ultimate width of the fibrils in vivo.

The human intervertebral disc does not contain dermatan sulphate but is rich in chondroitin sulphate/keratan sulphate proteoglycans and hyaluronic acid. Several observations suggest that interactions between these macromolecules and types I/II collagens are less specific, involving physical entrapment and excluded volume effects. On theoretical grounds it has been proposed that hyaluronic acid and chondroitin sulphate can each form *intra*molecular hydrogen bonds along the carbohydrate chain in preference to *inter*molecular bonds with other molecules, whereas dermatan sulphate has an increased tendency to form *inter*-molecular associations (for example with type I collagen).[252] Immunolocalization studies indicate that the distribution of chondroitin sulphate/keratan sulphate proteoglycans in the disc is different from that of types I and II collagens, particularly in the annulus fibrosus, and it has been suggested that proteoglycans and collagens form independent but possibly closely interwoven networks.[197] Proteoglycans are readily extracted at near neutral pH from the intervertebral disc, particularly from young disc,[228] which would indicate that no significant

interactions were occurring. However, protein- and keratan sulphate-rich proteoglycans which predominate on ageing are less readily extracted and may be more firmly bound to collagen, this possibly being due to protein core-collagen interactions.[253] It is also possible that interactions between proteoglycans and the major collagens may be mediated by non-collagenous glycoproteins as previously suggested.

The pericellular/territorial matrix around the chondrocytes of disc and cartilage contains a higher proportion of keratan sulphate-rich proteoglycans than the remaining matrix[254] and also contains the $[1\alpha2\alpha3\alpha]$ and type IX collagens.[152] It is therefore possible that a stronger interaction between these collagens and proteoglycans may occur in order to maintain the integrity of the pericellular capsule observed around these cells. It is interesting that when $[1\alpha2\alpha3\alpha]$ and type II collagens from bovine articular cartilage were applied to cartilage proteoglycan affinity columns, the $[1\alpha2\alpha3\alpha]$ collagen was more strongly bound than type II collagen.[255] Moreover, type IX collagen from chick cartilage has been reported to contain chondroitin sulphate covalently bound to one of its three chains,[246] and this form is almost certainly the same as a proteoglycan described by Noro et al,[245] although these workers identified the glycosaminoglycan as dermatan sulphate. It is still not quite certain whether type IX collagen is a true hybrid molecule or whether the glycosaminoglycan was originally linked to a larger proteoglycan prior to isolation. As type IX collagen is an integral component of the human intervertebral discs,[154,155] it can be tentatively concluded that similar covalent bonds will form between the type IX collagen molecules and glycosaminoglycans in this tissue.

Non-collagenous proteins and glycoproteins

The term non-collagenous proteins in essence describes all proteins other than the collagens and therefore includes the structural proteins of the cells themselves, and the enzymes involved in cellular metabolism and the biosynthesis and degradation of the extracellular matrix macromolecules. However, these account for only a small percentage of the non-collagenous pool, particularly in the disc, where the cellularity is low and the majority of the non-collagenous proteins have a structural or morphogenetic role.

Non-collagenous proteins and glycoproteins are emerging as an important class of macromolecules in their own right and, together with the collagens, proteoglycans and elastin play specific roles in the organization of cells and their extracellular matrices which ultimately defines tissue function.

The human disc is richer than most other connective tissues in its content of non-collagenous proteins which increases dramatically with age.[256,53,257] Analysis by Dickson et al[59] indicated that the amount of non-collagenous protein varied between 20–45% of the dry weight of the nucleus and 5–25% of the dry weight of the annulus, and there were compositional differences between the proteins in the two regions. Wide-angle X-ray diffraction studies focused on the proteins giving a 4.65 A reflection which is characteristic of β-proteins, and which increased in sharpness with age, indicating increased crystallinity. At least three different proteins were distinguished, all of which had an unoriented β-configuration, but whether this represented the native state or was due to denaturation of globular proteins was not established.[256–260] The proteins were rich in tyrosine,[59] which probably accounted for their ultra-violet fluorescence.[261] The relationship between these β-proteins and the many non-collagenous proteins which can be extracted from the disc[262] has not been established. One 'dense' β-protein was however equated with elastin;[263,261] others may represent the structural or matrix-associated glycoproteins.[264,265] Structural glycoproteins have been isolated from many tissues and are invariably highly insoluble, disulphide-bonded and acidic. They mediate cell-matrix interactions and interactions between the various extracellular-matrix macromolecules themselves, and also influence cell differentiation and morphogenesis.

Proteoglycan-associated glycoproteins

The link-protein which stabilizes the interaction between proteoglycans and hyaluronic acid in the formation of aggregates, has already been described and together with the core protein will contribute to the non-collagenous pool in the intervertebral disc. Recent studies indicate that the cartilage link-protein can also interact with collagen in vitro, suggesting that it may influence collagen fibrillo-genesis in vivo.[266] A close association between collagen and link-protein has in fact been demonstrated in articular cartilage by immuno-electron microscopy.[267]

Elastin-associated glycoproteins

The elastin-associated microfibrillar proteins are characteristic structural glycoproteins which act as a scaffold for elastin deposition. Their presence in discs will be described later (p. 121).

Collagen-associated glycoproteins

Biochemical studies[259,184] and electron microscopy[22] have indicated the strong association between glycoproteins and collagen in both the annulus and nucleus of the human disc. The glycoproteins were solubilized by trypsin digestion, resulting in a concomitant disappearance of the 4.65 A β-protein reflection.[259] The proportion of trypsin-soluble glycopeptides increased with age, particularly from the nucleus.[184] These proteins may be analogous to the structural glycoproteins which form a filamentous network around the type II collagen fibres in canine rib cartilage and which, on the basis of a low but consistent uronic acid and galactosamine content, have been postulated to mediate the interaction between the 'non-extractable' proteoglycans and the collagen fibrils.[268] It has also been suggested that these glycoproteins may act as a template for the subsequent deposition of correctly-oriented collagen fibrils,[264] that is analogous to the role of elastin-associated microfibrils in elastogenesis.

Glycoproteins in cell–matrix interactions

The term 'nectin' (from nectere, to bind, connect) describes a family of glycoproteins (nectins) which mediate the interaction between cells and the extracellular matrix. The most well-characterized is fibronectin, which occurs on the cell surface of many cells, particularly fibroblasts, as well as in the extracellular matrix.[269,270] It is comprised of 220–250 000 molecular mass subunits linked by disulphide bonds into dimeric and multimeric forms. Each subunit is divided into several functional domains which bind specifically to either collagen, fibrin, glycosaminoglycans or the cell surface.

Although fibronectin has not been reported in the intervertebral disc, it could be present in the annulus, particularly in the outer lamellae, where the cells have a more fibroblastic appearance, due possibly to the dedifferentiation of chondrocytes as discussed earlier.

Chondronectin is located at the interface between the chondrocytes and the cartilage extracellular matrix as well as on the chondrocyte surface.[271] It has a molecular weight of 180 000 and is composed of disulphide-bonded subunits of approximately 70 000. It specifically promotes the attachment of chondrocytes to type II collagen,[272] this interaction being enhanced in the presence of cartilage proteoglycans.[270] Since type II collagen and cartilage-specific proteoglycans are the major constituents of all three aspects of the human intervertebral disc and chondrocytes are the predominant cell type, it is highly probable that chondronectin will also be present.

A glycoprotein of molecular mass 31 000 has been isolated recently from chick chondrocyte membranes. This protein contains 30% carbohydrate, but is highly hydrophobic and has been shown to be an integral part of the chondrocyte membrane by its ability to insert into lecithin vesicles.[273] The isolated protein binds to several native collagens, but when inserted into liposomes is specific for native type II collagen.[274] Rotary shadowing indicates that binding occurs at the ends of the collagen molecules.[273] The glycoprotein was subsequently located to the surface of chondrocytes by immunofluorescence studies and named anchorin.[275] Antibodies to anchorin can immunoprecipitate similar proteins which have been produced by cell-free translation of mRNA from several other types of mesenchymal cells, suggesting that there may either be a family of anchorins which may show specificity for different collagen types,[276] or that anchorin is made by other cell types as well as chondrocytes. Anchorin provides an additional mechanism for chondrocyte–matrix interaction and possibly feedback control, and is likely to be present on the cell membrane of intervertebral disc chondrocytes.

Miscellaneous non-collagenous glycoproteins

Many non-collagenous proteins have been observed in the guanidinium chloride extracts of several bovine cartilages and intervertebral disc.[262] Link proteins were common to all, as was a glycoprotein of 36 000 M_r. This latter protein consists of a single highly hydrophobic chain (140 leucine residues/1000 residues), has a high turnover rate[277] but does not vary significantly in amount with age.[278] Other proteins were specific for the disc and articular cartilage, whereas the well-characterized 148 000 molecular weight cartilage matrix protein present in tracheal cartilage[279,280] was absent from articular cartilage and disc (annulus and nucleus). It was therefore suggested that non-collagenous proteins could be particularly important for the sub-differentiation among cartilages.[262]

Elastic fibres

Elastic fibres have been demonstrated as extracellular components of the intervertebral disc. Such fibres generally consist of two morphologically distinct components — an amorphous core of polymeric elastin and a peripheral mantle of microfibrils (10–12 nm diameter) which possess a bead-like periodicity[281,282] and are largely responsible for the reversible extensibility of tissues such as the nuchal ligament of ungulates, large blood vessels and the elastic cartilage of the ear. Both components of elastic fibres are therefore synthesized by a variety of cell types: fibroblasts (nuchal ligament), smooth muscle cells (aorta) and chondrocytes (ear cartilage), and coexist with different major collagen types — type I and III collagens in the nuchal ligament[132] and aorta[283] and type II collagen in the ear cartilage.[284] It is therefore not altogether surprising that elastic fibres should occur in the intervertebral disc.

As well as classical elastic fibres, two further morphological structures which exhibit some but not all of their characteristic histochemical staining properties have been described. These are (a) oxytalan fibres consisting of bundles of typical 10–12 nm microfibrils and no amorphous elastin, and (b) elaunin fibres consisting of bundles of microfibrils associated with small amounts of amorphous material.[285,286] These structures have not yet been characterized, and their relationship to each other and to elastin and its associated microfibrils has not been established. However, both oxytalan and elaunin fibres have been used synonymously with elastic microfibrils and elastic fibres, and it is probable that oxytalan fibres and elaunin fibres represent intermediate stages in elastogenesis.[285] During fetal development of classical elastic tissues, an accumulation of parallel bundles of microfibrils precedes the formation of, and acts as a template for, the deposition and polymerization of elastin to form the mature elastic fibre.[282,287]

Chemical characterization

The occurrence of elastic fibres and their intermediate forms as minor constituents of the intervertebral disc has been demonstrated largely by morphological studies at electron microscopic and light microscopic levels. There has only been one study in which elastic fibres have been extracted from discs. Although the chemical characterization of elastic fibres described below was obtained from classical elastic tissues and their cells in culture, it will certainly serve as a framework for the understanding of the elastic fibres of the disc.

Elastin-associated microfibrils

The chemistry of elastin-associated microfibrils is extremely controversial.[281] Early studies established that they consist of highly insoluble, disulphide-bonded glycoproteins which are acidic and exhibit an affinity for cationic stains.[288] Despite the use of proteinase inhibitors in the extraction procedure, molecular weights ranging from 14 000 to over 200 000 have been suggested for the microfibrillar protein! One particular glycoprotein (M_r approximately 34 000) however, is interesting since it exhibits enzyme activity similar to that of lysyl oxidase required for elastin cross-linking.[289] Biosynthetic studies, on the other hand, have shown that there are two glycoproteins with molecular weights of 150 000 and 300 000, the smaller of which is collagenous.[290,291] A definitive relationship between any glycoprotein and elastic microfibrils has yet to be established.

Elastin

Elastin is chemically distinct from the microfibrillar protein(s) and has an affinity for anionic stains. It consists predominantly of non-polar amino-acids, including approximately 33% glycine, 35–40% alanine plus valine, 12% proline and 1% hydroxyproline, which are present in unique sequences resulting in a β-spiral structure that is responsible for the rubber-like elasticity of elastin. No sulphur-containing amino-acid is present.[292-294]

Elastin is first synthesized as a soluble precursor of M_r 70–72 000, called tropoelastin, of which there are two forms — tropoelastin a and b. Whether they are initially secreted as a higher molecular weight proelastin analogous to procollagen has not been established.[295,296]

Insoluble elastin is formed extracellularly from tropoelastin monomers by a unique cross-linking mechanism, involving the oxidation of specific lysine residues by an enzyme lysyl oxidase, followed by the condensation of four oxidized residues to form the stable cross-links desmosine and isodesmosine.[297,89] Recent evidence suggests that the lysyl oxidase enzymes involved in collagen and elastin cross-linking may be different.[298] Once cross-linked, elastin is extremely resistant to both chemical and proteolytic degradation and can only be broken down in vivo by specific enzymes known as the elastases.

Elastic fibres and related structures of the intervertebral disc

Early studies failed to observe elastic fibres in the intervertebral disc both by electron microscopy and by specific histochemical stains using light microscopy.[299,300] Buckwalter et al[301] studied the human disc from birth to 56 years by electron microscopy and found elastic fibres in both the annulus and nucleus. In the very young annulus only bundles of microfibrils were observed, but as the annulus matured, increasing amounts of amorphous elastin were deposited, these changes being typical of normal elastogenesis observed in the major elastic tissues.[282,287] The fibres were generally cylindrical and oriented parallel to the collagen fibres with which they were closely associated. In the nucleus pulposus, however, only mature but irregular-shaped elastic fibres were seen at all ages, with no specific orientation to the collagen fibres. Hickey & Hukins[302] have confirmed that normal elastogenesis occurs in the human annulus. Other ultrastructural studies have concluded that elastic fibres are concentrated mainly at the annulus/nucleus junction.[22]

Renewed studies using specific histochemical stains and light microscopy have revealed the presence of elastic fibres in all lamellae of the canine cervical annulus fibrosus.[303] However, in the human annulus the elastic fibres were restricted to the annular lamellae at the interface between the disc and vertebral epiphysis.[304] The detection of elastic fibres and related structures by both light and electron microscopy was facilitated by pretreating the tissue sections with hyaluronidase to remove the proteoglycans. After this treatment, oxytalan and elaunin fibres could be distinguished in both the trachael hyaline cartilage and the annulus fibrosus of the young rat.[305] In the hyaline cartilage oxytalan fibres surrounded the chondrocytes in the deep zones, elaunin fibres were found at the cartilage/perichondrium interface and mature elastic fibres were found only in the perichondrium. In the annulus fibrosus, oxytalan and elaunin fibres were found along the periphery of collagen bundles.

There has been only one report describing the isolation and characterization of elastin from the intervertebral disc: this was by Keith et al[306] who analysed elastin extracted from the bovine nucleus pulposus. This elastin had a slightly different amino-acid composition from that isolated from the nuchal ligament or aorta, but was similar to that from elastic cartilage. In particular, it contained less valine and desmosines, and the sulphur-containing amino-acid methionine was shown to be present. It was therefore suggested by these workers that the elastin from cartilage and disc may represent a new genetic type. However, ear cartilage has recently been shown to synthesize a tropoelastin which is both chemically and immunologically identical to that of other elastic tissues,[307] and it is possible that the material obtained by Keith and co-workers was not pure or had been partially degraded.

It seems that, although elastin is present in disc, the elastic properties of the intervertebral disc are due rather to the hydrostatic nature of the nucleus combined with the ability of the collagen fibres in the lamellae of the annulus to change their orientation. Elastic fibres may, however, play a role by helping the disc recover its shape after deformation. This may be particularly important as the disc, particularly the nucleus, becomes more fibrous with age and loses its normal elasticity.

Connective tissue degrading enzymes

Interstitial collagenases and gelatinases

A general property of the collagen molecule is the triple helical configuration and, although in some collagen types the triple helix is interrupted with globular sequences (see Table 5.2), no true collagen can exist unless it has some triple helical conformation within its molecule. The collagen triple helices are resistant to the majority of proteinases and this resistance confers a great deal of stability on the molecule. However, in 1962 Gross & Lapiere[308] isolated an enzyme from the culture fluids of explants of metamorphosing tadpole tails which was capable of cleaving the native collagen helix of type I collagen. Subsequently enzymes with identical properties to the tadpole enzyme have been found in mesenchymal cells, epithelial cells and in polymorphonuclear leucocytes.[309,70] These enzymes, which are now known to be able to cleave types I, II and III collagens in the same manner, are generally referred to as the classical collagenases (E.C.3.4.24.7) or interstitial collagenases.[310] They are all metalloproteinases with an optimal pH similar to that of tissue fluids and blood. Although they all have an abolute requirement for calcium, other metals such as zinc are also needed for their catalytic function.

Classical collagenases cleave the native collagen helix at one single locus which is approximately three-quarters of the way along the molecule from the amino-terminal end. The resulting two fragments, a three-quarter fragment and a quarter fragment, denature at lower temperatures than the whole molecule. Since these melting temperatures are well below 37°C, the fragments form gelatins and can be degraded by a group of neutral proteolytic enzymes called gelatinases as well as by many other neutral proteinases.

The classical collagenases exert different activities towards types I, II and III collagens, and there is a relationship between the tissue source of the enzyme and its affinity for particular substrate collagens. However, whatever the tissue source, they are always less active against type II collagen than against types I and III collagens. It follows that the minor collagens of cartilage and disc, such as $[1\alpha2\alpha3\alpha]$ collagen and type IX collagen, are resistant to interstitial collagenase,[311] although a recent report has indicated that they are able to cleave type X collagen.[312]

Inhibitors of interstitial collagenase

The interstitial collagenases are secreted from the cells in an inactive or latent form and are laid down together with collagen fibres in either the latent form or as an enzyme inhibitor complex.[313] It is clear that all connective tissues synthesize inhibitors of collagenase. Cartilage, however, appears to be a particularly rich source of inhibitor. The first of these to be characterized was a cationic protein of M_r 11 000 from bovine articular cartilage.[314] Another inhibitor of metalloproteinases has been extracted from tissue culture medium conditioned by human synovial cells and cartilage explants.[315,316] This latter inhibitor, known as 'TIMP' (tissue inhibitor of metalloproteinases), is probably identical to a serum collagenase inhibitor.[317] It is a very stable protein, and this may be because of the large number of disulphide bonds present in the molecule.[318]

Collagen fibre bundles are themselves much more resistant to attack by collagenolytic enzymes than the soluble forms of collagen and, once cross-linked into insoluble polymers, collagen is very resistant to attack by collagenases.[310,319,320]

Elastase

Elastase, a neutral proteinase originally thought to be specific for elastin but now known to be capable of degrading many other connective tissue proteins, is able to break down the cross-linking areas of the collagen fibre and de-polymerize it.[321] It is also able to degrade proteoglycan.[322,323]

Proteoglycanases

Cultured tissue slices from immature rabbit articular cartilage have been shown to release, among other enzymes, a metalloproteinase capable of degrading proteoglycan at neutral pH.[324] Similar enzymes have been described in human cartilage.[325,326]

New collagenases

A new group of vertebrate collagenases is now being described which are capable of degrading types IV and V collagen.[327,328] The type V degrading enzyme, which like the interstitial collagenases is a metalloproteinase, has been extracted from culture medium of M50–76 murine reticulum cell sarcoma cells and has been shown to be capable of degrading the $1\alpha 2\alpha$ and 3α cartilage collagens, as well as type V collagen, and is also able to degrade type IX collagen.[329]

Enzymes of the intervertebral disc

There have been very few studies on the enzymes of the intervertebral disc. Sedowofia et al[323] reported the extraction of a group of collagenolytic enzymes from human intervertebral discs which included collagenase of the classical interstitial type, elastase and gelatinases. These three enzymes constitute a complete collagenolytic system, and it was pointed out that the human intervertebral disc contained enzymes capable of degrading the extracellular macromolecular matrix of the disc. Recently, Sedowofia & Weiss[330] have shown that the disc elastase, whilst not degrading type I collagen, was able to degrade partially type II and type IX collagen and completely degrade $[1\alpha 2\alpha 3\alpha]$ collagen. It is reasonable to surmise from these observations that the type I collagen synthesized during disc degeneration may be a defence against degradation by this elastinolytic enzyme. In the past the disc has generally been considered to be metabolically relatively inert; however, it is becoming more and more obvious that this is not the case and it is quite possible that activation of the enzymes capable of degrading the individual components of connective tissue could result in an altered composition of the disc, which may be very relevant to disc degenerative diseases and to age degenerative changes. However, although these enzymes have been found in the intervertebral disc, it should be pointed out that studies on chondrocytes themselves have shown that, although they do produce the collagenolytic enzymes described above, the amount of enzyme that they produce is remarkably small when compared to either synovial cells or fibroblasts. The amount of actual collagenase produced by chondrocytes is approximately 3% of that obtained from fibroblasts.[313]

Recently, a group of subjects with severe chronic back pain have been studied for the fibrinolytic activity in their blood, and shown to have evidence of defective fibrinolysis,[331] and the authors suggest that a deficiency of the enzymes capable of degrading fibrin or an excess of the inhibitors of these enzymes may account for persistent severe back pain. Plasmin, which is the enzyme which degrades fibrin, has not been looked for in the intervertebral disc, neither have plasminogen activators nor inhibitors of the plasminogen system such as $\alpha2$ macroglobulin and $\alpha2$ antiplasmin. Plasmin is known to be involved in connective tissue degradation, since not only is it able to activate latent collagenolytic enzymes[70,313] (Fig. 5.2), but it is also capable of cleaving type V collagen and probably $[1\alpha2\alpha3\alpha]$ collagen.[332] Paradoxically, we do not yet know whether an increase in levels of collagenolytic enzymes is advantageous or disadvantageous to the wellbeing of the intervertebral disc.

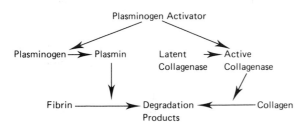

Fig. 5.2 Possible relationship between fibrinolysis and the degradation of collagen

AGE CHANGES, DEGENERATION AND DISEASE

The normal morphology and biochemistry of the intervertebral disc undergo changes during maturation and ageing processes. These natural phenomena differ from grossly exaggerated morphological changes observed in degenerative disc disease and also from the biochemical alterations, although these latter are apparently more subtle.

Whether the changes observed in disease are cause or effect has never been satisfactorily determined.

Age changes

Maturation

The neonatal disc shows the same basic morphological characteristics as the mature disc, except that the annulus fibrosus is completely distinguishable from the hydrated gelatinous nucleus pulposus. The collagen fibres of the annulus may become coarse during maturation, but the degree of hydration of the annulus itself remains unchanged (see Table 5.1). In contrast, the level of hydration in the nucleus decreases slightly during the first 20 years, and the annulus and nucleus begin to mesh with each other. During maturation the ratio of type II to type I collagen in the annulus increases slightly[189,187] and the immature 'reducible' cross-links are gradually replaced by more stable hydroxypyridinium cross-links, these being particularly pronounced in types II and IX collagens.[190,191] The amount of collagen in the annulus of individual discs increases progressively down the spine[228] and the collagen in the discs of the lower lumbar spine has the largest number of stable cross-links.[188]

Ageing

The number of cells in the cartilage end-plate, annulus fibrosus and nucleus pulposus increases slightly with age (Table 5.1), suggesting that they play an active role in the synthesis and degradation of the extracellular matrix throughout life. However, not all cells may be equally active, as many appear to be necrotic.[21,22] Both quantitative and qualitative changes in the extracellular matrix macromolecules occur with age, and this must be due to an alteration in cellular activity. The quantitative changes have already been described (Table 5.1). The nucleus pulposus gradually becomes more fibrous as the amount of proteoglycans and accompanying water decreases and the proportion of non-collagenous proteins increases. The demarcation between the annulus and nucleus becomes less distinct and the two regions gradually merge completely. The disc also becomes discoloured due to a brown 'age pigment', lipofuscin, which is believed to originate from the slow peroxidation of lipids.[333] Lipofuscin is more concentrated in the nucleus than in the annulus.[333]

No apparent change in either the total collagen content (Table 5.1) or ratio of type I to II collagen[187] occurs after maturity. The relative amounts of the minor $[1\alpha2\alpha3\alpha]$ and type IX collagens which are also present in the adult disc have not been assessed at different ages, but it is possible that they may decrease on ageing, particularly in the end-plate, as has been observed in human articular cartilage.[334] It is generally believed that the desiccation of the disc (particularly nucleus pulposus) with increasing age is due to loss of proteoglycans, specifically those rich in chondroitin sulphate. The ratio of keratan sulphate to chondroitin sulphate increases with age[228,52,53] and this is seen more clearly in the less easily extracted or non-extractable proteoglycans.[228] The chondroitin-6-sulphate to chondroitin-4-sulphate ratio also increases with age, chondroitin-6-sulphate becoming the only isomer present in later life.[231,232]

Because, with age, proteoglycans have a smaller hydrodynamic size and show a decreased tendency to form stable aggregates with hyaluronic acid, they are more easily extracted from the tissue.[228] These age changes may result from increased proteolytic degradation of the same parent molecules or the preferential removal of one of two or more chemically distinct pools. Alternatively, the chondrocytes could synthesize a different cellular product on ageing. Recent studies by Plaas & Sandy[335] have shown that the percentage proteoglycan subunits present as link-stabilized aggregates, in cultures of rabbit articular chondrocytes, decreases with increasing time in culture, the synthesis of link protein being the limiting factor. Disc link protein is inherently less effective in stabilizing the aggregates than the cartilage protein.[241] This, together with a decrease in total amount of link protein synthesized in vivo in the ageing disc, could account for the diminished aggregation of the proteoglycans on ageing.

The proportion of non-collagenous protein increases remarkably with age (Table 5.1). However, it is not known whether this is due to a general increase in all types of proteins or whether specific proteins are selectively increased,or whether this merely reflects a diminution in synthesis of the other disc macromolecules.

Degeneration

It has been suggested that the high incidence of degenerative disease of the spine and other weight-bearing joints is a consequence of the inadequate adaptation by the axial and appendicular skeleton of humans on assuming an upright position.[260] Most human spines show signs of degenerative changes by the end of the third decade. However, in some spines degeneration occurs earlier, while in others no degenerative changes are observed even as late as the 6th decade. The physiochemical changes observed in degenerated discs, particularly with respect to proteoglycans, are similar to those found on normal ageing but are more pronounced.[228,52,55,336] However, most of these observations were made on *whole* discs which had been obtained as surgical or postmortem specimens *at a specific point in time* during degeneration. Neither sequential changes nor changes occurring at specific foci were therefore assessed. Some of these problems were overcome by the use of an animal model in which disc degeneration was induced in the rabbit by surgical disc herniation and the total and newly synthesized proteoglycans assessed by chemical analysis and radioactive labelling respectively.[337] The results of this study showed that the morphological changes paralleled those seen in human degenerated discs and correlated well with the decreased aggregating properties of the proteoglycans with hyaluronic acid. In particular there were two periods during the early course of degeneration when the ability of the proteoglycans to aggregate with hyaluronic acid was recovered. These times were correlated with (a) the original loss of nuclear material and (b) the proliferation of fibro-cartilaginous material respectively and suggested the operation of a repair mechanism. However, degeneration progressed rapidly in the later stages after injury.

Disc degeneration resembles osteoarthrosis in several respects, including the loss of proteoglycans,[338] the presence of smaller proteoglycan aggregates[339] and the attempt to repair tissue damage by an increased synthesis of new tissue. Type III collagen has recently been demonstrated in the outer annulus fibrosus of the human degenerated disc, both by its isolation and chemical characterization and by immunofluorescence studies.[340] This collagen also had a relatively high content of hydroxylysine which, although characteristic of embryonic or granulation tissue,[341] may simply reflect the tendency towards a higher hydroxylation observed in other disc collagens.

A reversion to the immature stage of hyaline cartilage synthesis has recently been demonstrated in specific regions of human osteo-arthrotic cartilage showing evidence of repair, with an increased synthesis of both the $[1\alpha 2\alpha 3\alpha]$ and type IX collagens compared to aged controls, which normally contains less of these minor collagens.[334] It would be interesting to ascertain whether the reparative regions of the intervertebral disc, particularly those of the cartilage end-plate, showed analogous changes during degeneration.

Synthesis of new collagen during disc degeneration was also observed by Herbert et al.[188] The new collagen was predominantly type I in both the annulus and nucleus and was rich in immature 'reducible' cross-links. This new collagen rather surprisingly was present in the disc above the degenerated one, and not in the degenerated disc itself. It was therefore suggested that the normal disc had compensated for the defective disc below by synthesizing type I collagen, which in general forms stronger fibrils than type II collagen. It is obvious that the degenerative process is unevenly distributed throughout the disc tissue, and hence different cellular mechanisms are expected in different regions. As described earlier, the nutritional status of the disc is extremely important, and inadequate nutrition may lead to impaired cell function and can be a contributing factor in degeneration.[34] The possible role of degradative enzymes in degeneration has already been discussed (p. 123).

Degenerated discs often calcify as mineral is deposited in clefts which appear in the annulus fibrosus and in the perilacunar regions around the chondrocytes of the cartilage end-plates.[19] These mineral deposits may accelerate degeneration by blocking the normal diffusion of nutrients.

Diseases of the intervertebral disc

Prolapse

The tears and fissures which are frequently observed in the tissues of the degenerated disc are more commonly present and more severe when there is also evidence of true disc prolapse of the nucleus pulposus through the posterior annulus into the spinal column or through the cartilage end-plate into the vertebral bone (end-plate lesions or Schmorl's nodes). The distribution of such end-plate lesions and also of annular tears and their relationship to disc degeneration has been extensively studied in the dorsolumbar spine.[342,343] Taylor & Akeson[260] have reviewed the biochemical changes in prolapsed disc and have proposed some hypothetical ideas as to the possible underlying abnormalities.

The presence of nerve fibres in the disc tissues rather than in the longitudinal ligaments has been the subject of some dispute.[344,345] Nerve fibres have been reported in the nucleus, but by one worker only,[346] whereas other workers have shown nerve fibres in the posterior area of the outer surface of the annulus.[344] A recent report by Yoshizawa et al[347] confirms the findings of nerve fibres in the outer half of the annulus but not in the nucleus pulposus. The axonal network in the ligaments and annulus had abundant free-lying terminals often arranged in complex branched formation. These findings suggest that partial herniation of nucleus pulposus into the outer half of annulus could produce pain. However, herniation of the nucleus pulposus into the spinal cord will also give rise to secondary inflammatory changes as the tissue is invaded by capillaries and is probably the major factor when the end-plates have been breached by Schmorl's nodes and the nucleus pulposus has come in contact with the immune system.

It has been suggested that chronic inflammation in degenerative disc disease is an auto-immune phenomenon, with antibodies directed against the 'foreign' components of the nucleus pulposus. A number of studies on patients with degenerative disc disease give credence to this hypothesis. In one study a cellular immune response, evaluated by a leucocyte migration-inhibition test, was observed in patients whose discs were considered to have become vascularized as compared to others which were contained within the annulus fibrosus and posterior longitudinal ligament.[348] In other studies significantly elevated levels of immunoglobulin M have been reported in patients with proven Schmorl's nodes.[349]

Scoliosis

Scoliosis, or lateral curvature of the spine, often develops during the adolescent growth phase in otherwise normal individuals and is called idiopathic. Idiopathic scoliosis is a familial disorder,[350] but its aetiology remains obscure. Although it is not believed to result from a generalized connective tissue disorder, several lines of evidence suggest that the metabolism of both collagens and proteoglycans in the scoliotic spine is abnormal. The extent of these abnormalities varies in the different regions of the affected discs. Most studies agree that the amount of collagens in nucleus pulposus is increased in idiopathic scoliosis.[351,232,352] However, this increase is only statistically significant for those discs at the apex of curvature.[351] In the case of the annulus fibrosus, the collagen content of the lateral half nearest the convex aspect of the scoliotic curve is generally higher than that from the segment nearest the concave aspect. This abnormal distribution is again found only in those discs encompassed by the curve.[351] More recent studies on the distribution of the major types I and II collagens across the annulus of the scoliotic spine have indicated an increase in the type I to type II collagen ratio in segments convex to the curvature but a decrease in the same ratio in the segment concave to the curvature.[353] Immuno-fluorescence studies have also shown an enhanced staining for type I collagen as well as the appearance of type III collagen, the latter being particularly apparent in the inner annulus when secondary scoliotic changes involving marked vascularization occur.[197]

Differences in the *extractability* of collagen from the nucleus and annulus of scoliotic spines compared with controls have also been observed, but these differences are apparently independent of location, convex or concave aspect, of the scoliosis.[351] The amount of newly synthesized collagen is significantly decreased for the nucleus, but not the annulus, of scoliotic discs. Conversely, the amount of insoluble collagen is only markedly decreased in the inner annulus and transition zone. These changes may be due to an increase in cross-linking of collagen or increased stability of the cross-links. However, it is more likely that they are a reflection of the increased type I collagen content of the disc.

The increased collagen content of the scoliotic nucleus pulposus is accompanied by a decrease in both sulphated and non-sulphated glycosamino-glycans, but the relative proportions of chondroitin sulphate, keratan sulphate and hyaluronic acid generally remain the same.[232] In some patients, however, the solubility and chromatographic behaviour of the sulphated glycosaminoglycans is abnormal and indicates a shorter chain length. It has been suggested that this is the result of excessive enzymatic degradation.[232] The glycosaminoglycans of the scoliotic annulus fibrosus are not significantly lower than in normal adolescents, except in patients with severe juvenile scoliosis.

Recent studies by Pedrini-Mille et al[354] have assessed the proportion of proteoglycan monomers and their aggregates in the nucleus pulposus, inner regions of the annulus fibrosus and end-plates of scoliotic spines. Both the nucleus and inner annulus contain normal amounts of aggregates and monomers, but the proportion of glycosaminoglycans in the nucleus was decreased, as previously observed.[232] In contrast, marked changes were observed in the cartilage end-plates. The growth-plate portion of the end-plate from the concave side disappeared, but the proteoglycans of the remaining hyaline cartilage were normal. The convex portion of the end-plate, although morphologically normal, contained virtually no proteoglycan aggregates and the non-aggregated proteoglycans were smaller than the proteoglycan subunits of normal tissue. Whether this is due to degradation and the alteration of the hyaluronic acid binding site of normal monomers or the synthesis of different proteoglycan species is not known. The absence of aggregates will be deleterious to the function of both hyaline and growth plate cartilages, since monomers do not adequately resist com-pression or control mineralization.[355]

Scoliosis often occurs secondary to several in-herited connective tissue disorders such as Ehlers-Danlos syndrome (particularly subtype VI) and Marfan's syndrome, or in association with cerebral palsy and paralysis resulting from poliomyelitis.[356] Specific biochemical defects have been identified in many of the inherited disorders. In Ehlers-Danlos syndrome sub-type VI the enzyme involved in lysine hydroxylation is deficient or absent, which results in defective intermolecular cross-linking of type I collagen in skin, bone and other tissues.[357,358] The type I collagen of the intervertebral disc is also abnormal, but the type II collagen is normal.[359] Similarly, Ihme et al[357] showed that no abnormal hydroxylation of type II collagen was observed in articular cartilage. This suggests that independent enzymes hydroxylate types I and II collagens in disc. It also suggests that the primary abnormality causing the scoliosis is in the annulus fibrosus and not in the nucleus.

CONCLUSION

Increased interest is being taken in studying the matrix components of the intervertebral disc and the enzymes responsible for their degradation. Nevertheless, it is obvious that we are still a long way from understanding the relationship between biochemical changes in the disc and back pain.

ACKNOWLEDGEMENTS

We would like to thank Mrs Sarah Lawrence for her excellent secretarial help and unfailing good humour.

REFERENCES

1   Hay E D 1968 Organisation and fine structure of epithelium and mesenchyme in the developing chick embryo. In: Fleischmajer R, Billingham R E (eds) Epithelial-mesenchymal interactions. Williams & Wilkins, Baltimore, p 31–55
2   Balinsky B I 1975 An introduction to embryology, 4th edn. Saunders, Philadelphia
3   Peacock A 1951 Observations on the pre-natal development of the intervertebral disc in man. J. Anat. 85: 260–274
4   Prader A 1947 Die fruchembryonal Entwicklung der menschlichen Zwischenwirbelscheibe. Acta Anat. 3: 68–83
5   Prader A 1974 Die Entwicklung der Zwischenwirbelscheibe beim menschlichen Keimling. Acta Anat. 3: 115–52
6   Walmsley R 1953 The development and growth of the intervertebral disc. Edinb. Med. J. 60: 341–364
7   Levitt D, Dorfman A 1974 Concepts and mechanisms of cartilage differentiation. Curr. Top. Devel. Biol. 8: 103–150
8   Stockwell R A 1979 Biology of cartilage cells. Cambridge University Press
9   Von der Mark K, Conrad G 1979 Cartilage cell differentiation. Clin. Orth. Rel. Res. 139: 185–205
10   Bancroft M, Bellairs R 1976 The development of the notochord in the chick embryo, studied by scanning and transmission electron microscopy. J. Embryol. Exp. Morph. 35: 383–401
11   Kosher R A, Lash J W 1975 Notochordal stimulation of in vitro somite chondrogenesis before and after enzymatic removal of perinotochordal materials. Devel. Biol. 42: 362–378
12   Linsenmayer T F, Trelstad R L, Gross J 1973 The collagen of chick embryonic notochord. Biochem. Biophys. Res. Commun. 53: 39–45
13   Kosher R A, Lash J W, Minor R R 1973 Environmental enhancement of in vitro chondrogenesis. IV stimulation of somite chondrogenesis by exogenous chondromucoprotein. Devel. Biol. 35: 210–220
14   Kosher R A, Church R L 1975 Stimulation of in vitro somite chondrogenesis by procollagen and collagen. Nature (London) 258: 327–330
15   Kosher R A, Savage M P 1979 The effect of collagen on the cyclic AMP content of embryonic somites. J. Exp. Zool. 208: 35–40
16   Adamson E D 1982 The effect of collagen on cell division, cellular differentiation and embryonic development. In: Weiss J B, Jayson M I V (eds) Collagen in health and disease. Churchill Livingstone, Edinburgh, p 218–243
17   Hukins D W L 1982 Biochemical properties of collagen. In: Weiss J B, Jayson M I V (eds) Collagen in health and disease. Churchill Livingstone, Edinburgh, ch 4
18   Maroudas A, Stockwell R A, Nachemson A, Urban J 1975 Factors involved in the nutrition of the human intervertebral disc: cellularity and diffusion of glucose in vitro. J. Anat. 120: 113–130
19   Pritzker K P H 1977. Ageing and degeneration in the lumbar intervertebral disc. Orthop. Clinic N. America 8: 65–77
20   Meachim G 1972 Meshwork patterns in the ground substance of articular cartilage and nucleus pulposus. J. Anat. III: 219–227
21   Meachim G, Cornah M S 1970 Fine structure of juvenile human nucleus pulposus. J. Anat. 107: 337–350
22   Sylvest J, Hentzer B, Kobayasi T 1977 Ultrastructure of prolapsed disc. Acta Orthop. Scand. 48: 32–40
23   Poole C A, Flint M H, Beaumont B W 1984 Morphological and functional inter-relationships of articular cartilage matrices. J. Anat. 138: 113–138
24   Bijlsma F, Copius Peereboom J W 1972 The ageing pattern of human intervertebral disc. Gerontologia 18: 157–168
25   Happey F, Pearson C H, Naylor A, Turner R L 1969 The ageing of the human intervertebral disc. Gerontologia 15: 174–188
26   Knese K-H 1978 Kristallisation und Auflosung von Kollagen Fibrillen während der Histogenese der Zwischenwerbelscheibe. Acta Anat. 100: 328–346
27   Mayne R, Von der Mark K 1983 Collagens of cartilage. In: Hall B K (ed) Cartilage, vol 1. Academic Press, New York, p 181–214
28   Dessau W, Sasse J, Timpl R, Jilek F, Von der Mark K 1978 Synthesis and extracellular deposition of fibronectin in chondrocyte cultures. Responses to the removal of extracellular cartilage matrix. J. Cell Biol. 79: 342–355
29   Von der Mark K, Gauss V, Von der Mark H, Muller P 1977 Relationship between cell shape and type of collagen synthesised as chondrocytes lose their cartilage phenotype in culture. Nature (London) 267: 531–532
30   Dessau W, Vertel B M, Von der Mark H, Von der Mark K 1981 Extracellular matrix formation by chondrocytes in monolayer culture. J. Cell Biol. 90: 78–83
31   Schilz J R, Mayne R, Holtzer H 1973 The synthesis of collagen and glycosaminoglycans by dedifferentiated chondroblasts in culture. Differentiation 1: 97–108
32   Mayne R, Elrod B W, Mayne P M, Sanderson R D, Linsenmayer T F 1984 Changes in the synthesis of minor cartilage collagens after growth of chick chondrocytes in 5-bromo-2^1-deoxyuridine or to senescence. Exp. Cell Res. 151: 171–182
33   Bohmig R 1930 Die Blutgefassversorgung der Wirbelandscheiben, das Verhalten des intervertebralen

Chordasegmente. Archiv für Klinische Chirurgie 158: 374–424

34 Nachemson A, Lewin T, Maroudas A, Freeman M A R 1970 In vitro diffusion of dye through the end-plates and the annulus fibrosus of human lumbar intervertebral discs. Acta Orthop. Scand. 41: 589–607

35 Brodin H 1955 Paths of nutrition in articular cartilage and intervertebral discs. Acta Orthop. Scand. 24: 177–183

36 Urban J P G, Holm S, Maroudas A, Nachemson A 1977 Nutrition of the intervertebral disc. An in vivo study of solute transport. Clin. Orthop. Relat. Res. 129: 101–114

37 Bywaters E G L 1973 The metabolism of joint tissues. J. Pathol. Bacteriol. 44: 247–268

38 Lane L M, Brighton C T, Menkowitz B, Cochran W, Robinson M A 1976 Aerobic vs anaerobic metabolism of articular cartilage. American Orthopaedics Research Society 22nd Meeting, New Orleans (abstr), p 90

39 Holm S, Maroudas A, Urban J P G, Selstam G, Nachemson A 1981 Nutrition of the intervertebral disc: solute transport and metabolism. Connect. Tissue Res. 8: 101–119

40 Hansen H J, Ullberg S 1960 Uptake of S^{35} in the intervertebral discs after injection of S^{35}-sulphate. An autoradiographic study. Acta Orthop. Scand. 30: 84–90

41 Souter W A, Taylor T K F 1970 Sulphated acid mucopolysaccharide metabolism in the rabbit intervertebral disc. J. Bone Jt. Surg. 52B: 371–384

42 Szirmai J A 1970 Structure of the intervertebral disc. In: Balazs E A (ed) Chemistry and molecular biology of the intercellular matrix, vol 3. Academic Press, New York, p 1279–1308

43 Happey F 1976 A biophysical study of the human intervertebral disc. In: Jayson M I V (ed) The lumbar spine and back pain, 1st edn. Pitman Medical, Tunbridge Wells, p 293–316

44 Happey F 1980 Studies of the structure of the human intervertebral disc in relation to its function and ageing processes. In: Sokoloff L (ed) The joints and synovial fluid, vol II. Academic Press, New York, p 95–137

45 Inoue H, Takeda T 1975 Three-dimensional observation of collagen framework of lumbar intervertebral discs. Acta Orthop. Scand. 46: 949–956

46 Happey F 1973 A study of the changes in collagen and allied polysaccharides and proteins in ageing of the human intervertebral disc. J. Polymer Sci. Symposium 42: 1481–1492

47 Buckwalter J A, Maynard J A, Cooper R R 1978 Sheathing of collagen fibrils in human intervertebral discs. J. Anat. 125: 615–618

48 Marchini M, Strocch R, Castellani P P, Riva R 1979 Ultrastructural observations on collagen and proteoglycans in the annulus fibrosus of the intervertebral disc. Basic and Applied Histochem. 23: 137–148

49 Sylven B, Paulson S, Hirsch C, Snellman O 1951 Biophysical and physiological investigations on cartilage and other mesenchymal tissues: II the ultrastructure of bovine and human nuclei pulposi. J. Bone Jt. Surg. 33A: 333–340

50 Buckwalter J A, Maynard J A, Cooper R R 1979 Banded structures in human nucleus pulposus. Clin. Orthop. Rel. Res. 139: 259–266

51 Cornah M S, Meachim G, Parry E W 1970 Banded

52 Gower W E, Pedrini V 1969 Age-related variations in protein polysaccharides from human nucleus pulposus, annulus fibrosus and costal cartilage. J. Bone Jt. Surg. 51A: 1154–1162

53 Hallen A 1962 The collagen and ground substance of human intervertebral disc at different ages. Acta Chim. Scand. 16: 705–710

54 Hirsch C, Nachemson A 1954 New observations on mechanical behaviour of lumbar discs. Acta Orthop. Scand. 23: 254–283

55 Hirsch C, Paulson S, Sylven B, Snellman O 1952 Biophysical and physiological investigations on cartilage and other mesenchymal tissues. Acta Orthop. Scand. 22: 175–181

56 Venn M, Maroudas A 1977 Chemical composition and swelling of normal and osteoarthrotic femoral head cartilage. I. chemical composition. Ann. Rheum. Dis. 36: 121–129

57 Sewell A C, Pennock C A 1976 The chemistry of human neonatal femoral epiphysial cartilage. Clin. Chim. Acta 68: 123–126

58 Adams P, Eyre D R, Muir H 1977 Biochemical aspects of development and ageing of human lumbar intervertebral discs. Rheum. Rehab. 16: 22–29

59 Dickson I R, Happey F, Pearson C H, Naylor A, Turner R L 1967 Variations in the protein components of human intervertebral disc with age. Nature (London) 215: 52–53

60 Uitto J 1979 Collagen polymorphism. Isolation and partial characterisation of $\alpha 1(I)$ trimer molecules in normal human skin. Arch. Biochem. Biophys. 192: 371–379

61 Bentz H, Morris N P, Murray L W, Sakai L Y, Hollister D W, Burgeson R E 1983 Isolation and partial characterisation of a new human collagen with an extended triple-helical structural domain. Proc. Nat. Acad. Sci. USA 80: 3168–3172

62 Sage H, Trueb B, Bornstein P 1983 Biosynthesis and structural properties of endothelial cell type VIII collagen. J. Biol. Chem. 258: 13391–13401

63 Fietzek P P, Kuhn K 1976 The primary structure of collagen. Int. Rev. Connect. Tissue. Res. 7: 1–60

64 Piez K A 1976 Primary structure. In: Ramachandran G N, Reddi A H (eds) Biochemistry of collagen. Plenum Press, New York, p 1–44

65 Ramachandran G N, Ramakrishnan C 1976 Molecular structure. In: Ramachandran G N, Reddi A H (eds) Biochemistry of collagen. Plenum Press, New York, p 45–84

66 Bansal M, Ramakrishnan C, Ramachandran G N 1975 Stabilisation of the collagen structure by hydroxyproline residues. Proc. of the Indian Academy of Sciences, Section A82: 152–164

67 Ramachandran G N, Bansal M, Ramakrishnan C 1975 Hydroxyproline stabilises both intra-fibrillar structure as well as inter-protofibrillar linkages in collagen. Current Science 44: 1–3

68 Bornstein P, Sage H 1980 Structurally distinct collagen types. Annual Review of Biochemistry 49: 957–1003

69 Miller E J, Gay S 1982 Collagen: an overview. In: Colowick S P, Kaplan O (eds) Methods in enzymology, vol 82A. Academic Press, New York, p 3–32

70 Weiss J B 1984 Collagens and collagenolytic enzymes.

In: Hukins D W L (ed) Connective tissue matrix. Macmillan, London, p 17–54

71   Weiss J B, Ayad S 1982 An introduction to collagen. In: Weiss J B, Jayson M I V (eds) Collagen in health and disease. Churchill Livingstone, Edinburgh, p 1–17

72   Miller E J, Matukas V J 1969 Chick cartilage collagen. A new type of $\alpha 1$ chain not present in bone or skin of the species. Proc. Nat. Acad. Sci. USA 65: 1264–1268

73   Miller E J, Epstein E H, Piez K A 1971 Identification of three genetically distinct collagens by cyanogen bromide cleavage of insoluble human skin and cartilage collagen. Biochem. Biophys. Res. Commun. 42: 1024–1029

74   Kuhn K, Glanville R W 1980 Molecular structure and higher organization of different collagen types. In: Viidik A, Vuust J (eds) Biology of collagen. Academic Press, New York, p 1–14

75   Miller E J 1976 Biochemical characteristics and biological significance of the genetically distinct collagens. Mol. Cell. Biochem. 13: 165–192

76   Schneir M, Miller E J 1976 Studies on the sulphydryl groups in type III collagen. Biochim. Biophys. Acta 446: 240–244

77   Walter P, Gilmore R, Blobel G 1984 Protein translocation across the endoplasmic reticulum. Cell 38: 5–8

78   Kivirikko K I, Myllyla R 1982 Post-translational modifications. In: Weiss J B, Jayson M I V (eds) Collagen in health and disease. Churchill Livingstone, Edinburgh, p 101–120

79   Kivirikko K I, Myllyla R 1979 Collagen glycosyl transferases. Int. Rev. Connect. Tissue Res. 8: 23–72

80   Brandt A, Glanville R W, Horlein D, Bruckner P, Timpl R, Fietzek P P, Kuhn K 1984 Complete amino acid sequence of the N-terminal extension of calf skin type III collagen. Biochem. J. 219: 625–634

81   Curran S, Prockop D J 1982 Isolation and partial characterisation of the amino-terminal propeptide of type II procollagen from chick embryos. Biochemistry 21: 1482–1487

82   Galloway D 1982 The primary structure of collagen. In: Weiss J B, Jayson M I V (eds) Collagen in health and disease. Churchill Livingstone, Edinburgh, p 528–557

83   Horlein D, Fietzek P, Wachter E, Lapiere C M, Kuhn K 1979 Amino acid sequence of the amino terminal segment of dermatosparactic calf skin procollagen type I. Eur. J. Biochem. 99: 31–38

84   Kuhn K 1984 Structural and functional domains of collagen: a comparison of the protein with its gene. Collagen Rel. Res. 4: 309–322

85   Hayashi F, Curran-Patel S, Prockop D J 1979 Thermal stability of the triple helix of type I procollagen and collagen. Precautions for minimizing ultraviolet damage to proteins during circular dichroism studies. Biochemistry 18: 4182–4187

86   Trelstad R L, Hayashi K 1979 Tendon collagen fibrillogenesis: intracellular subassemblies and cell surface changes associated with fibril growth. Devel. Biol. 71: 228–242

87   Paglia L, Wilczek J, de Leon L D, Martin G R, Horlein D, Muller P 1979 Inhibition of procollagen cell-free synthesis by amino terminal extension peptides. Biochemistry 18: 5030–5034

88   Light N D, Bailey A J 1980 Molecular structure and stabilization of the collagen fibre. In: Viidik A, Vuust J (eds) Biology of collagen. Academic Press, New York, p 15–38

89   Siegel R C 1979 Lysyl oxidase. Int. Rev. Connect. Tissue Res. 8: 73–118

90   Robins S P 1982 Turnover and crosslinking of collagen. In: Weiss J B, Jayson M I V (eds) Collagen in health and disease. Churchill Livingstone, Edinburgh, p 160–178

91   Grant M E, Freeman I L, Schofield J D, Jackson D S 1969 Variations in the carbohydrate content of human and bovine polymeric collagens from various tissues. Biochim. Biophys. Acta 177: 682–685

92   Obrink B, Laurent T C, Carlsson B 1975 The binding of chondroitin sulphate to collagen. FEBS Letters 56: 166–169

93   Scott J E 1984 The periphery of the developing collagen fibril. Quantitative relationships with dermatan sulphate and other surface-associated species. Biochem. J. 218: 229–233

94   Fleischmajer R, Olsen B R, Timpl R, Perlish J S, Lovelace O 1983 Collagen fibril formation during embryogenesis. Proc. Nat. Acad. Sci. USA 80: 3354–3358

95   Hulmes D J S 1983 A possible mechanism for the regulation of collagen fibril diameter in vivo. Collagen Rel. Res. 3: 317–321

96   Heathcote J G, Bailey A J, Grant M E 1980 Studies on the assembly of rat lens capsule. Biosynthesis of a cross-linked collagenous component of high molecular weight. Biochem. J. 190: 229–237

97   Heathcote J G, Sear C H, Grant M E 1978 Studies on the assembly of rat lens capsule. Biosynthesis and partial characterisation of the collagenous components. Biochem. J. 176: 283–294

98   Tryggvason K, Gehron-Robey P, Martin G R 1980 Biosynthesis of type IV procollagens. Biochemistry 19: 1284–1289

99   Grant M E, Heathcote J G 1981 The molecular organization of basement membranes. Int. Rev. Connect. Tissue Res. 9: 191–264

100   Timpl R, Wiedemann H, Van Delden V, Furthmayr H, Kuhn K 1981 A network model for the organisation of type IV collagen molecules in basement membranes. Eur. J. Biochem. 120: 203–211

101   Weber S, Engel J, Wiedemann H, Glanville R W, Timpl R 1984 Sub-unit structure and assembly of the globular domain of basement-membrane collagen type IV. Eur. J. Biochem. 139: 401–410

102   Bailey A J, Sims T J, Light N 1984 Cross-linking in type IV collagen. Biochem. J. 218: 713–723

103   Kuhn K, Wiedemann N H, Timpl R, Risteli J, Dieringer H, Voss T, Glanville R W 1981 Macromolecular structure of basement membrane collagens. Identification of 7S collagen as a crosslinking domain of type IV collagen. FEBS Letters 125: 123–128

104   Schuppan D, Timpl R, Glanville R W 1980 Discontinuities in the triple helical sequence Gly-X-Y of basement membrane (type IV) collagen. FEBS Letters 115: 297–300

105   Hofman H, Voss T, Kuhn K, Engel J 1984 Localization of flexible sites in thread-like molecules from electron micrographs. Comparison of interstitial, basement membrane and intima collagens. J. Mol. Biol.

172: 325–343

106 Taylor C M, Grant M E 1985 Assembly of chick and bovine lens capsule collagen. Biochem. J. 226: 527–536

107 Trueb B, Grobil B, Spiess M, Odermatt B F, Winterhalter K H 1982 Basement membrane (type IV) collagen is a heteropolymer. J. Biol. Chem. 257: 5239–5245

108 Epstein E H 1974 [α1(III)]₃ human skin collagen. Release by pepsin digestion and preponderance in fetal life. J. Biol. Chem. 249: 3225–3231

109 Ayad S, Evans H B, Holt P J L, Weiss J B 1984 Type VI collagen but not type V collagen is present in cartilage. Coll. Rel. Res. 4: 165–168

110 Von der Mark K, Ocalan M 1982 Immunofluorescent localization of type V collagen in chick embryo with monoclonal antibodies. Coll. Rel. Res. 2: 541–555

111 Gay S, Rhodes R K, Gay R, Miller E J 1981 Collagen molecules comprised of α1(V)-chains (B chains): an apparent localization in the exocytoskeleton. Collagen Rel. Res. 1: 53–58

112 Rhodes R K, Miller E J 1978 Physical characterisation and molecular organisation of collagen A and B chains. Biochemistry 17: 3442–3448

113 Gay S, Martinez-Hernandez A, Rhodes R K, Miller E J 1981 The collagenous exocytoskeleton of smooth muscle cells. Collagen Rel. Res. 1: 377–384

114 Sano J, Fujiwara S, Sato S, Ishizaki M, Sugisaki Y, Yajima G, Nagai Y 1981 AB (type V) and basement membrane (type IV) collagens in the bovine lung parenchyma: electron microscopic localization by the peroxidase-labelled antibody method. Biomed. Res. 2: 20–29

115 Haralson M A, Mitchell W M, Rhodes R K, Kresina T F, Gay R, Miller E J 1980 Chinese hamster lung cells synthesize and confine to the cellular domain a collagen composed solely of B chains. Proc. Nat. Acad. Sci. USA 77: 5206–5210

116 Sage H, Pritzl P, Bornstein P 1981 Characterisation of cell matrix associated collagens synthesised by aortic endothelial cells in culture. Biochemistry 20: 436–442

117 Gay S, Gay R, Miller E J 1980 The collagens of the joint. Arth. Rheum. 23: 937–941

118 Martinez-Hernandez A, Gay S, Miller E J 1982 Ultrastructural localization of type V collagen in rat kidney. J. Cell Biol. 92: 343–349

119 Burgeson R E, El Adli F A, Kaitila I I, Hollister D W 1976 Fetal membrane collagens: identification of two new collagen alpha chains. Proc. Nat. Acad. Sci. USA 73: 2579–2583

120 Chung E, Rhodes R K, Miller E J 1976 Isolation of three collagenous components of probable basement membrane origin from several tissues. Biochem. Biophys. Res. Commun. 71: 1167–1174

121 Abedin M Z, Ayad S, Weiss J B 1981 Type V collagen: the presence of appreciable amounts of α3(V) chain in uterus. Biochem. Biophys. Res. Commun. 102: 1237–1245

122 Abedin M Z, Ayad S, Weiss J B 1982 Isolation and native characterization of cysteine-rich collagens from bovine placental tissues and uterus and their relationship to types IV and V collagens. Biosci. Rep. 2: 493–502

123 Browns R A, Shuttleworth C A, Weiss J B 1978 Three new alpha chains of collagen from a non-basement membrane source. Biochem. Biophys. Res. Commun.

80: 866–872

124 Sage H, Bornstein P 1979 Characterisation of a novel collagen chain in human placenta and its relation to AB collagen. Biochemistry 18: 3815–3822

125 Bentz H, Bachinger H P, Glanville R, Kuhn K 1978 Physical evidence for the assembly of A and B chains in human placental collagen in a single triple helix. Eur. J. Biochem. 92: 563–569

126 Rhodes R K, Miller E J 1981 Evidence for the existence of an α1(V)α2(V)α3(V) collagen molecule in human placental tissue. Collagen Rel. Res. 1: 337–343

127 Fessler L I, Robinson W J, Fessler J H 1981 Biosynthesis of procollagen [(proα1 V)₂ (proα2 V)] by chick tendon fibroblasts and procollagen (proα1 V)₃ by hamster lung cell cultures. J. Biol. Chem. 256: 9646–9651

128 Fessler L I, Kumamoto C A, Meis M E, Fessler J M 1981 Assembly and processing of procollagen V (AB) in chick blood vessels and other tissues. J. Biol. Chem. 256: 9640–9645

129 Kumamoto C A, Fessler J H 1981 Propeptides of procollagen V (A,B) in chick embryo crop. J. Biol. Chem. 256: 7053–7058

130 Chiang T M, Mainardi C L, Seyer J M, Kang A H 1980 Collagen platelet interaction. Type V (AB) collagen induces platelet aggregation. J. Lab. Clin. Med. 95: 99–107

131 Weiss J B Personal observations

132 Chambers C A, Shuttleworth C A, Ayad S, Grant M E 1984 Collagen heterogeneity and quantification in developing bovine nuchal ligament. Biochem. J. 220: 385–394

133 Furuto D K, Miller E J 1980 Isolation of a unique collagenous fraction from limited pepsin digests of human placental tissue. J. Biol. Chem. 255: 290–295

134 Furuto D K, Miller E J 1981 Characterisation of a unique collagenous fraction from limited pepsin digests of human placental tissue: molecular organisation of the native aggregate. Biochemistry 20: 1635–1640

135 Jander R, Rauterberg J, Glanville R W 1983 Further characterization of the three polypeptide chains of bovine and human short-chain collagen (intima collagen). Eur. J. Biochem. 133: 39–46

136 Jander R, Rauterberg J, Voss B, von Bassewitz D B 1981 A cysteine-rich collagenous protein from bovine placenta. Isolation of its constituent polypeptide chains and some properties of the non-denatured protein. Eur. J. Biochem. 114: 17–25

137 Laurain G, Delvincourt T, Szymanowicz A G 1980 Isolation of a macromolecular fraction and AB₂ collagen from calf skin. FEBS Letters 120: 44–48

138 Odermatt E, Risteli J, Van Delden V, Timpl R 1983 Structural diversity and domain composition of a unique collagenous fragment (intima collagen) obtained from human placenta. Biochem. J. 211: 295–303

139 Rojkind M, Giambrone M-A, Biempica L 1979 Collagen types in normal and cirrhotic liver. Gastroenterology 76: 710–719

140 Furthmayr H, Wiedemann H, Timpl R, Odermatt E, Engel J 1983 Electron-microscopical approach to a structural model of intima collagen. Biochem. J. 211: 303–311

141 Ayad S, Shuttleworth C A, Grant M E 1984 Isolation of a type VI collagen precursor from bovine elastic tissue. Biochem. Soc. Trans. 12: 1052–1053

142 Heller-Harrison R A, Carter W G 1984 Pepsin-generated type VI collagen is a degradation product of GP140. J. Biol. Chem. 259: 6858–6864

143 Hessle H, Engvall E 1984 Type VI collagen. Studies on its localization, structure and biosynthetic form with monoclonal antibodies. J. Biol. Chem. 259: 3955–3961

144 Jander R, Troyer D, Rauterberg J 1984 A collagen-like glycoprotein of the extracellular matrix is the undegraded form of type VI collagen. Biochemistry 23: 3675–3680

145 Knight K R, Ayad S, Shuttleworth C A, Grant M E 1984 A collagenous glycoprotein found in dissociative extracts of foetal bovine nuchal ligament. Evidence for a relationship with type VI collagen. Biochem J. 220: 395–403

146 Trueb B, Bornstein P 1984 Characterization of the precursor form of type VI collagen. J. Biol. Chem. 259: 8597–8604

147 Von der Mark K, Aumailley M, Wick G, Fleischmajer R, Timpl R 1984 Immunochemistry, genuine size and tissue localisation of collagen VI. Eur. J. Biochem. 142: 493–502

148 Burgeson R E, Hollister D W 1979 Collagen heterogeneity in human cartilage: indentification of several new collagen chains. Biochem. Biophys. Res. Commun. 87: 1124–1131

149 Burgeson R E, Hebda P A, Morris N P, Hollister D W 1982 Human cartilage collagens. Comparison of cartilage collagens with human type V collagen. J. Biol. Chem. 257: 7852–7856

150 Ayad S, Weiss J B 1984 A new look at vitreous humour collagen. Biochem. J. 218: 835–840

151 Smith G N, Williams J M, Brandt K D 1985 Interaction of proteoglycans with pericellular $(1\alpha,2\alpha,3\alpha)$ collagens of cartilage. J. Biol. Chem. 260: 10761–10767

152 Evans H B, Ayad S, Abedin M Z, Hopkins S, Morgan K, Walton K W, Weiss J B, Holt P J L 1983 Localisation of collagen types and fibronectin in cartilage by immunofluorescence. Ann. Rheum. Dis. 42: 575–581

153 Weiss J B, Ayad S Unpublished observations

154 Ayad S, Abedin M Z, Grundy S, Weiss J B 1981 Isolation and characterisation of an unusual collagen from hyaline cartilage and intervertebral disc. FEBS Letters 123: 195–199

155 Ayad S, Abedin M Z, Weiss J B, Grundy S M 1982 Characterisation of another short-chain disulphide-bonded collagen from cartilage, vitreous and intervertebral disc. FEBS Letters 139: 300–304

156 Reese C A, Mayne R 1981 Minor collagens of chicken hyaline cartilage. Biochemistry 20: 5443–5448

157 Reese C A, Wiedemann H, Kuhn K, Mayne R 1982 Characterisation of a highly soluble collagenous molecule isolated from chicken hyaline cartilage. Biochemistry 21: 826–830

158 Ricard-Blum S, Hartman D J, Herbage D, Payen-Meyran C, Ville G 1982 Biochemical properties and immunolocalization of minor collagens in foetal calf cartilage. FEBS Letters 146: 343–347

159 Shimokomaki M, Duance V C, Bailey A J 1980 Identification of a new disulphide bonded collagen from cartilage. FEBS Letters 121: 51–54

160 Shimokomaki M, Duance V C, Bailey A J 1981 Identification of two further collagenous fractions from articular cartilage. Biosci. Rep. 1: 561–570

161 Mayne R, Van der Rest M, Weaver D C, Butler W T 1985 The structure of a small collagenous fragment isolated from chicken hyaline cartilage. J. Cell. Biochem. 27: 133–141

162 Von der Mark K, Van Menxel M, Wiedemann H 1982 Isolation and characterization of new collagens from chick cartilage. Eur. J. Biochem. 124: 57–62

163 Ayad S, Weiss J B Unpublished results

164 Bruckner P, Mayne R, Tuderman L 1983 p-HMW-collagen, a minor collagen obtained from chick embryo cartilage without proteolytic treatment of the tissue. Eur. J. Biochem. 136: 333–339

165 Gibson G J, Kielty C M, Garner C, Schor S L, Grant M E 1983 Identification and partial characterisation of 3 low molecular weight collagenous polypeptides synthesised by chondrocytes cultured within collagen gels in the absence and presence of fibronectin. Biochem. J. 211: 417–426

166 Von der Mark K, Van Menxel M, Wiedemann H 1984 Isolation and characterization of precursor form of M collagen from embryonic chicken cartilage. Eur. J. Biochem. 138: 629–633

167 Ninomiya Y, Olsen B R 1984 Synthesis and characterization of cDNA encoding a cartilage-specific short collagen. Proc. Nat. Acad. Sci. USA 81: 3014–3018

168 Grant M E, Kielty C M, Kwan A P L, Holmes D F, Schor S L 1986 Partial characterization of collagen types IX and X synthesized by embryonic chick chondrocytes. Ann. NY Acad. Sci. in press

169 Mayne R, Van der Rest M, Ninomiya Y, Olsen B R 1984 Structure of type IX collagen. Abstract NY Academy of Sciences, 17–19 Oct, NY, USA

170 Duance V C, Shimokomaki M, Bailey A J 1982 Immunofluorescence localisation of type M collagen in articular cartilage. Biosci. Rep. 2: 223–227

171 Hartman D J, Maglioire H, Ricard-Blum S, Joffre A, Couble M-L, Ville G, Herbage D 1983 Light and electron immunoperoxidase localization of minor disulphide-bonded collagens in fetal calf epiphysial cartilage. Collagen Rel. Res. 3: 349–357

172 Olsen B R, Ninomiya Y, Lozano G, Konomi H, Gordon M et al 1984 Short chain collagen genes and their expression in cartilage. Abstr. No 11, NY Acad. Sci. 17–19 Oct

173 Yamada Y, Kohno K, Sakurai Y, Fernandez P, Nunez A et al 1984 Gene structure. Cartilage and basement membrane collagen genes. Abstr. NY Acad. Sci. 17–19 Oct

174 Gibson G J, Schor S L, Grant M E 1982 Effects of matrix macromolecules on chondrocyte gene expression: synthesis of a low molecular weight collagen species by cells cultured within collagen gels. J. Cell Biol. 93: 767–774

175 Kielty C M, Hulmes D J S, Schor S L, Grant M E 1984 Embryonic chick cartilage collagens: differences in low-M_r species present in sternal cartilage and tibiotarsal articular cartilage. FEBS Letters 169: 179–184

176 Remington M C, Bashey R I, Brighton C T, Jimenez S A 1983 Biosynthesis of a low molecular weight collagen by rabbit growth plate cartilage organ cultures. Collagen Rel. Res. 3: 271–278

177 Schmid T M, Conrad H E 1982 A unique low molecular weight collagen secreted by cultured chick embryo chondrocytes. J. Biol. Chem. 257: 12444–12450

178 Schmid T M, Conrad H E 1982 Metabolism of low molecular weight collagen by chondrocytes obtained from histologically distinct zones of the chick embryo tibiotarsus. J. Biol. Chem. 257: 12451–12457

179 Schmid T M, Linsenmayer T F 1983 A short chain (Pro) collagen from aged endochondral chondrocytes. Biochemical characterisation. J. Biol. Chem. 258: 9504–9509

180 Gibson G J, Beaumont B W, Flint M H 1984 Synthesis of a low molecular weight collagen by chondrocytes from the presumptive calcification region of the embryonic chick sterna: the influence of culture with collagen gels. J. Cell Biol. 98: 208–216

181 Kielty C M, Kwan A P L, Holmes D F, Schor S L, Grant M E 1985 Type X collagen a product of hypertrophic chondrocytes. Biochem. J. 227: 545–554

182 Steven F S, Jackson D S, Broady K 1968 Proteins of the human intervertebral disc. The association of collagen with a protein fraction having an unusual amino acid composition. Biochim. Biophys. Acta 160: 435–446

183 Steven F S, Knott J, Jackson D S, Podrazky V 1969 Collagen-protein-polysaccharide interactions in human intervertebral disc. Biochim. Biophys. Acta 188: 307–313

184 Pearson C H, Happey F, Naylor A, Turner R L, Palframen J, Shentall R D 1972 Collagens and associated glycoproteins in the human intervertebral disc. Variations in sugar and amino acid composition in relation to location and age. Ann. Rheum. Dis. 31: 45–53

185 Eyre D R, Muir H 1974 Collagen polymorphism: two molecular species in pig intervertebral disc. FEBS Letters 42: 192–196

186 Eyre D R, Muir H 1976 Types I and II collagens in intervertebral disc. Interchanging radial distributions in annulus fibrosus. Biochem. J. 157: 267–270

187 Eyre D R, Muir H 1977 Quantitative analysis of types I and II collagens in human intervertebral discs at various ages. Biochim. Biophys. Acta 492: 29–42

188 Herbert C M, Lindberg K A, Jayson M I V, Bailey A J 1975 Changes in the collagen of human intervertebral discs during ageing and degenerative disc disease. J. Molec. Med. 1: 79–91

189 Eyre D R 1979 Biochemistry of intervertebral disc. Int. Rev. Connect. Tissue Res. 8: 227–291

190 Wu J J, Eyre D R 1984 Identification of hydroxypyridinium cross-linking sites in type II collagen of bovine articular cartilage. Biochemistry 23: 1850–1857

191 Wu J J, Eyre D R 1984 Cartilage type IX collagen is crosslinked by hydroxypyridinium residues. Biochem. Biophys. Res. Commun. 123: 1033–1039

192 Osebold W R, Pedrini V 1976 Pepsin-solubilised collagen of human nucleus pulposus and annulus fibrosus. Biochim. Biophys. Acta 435: 390–405

193 Lee-Own V, Anderson J C 1976 Interaction between proteoglycan subunit and type II collagen from bovine nasal cartilage and the preferential binding of proteoglycan subunit to type I collagen. Biochem. J. 153: 259–264

194 Eyre D R, Wu J J 1983 Collagen of fibrocartilage: a distinctive molecular phenotype in bovine meniscus. FEBS Letters 158: 265–270

195 Beard H K, Stevens R L 1980 Biochemical changes in the intervertebral disc. In: Jayson M I V (ed) The lumbar spine and back pain, 2nd edn. Pitman Medical, Tunbridge Wells, p 407–436

196 Beard H K, Ryvar R, Brown R, Muir H 1980 Immunochemical localization of collagen types and proteoglycan in pig intervertebral discs. Immunology 41: 491–501

197 Beard H K, Roberts S, O'Brien J P 1981 Immunofluorescent staining for collagen and proteoglycans in normal and scoliotic intervertebral discs. J. Bone Jt. Surg. 63B: 529–534

198 Wick G, Nowack H, Hahn E, Timpl R, Miller E J 1976 Visualisation of type I and II collagens in tissue sections by immunohistologic techniques. J. Immunol. 117: 298–303

199 Balazs E A, Gibbs D A 1970 The rheological properties and biological function of hyaluronic acid. In: Balazs E A (ed) Chemistry and molecular biology of the intercellular matrix, vol 3. Academic Press, London, p 1241–1253

200 Hamerman D, Rosenberg L C, Schubert M 1970 Diarthrodial joints revisited. J. Bone Jt. Surg. 52A: 725–774

201 Hardingham T E 1981 Proteoglycans: their structure, interactions and molecular organization in cartilage. Biochem. Soc. Trans. 9: 489–497

202 Muir H 1983 Proteoglycans as organizers of the intercellular matrix. Biochem. Soc. Trans. 11: 613–622

203 Hascall V C, Sajdera S W 1970 Physical properties and polydispersity of proteoglycan from bovine nasal cartilage. J. Biol. Chem. 245: 4920–4930

204 Mathews M B, Lozaityte I 1958 Sodium chondroitin sulfate-protein complexes of cartilage. I. Molecular weight and shape. Arch. Biochem. Biophys. 74: 158–174

205 Hascall V C, Sajdera S W 1969 Protein-polysaccharide complex from bovine nasal cartilage. The function of glycoprotein in the formation of aggregates. J. Biol. Chem. 244: 2384–2396

206 Sajdera S W, Hascall V C 1969 Proteinpolysaccharide complex from bovine nasal cartilage. A comparison of low and high shear extraction procedures. J. Biol. Chem. 244: 77–87

207 Heinegard D, Hascall V C 1974 Characterization of chondroitin sulphate isolated from trypsin-chymotrypsin digests of cartilage proteoglycans. Arch. Biochem. Biophys. 165: 427–441

208 Heinegard D 1977 Polydispersity of cartilage proteoglycans. Structural variations with size and buoyant density of the molecules. J. Biol. Chem. 252: 1980–1989

209 Heinegard D, Axelsson I 1977 Distribution of keratan sulphate in cartilage proteoglycans. J. Biol. Chem. 252: 1971–1979

210 Helting T, Roden L 1968 The carbohydrate-protein linkage region of chondroitin-6-sulphate. Biochim. Biophys. Acta 170: 301–308

211 Bray B A, Lieberman R, Meyer K 1967 Structure of human skeletal keratosulphate. The linkage region. J. Biol. Chem. 242: 3373–3380

212 Hopwood J J, Robinson H C 1974 The structure and composition of cartilage keratan sulphate. Biochem. J. 141: 517–526

213 Lohmander L S, DeLuca S, Nilsson B, Hascall V C, Caputo C B, Kimura J H, Heinegard D 1980 Oligosaccharides on proteoglycans from the swarm rat chondrosarcoma. J. Biol. Chem. 255: 6084–6091

214 Thonar E J M A, Sweet M B E 1979 An oligosaccharide component in proteoglycans of articular cartilage. Biochim. Biophys. Acta 584: 353–357

215 Tsiganos C P, Muir H 1969 Studies on protein-polysaccharides from pig laryngeal cartilage. Heterogeneity, fractionation and characterisation. Biochem. J. 113: 885–894

216 Rosenberg L, Hellmann W, Kleinschmidt A K 1975 Electron microscopic studies of proteoglycan aggregates from bovine articular cartilage. J. Biol. Chem. 250: 1877–1883

217 Thyberg J, Lohmander S, Heinegard D 1975 Proteoglycans of hyaline cartilage. Electron microscope studies on isolated molecules. Biochem. J. 151: 157–166

218 Hardingham T E, Ewins R J F, Muir H 1976 Cartilage proteoglycans. Structure and heterogeneity of the protein core and effects of specific protein modifications on the binding to hyaluronate. Biochem. J. 157: 127–143

219 Hardingham T E, Muir H 1972 The specific interaction of hyaluronic acid with cartilage proteoglycans. Biochim. Biophys. Acta 279: 401–405

220 Hardingham T E, Muir H 1973 Binding of oligosaccharides of hyaluronic acid to proteoglycans. Biochem. J. 135: 905–908

221 Hascall V C, Heinegard D 1974 Aggregation of cartilage proteoglycans. II oligosaccharide competition of the proteoglycan-hyaluronic acid interaction. J. Biol. Chem. 249: 4242–4249

222 Baker J R, Caterson B 1979 The isolation and characterisation of the link proteins from proteoglycan aggregates of bovine nasal cartilage. J. Biol. Chem. 254: 2387–2393

223 Gregory J D 1973 Multiple aggregation factors in cartilage proteoglycans. Biochem. J. 133: 383–386

224 Christner J E, Baker J R, Caterson B 1983 Studies on the properties of the inextractable proteoglycans from bovine nasal cartilage. J. Biol. Chem. 258: 14335–14341

225 Kleine T O 1981 Biosynthesis of proteoglycans: an approach to locate it in different membrane systems. Int. Rev. Connect. Tissue Res. 9: 27–98

226 Geetha-Habib M, Campbell S C, Schwartz N B 1984 Subcellular localization of the synthesis and glycosylation of chondroitin sulphate proteoglycan core protein. J. Biol. Chem. 259: 7300–7311

227 Kimura J H, Hardingham T E, Hascall V C, Solursh M 1979 Biosynthesis of proteoglycans and their assembly into aggregates in cultures of chondrocytes from the swarm rat chondrosarcoma. J. Biol. Chem. 254: 2600–2609

228 Adams P, Muir H 1976 Quantitative changes with age of proteoglycans of human lumbar discs. Ann. Rheum. Dis. 35: 289–296

229 Emes J H, Pearce R H 1975 The proteoglycans of the human intervertebral disc. Biochem. J. 145: 549–556

230 Stevens R L, Ewins R J F, Revell P A, Muir H 1979 Proteoglycans of the intervertebral disc. Homology of structure with laryngeal proteoglycans. Biochem. J. 179: 561–572

231 Pearce R H, Grimmer B J 1976 The chemical constitution of the proteoglycan of human intervertebral disc. Biochem. J. 157: 753–763

232 Pedrini V A, Ponseti I V, Dohrman S C 1973 Glycosaminoglycans of intervertebral disc in idiopathic scoliosis. J. Lab. Clin. Med. 82: 938–950

233 Heinegard D, Gardell S 1967 Studies on protein-polysaccharide complex (proteoglycan) from human nucleus pulposus. I. Isolation and preliminary characterization. Biochim. Biophys. Acta 148: 164–171

234 Hopwood J J, Robinson H C 1974 The alkali-labile linkage between keratin sulphate and protein. Biochem. J. 141: 57–69

235 Habuchi H, Yamagata T, Iwata H, Suzuki S 1973 The occurrence of a wide variety of dermatan sulfate-chondroitin sulfate copolymers in fibrous cartilage. J. Biol. Chem. 248: 6019–6028

236 Butler W F, Wels C M 1971 Glycosaminoglycans of cat intervertebral disc. Biochem. J. 122: 647–652

237 Scott J E, Haigh M 1984 Proteoglycan — type I collagen fibril interactions in calcifying and non-calcifying connective tissues. Biochem. Soc. Trans. 13: 933

238 Pedrini V A, Pedrini-Mille A 1977 Aggregation of proteoglycans of human intervertebral disc. Trans. Orthop. Res. Soc. 2: 18

239 Hardingham T E, Muir H 1974 Hyaluronic acid in cartilage and proteoglycan aggregation. Biochem. J. 139: 565–581

240 Hardingham T E, Adams P 1976 A method for determination of hyaluronate in the presence of other glycosaminoglycans and its application to human intervertebral disc. Biochem. J. 159: 143–147

241 Tengblad A, Pearce R H, Grimmer B J 1984 Demonstration of link protein in proteoglycan aggregates from human intervertebral disc. Biochem. J. 222: 85–92

242 Stevens R L, Dondi P G, Muir H 1979 Proteoglycans of the intervertebral disc. Absence of degradation during the isolation of proteoglycans from the intervertebral disc. Biochem. J. 179: 573–578

243 Oegema T R, Bradford D S, Cooper K M 1979 Aggregated proteoglycan synthesis in organ cultures of human nucleus pulposus. J. Biol. Chem. 254: 10579–10581

244 Shinomura T, Kimata K, Oike Y, Noro A, Hirose N, Tanabe K, Suzuki S 1983 The occurrence of three different proteoglycan species in chick embryo cartilage. Isolation and characterization of a second proteoglycan (PG-Lb) and its precursor form. J. Biol. Chem. 258: 9314–9322

245 Noro A, Kimata K, Oike Y, Shinomura T, Maeda N, Yano S, Takahashi N, Suzuki S 1983 Isolation and characterization of a third proteoglycan (PG-Lt) from chick embryo cartilage which contains disulphide bonded collagenous polypeptides. J. Biol. Chem. 258: 9323–9331

246 Bruckner P, Winterhalter K H, Vaughan L 1984 Type IX collagen is identical to proteoglycan-Lt. Abstract New York Academy of Sciences 17–19 Oct, NY, USA

247 Obrink B 1973 The influence of glycosaminoglycans on the formation of fibres from monomeric tropocollagen in vitro. Eur. J. Biochem. 34: 129–137

248 Toole B P, Lowther D A 1968 The effect of chondroitin sulphate-protein in the formation of collagen fibrils in vitro. Biochem. J. 109: 857–866

249 Wood G C 1960 The formation of fibrils from collagen solutions. 3. Effect of chondroitin sulphate and some other naturally occurring polyanions on the rate of formation. Biochem. J. 75: 605–612

250 Scott J E, Orford C R 1981 Dermatan sulphate-rich

proteoglycan associates with rat tail-tendon collagen at the d-band in the gap region. Biochem. J. 197: 213–216

251   Scott J E, Orford C R, Hughes E W 1981 Proteoglycan-collagen arrangements in developing rat-tail tendon. An electron-microscopical and biochemical investigation. Biochem. J. 195: 573–581

252   Scott J E, Tigwell M 1978 Periodate oxidation and the shapes of glycosaminoglycuronans in solution. Biochem. J. 173: 103–114

253   Hallen A 1970 On the differences in extractability of the proteoglycans. In: Balazs E A (ed) Chemistry and molecular biology of the intercellular matrix, vol 2. Academic Press, New York, p 903–906

254   Evans H Personal communication

255   Smith G N, Brandt K D 1983 Interactions of cartilage proteoglycans (PG) with the minor collagens of cartilage. Arth. Rheum. 26: (suppl): S30

256   Blakey P R, Happey F, Naylor A, Turner R L 1962 Protein in the nucleus pulposus of the intervertebral disc. Nature (London) 195: 73

257   Taylor T K, Little K 1965 Intercellular matrix of the intervertebral disc in ageing and in prolapse. Nature (London) 208: 384–386

258   Naylor A, Happey F, MacRae T 1954 The collagenous changes in the intervertebral disc with age and their effect on its elasticity. An X-ray crystallographic study. Br. Med. J. 2: 570–573

259   Pearson C H, Happey F, Shentall R D, Naylor A, Turner R L 1969 The non-collagenous proteins of the human intervertebral disc. Gerontologia 15: 189–202

260   Taylor T K, Akeson W H 1971 Intervertebral disc prolapse: a review of morphologic and biochemic knowledge concerning the nature of prolapse. Clin. Orthop. Relat. Res. 76: 54–79

261   Moschi A, Little K 1966 Fluorescent properties of the non-collagenous components of the intervertebral disc. Nature (London) 212: 722

262   Paulsson M, Heinegard D 1984 Non-collagenous cartilage proteins. Current status of an emerging research field. Collagen Rel. Res. 4: 219–229

263   Little K 1973 Observations on the nature and production of proteins in the intercellular matrices of connective tissue. J. Path. 110: 1–12

264   Anderson J C 1976 Glycoproteins of the connective tissue matrix. Int. Rev. Connect. Tissue Res. 7: 251–322

265   Robert L, Moczar M 1982 Structural glycoproteins. In: Colowick S P, Kaplan N O (eds) Methods in enzymology, vol 82, part A. Academic Press, New York, p 839–852

266   Chandrasekhar S, Kleinman H K, Hassell J R 1983 Interaction of link protein with collagen. J. Biol. Chem. 258: 6226–6231

267   Poole A R, Pidoux I, Reiner A, Rosenberg L 1982 An immunoelectron microscope study of the organisation of proteoglycan monomer, link protein and collagen in the matrix of articular cartilage. J. Cell Biol. 93: 921–937

268   Shipp D W, Bowness J M 1975 Insoluble non-collagenous cartilage glycoproteins with aggregating sub-units. Biochim. Biophys. Acta 379: 282–294

269   Kleineman H K, Klebe R J, Martin G R 1981 Role of collagenous matrices in the adhesion and growth of cells. J. Cell Biol. 88: 473–485

270   Yamada K 1983 Cell surface interactions with extracellular materials. Annual Rev. of Biochem. 52: 761–799

271   Hewitt A T, Varner H H, Silver M H, Dessau W, Wilkes C M, Martin G R 1982 The isolation and partial characterization of chondronectin, an attachment factor for chondrocytes. J. Biol. Chem. 257: 2330–2334

272   Hewitt A T, Kleinman H K, Pennypacker J P, Martin G R 1980 Identification of an adhesion factor for chondrocytes. Proc. Nat. Acad. Sci. USA 77: 385–388

273   Mollenhauer J, Von der Mark K 1983 Isolation and characterization of a collagen-binding glycoprotein from chondrocyte membranes. EMBO J. 2: 45–50

274   Von der Mark K, Mollenhauer J, Kuhl U, Bee J, Lesot H 1984 Anchorins, a new class of membrane proteins involved in cell matrix interactions. (Ed. Trelstad R) 42nd annual meeting of the American Society of Developmental Biology

275   Mollenhauer J, Bee J A, Lizarbe M A, Von der Mark K 1984 Role of anchorin C11, a 31 000-mol-wt membrane protein, in the interaction of chondrocytes with type II collagen. J. Cell Biol. 98: 1572–1578

276   Mollenhauer J, Van Menxel M, Muller P, Von der Mark K 1984 Interaction of collagen with the cell surface. Abstract presented at the British Connective Tissue Society Meeting in Lancaster, 12–13 April

277   Paulsson M, Sommarin Y, Heinegard D 1983 Metabolism of cartilage proteins in cultured tissue sections. Biochem. J. 212: 659–667

278   Paulsson M, Inerot S, Heinegard D 1984 Variation in quantity and extractability of the 148-kilodalton protein with age. Biochem. J. 221: 623–630

279   Paulsson M, Heinegard D 1981 Purification and structural characterization of a cartilage matrix protein. Biochem. J. 197: 367–375

280   Paulsson M, Heinegard D 1982 Radioimmunoassay of the 148-kilodalton cartilage protein. Distribution of the protein among bovine tissues. Biochem. J. 207: 207–213

281   Cleary E G, Gibson M A 1983 Elastin-associated microfibrils and microfibrillar proteins. Int. Rev. Connect. Tissue Res. 10: 97–209

282   Ross R 1983 The elastic fibre. A review. J. Histochem. Cytochem. 21: 199–208

283   Burke J M, Ross R 1979 Synthesis of connective tissue macromolecules by smooth muscle. Int. Rev. Connect. Tissue Res. 8: 119–157

284   Eyre D R, Muir H 1975 The distribution of different molecular species of collagen in fibrous, elastic and hyaline cartilages of the pig. Biochem. J. 151: 595–602

285   Cotta-Pereira G, Rodrigo F G, David-Ferreira J F 1977 The elastic system fibres. In: Sandberg L B, Gray W R, Franzblau C (eds) Advances in experimental medicine and biology, vol 79, Elastin and elastic tissue. Plenum Press, New York, p 19–30

286   Fullmer H M, Sheetz J H, Narkates A J 1974 Oxytalan connective tissue fibers: a review. J. Oral Pathol. 3: 291–316

287   Greenlee T K, Ross R, Hartman J L 1966 The fine structure of elastic fibers. J. Cell Biol. 30: 59–71

288   Ross R, Bornstein P 1969 The elastic fiber. I. The separation and partial characterization of its macromolecular components. J. Cell Biol. 40: 366–381

289   Serafini-Fracassini A, Ventrella G, Field M J, Hinnie J, Onyezili N I, Griffiths R 1981 Characterization of a structural glycoprotein from bovine ligamentum nuchae

exhibiting dual amine oxidase activity. Biochemistry 20: 5424–5429

290 Sear C H J, Grant M E, Jackson D S 1981 The nature of the microfibrillar glycoproteins of elastic fibres. A biosynthetic study. Biochem. J. 194: 587–598

291 Sear C H J, Kewley M A, Jones C J P, Grant M E, Jackson D S 1978 The identification of glycoproteins associated with elastic-elastic-tissue microfibrils. Biochem. J. 170: 715–718

292 Sandberg L B 1969 Elastin structure in health and disease. Int. Rev. Connect. Tissue Res. 7: 159–210

293 Sandberg L B, Soskel N T, Leslie J G 1981 Elastin structure, biosynthesis and relation to disease states. New Engl. J. Med. 304: 566–579

294 Urry D M 1982 Characterization of soluble peptides of elastin by physical techniques. In: Colowick S P, Kaplan N O (eds) Methods in enzymology, vol 82, part A. Academic Press, New York, p 673–716

295 Foster J A 1982 Elastin structure and biosynthesis: an overview. In: Colowick S P, Kaplan N O (eds) Methods of enzymology, vol 82, part A. Academic Press, New York, p 559–570

296 Rosenbloom J 1982 Biosynthesis of soluble elastin in organ and cell culture. In: Colowick S P, Kaplan N O (eds) Methods in enzymology, vol 82, part A. Academic Press, New York, p 716–731

297 Kagan H M, Sullivan K A 1982 Lysyl oxidase: preparation and role in elastin biosynthesis. In: Colowick S P, Kaplan M O (eds) Methods in enzymology, vol 82, part A. Academic Press, New York, p 637–650

298 Faris B, Ferrera R, Toselli P, Nambu I, Gonnerman W A, Franzblau C 1984 Effect of varying amounts of ascorbate on collagen, elastin and lysyl oxidase synthesis in aortic smooth muscle cell cultures. Biochim. Biophys. Acta 797: 71–75

299 Vasilev V, Ruseva M 1969 Electron microscopic investigations of the annulus fibrosus in mammals. Acta Med. Inst. Super. Medici. Sofia 48: 69–80

300 Vasilev V, Ruseva M 1969 Electron microscopic investigations of nucleus pulposus in cat. Acta Med. Inst. Super. Medici. Sofia 48: 81–89

301 Buckwalter J, Cooper R, Maynard J 1976 Elastic fibres in human intervertebral disc. J. Bone Jt. Surg. 58A: 73–76

302 Hickey D S, Hukins D W L 1981 Collagen fibril diameters and elastic fibres in the annulus fibrosus of human fetal intervertebral disc. J. Anat. 133: 351–357

303 Johnson E F, Caldwell R W, Berryman H E, Miller A, Chetty K 1984 Elastic fibres in the annulus fibrosus of the dog intervertebral disc. Acta Anat. 118: 238–242

304 Johnson E, Chetty C, Moore I, Stewart T A, Jones W 1982 The distribution and arrangement of elastic fibers in the intervertebral disc of the adult human. J. Anat. 135: 301–309

305 Cotta-Pereira G, Del-Caro L M, Montes G S 1984 Distribution of elastic system fibres in hyaline and fibrous cartilages of the rat. Acta Anat. 119: 80–85

306 Keith D A, Paz M A, Gallop P M, Glimcher M J 1977 Histological and biochemical identification and characterization of an elastin in cartilage. J. Histochem. Cytochem. 25: 1154–1162

307 Heeger P, Rosenbloom J 1980 Biosynthesis of tropoelastin by elastic cartilage. Connect. Tissue Res. 8: 21–25

308 Gross J, Lapiere C M 1962 Collagenolytic activity in amphibian tissues: a tissue culture assay. Proc. Nat. Acad. Sci. USA 48: 1014–1022

309 Harris E D Jr, Vater C A 1982 Vertebrate collagenases. In: Colowick S P, Kaplan N O (eds) Methods in enzymology, vol 82, part A. Academic Press, New York, p 423–452

310 Harris E D Jr, Welgus H G, Krane S M 1984 Regulation of the mammalian collagenases. Collagen Rel. Res. 4: 493–512

311 Eyre D R, Wu J J, Woolley D E 1984 All three chains of $1\alpha2\alpha3\alpha$ collagen from hyaline cartilage resist human collagenase. Biochem. Biophys. Res. Commun. 118: 724–729

312 Woolley D E, Gadher S, Duance V C, Wu J J, Eyre D R 1984 Susceptibility of various collagens to human collagenase. Abstr. British Connective Tissue Society meeting, Oxford, 1–2 October

313 Werb Z 1982 Degradation of collagen. In: Weiss J B, Jayson M I V (eds) Collagen in health and disease. Churchill Livingstone, Edinburgh, p 121–134

314 Kuettner K E, Hiti J, Eisenstein R, Harper E 1976 Collagenase inhibition by cationic proteins derived from cartilage and aorta. Biochem. Biophys. Res. Commun. 72: 40–46

315 McGuire M B, Murphy G, Reynolds J J, Russell R G G 1981 Production of collagenase and inhibitor (TIMP) by normal, rheumatoid and osteoarthritic synovium in vitro: effects of hydrocortisone and indomethacin. Clin. Sci. 61: 703–710

316 Murphy G, McGuire M B, Russell R G G, Reynolds J J 1981 Characterisation of collagenase, other metalloproteinases and an inhibitor (TIMP) produced by synovium and cartilage in culture. Clin. Sci. 61: 711–716

317 Woolley D E, Roberts D R, Evanson J M 1976 Small molecular weight β serum protein which specifically inhbibits human collagenases. Nature 261: 325–327

318 Stricklin G P, Welgus H G 1983 Human skin fibroblast collagenase inhibitor: purification and chemical characterisation. J. Biol. Chem. 258: 12252–12258

319 Leibovich S J, Weiss J B 1971 Failure of human rheumatoid synovial collagenase to degrade either normal or rheumatoid arthritic synovial polymeric collagen. Biochim. Biophys. Acta 251: 109–118

320 Weiss J B 1976 Enzymic degradation of collagen. Int. Rev. Conn. Tiss. Res. 7: 101–149

321 Burleigh M C 1979 Degradation of collagen by non-specific proteinases. In: Barratt A J (ed) Proteinases in mammalian cells and tissues. North Holland, Amsterdam, p 285–309

322 Barratt A J 1975 The enzymic degradation of cartilage matrix. In: Burleigh M C, Poole A E (eds) Dynamics of connective tissue macromolecules. North Holland, Amsterdam, p 189–226

323 Sedowofia K A, Tomlinson I W, Weiss J B, Hilton R C, Jayson M I V 1982 Collagenolytic enzyme systems in human intervertebral disc: their control, mechanism and their possible role in the initiation of biomechanical failure. Spine 7: 213–221

324 Cartwright E C, Campbell I K, Britz M L, Sandy J D, Lowther D A 1983 Characterisation of latent and active forms of cartilage proteinases produced by normal

immature rabbit articular cartilage in tissue culture. Arthr. Rheum. 26: 984–993

325   Sandy J D, Brown H L G, Lowther D A 1978 Degradation of proteoglycan in articular cartilage. Biochem. Biophys. Acta 543: 536–544

326   Sapolsky A, Keiser H, Howell D S, Woessner J F Jr 1976 Metalloproteinases of human articular cartilage that digest cartilage proteoglycan at neutral pH. J. Clin. Invest. 58: 1030–1041

327   Liotta L A, Lanzer W L, Garbisa S 1981 Identification of a type V collagenolytic enzyme, Biochem. Biophys. Res. Commun. 98: 184–190

328   Liotta L A, Abe S, Robey P G, Martin G R 1979 Preferential digestion of basement membrane collagen by an enzyme derived from a metastatic murine tumour. Proc. Nat. Acad. Sci. USA 76: 2268–2272

329   Liotta L A, Kalebic T, Reese C A, Mayne R 1982 Protease susceptibilities of HMW, $1\alpha2\alpha3\alpha$ cartilage collagens are similar to type V collagen. Biochem. Biophys. Res. Commun. 104: 500–506

330   Sedowofia K A, Weiss J B Unpublished observation

331   Jayson M I V, Million R, Keegan A, Tomlinson I 1984 A fibrinolytic defect in chronic back pain syndromes. Lancet (24 Nov. 1984): 1186–1187

332   Abedin M Z, Weiss J B Unpublished results

333   Banga I 1975 Investigations of fluorescent peptides and lipofuscins of human intervertebral disc relating to atherosclerosis. Atherosclerosis 22: 533–541

334   Nemeth-Csoka M, Meszaros T 1983 Minor collagens in arthrotic human cartilage. Change in content of $1\alpha2\alpha3\alpha$ and M-collagen with age and in osteoarthrosis. Acta Orthop. Scand. 54: 613–619

335   Plaas A H K, Sandy J D 1984 Age related decrease in the link-stability of proteoglycan aggregates formed by articular chondrocytes. Biochem. J 220: 337–340

336   Lyons H, Jones E, Quinn F E, Sprunt D H 1966 Changes in the protein-polysaccharide fraction of nucleus pulposus from human intervertebral disc with age and disc herniation. J. Lab. Clin. Med. 68: 930–939

337   Lipson S J, Muir H 1981 Experimental intervertebral disc degeneration. Morphologic and proteoglycan changes over time. Arth. Rheum. 24: 12–21

338   Mankin H J, Lippiello L 1970 Biochemical and metabolic abnormalities in articular cartilage from osteoarthritic human hips. J. Bone Jt. Surg. 52A: 424–434

339   Altman R D, Pita J C, Howell D S 1973 Degradation of proteoglycans in human osteoarthritic cartilage. Arth. Rheum. 16: 179–185

340   Adam M, Deyl Z 1984 Degenerated annulus fibrosus of the intervertebral disc contains collagen type III. Ann. Rheum. Dis. 43: 258–263

341   Bailey A J, Bazin S, Delauney A 1973 Changes in the nature of the collagen during development and resorption of granulation tissue. Biochim. Biophys. Acta 328: 383–389

342   Hilton R C, Ball J, Benn R T 1976 Vertebral end-plate lesions (Schmorl's nodes) in the dorsolumbar spine. Ann. Rheum. Dis. 35: 127–132

343   Hilton R C, Ball J. Benn R T 1980 Annular tears in the dorsolumbar spine. Ann. Rheum. Dis. 39: 533–538

344   Malinsky J 1959 The ontogenetic development of nerve terminations in the intervertebral discs of man. Acta Anat. 38: 96–113

345   Pederson H E, Blunck C F J, Gardner E 1956 The anatomy of lumbosacral posterior remi and meningeal branches of spinal nerves (sinu-vertebral nerves): with an experimental study of their functions. J. Bone Jt. Surg. 38A: 377–391

346   Tsukada K 1939 Histologische Studien uber die Zwischenwirbelscheibe des Menschen. Altersveranderungen. Mitt. a.d. Med. Akad. zu. Kioto 25: 207

347   Yoshizawa H, O'Brien J P, Smith W T, Trumper M 1980 The neuropathology of intervertebral discs removed for low back pain. J. Path. 132: 95–104

348   Gertzbein S D, Tait J H, Devlin S R 1977 The stimulation of lymphocytes by nucleus pulposus in patients with degenerative disc disease of the lumbar spine. Clin. Orthop. Relat. Res. 123: 149–154

349   Bisla R S, Marchisello P J, Lockshin M D, Hart D M, Marcus R E, Granda J 1976 Auto-immunological basis of disc degeneration. Clin. Orthop. Relat. Res. 121: 205–211

350   Riseborough E J, Wynne-Davies R 1973 A genetic survey of idiopathic scoliosis in Boston, Massachusetts. J. Bone Jt. Surg. 55A: 974–982

351   Bushell G R, Ghosh P, Taylor T K F, Sutherland J M 1979 The collagen of the intervertebral disc in adolescent idiopathic scoliosis. J. Bone Jt. Surg. 61B: 501–508

352   Taylor T K, Ghosh P, Bushell G R, Sutherland J M 1976 In: Zorab P A (ed) Scoliosis. Academic Press, London, p 231–246

353   Parsons D B, Brennan M B, Glimcher M J, Hall J 1982 Scoliosis: collagen defect in the intervertebral disc. Trans. Orthop. Res. Soc. 7: 52

354   Pedrini-Mille A, Pedrini V A, Tudisio C, Ponseti I V, Weinstein S L, Maynard J A 1983 Proteoglycans of human scoliotic intervertebral disc. J. Bone Jt. Surg. 65A: 815–823

355   Pita J C, Muller F J, Howell D S 1979 Structural changes of sulphated proteoglycans of the growth cartilage of rats during endochondral calcification. In: Gregory J D, Jeanloz R W (eds) Glycoconjugate research, vol 2. Academic Press, New York, p 743–746

356   Ponseti I V, Pedrini V, Wynne-Davies R, Duval-Baupere G 1976 Pathogenesis of scoliosis. Clin. Orthop. Rel. Res. 120: 268–280

357   Ihme A, Krieg T, Nerlich A, Feldmann U, Rauterberg J, Glanville R W, Edel G, Muller P K 1984 Ehlers-Danlos syndrome type VI: collagen type specificity of defective lysyl hydroxylation in various tissues. J. Invest. Dermatology 83: 161–166

358   Pinnell S R, Krane S M, Kenzora J E, Glimcher M J 1972 A heritable disorder of connective tissue. Hydroxylysine-deficient collagen disease. New Engl. J. Med. 286: 1013–1020

359   Eyre D R, Glimcher M J 1972 Reducible crosslinks in hydroxylysine-deficient collagens of a heritable disorder of connective tissue. Proc. Nat. Acad. Sci. USA 69: 2594–2598

Properties of spinal materials

INTRODUCTION

Mechanical damage to the spine is generally believed to be a major cause of low back pain. It is therefore important to understand spinal mechanics for two reasons: firstly, in order to avoid injury which might lead to pain and, secondly, to provide a rational basis for the treatment of the damaged spine.

When designing a structure it is essential to choose appropriate materials for its construction. If the materials used are inappropriate, the forces to which they are subjected will lead to failure of the structure; conversely, if unexpected or unduly large forces are applied, even well-chosen materials will be unable to withstand them. The spine is a highly sophisticated mechanical system of which the tissues are presumably well suited to withstanding the forces to which they are normally subjected. Nevertheless, if the tissues are abused, they will be damaged and act as sources of pain either directly, through their own nerve supply, or indirectly, because they become distorted and compress nerve roots.

The tissues of the spine are biological examples of composite materials. With the exception of muscle and nerve, they consist largely of connective tissues. Connective tissues contain relatively few cells and their extracellular matrices have a limited number of components which are combined in different proportions to make materials with widely differing mechanical properties. A difference in mechanical properties implies that tissues are intended to be subjected to different stresses.

In the first part of this chapter the constituents of the extracellular matrix are considered not from a biochemical viewpoint but as components from which mechanically stable materials are to be fabricated. The constituents considered are the gel-like ground substance, collagen, elastic fibres and the mineral which is so evidently important for the behaviour of bone. In the next part of the chapter the ways in which these components are combined in specific tissues will be described. Attention is given not only to the more obvious parts of the spine (intervertebral discs, vertebrae, ligaments) but also to the tissues of the apophyseal joints, tendon, etc. of which the properties may be relevant to mechanical damage and back pain. Mechanical properties of muscle and nerve are also described briefly. The chapter concludes with some general considerations on how spinal tissues become damaged and the mechanisms by which they might recover or be repaired.

COMPONENTS

Ground substance

The fibres of the extracellular matrix are surrounded by a weak gel, known as 'ground substance', which consists mostly of water. All the tissues of the spine contain some reinforcing fibres, and so their cells are never surrounded purely by ground substance. However, the proportion of this weak component is very high in the nucleus pulposus which is about 80% water.[1,2] Thus until the onset of fibrotic changes which accompany ageing (from around 30 years of age), the nucleus pulposus is distinctly mucoid in properties and appearance.[3]

Water is attracted to the ground substance because it contains glycosaminoglycans. Glycosaminoglycans are linear polymers which have a large number of sulphate and carboxylate groups, i.e. they are polyanions.[4-6] In tissues these negative charges are balanced by the positive charges of small cations, e.g. Ca^{2+} and Na^+. Thus to a first approx-imation the ground substance can be considered to contain a polymer network with fixed negative charges which smaller ions can diffuse into,[7-9] as shown in Figure 6.1.

These fixed negative charges lead to an uneven partition of small ions between the ground substance and the surrounding body fluids by the Donnan effect.[8,10] Small anions, e.g. PO_4^{3-}, are able to diffuse into the ground substance, but the very much larger polyanions are unlikely to diffuse out. Thus small anions will tend to be distributed between the ground substance and the surrounding fluid, where-as the polyanions will be confined to the ground substance. In Figure 6.1 the ground substance contains both fixed negative charges and small polyanions, denoted by X^-; the only anions in the surrounding fluid are the small X^- ions. However, since the ground substance and body fluids are electrically neutral, their negative charges must be balanced by the positive charges of cations, marked M^+ in Figure 6.1. Because there are more negative charges in the ground substance, there are more of the mobile M^+ ions. As a consequence of its higher concentration of ions, the ground substance has a higher osmotic pressure than the surrounding body fluids and attracts water from them. The tendency of a charged polymer network to partition smaller ions unevenly in this way and hence attract water by osmosis is known as the Donnan effect.[11]

The high osmotic pressure of the ground sub-stance allows tissues to withstand compressive loads.[7,8] Osmosis leads to a high internal fluid pressure which can support a load just as the pressure of air in a tyre supports the weight of a car. Gel-like tissues, such as nucleus pulposus, which contain a higher proportion of glycosaminoglycans, are better suited to withstanding compression, but there are also glycosaminoglycans in more fibrous tissues, such as annulus fibrosus, so that they can have some ability to withstand compressive loads.

This osmotic 'swelling pressure' has been mea-sured for solutions of glycosaminoglycans and the experimental results compared with predictions based on the theory of the Donnan effects.[8,9] Glycosaminoglycans were extracted from inter-vertebral disc and various cartilaginous tissues. They were then dissolved in physiological saline at a concentration comparable to that occurring in vivo. Osmotic pressures of these solutions were close to those predicted by the Donnan effect, indicating that this must indeed provide the explanation for the swelling pressure of tissues.

Ground substance contains several macromole-cular components. Further details of its composition are given elsewhere;[4-6,12] this account is included merely to make the explanation of physical proper-ties comprehensible. Sulphated glycosaminoglycans are covalently bound to protein; the result is called a proteoglycan. Each proteoglycan consists of a single

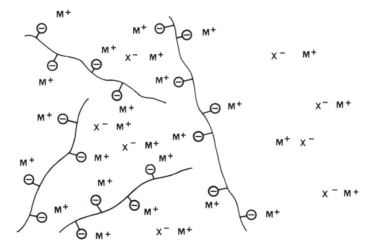

Fig. 6.1 Schematic diagram to show the partition of mobile M^+ and X^- ions between a polyelectrolyte gel and its surrounding fluid

rod-like protein core with about a hundred sulphated glycosaminoglycan side chains.[5] At least some of these proteoglycans form aggregates with hyaluronic acid, which is a very high-molecular-weight, non-sulphated glycosaminoglycan.[5,13] Although the purpose of these complex structures is not really known, it seems likely that they exist, at least in part, to ensure that the negatively-charged glycosaminoglycans, which are essential for the mechanical properties, are not leached out of the ground substance.

Ground substance is weak in shear, i.e. it is readily pulled apart like putty. This weakness is not surprising, given its high water content, since fluids simply flow when sheared. (Putty depends on a very high proportion of linseed oil for its mechanical properties.) It is not easy to measure the shear strength because no tissue has an extracellular matrix which consists solely of ground substance. Solutions which contain glycosaminoglycans at similar concentrations have a shear strength of around only $10 \, N \, m^{-2}$.[14] However, intact ground substance may well be stronger because of the interactions between its macromolecular components. An analysis of the behaviour of tendon suggests that its ground substance alone would have a shear strength of around $10^5 \, N \, m^{-2}$.[15] This estimate is likely to be reasonable for other tissues too, because their ground substances have similar compositions.

Weakness in shear means that, on its own, ground substance is not suitable for withstanding compression. At atmospheric pressure the compressibility of water is only $4.5 \times 10^{-10} \, N^{-1} \, m^2$,[16] which means that, if it is contained within a rigid vessel, it is virtually incompressible; thus the ground substance is well suited to withstanding compression, provided it is contained. If it is not contained, a hydrated gel will squeeze sideways when compressed — like toothpaste out of a tube (because shear stresses are generated at 45° to the direction of the applied pressure[17]). Thus ground substance alone is weak in tension, because it can be pulled apart, and in compression, because it can be squeezed away.

Collagen

Collagen fibrils are able to reinforce the weak ground substance because of their much great stiffness and strength in tension.[14,18,19] Furthermore, the combination of strong fibrils with a weak gel leads to a composite material which is less susceptible than a homogeneous material to mechanical damage and in particular to sudden failure; this principle is widely exploited in engineering to make fibre-reinforced composite materials in which weak plastics are reinforced by, for example, glass or carbon fibres.[20,21]

Fibrils of collagen have a characteristic appearance and can be easily identified in electron micrographs of sectioned tissue. Their lengths (at least several micrometres) are considerably greater than their diameters (typically around 30 nm) and they have a banded appearance with a 67 nm periodicity.[12,22] Each fibril is a rope of thread-like molecules which are covalently cross-linked to give it tensile strength.[23,24] In many tissues, e.g. tendon and annulus fibrosus, the fibrils aggregate into fibres which can have diameters of around 100 μm, but even in these fibres the individual fibrils are surrounded by ground substance.

The function of both dispersed fibrils and fibres which consist of aggregates of fibrils must be to withstand axial tension.[18] Whenever a fibre is pulled, its length increases. This length increase, usually expressed as a fraction of the original length or strain, leads to a restoring force in the fibre which balances the applied force. (The fibre behaves like a stretched spring which tends to return to its relaxed length and is thus able to support a load.) Similarly, collagen fibrils and fibres are able to reinforce a tissue, provided that they are oriented so that an applied force tends to stretch them.[18]

Most information on the properties of collagen has been inferred from experiments on tendon. Although tendon contains a relatively high proportion of collagen, the fibrils are surrounded by ground substance, and most of the experiments which have been performed really provide information on the behaviour of ground substance reinforced by collagen fibrils. Tendon provides the simplest example of such a system.

Figure 6.2 shows the stress–strain curve for tendon. In order to obtain this curve, the tendon is subjected to a force which tends to stretch it; this force divided by the cross-sectional area of the tendon yields the tensile stress. As the stress is increased, the tendon gets longer; the fractional increase in length is the strain. The steepness of a stress–strain curve is a measure of the stiffness of a

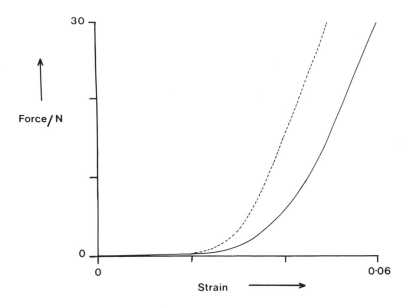

Fig. 6.2 Force required to produce a given strain in a tendon. The two nerves correspond to very slow loading (continuous line) and a faster strain rate of 0.01 s⁻¹ (dashed line). Drawn from data published by Kenedi et al[137]

material. Figure 6.2 shows that the stiffness of tendon increases rapidly at a strain of around 0.3, which corresponds to a stress of roughly 10^7 N m⁻².[25] Since tendons are believed to function at strains of at least up to about 0.3,[26] it is clear that they are subjected to stresses which are about 100 times greater than those needed to shear the ground substance.

Tendons contain crimped collagen fibrils; the initial stages of tendon extension involve straightening the crimp.[27,28] The crimp arises because the fibrils bend at certain points along their length.[29] Initial elongation of the tendon requires a relatively low stress, because it simply involves removal of the crimp, as shown in Figure 6.3. When the crimp is removed, the collagen itself has to be stretched and the tendon becomes much stiffer. Thus the crimped structure of the tendon accounts for the shape of the stress–strain curve in Figure. 6.2.

While the crimped collagen fibres are being straightened, the weak ground substrate must be sheared; the result is that tendons are viscoelastic, i.e. their mechanical properties depend on the rate at which a force is applied — as shown in Figure 6.2. It has already been indicated that tendons function at stresses of up to at least 10^7 N m⁻², while the ground substance shears at around 10^5 N m⁻². Thus when the tendon is stretched, the ground substance

is sheared and begins to flow. However, the gel does not immediately move to an equilibrium position when the stress is applied, neither does it immediately spring back to its original position when the stress is removed. In consequence, tendon does not behave like a steel cable, of which the strain depends on stress alone, but instead its mechanical properties depend also on how long the stress is applied for.

Viscous forces exerted by the flowing ground substance will tend to stretch the collagen fibrils; it is because the flow tends to stretch them that the fibrils are able to provide reinforcement.[18,30] Flow will tend

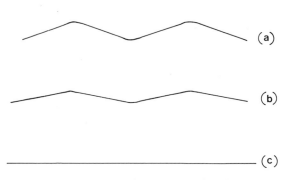

Fig. 6.3 Schematic diagram of three stages of tendon extension: (a) unstretched, (b) with the crimp partially removed by stretching, and (c) stretched sufficiently to remove the crimp

to orient the collagen fibrils which are not already aligned in its direction, in the same way as sticks are aligned by the flow of water in a river. If the fibrils are already highly aligned in this direction, the flowing gel will tend to stretch them immediately and the tissue will be stiffer than if reorientation had to occur first.[31]

The time dependence in the mechanical properties, or viscoelasticity, of connective tissues has a number of important implications. First of all, when a tendon is subjected to a fixed tensile stress it is rapidly strained, but this strain does not remain constant; instead, it gradually increases, tending slowly to an equilibrium value. Thus tissues continue to stretch slowly for some time under the influence of a fixed stress — they exhibit creep. Secondly, a tendon which is being stretched follows a different path on a stress–strain curve like Figure 6.2 than one which is relaxing after the stress has been removed — tissues are said to exhibit hysteresis in their mechanical properties. Finally, the mechanical response of a tissue will depend on the rate at which a stress is applied — a rapidly loaded viscoelastic material is stiffer than one which is slowly loaded.

If the applied stress is sufficiently high, the tissue will be damaged. When the tissue is being stretched, work is being done on it, so its energy increases (energy being simply stored work). Because tissues are viscoelastic, they dissipate some of this energy to their surroundings and store the rest. (All the energy used to initiate flow in a viscous fluid is dissipated, while all that used to deform a purely elastic solid is stored.) Stored energy can be used to break bonds within a material.

In a fibre-reinforced composite material there are several different kinds of bonds that can break, so that damage can occur in different ways;[20] biological tissues are more complicated than engineering composites because of the chemical complexity of their components, the complexity of their internal structures and because of the possibility of repair. It is likely that the weak ground substance will crack before the collagen fibrils. Since collagen fibrils are supposed to be stronger than the ground substance, such a crack is not likely to spread into a fibril — it is more likely to be deflected, as shown in Figure 6.4. Thus a large crack could be propagated, leading to release of considerable energy, without it spreading right across the tissue and causing complete fracture.

Further damage could occur in three different ways, depending on the exact structure of the tissue and the properties of its components. The collagen fibrils themselves can break, although since the fibrils are separated by ground substance they are unable to transfer energy directly to each other and so are unlikely to all break together. A second way in which the tissue could be damaged involves spread of a very large crack down the edge of a fibril, around the bottom and up the other side. The result is a fibril with one end which is no longer firmly secured in the ground substance — this is called fibre debonding.

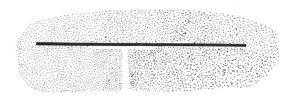

Fig. 6.4 Deflection of a crack in the weak ground substance by a collagen fibril

In a layered structure, such as annulus fibrosus, the layers could be separated by cracks known as delamination cracks. Finally, it has also been repeatedly suggested that denaturation of collagen might be implicated in degeneration of the intervertebral disc,[32] but the evidence for this suggestion is not convincing.[33]

It appears that tendon and, by implication, other tissues with similar compositions can continue to withstand a stress long after they have been damaged but, of course, before complete fracture occurs.[34,35] This additional stress will continue to strain the tissue. However, since damage implies an irreversible change (until the process of biological repair begins), the tissue cannot return to its original dimensions when the stress is removed; irreversible strain of this kind is called plastic deformation. The combination of collagen fibrils with weak ground substance leads to tissues which do not often fail catastrophically.[36]

Elastic fibres

Many of the tissues in the spine contain elastic fibres which consist of two components — elastic fibre microfibrils and the rubber-like protein, elastin. The microfibrils have diameters of 10 to 12 nm and consist of glycoproteins.[37] Immature elastic fibres have a distinctly fibrous appearance because of the high proportion of these microfibrils but, as a tissue matures, the proportion of elastin in its elastic fibres increases.[37]

Elastic fibres are highly extensible, they do not creep and their extension is reversible even at high strains.[38] Their mechanical properties are thus quite different from those of collagen. Most of our knowledge of their mechanical properties is derived from experiments on ligamentum nuchae (from the cervical spine) which is about 25% elastin, or on the elastin extracted from this tissue;[39] it is therefore much more extensible than collagen which fractures at strains of about 0.1.[34] When the strain is less than about 0.6, elastin is readily extensible, but at higher strains it is stiffer.[39]

Elastin closely resembles rubber in many respects. Its mechanical properties are certainly very similar.[38] Also, the energy changes involved in its extension can be explained by a similar mechanism to that which is used to explain the behaviour of rubber.[40] However, elastin has a much more complex chemical structure than rubber, and its complexities are often emphasized in explanation of its behaviour[41] rather than the important underlying idea of its rubber-like elasticity.[12]

Some ligaments, e.g. ligamentum flavum, have a high proportion of elastin, while other tissues, such as annulus fibrosus, may contain only a few elastic fibres. It is not surprising that those ligaments which are subject to high strains need to contain a high proportion of this protein because it can withstand high strains without fracture.[19] Collagen fibrils in such ligaments are sufficiently disorientated so that they do not become aligned to stiffen the tissue until high strains are attained — they may then provide a protective mechanism[19,31] (see later).

The presence of a small number of elastic fibres in relatively inextensible tissues, such as annulus fibrosus or tendon, is less easy to explain. A clue is provided by the properties of those synthetic hybrid composite materials which contain two different kinds of reinforcing fibres.[20] Here a small proportion of high-strength but low-stiffness fibres are added to the composite; the effect is to produce a material which is better able to withstand the sudden application of stress than one which contains only the stiffer fibres, i.e. the incorporation of the low-stiffness fibres makes the material less brittle. It may well be that elastin serves a similar purpose in some of the soft tissues of the spine; certainly both annulus fibrosus and tendon are likely to be subjected to sudden high stress and would be expected to benefit from the protection which incorporation of low-stiffness fibres might provide.

Mineral

Bone is much stiffer than the other tissues of the spine because it is calcified. Compression tests show that decalcification leads to a decrease in bone stiffness.[42] Bone mineral closely resembles hydroxyapatite, $Ca_5(PO_4)_3OH$, although it contains other ions, especially carbonate,[43] and is poorly crystalline,[43,44] especially in immature bone.[45,43] Despite reports to the contrary, there is no evidence for extensive crystals of the mineral brushite, $CaHPO_4.2H_2O$ in fetal bone; however, ^{31}P nmr spectroscopy indicates that it may contain some small domains of mineral which resembles brushite.[46]

Calcification stiffens tissues because of its effect on the properties of collagen. Calcium ions bind to collagen rather than to elastin of aorta in vitro; as a result the tissue becomes stiffer but more brittle.[47] Lees & Davidson[48] measured the velocity of sound in bone and showed that their results were consistent with comparable stresses being developed in both collagen and mineral phases; i.e. bone appears to behave as a so-called Reuss solid. Their measurements are supported by subsequent experiments[49] and indicate that collagen must be stiffened by calcification. They supposed that crystals stiffened collagen because they restricted the movement and flexibility of its thread-like molecules;[48] it has also been suggested that the mechanism involves the covalent cross-links which hold the molecules together in a collagen fibril becoming embedded in mineral.[50,48]

The compressive stiffness of bone may arise, in part, because calcification leads to greater adhesion of ground substance to the collagen fibrils and effectively cements them together.[51] A simple fibre-reinforced composite has little strength when it is compressed along the fibre axis direction, as shown in Figure 6.5(a); it fails because the fibres buckle independently (Fig. 6.5(b)) or cooperatively (Fig. 6.5(c)).[20] Bone contains mineral between, as well as within, its collagen fibrils.[50] If mineral then cements fibrils together, they effectively become a large-diameter pillar rather than a number of slender filaments; they are then much less prone to buckling.[51] Of course the structure of bone is sufficiently complicated that its collagen fibrils are unlikely to be subjected to simple compression in quite this way. Nevertheless, the idea goes some way towards explaining the compressive stiffness of bone.

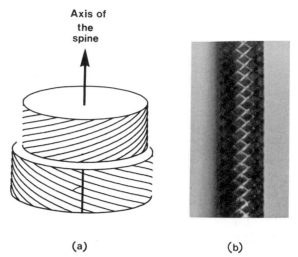

Axis of the spine

(a)　　　　　(b)

Fig. 6.6 Comparison of (a) an exploded view of two consecutive lamellae of the annulus showing the orientations of its collagen fibres with (b), a reinforced hose-pipe

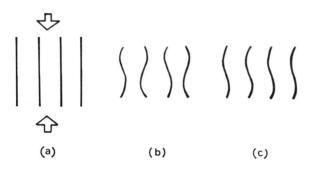

(a)　　　　(b)　　　　(c)

Fig. 6.5 Parallel fibres (a) subjected to axial compression and, as a result, buckling (b) independently and (c) cooperatively

Calcification can occur in the intervertebral disc. Both the nucleus pulposus and the annulus fibrosus may be calcified, and the mineral deposited can be either hydroxyapatite or calcium pyrophosphate dihydrate, $Ca_2P_2O_7.2H_2O$.[52] Calcification will stiffen the affected tissue site, which could lead to stress concentrations that might damage the surrounding soft tissue.[18] Thus the incorporation of mineral into the fibre-reinforced ground substance leads to a stiffening of the material, which is obviously an advantage in hard tissues, but the resulting brittleness and the possibility of stress concentrations in surrounding soft tissues may prove a problem.

INTERVERTEBRAL DISC

Structure

Figure 6.6 provides a schematic view of the structure of the intervertebral disc in which the nucleus pulposus (or nucleus) is surrounded by the roughly cylindrical lamellae of the annulus fibrosus (or annulus). In children and young adults the nucleus is gel-like and consists of over 80% water,[1] with only 5% by weight of collagen[53] in contrast to the more fibrous laminated annulus. However, the boundary between the nucleus and the annulus is not clearly defined, especially in older discs. There is also a gradual change in the composition of the annulus, going from the inner to the outer lamellae. Its water content gradually decreases from over 80% in the inner lamellae to around 65% in the outer, while there is a corresponding increase in collagen from 5% to 30%.[53] Thus the outer annulus is more highly reinforced. The annulus also contains some elastic fibres,[33,54,55] perhaps to ensure that it is not too brittle, as discussed previously.

Inner and outer lamellae of the annulus differ in several respects. Not only is the overall proportion of collagen different, but there are also differences in its detailed composition. Although human annulus contains about twice as much type II collagen as type I,[56] the proportion of type I increases from the inner to the outer lamellae.[57,56] (See Chapter 5 for information on collagen types). But, more importantly, there are clear anatomical differences. The outer lamellae are joined to the bone of the vertebral bodies.[3] In complete contrast, the inner lamellae merge into the cartilage end-plates, which separate the disc from the vertebrae, as shown in Figure

6.7.[58,59] Thus the inner lamellae and the end-plates together form a vessel which encloses the nucleus.

Collagen fibres in the annulus are arranged in a definite geometric pattern, while the nucleus contains a few randomly-dispersed collagen fibrils. Annular fibres are aggregates of collagen fibrils which closely resemble tendon fibres; when the tissue is dissected under a microscope, the crimp, which has been vividly demonstrated by scanning electron microscopy,[60] can be clearly seen. In a single lamella the fibres are parallel and tilted with respect to the axis of the spine by about 65°; the direction of tilt alternates in successive lamellae as shown in Figure 6.6[33,61-64]

Mechanical tests have been performed to determine the tensile strength of the annulus, but the results are not easy to interpret because each lamella is stiffer and stronger in the direction in which its reinforcing fibres are aligned. The earlier tests involved measuring the strength of strips of annulus in the direction of the spinal axis;[65] however, these results are especially difficult to interpret as the tilted fibres tend to reorient in the direction of the applied stress during the course of the test.[66] Later tests attempted to overcome this problem by testing 'along the fibre axis'.[67] However, the contribution of fibres in alternate lamellae which were not aligned in this direction but would nevertheless be able to contribute to the overall stiffness and strength was ignored. An analysis of all these results suggests that the tensile strength provided by annular fibres is about half that of tendon, which is consistent with

annulus containing, on average, about half as much collagen.[68]

Ageing changes occur in the composition and hence in the properties of the nucleus. It loses water and becomes fibrotic, so that by around 30 years of age its consistency has changed to a much firmer tissue.[3] Although this change appears to be perfectly normal, it is probably more useful to consider the younger disc when trying to understand the relationship between structure and function. The change in the texture of the nucleus continues, and it is not completely fibrotic until about 40 years of age.[3] This is relatively late in life and suggests that like, for example, the appearance of wrinkles in the skin at about the same age, the fibrotic nucleus confers no functional advantage. Increased deposition of fibrous material presumably requires the expression of genes which would have to be late-acting; they would thus be passed on, during reproduction, before any disadvantages had made themselves felt and their possessor been disadvantaged by natural selection.[69]

Changes in the ageing annulus are far less marked. Early measurements, based on a very small number of samples, suggested that the tilt of the collagen fibres changed during ageing;[32] later results indicated that the fibre tilt does not change from the time when the collagen is first laid down in the fetal annulus to old age.[33,61] However, the distribution of collagen fibril diameters in the annulus does appear to change during ageing; the presence of some larger-diameter fibrils might make the annulus more

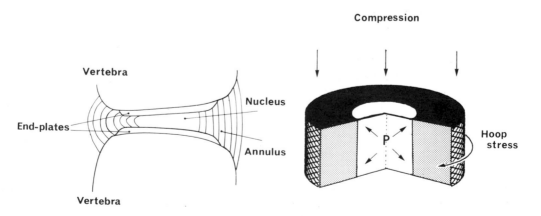

Fig. 6.7 (a) The structure of the intervertebral disc and (b) how it could be considered to act as a pressure vessel

susceptible to tearing.[33] (Details of the influence of fibril diameters on mechanical properties are explained elsewhere.)[18,30] Appearance of larger-diameter fibrils could be linked to the increased proportion of type I collagen in the ageing annulus.[56]

Some of the changes which occur in the disc are more obviously linked to degenerative or pathological changes. Loss of ground substance from the anterior annulus of degenerate discs has been observed, while in some individuals there is also loss of collagen and an increased water content; these observations were based on degenerative discs removed during surgery.[2] Changes in water content also occur in rabbit discs when incisions are made in the annulus to simulate the effects of tearing.[70,71] Discs from scoliotic spines show some differences in composition, but these are generally believed to be a consequence rather than a cause of the condition.[72]

In order to relate changes in composition to mechanical failure, it will be essential to understand how the normal disc functions. This understanding requires insight into how the materials of the disc are suited to withstanding the forces to which they are subjected. But it is also essential to know what the function of the disc is.

Function

The primary function of the intervertebral disc is to allow the spine to twist and bend to an almost continuously variable range of postures. It is often stated, without any evidence, that it is primarily a shock-absorber. However, there is no reason to suppose that the spine needs to be regularly punctuated by shock-absorbers any more than, for example, does the femur. In any case, shock absorption normally appears to be accomplished by the musculature.[73]

However, as a result of their positions in the spine, the discs are subjected to compressive forces; these arise from tension in the ligaments and muscles.[8] Forces exerted by the back muscles, during twisting and bending, will have a considerable axial component which will tend to compress the disc. The idea that disc prolapse could be caused by upright stance is implausible, not least because the same compressive forces will be exerted on the discs of quadrupeds; indeed, quadruped discs show evidence

of degenerative change.[74] Furthermore, Farfan[75] has provided theoretical arguments for human spines being better suited to bipedal locomotion than those of other primates. Thus it appears that (a) the disc is not primarily a shock-absorber, (b) it is an important element in the intervertebral joint, allowing postural changes, and (c) as a consequence of this function it has to withstand compression. The way in which the properties of its materials allow it to perform these functions will now be considered.

Compression and the ground substance

The swelling pressure of the ground substance enables the disc to withstand axial compression.[8] Furthermore, its high water content means that the ground substance is not very compressible and so can withstand applied pressure, provided that it is suitably contained — the analogy with a tyre was drawn earlier. Thus the internal swelling pressure exerted by the ground substance balances the applied axial pressure in the resting spine, when it is low (0.8 MN m_2), and in the exercised spine, when it is much higher (5 MN m_2).[8]

This idea suggests that it is the nucleus, the most highly hydrated part of the disc, which contributes the majority of the internal pressure needed to balance the applied pressure. The distribution of fixed charge density across a 28-year-old lumbar disc, as measured by Urban & Maroudas,[9] appears consistent with this conclusion — remembering that fixed-charge density is directly related to swelling pressure. Figure 6.8 summarizes their results and shows that the fixed charge density is roughly constant across the centre of the disc, where it is at its highest, (the nucleus) then decreases (inner annulus) to its lowest value at the periphery of the disc (outer annulus). However, Figure 6.8 also shows that, for a 78-year-old, the fixed-charge density in the nucleus is considerably decreased, indicating that compressive load is distributed more evenly across the disc. It has already been argued that it is more profitable to consider the discs of younger people when attempting to relate structure to function. Thus it appears reasonable to suppose that the nucleus provides most of the resistance of a healthy disc to compression — a simple calculation suggests that its contribution is about 70% (see Appendix). Even in the 78-year-old disc (Fig. 6.8), the fixed-charge density is much less

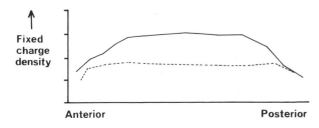

Fixed charge density

Anterior   Posterior

Fig. 6.8 Fixed-charge density across a lumbar intervertebral disc (sagittal section) of (a) a 28-year-old (continuous line), and (b) a 78-year-old (dashed line). Drawn from data published by Urban & Maroudas[9]

in the outer annulus. However, the importance of the nucleus in resisting compression is disputed by Farfan[76] — the controversy will be discussed in the next section where the disc is considered as a thick-walled pressure vessel.

Changes in the types and proportion of glyco-saminoglycans as well as direct loss of fluid may be implicated in diurnal variation of height and loss of height during ageing. Loss of glycosaminoglycans during ageing leads to a decrease in swelling pressure, which means not only that the disc is less highly hydrated, but also that it is less able to withstand compression.[8] The disc is generally considered to be the most 'leak-proof' component of the spinal column.[76] Nevertheless, some loss of fluid may be implicated in diurnal height variation[8] — we are at our tallest when we get out of bed in the morning.[77] Indeed, Adams & Hutton[78] have shown that sustained compression, especially when coupled with flexion, leads to fluid loss from excised cadaveric discs and consequent height decrease. However the cause of height changes, whether in the course of a day or a lifetime, are not simple, because postural changes, perhaps associated with loss of muscle tone, viscoelasticity and damage to ligaments etc., are all likely to contribute.

Annulus as the wall of a pressure vessel

Swelling pressure has a radial component, which must be balanced if the disc is in equilibrium, as well as the axial component which is balanced by compression. Returning to an earlier analogy, the swelling pressure supports a compressive load like the air pressure in a tyre — but, like air, the fluid will leak away if it is not contained. The structure of the annulus suggests that its function is similar to that of the wall of a tyre.

Figure 6.7(b) shows that the radial component of the swelling pressure must be balanced by tensile stress acting tangentially to the annulus — this tangential stress is sometimes called 'hoop stress' (metal hoops provide reinforcement for wooden barrels so that they can withstand the internal pressure of the beer). Thus it is often supposed that the annulus resembles a 'pressure vessel'[63] in which internal pressure is balanced by tension in its walls — like a tyre.[17,79] The idea is that internal pressure stretches the walls of the vessel — the restoring stress in the stretched walls thus balances the pressure and the system is in equilibrium. (If the pressure is too high, the walls are stretched to failure and the vessel bursts.)

Of course this is a very simple model for a complex system — because it cannot explain every detail, it has been challenged, but it is useful because it provides insights into the relationship between disc structure and function. Farfan[76] believes that the nucleus plays no part in resisting compression, in part because some experiments have shown that its removal leaves the response of the disc unchanged in vitro;[80] however, Quandieu et al[81] show that removal of the nucleus from living baboon discs changes the response of the intervertebral joint to oscillating compression. Injection of extra fluid into the nucleus of cadaveric discs increases their stiffness — in support of the simple pressure-vessel model.[82,83] Measurements of pressure in the nucleus, both in vivo and in vitro, by Nachemson[84] also add support. Ranu & King[85] showed that pressure in the nucleus was higher than in the annulus of a disc compressed in vitro, although the ratio was not as high as expected from Nachemson's results. Sonnerup[86] found a peak pressure in the annulus with a decrease in the nucleus and outer annulus, but believed that his results were not very reliable. Horst & Brink-mann[87] showed that the pressure was even across the cartilage end-plates, but this result could be explained by its being distorted by their pressure transducers.[88] Quinnel et al[89] concluded from their in vitro pressure measurements that the nucleus was not simply hydrostatic. On balance it appears that, although the nucleus is not just a simple fluid and the annulus is not merely a container, the pressure-vessel idea permits us to gain a considerable understanding of how the materials of the disc enable it to be mechanically stable. In particular, the fibres of the annulus would not be able to withstand direct compression (Fig. 6.5).

Tensile reinforcing of the annulus, which allows it to withstand nuclear pressure, is provided by its collagen fibres. However, they can only provide reinforcement if they tend to be stretched by the internal pressure. In a simple model for disc compression the radius increases uniformly as the height decreases — the fibres will then be stretched, provided they are tilted by at least 54.7° with respect to the axis of the spine (Fig. 6.6).[90] The pressure vessel then resembles a short length of reinforced pipe in which the two directions of tilted fibres make an appropriate angle with the axis to withstand internal pressure (Fig. 6.6). Calculations show that, if the fibres are stretched, they must reorient;[90,91] reorientation of collagen fibres has been measured during in vitro compression of rabbit discs and the results are in good agreement with theory.[92] However, the disc differs from a pipe in that its height is comparable with its radius — as a result, an increase in internal pressure leads to a visible bulging (Fig. 6.9). The critical tilt angle for the fibres to be stretched then depends on some further factors which explains why experimentally determined

values are more commonly around 65–70°.[93] These factors are the shape of the disc and other mechanisms for accommodating displaced fluid — particularly bulging of the end-plate into the cancellous bone of the vertebral body (see later).

It has been argued that the inner lamellae of the annulus and the end-plates together form a vessel which contains the nucleus, as shown in Figure 6.7(a), and that as a result it is the inner region of the vertebral column, including the cancellous bone, which is best suited for response to compression.[94] Collagen fibre strain in the outer lamellae of the annulus is negligible, even when the disc is compressed to failure.[93] Thus tension in the fibres of the inner lamellae provides most of the resistance to nuclear pressure — this would indeed be expected if the disc acts as a thick-walled pressure vessel for which tangential stress is greater on the inner surface of the wall and falls to zero on the outer surface.[93] Furthermore, the inner lamellae are joined to the end-plates, of which the collagen fibrils are oriented so that they will be stretched by increased pressure in the nucleus.[58] When the intervertebral joint is compressed in vitro, blood is lost by the cancellous bone, showing that it is compressed.[95] Compression of the bone could arise by the end-plates bulging into it,[94,95] leading to a mechanically coupled system of

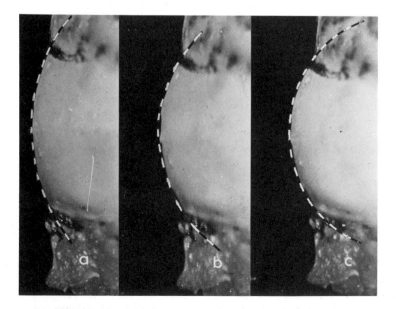

Fig. 6.9 Profile of a rabbit lumbar intervertebral disc (a) uncompressed, (b) compressed and (c) further compressed. Each profile can be closely matched by an arc of a circle (superimposed on the photograph)

inner disc and cancellous bone which provides resistance to compression of the spine.[94] However, Reuber et al[96] have argued that end-plate bulge is small compared to annular bulge and may be negligible; in contrast radiographs[95] and calculations based on the results of Klein et al[93] suggest that end-plate bulging may be important.

The response of the disc to compression depends on the rate at which it is loaded, i.e. it is viscoelastic.[97] An intact intervertebral joint is very stiff when it is loaded suddenly, and it stores nearly all the energy used to deform it; when a fixed load is applied for a longer period, it does not immediately deform to an equilibrium position but gradually creeps towards one over a period of about nine hours.[98] The mechanism of the time-dependent behaviour might involve fluid flow, it might arise simply from the viscoelasticity of the component materials of the disc or it might be a combination of the two.[97] Furthermore, fluid flow need not be directly from the disc — the end-plate could bulge into the cancellous bone of the vertebral body, leading to loss of blood via the vertebral veins; absence of valves in these veins could also allow the blood supply to be replenished when the load is removed.[94] Since such mechanisms appear to exist for fluid flow and the materials themselves are viscoelastic (as discussed earlier), it seems likely that a combination of factors would lead to time dependence in the response to compression of the living intervertebral disc.

Finally, in vitro mechanical testing shows that compression of a healthy disc does not cause the nucleus to burst out through the annulus — instead the end-plate fractures and the cancellous bone of the vertebral bodies is damaged.[65,95,99–101] Failure of the cancellous bone in compression will be described later. The problem is, what form of mechanical abuse can tear the annulus and lead to the posterio-lateral protrusion of nucleus which is a common cause of low back pain?

Torsion

Collagen fibres are also able to reinforce the annulus during torsion of the disc. Figure 6.10 shows how torsion stretches a fibre in a lamella of the annulus. However, the fibres in the adjacent lamellae are tilted in the opposite direction and so are not stretched; they are only able to provide reinforce-

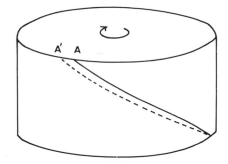

Fig. 6.10 Effect of disc torsion, in the direction indicated, on a fibre in one lamella of the annulus. As a result of torsion the fibre end moves from A to A'; it is thus stretched as it moves from its original position (continuous line) to its final position (dashed line)

ment when the disc is twisted in the other direction. It can also be seen from Figure 6.10 that, as the disc is twisted, those fibres which are stretched are tilted further from the spinal axis direction. This tilt increase has been calculated theoretically[90,91] and compared with experimental measurements on rabbit discs twisted in vitro;[102] the experimental results were in good agreement with theoretical predictions, indicating that the fibres respond to torsion and reinforce the annulus as supposed.[102]

Torsion is potentially damaging for the annulus. One reason is simply that only half of the total number of fibres is able to provide reinforcement during torsion in a given direction, as already explained. Another is that, for a disc of constant height, the fibres of the outer lamellae are stretched more than those of the inner lamellae. This is the reverse of what happens in compression and suggests a difference in function between inner and outer lamellae, which reflects their differences in composition and attachments to the vertebrae described previously.[94] It also means that not all the fibres which are appropriately oriented will be stretched equally — the outer fibres will be stretched more and so are more likely to be damaged. Furthermore, because of the cross-sectional shapes of lumbar discs, the stress induced by torsion is not evenly distributed around the circumference. This stress distribution would be even for a circular cross-section twisted about an axis which passed through its centre. But lumbar discs do not have circular cross-sections, and the position of the torsion axis appears to be somewhat posterior to its geometric centre.[103,104] An electrical analogue technique shows that for the cross-sectional shapes of lumbar discs, the torsional stress is concentrated posteriorly.[105]

Failure of the disc in torsion need not involve direct damage to the fibres — the shear stress resulting from torsion can also lead to delamination fractures (defined previously). Farfan[76] noted that the earliest signs of disc degeneration involved the appearance of cracks tending to separate the lamellae of the annulus. Hickey[68] has pointed out that these are typical of the delamination fractures which occur in laminated fibre composites.[20] When the disc is twisted, the outer lamellae will tend to move further than the inner lamellae, i.e. the annulus will be subjected to a shear stress. Thus the appearance of circumferential cracks is exactly what would be expected in torsional failure. Farfan et al[105] found that radial cracks appear in later stages of degeneration. Once again Hickey[68] has pointed out that similar cracks occur in synthetic fibre-reinforced composite materials, where they are a sign of fatigue damage.[20]

It has been argued that the apophyseal joints limit torsion so much that it cannot lead to damage of the disc.[106] However, the observation that these joints are often asymmetric[105] suggests that this protection mechanism might sometimes fail.[99] In any case, the pattern of disc injury is consistent with torsion being one possible cause, as described above.

Bending

Collagen fibres reinforce the annulus during flexion, extension and lateral bending of the disc, but they are likely to be damaged only by flexion. Bending implies that one surface of the disc tilts with respect to the other, as shown in Figure 6.11. As a result, flexion stretches the posterior fibres, which then provide reinforcement, but slackens the anterior fibres.[90] The exact value of strain in the stretched fibres depends on the position of the flexion axis about which one surface of the disc is considered to rotate. It appears that in flexion the axis passes through the nucleus[107,108] — the anterior fibres are stretched and are sufficiently far from this axis that the strain may be high enough to cause damage.[90] Adams & Hutton[109] demonstrated that, if an offset compression was applied to cadaveric intervertebral joints to simulate flexion, posterior tears appeared in the annulus if the disc was bent only a few degrees

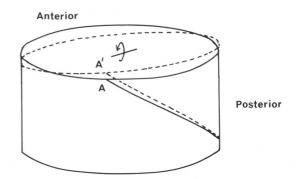

Fig. 6.11 Effect of disc flexion on a posterior fibre in one lamella of the annulus. As a result of flexion the fibre end moves from A to A′; it is thus stretched as it moves from its original position (continuous line) to its final position (dashed line)

more than normally occurs in vivo. However, extension is far less likely to cause damage, not only because the bending angles involved are more limited, but also because the bending axis shifts anteriorly[107,108] — the fibre strain is then reduced.[90] Lateral bending is also more limited than flexion and so less likely to lead to damage.

The inescapable conclusion is that the annulus can be damaged during either torsion or flexion of the disc. This damage could involve tearing, or one of the other forms of fracture described previously, but might merely take the form of plastic deformation in which the annular fibres are stretched irreversibly. In any case, the mechanical properties of the disc will then be impaired. Furthermore, the damage caused by either torsion or flexion is likely to be located posteriorly, as is observed during necropsy of lumbar discs.[52]

OTHER TISSUES

Bone

There is an extensive literature on the properties of bone which has been reviewed by Katz.[110] Calcification leads to stiffening of collagen, as described previously, with the result that bone is more rigid and brittle than the other tissues of the spine, but nevertheless has some viscoelastic properties. The purpose of this section is not to provide an exhaustive review of its properties, but merely to indicate some aspects which are relevant to the function of the spine.

Vertebrae consist mostly of cancellous bone surrounded by a layer of cortical bone. Cortical bone is denser and stronger than cancellous bone. Because of its high density a vertebra which consisted solely of cortical bone would be excessively heavy.[38] A hollow tube of cortical bone would be nearly as strong as a cylindrical rod in torsion, but would tend to buckle because of the bending moments and compressive stress to which it would be subjected. A filling of cancellous bone will guard the cortical bone tube against buckling so that it is strong in torsion, bending and compression without being too heavy. Vertebrae resemble the 'sandwich materials' used in engineering; these materials are combinations of a light cellular component (like cancellous bone) surrounded by a stiffer, denser component (like cortical bone) to produce a combination which is rigid yet light.[17] The trabeculae of cancellous bone prevent the surrounding tube of cortical bone from deflecting inwards — thus the tube cannot readily buckle. Even though cancellous bone is much weaker than cortical bone, it is essential for the mechanical stability of a vertebra.

Although bone is stiffer than the other tissues of the spine, its flexibility is not negligible — indeed, it has been suggested that the compressibility of cancellous bone may be implicated in the viscoelastic behaviour of the intervertebral joint.[94,95] When an intervertebral joint is compressed in vitro, blood flows from the bone.[95] Therefore compression of the joint must involve a decrease in volume of the cancellous bone, otherwise the blood would not be squeezed out. Blood which flowed out of the vertebral veins in vivo would not return instantaneously, so that the flow could contribute to the time-dependence in the mechanical behaviour of the intervertebral joint. Furthermore, compression of a vertebra increases its energy; the stored energy could lead to fracture unless there were some other mechanism available to dissipate it. Fluid flow provides an alternative, non-damaging mechanism for energy dissipation; hence blood flow from compressed cancellous bone of a vertebra might provide some protection against fracture.[94]

Cancellous bone is susceptible to fracture by excessive or suddenly applied compressive loads. Intervertebral joints invariably fail during in vitro compression tests by the end-plates cracking and fracture of the cancellous bone of the verte-brae.[65,80,95,99,100] Sudden impact along the axis of the spine is a common cause of vertebral body fractures in vivo.[111] Trabecular microfractures have been observed in macerated lumbar vertebrae,[112] and radiographs have indicated the presence of micro-fractures in the vertebrae of some patients with 'non-specific' back pain.[113]

Protrusions of the nucleus into the vertebral body are known as Schmorl's nodes, but this term appears to be loosely and variously applied. Hansson & Roos[114] compressed lumbar vertebrae to failure in vitro. They obtained irregular mushroom-like nodes as a result of fracture which were especially prevalent where the mineral content of the bone was low; a second, more regular, type of Schmorl's node was considered to be congenital or developmental in origin as suggested by Ball.[52]

Ligaments

Ligaments act together with the intervertebral disc to achieve a mechanically stable joint. Some limit the mobility of the joint and hence protect the disc — the anterior longitudinal ligament is believed to limit extension, while supraspinous, interspinous and posterior longitudinal ligaments limit flexion.[76] These ligaments have a nerve supply and are therefore potential sources of pain. Their properties have been extensively studied by in vitro mechanical tests, including combined investigations of structure and properties.

Examination of a large number of post-mortem specimens by Ball[115] has shown that when ligaments tear it is usually at their junctions to bone. He has shown that at these junctions the fibres of the ligament become more compact, then cartilaginous and then calcified, before they finally merge into the bone. This complexity of structure presumably reflects the difficulty of making a joint between a tough flexible material and a stiff brittle one while minimizing the likelihood of potentially damaging stress concentrations. The problems associated with such a joint are emphasized by the common failure of even such a sophisticated structure. However, the fractured junctions can heal by deposition of woven bone which penetrates any cracks in the cortical bone and hence joins the cancellous bone to the end of the ligament; thus a new junction is made on top of the original surface of the vertebra.[115] Sometimes the trabeculae of the cancellous bone are thickened in the region of the repair.[115]

The properties of the longitudinal ligaments resemble those of tendon. Shah et al[116] showed that initial extension of an excised ligament involved straightening the crimp, as described previously, after which the ligament became much stiffer — crimps disappeared at a strain of about 0.01 for the anterior longitudinal ligament. X-ray diffraction patterns have been recorded from rabbit longitudinal ligaments at various stages of extension and while still attached to the bone in vitro; the results show that the collagen fibres become more highly oriented as the ligament is extended, in agreement with the results of Shah et al,[116] and that the degree of orientation is consistent with the ligament being strained when it is attached to the bone. Thus the ligament must normally be stretched in vivo even when the intervertebral joint is relaxed — which is why it rapidly contracts when cut.

Tkaczuk[117] has published a detailed account of the mechanical properties of human longitudinal ligaments. They are viscoelastic, i.e. they are stiffer when loaded rapidly than when a load is applied gradually, and they exhibit hysteresis because they do not store all the energy used to stretch them. When they are subjected to repetitive loading they become stiffer and the hysteresis is less marked, as shown in Figure 6.12, i.e. a higher proportion of the energy transferred to the ligament is stored by it. As a result the longitudinal ligaments might be expected to be prone to fatigue failure.

Interspinous ligaments are more extensible, as presumably are the supraspinous ligaments to which they are attached. Extension of both ligaments involves crimp removal which, at least for the supraspinous ligament, occurs at a higher strain (0.03) than for the longitudinal ligaments.[116] Waters & Morris[118] observed no difference in the mechanical properties of interspinous ligaments from normal and scoliotic spines. Fibres in the interspinous ligaments are angled at roughly 45° to the axis of the spine; they are therefore expected to reorient as they are stretched by flexion. Since the supraspinous and interspinous ligaments are further from the flexion axis of the intervertebral joint, they need to stretch more than the posterior longitudinal ligament if all three are to contribute resistance to flexion. Thus the difference in mechanical properties is consistent with the function attributed to these ligaments by Farfan.[76]

Ligamentum flavum contains nearly twice as much elastin as collagen, and hence has very different mechanical properties from those of tendon.[119] Although it is viscoelastic, the time-dependence of mechanical properties is much less marked for ligamentum flavum than for tendon, which would be expected because extension of

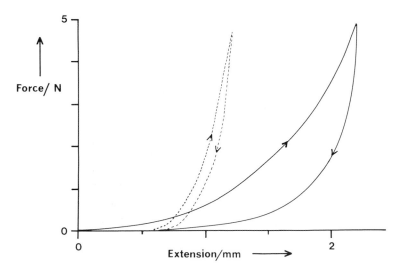

Fig. 6.12 Force required to maintain a longitudinal ligament in an extended position during extension (up arrow) and relaxation (down arrow). The dashed line corresponds to a second cycle of extension and relaxation after an interval of 35 s. Drawn from data published by Tkaczuk[117]

elastic fibres is reversible (as described earlier). Ligaments from a young person did not break until the strain reached 0.7, i.e. until the ligament had nearly doubled in length; this decreased to 0.3 in the ligament from a 79-year-old, indicating loss of function during ageing.[119] The ligament is normally stretched in the young spine, and the restoring force in the stretched ligament can be as high as 15 N; this tension would be balanced by a swelling pressure of about 0.07 MN m^{-2} within the nucleus,[119] which is comparable with the nuclear pressure in cadaveric spines (see Chapter 9).

Nachemson & Evans[119] suggested that collagen probably acted to prevent extension of the ligamentum flavum. Their suggestion is consistent with the idea that collagen fibrils in such ligaments are highly disoriented but become aligned by tension, as discussed previously, and with the observation that the ligament is easily stretched at low strains but becomes much stiffer when the strain reaches about 0.6 (Fig. 6.13). Recent X-ray diffraction experiments on rabbit ligamentum flavum have demonstrated this reorientation of collagen fibrils during in vitro extension; furthermore, comparison of these results with those obtained from a ligament still attached, at both ends, to bone are consistent with it

being under tension in vivo as suggested by Nachemson & Evans.[119] When the ligament is relaxed, the collagen fibril orientations are effectively random, but some alignment is noticeable when a strain of around 0.4 is attained. A decrease in the spread of orientations continues to occur as the ligament is stretched (Fig. 6.14), so that by the time the strain reaches 0.6 the collagen fibrils are highly aligned. (Further information on the interpretation of orientation distribution functions like those of Fig. 6.14 is given elsewhere.[31]) When the collagen fibrils are aligned, the tissue stiffens so that the results of Figure 6.14 explain the form of the stress–strain curve for ligamentum flavum in Figure 6.13.

Apophyseal joint tissue

The tissues of the apophyseal joints are subject to the same kinds of degenerative change as those of the other synovial joints. These changes are expected to impair the mechanical function of the spine and can be a source of back pain.

Articular cartilage presumably has its usual function of providing a resilient coating to the ends of bones where they come into contact; at the same time it acts, together with synovial fluid, to keep the frictional forces low when the surfaces slide over each other. Mechanical tests on cadaveric material indicate that sustained compression reduces the height of the intervertebral disc, so that the apophyseal joints will then resist about 16% of the compressive forces when the joint is angled to mimic its position in upright stance.[120] In the upper lumbar spine this will force the cartilage-coated surfaces closer together.[75]

The cartilage is able to withstand compression because of the internal swelling pressure exerted by its glycosaminoglycan gel.[121] In the resting tissue this internal pressure must be balanced by tension in the collagen fibrils of the cartilage[14,121] and, in order to perform this function, they must be appropriately oriented.[30] Collagen fibrils are oriented parallel to the articular surface, so that they are stretched by the internal pressure of the tissue; the restoring force in the stretched fibrils then balances this swelling pressure, so that the tissue remains in equilibrium when no external pressure is applied. The deep zone of articular cartilage is tethered to the subchondral

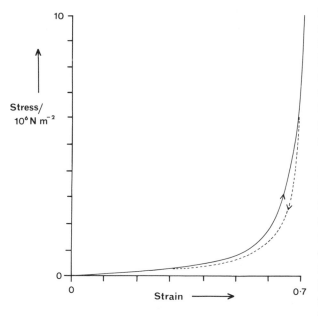

Fig. 6.13 Stress–strain curve for ligamentum flavum during extension (continuous curve) and relaxation (dashed curve). Drawn from data published by Nachemson & Evans[119]

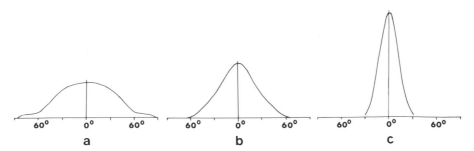

Fig. 6.14 Spread of collagen fibril orientations during extension of rabbit ligamentum flavum at strains of (a) 0.41, (b) 0.54 and (c) 0.65 as measured by X-ray diffraction

bone by collagen fibrils which are perpendicular to their direction at the surface and an intermediate zone, where the fibril orientations are effectively random, ensures that there is no mechanical discontinuity.[30,122]

Ligaments of the joint capsule provide some resistance to flexion and compression of the spine, as well as to torsion. Adams & Hutton[78] have stated that these capsular ligaments 'play a dominant role in resisting flexion of the intervertebral joint'. They believe that the collagen fibres of the capsule are oriented to resist flexion, i.e. so that they are stretched when the intervertebral joint is flexed. Furthermore, Cyron & Hutton[123] have demonstrated that, when cadaveric intervertebral joints are simultaneously compressed and sheared, the capsular ligaments stretch and provide some resistance. They also showed that the ligaments were viscoelastic and noted a marked change in their mechanical properties over a period of time when the intervertebral joint was repeatedly loaded and relaxed at a frequency of 1.2 Hz (i.e. 1.2 times a second). The ability of the apophyseal joints to limit torsion and hence, to some extent, protect the intervertebral disc, has already been discussed.

Muscle, tendon and nerve

Farfan[124] has clearly drawn the distinction between the active, contractile properties of muscle and the passive mechanical properties of the other tissues of the spine. Stability of the spine during movement then depends on how the passive tissues respond to the forces generated by muscular contraction; the stability of such a system is analogous to the behaviour of an electronic circuit of which the properties are determined by the combination of active devices (amplifiers) and passive components (resistors, capacitors and inductors). However, muscles can also be stretched passively by movement of the body.[124,125] Thus they have to withstand the forces that they themselves generate in contraction and forces transmitted to them arising from contraction of other muscles or external loads on the body.

Muscle contraction, controlled by the nervous system, occurs when the thin filaments (composed of the protein, actin) slide between the thick filaments (composed of the protein, myosin);[126] the contractile cells are surrounded by connective tissue which reinforce the muscle, both in passive stretch and active contraction.[124] The structure of the connective tissue in various animal skeletal muscles has been investigated by scanning electron microscopy.[125,127] It consists of epimysium (surrounding the whole muscle), perimysium (surrounding several muscle cells and hence delineating them as fibres) and endomysium (surrounding individual muscle cells). Endomysium contains collagen fibrils with no obvious preferred orientation and merges into a similar zone of the perimysium.[127] Perimysium also contains crimped collagen fibres, aggregates of fibrils, which are oriented at about 45° to the axis of the muscle; as the muscle elongates this angle decreases, and when the muscle contracts it increases.[127,128] Connective tissue in which collagen fibrils are randomly oriented is expected to be highly extensible and so will allow the muscle which it surrounds to change shape during contraction. More oriented regions presumably reinforce the muscle and in some way guide the forces generated by contraction into the tendons,[127] although the relationship between the function of this tissue and the orientations of its collagen fibres is not clear.

The structure of tendon is obviously well suited to transmitting forces generated by muscular contraction to bone. Collagen fibrils in tendon are aggregated to form crimped fibres, as described previously. When a contracting muscle pulls on a tendon, the crimp is removed, the collagen fibrils become oriented along the direction of the contractile force and the tendon stiffens as shown in Figures 6.2 and 6.3. The initially low stiffness provides resilience which guards against the tendon being torn by suddenly applied forces; however, the tendon needs to stiffen so that it can transmit force to the skeletal system rather than merely being stretched by muscular contraction. When the crimp is removed the tendon is stiff and strong, with its collagen fibrils oriented in the direction of the tensile stress generated by the muscle.

Tendon can withstand much higher tensile stress than muscle, so that a tendon can be much thinner than the muscle to which it is attached. This greater strength arises from its higher collagen content and from the alignment of its collagen fibrils once the crimp is removed. Many of the muscles attached to the spine need to have large cross-sectional areas to generate the considerable forces required, e.g. for lifting, but several different muscles need to be attached to relatively small areas of vertebra in order to produce a wide variability of motion. Attachment of thick muscles via thinner (but equally strong) tendons then allows them to act on selected small areas of the skeletal system.

Nerves which control the musculature also have to withstand some mechanical stress; for example, the spinal cord is stretched by flexion.[129] Furthermore, protrusion of the nucleus from a ruptured disc an exert pressure on nerve roots (see Chapter 19). Most investigations of the mechanical properties of spinal cord have been intended to simulate trauma. Panjabi et al[130] have shown that the extent of injury incurred in impact loading depends on the rate of application, i.e. the spinal cord is viscoelastic; Wennerstrand et al[131] investigated the histological effects of impact. Tensile testing of spinal cord in living cats and dogs showed that it was viscoelastic, with pronounced hysteresis.[132,133] Loss of motor function in the hind limbs of cats occurred when the nerve was slowly stretched to between 10 and 50% of its original length, but function was regained after five days. It is likely that this slow recovery arises because the nerve is first damaged by the applied mechanical stress and does not regain its function until biological repair processes have taken place.

CONCLUSIONS

The tissues of the spine are viscoelastic — they do not store all of the energy used to deform them but dissipate some to their surroundings. Because they dissipate energy they exhibit hysteresis, i.e. a longitudinal ligament does not follow the same path on the stress–strain diagram of Figure 6.12 when it is being stretched as when it is relaxing. The area between the two paths is a measure of the energy dissipated. Ligamentum flavum dissipates relatively little of its deformation energy (Fig. 6.13) because of its high elastin content. Since energy dissipation mechanisms require a finite time, the response of a tissue to an applied force depends on its rate of application (see Fig. 6.2).

Both rapid and repetitive application of a force are more likely to damage tissues. When a tissue is loaded rapidly, more energy is stored because it is supplied more quickly than it can be dissipated. If the stored energy is sufficiently high, the tissue may fracture. Fracture involves formation of new surfaces and provides a mechanism for a material to rid itself of stored energy, i.e. it is an alternative mechanism for energy dissipation.[17,36] Repetitive loading can also lead a tissue to store an increasing proportion of its deformation energy, as exemplified by the behaviour of longitudinal ligament in Figure 6.12. Exactly how much energy is stored depends on the frequency at which the load is applied, but repetitive loading at some frequencies can lead to fatigue failure.

Damage to the soft tissues of the spine is unlikely to be as simple as the fracture of bone. Bone is more brittle than the other tissues and so breaks more like a ceramic — formation of a brittle fracture. Softer materials tend to become irreversibly strained before they break — formation of a ductile fracture.[36] This irreversible strain is known as 'plastic deformation'. When the stress is removed from a plastically deformed material, it does not return to its original length and so its properties are irreversibly altered. It is therefore damaged but not fractured.

Back pain indicates that the tissues of the spine no

longer have their normal mechanical properties. These properties may be altered by damage or by creep under sustained load or because of stiffening caused by repetitive loading. Fracture of the vertebrae is likely to be caused by compression, while the annulus of the disc is likely to be torn, with the possibility of protrusion of the nucleus, by torsion and flexion. It is also possible that sudden hyperflexion could damage those ligaments which are supposed to limit flexion. When ligaments are torn, it is usually at their attachments to bone. However, damage need not be so obvious — soft tissues may be plastically deformed, so that the intervertebral joint no longer responds to applied force in the same way as previously. The damaged joint may then move in a manner which gives rise to pain, but the underlying cause could be very difficult to diagnose. Furthermore, either sustained or cyclic loading could alter the mechanical properties of tissues, leading to pain without real damage; after rest the tissues would regain their original mechanical properties. For example, the effect of sustained compression in bringing the surfaces of the apophyseal joints closer together has already been described. However, if the activity which causes pain is continued, more permanent damage might result because a tissue was no longer able to provide the usual stability to the intervertebral joint and other tissues might be inappropriately loaded.

Rest is important in the treatment of back pain for two reasons: (a) because tissues are viscoelastic and (b) to allow time for biological repair mechanisms to operate. Biological repair will be more rapid in highly vascular tissues. Healing microfractures have been observed in macerated lumbar vertebrae[112] and torn ligamentous attachments can repair.[115] In the disc the outer lamellae of the annulus have some blood supply. These outer lamellae are responsible for strength in flexion and torsion and so are more likely to be torn,[94] but a supply of blood indicates that they can heal more readily than the inner lamellae. However, if a damaged disc continues to be used strenuously, further damage may occur to the inner region which is avascular and hence expected to repair more slowly.

Healing of the annulus in torn discs is indicated by the appearance of scar tissue.[134] Harkness[34] suggested that scars have similar mechanical properties wherever they form — therefore their properties are not necessarily the same as those of the tissues they join. Indeed, O'Brien[135] has stated that scars in disc are prone to damage and that this could explain the recurrent nature of many attacks of low back pain. Furthermore, scars acquire tensile strength more slowly as we get older.[34]

Immobilized tissues tend to stiffen; manipulation is intended to reduce stiffness.[136] Confusingly, different manipulators specify different contra-indications — Paris[136] lists prolapsed disc, instability, etc. Any manipulation which simply restored congruity of joints would be expected to alleviate problems for a short while — but if the tissues are not fully repaired, their mechanical properties will not be restored and so the joint may not regain its stability. The function of the pain is to warn that damage has occurred so that inappropriate physical activity will not aggravate the problem or interfere with natural repair processes. Treatment of low back pain involves repairing a structure in which the materials are damaged — or leaving it to repair itself.

ACKNOWLEDGMENTS

Many ideas in this chapter were developed in collaboration with Drs D. S. Hickey and J. A. Klein, in the course of research on the spine, and with Dr R. M. Aspden, during research on fibre reinforcing in connective tissues. Some of the experiments on ligaments described here were performed with the help of Mr G. J. Chapman. I am grateful to Professor J. Ball, Drs J. H. Evans, S. Lees and P. P. Purslow for information and Mrs C. E. Hukins for help with the literature; Dr Y. E. Yarker assisted with production of the manuscript and Miss K. E. Davies helped produce the figures. But any mistakes or misunderstandings are my own.

APPENDIX

This calculation shows that the nucleus contributes about 72% of the resistance to compression for a healthy lumbar disc.

Consider the nucleus to have an elliptical cross-section of semi-minor axis 1.20 cm and semi-major axis 1.95 cm.[76] Then its cross-sectional area is

$$1.95 \times 1.20\pi = 7.35 \text{ cm}^2$$

Similarly, consider the disc cross-section also to be elliptical with semi-minor axis 1.70 cm and semi-major axis 2.45 cm.[76] Then the cross-sectonal area of the annulus is

$$(2.45 \times 1.7\pi) - 7.35 = 5.73 \text{ cm}^2$$

Since the fixed-charge density of the nucleus is on average about twice that of the annulus,[9] its internal swelling pressure will be about twice as high. Let the annular swelling pressure be p so that the nuclear swelling pressure is $2p$. Thus the axial force

(pressure × cross-sectional area) exerted by the annulus will be $5.73p$ and by the nucleus $7.35 \times 2p = 1.47p$. The force exerted by the nucleus, expressed as a percentage of the total for the entire disc, is then

$$\frac{14.7p \times 100}{(14.7p + 5.73p)} = 72\%$$

Even if we assume that the nucleus and annulus have the same cross-sectional area, a similar calculation shows that the nucleus will still provide about 67% of the total resistance to compression.

REFERENCES

1 Gower W E, Pedrini V 1969 Age-related variations in protein-polysaccharide from human nucleus pulposus, annulus fibrosus and costal cartilage. J. Bone Jt Surg. 51A: 1154–1162
2 Stevens R L, Ryvar R, Robertson W R, O'Brien J P, Beard H K 1982 Biological changes in the annulus fibrosus in patients with low back pain. Spine 7: 22–233
3 Peacock A 1953 Observations on post-natal structure of intervertebral disc in man. J. Anat. 86: 162–179
4 Bayliss M T 1984 Proteoglycans: structure and molecular organization in cartilage. In: Hukins D W L (ed) Connective tissue matrix. Macmillan, London, p 55–88
5 Eyre D R 1979 Biochemistry of the intervertebral disc. Intern. Review of Conn. Tissue Res. 8: 227–291
6 Hardingham T E 1981 Proteoglycans: their structure, interactions and molecular organisation in cartilage. Biochem. Soc. Trans. 9: 489–497
7 Maroudas A 1975 Biophysical chemistry of cartilaginous tissues with special reference to solute and fluid transport. Biorheology 12: 233–248
8 Maroudas A, Urban J P G 1980 Swelling pressures of cartilaginous tissues. In: Maroudas A, Holborrow E J (eds) Studies in joint diseases, vol 1. Pitman Medical, Tunbridge Wells, p 87–116
9 Urban J P G, Maroudas A 1979 Measurement of fixed charge density in the intervertebral disc. Biochim. Biophys. Acta 586: 116–178
10 Urban J P G, Maroudas A, Bayliss M T, Dillon J 1979 Swelling pressures of proteoglycans at the concentrations found in cartilaginous tissues. Biorheology 16: 337–464
11 Shaw D J 1980 Introduction to surface and colloid chemistry, 3rd edn. Butterworth, London, p 40–42
12 Hukins D W L 1984 Tissue components. In: Hukins D W L (ed) Connective tissue matrix. Macmillan, London, p 1–16
13 Hardingham T E, Adams P 1976 A method for the determination of hyaluronate in the presence of other glycosaminoglycans and its application to human intervertebral disc. Biochem. J. 159: 143–147
14 Myers E R, Armstrong C G, Mow V C 1984 Swelling pressure and collagen tension. In: Hukins D W L (ed)
Connective tissue matrix. Macmillan, London, p 161–186
15 Hooley C J, Cohen R E 1979 A model for the creep behaviour of tendon. Intern. J. Biol. Macromol. 1:
16 Kell G S 1967 Precise representation of volume properties of water at one atmosphere. J. Chem. Eng. Data 12: 66–69
Tissue Mechanics. Phys. Med. Biol. 20: 699–717
17 Gordon J E 1978 Structures. Penguin, Harmondsworth
18 Hukins D W L 1982 Biomechanical properties of collagen. In: Weiss J B, Jayson M I V (eds) Collagen in health and disease. Churchill Livingstone, Edinburgh, p 49–72
19 Minns R J, Soden P D, Jackson D S 1973 The role of the fibrous components and ground substance in the mechanical properties of biological tissues: a preliminary investigation. J. Biomech. 6: 153–165
20 Agarwal B D, Broutman L J 1980 Analysis and performance of fibre composites. Wiley, Chichester
21 Krenchel H 1964 Fibre reinforcement. Akademisk Forlag,
22 Woodhead-Galloway J 1980 Collagen: the anatomy of a protein. Edward Arnold, London
23 Chapman J A 1984 Collagen fibril structure. In: Hukins D W L (ed) Connective tissue matrix. Macmillan, London, p 89–132
24 Woodhead-Galloway J 1982 Structure of the collagen fibril: an interpretation. In: Weiss J B, Jayson M I V (eds) Collagen in health and disease. Churchill Livingstone, Edinburgh, p 28–48
25 Elliott D H 1965 Structure and function of mammalian tendon. Biol. Reviews 40: 392–421
26 Haut R C, Little R W 1972 A constitutive equation for collagen fibres. J. Biomech. 5: 423–430
27 Buckley C P, Lloyd D W, Konopasek M 1980 On the deformation of slender filaments with planar crimp: theory, numerical solution and application to tendon and textile materials. Proc. Roy. Soc. A372: 33–64
28 Diamant J, Keller A, Baer E, Litt M, Arridge R G C 1972 Collagen: ultrastructure and its relationship to mechanical properties as a function of ageing. Proc. Roy. Soc. B180: 293–315
29 Dlugosz J, Gathercole L J, Keller A 1978 Transmission electron microscope studies and their relation to polarizing optical microscopy in rat tail tendon. Micron 9: 71–81
30 Hukins D W L, Aspden R M, Yarker Y E 1984 Fibre

reinforcement and mechanical stability in articular cartilage. Engng in Med. 13: 153–156

31 Hukins D W L 1984 Collagen orientations. In: Hukins D W L (ed) Connective tissue matrix. Macmillan, London, p 211–240

32 Happey F 1980 Studies of the structure of the human intervertebral disc in relation to its function and aging processes. In: Sokoloff L (ed) The joints and synovial fluid, vol 2. Academic Press, New York, p 95–137

33 Hickey D S, Hukins D W L 1982 Aging changes in the macromolecular organization of the intervertebral disc: an X-ray diffraction and electron microscopic study. Spine 7: 234–242

34 Harkness R D 1968 Mechanical properties of collagenous tissues. In: Gould B S (ed) Treatise on collagen, vol 2, part A. Academic Press, New York, p 248–310

35 Rigby B J, Hirai N, Spikes J D, Eyring H 1959 The mechanical properties of rat tail tendon. J. Gen. Phys. 43: 265–283

36 Vincent J F V 1982 Structural biomaterials. Macmillan, London, p 27–33

37 Ross R 1973 The elastic fiber: a review. J. Histochem. Cytochem. 21: 199–208

38 Wainwright S A, Biggs W D, Currey J D, Gosline J M 1976 Mechanical design in organisms. Edward Arnold, London

39 Minns R J, Steven F S 1976 The tensile properties of developing fetal elastic tissue. J. Biomech. 9: 9–11

40 Hoeve C A J, Flory P J 1974 The elastic properties of elastin. Biopolymers 13: 677–686

41 Partridge S M 1966 Elastin. In: Trautman J C (ed) The physiology and biochemistry of muscle as food. University of Wisconsin Press, p 327–339

42 Minns R J, Atkinson A, Steven F S 1983 The role of calcium in the mechanical behaviour of bone. Phys. Med. Biol. 28: 1057–1066

43 Boskey A L 1980 Current concepts of the physiology and biochemistry of calcification. Clin. Orth. Rel. Res. 157: 225–257

44 Miller R M, Hukins D W L, Hasnain S S, Lagarde P 1981 Extended X-ray absorption fine structure (EXAFS) studies of the calcium ion environment in bone mineral and related calcium phosphates. Biochem. Biophys. Res. Commun. 99: 102–106

45 Binsted N, Hasnain S S, Hukins D W L 1982 Developmental changes in bone material demonstrated by extended X-ray absorption fine structure (EXAFS) spectroscopy. Biochem. Biophys. Res. Commun. 107: 89–92

46 Bonar L C, Grynpas M, Glimcher M J 1984 Failure to detect crystalline brushite in embryonic chick and bovine bone by X-ray diffraction. J. Ultrastructure Res. 86: 93–99

47 Minns R J, Steven F S 1977 The effect of calcium on the mechanical behaviour of aorta media elastin and collagen. Br. J. Exp. Path. 58: 572–579

48 Lees S, Davidson C L 1977 The role of collagen in the elastic properties of calcified tissues. J. Biomech. 10: 473–486

49 Lees S, Ahern J M, Leonard M 1983 Parameters influencing the sonic velocity in compact calcified tissues of various species. J. Acoust. Soc. Am. 74: 28–33

50 Lees S 1979 A model for the distribution of HAP crystallites in bone — an hypothesis. Calc. Tissue Intern. 27: 53–56

51 Jeronimidis G, Vincent J F V 1984 Composite materials. In: Hukins D W L (ed) Connective tissue matrix. Macmillan, London, p 187–210

52 Ball J 1978 New knowledge of intervertebral disc disease. J. Clin. Path. 31 (Suppl Roy. Coll. Path. 12): 200–204

53 Lyons G, Eisenstein S M, Sweet M B E 1981 Biochemical changes in intervertebral disc generation. Biochim. Biophys. Acta 673: 443–453

54 Buckwalter J A, Cooper R R, Maynard J A 1976 Elastic fibres in human intervertebral disc. J. Bone Jt Surg. 58A: 73–76

55 Hickey D S, Hukins D W L 1981 Collagen fibril diameters and elastic fibres in human fetal intervertebral disc. J. Anat. 133: 351–357

56 Herbert C M, Lindberg K A, Jayson M I V, Bailey A J 1975 Changes in the collagen of human intervertebral discs during ageing and degenerative joint disease. J. Mol. Med. 1: 79–91

57 Eyre D R, Muir H 1976 Type I and II collagens in intervertebral disc. Biochem. J. 157: 267–270

58 Aspden R M, Hickey D S, Hukins D W L 1981 Determination of collagen fibril orientation in the cartilage of vertebral end plate. Conn. Tissue Res. 9: 83–87

59 Inoue H 1981 Three-dimensional architecture of lumbar intervertebral discs. Spine 6: 139–146

60 Gathercole L J, Keller A 1975 Light microscopic waveforms in collagenous tissues and their structural implications. In: Atkins E D T, Keller A (eds) Structure of fibrous biopolymers. Butterworth, London, p 153–187

61 Hickey D S, Hukins D W L 1980 X-ray diffraction studies of the arrangement of collagenous fibres in human fetal intervertebral disc. J. Anat. 131: 81–90

62 Horton G W 1958 Further observations on the elastic mechanism of the intervertebral disc. J. Bone Jt Surg. 40B: 552–557

63 Naylor A, Happey F, Macrae T 1954 The collagenous changes in the intervertebral disc with age and their effects on its elasticity, an X-ray crystallographic study. Br. Med. J. ii: 570–573

64 Walmsley R 1953 The development and growth of the intervertebral disc. Edin. Med. J. 60: 341–365

65 Brown T, Hansen R J, Yorra A J 1957 Some mechanical tests on the lumbo-sacral spine with particular reference to the intervertebral disc. J. Bone J Surg. 39A: 1135–1164

66 Wu H-C, Yao R-F 1976 Mechanical behaviour of the human annulus fibrosus. J. Biomech. 9: 1–7

67 Galante J O 1967 Tensile properties of the human lumbar annulus fibrosus. Acta Orth. Scand. Suppl 100

68 Hickey D S 1983 Arrangement and structure of collagenous fibres in the annulus fibrosus of lumbar intervertebral discs: relationship to mechanical function, development and ageing. PhD thesis, University of Manchester

69 Dawkins R 1976 The selfish gene. Oxford University Press, Oxford, p 43–45

70 Lipson S J, Muir H 1981 Experimental intervertebral disc degeneration. Arth. Rheum. 24: 12–21

71 Lipson S J, Muir H 1981 Proteoglycans in experimental intervertebral disc degeneration. Spine 6: 194–210

72 Beard H K, Stevens R L 1980 Biochemical changes in the intervertebral disc. In: Jayson M I V (ed) The lumbar spine and back pain, 2nd edn. Pitman Medical, Tunbridge Wells, p 407–436

73 Smeathers J E, Biggs W D 1980 Mechanics of the spinal column. In: Engineering aspects of the spine. Institution of Mechanical Engineers Conference Publications, p 103–109

74 Wood P H N, Badley E M 1980 Epidemiology of back pain. In: Jayson M I V (ed) The lumbar spine and back pain, 2nd edn. Pitman Medical, Tunbridge Wells, p 29–55

75 Farfan H F 1978 The biomechanical advantage of lordosis and hip extension for upright activity. Spine 3: 336–342

76 Farfan H F 1973 Mechanical disorders of the low back. Lead & Febiger, Philadelphia

77 Goode J D, Theodore B M 1983 Voluntary and diurnal variation in height and associated surface contour changes in spinal curves. Eng. Med. 12: 99–101

78 Adams M A, Hutton W C 1983 the mechanical function of the lumbar apophyseal joints. Spine 8: 327–330

79 Higdon A, Ohlsen E H, Stiles W B, Weese J A, Riley W F 1976 Mechanics of materials. Wiley, Chichester, p 147–239

80 Virgin W J 1951 Experimental investigation into the physical properties of the intervertebral disk. J. Bone Jt Surg. 33B: 607–61

81 Quandieu P, Pellieux L, Lienhard F, Valezy B 1983 Effects of the ablation of the nucleus pulposus on the vibrational behaviour of the lumbosacral hinge. J. Biomech. 16: 777–784

82 Anderson G B, Schultz A B 1979 Effects of fluid injection on the mechanical properties of intervertebral discs. J. Biomech. 12: 453–458

83 Tencer A F, Ahmed A M 1981 The role of secondary variables in the measurement of the mechanical properties of the lumbar intervertebral joint. J. Biomech. Engng 103: 129–137

84 Nachemson A 1975 Towards a better understanding of low back pain: a review of the mechanics of the lumbar disc. Rheum. Rehab. 14: 129–143

85 Ranu H S, King A J 1980 Correlation of intradiscal pressure with vertebral end plate pressure. In: Engineering aspects of the spine. Institute of Mechanical Engineers Conference Publications, p 37–42

86 Sonnerup L 1972 Semiexperimental stress analysis of the human intervertebral joint. J. Soc. Exp. Stress Anal. 29: 142–149

87 Horst P, Brinckmann P 1981 Measurement of the distribution of axial stress on the end-plate of the vertebral body. Spine 6: 217–232

88 Klein J A 1982 Mechanics of the intervertebral disc: implications for the response of the lumbar spine to loading. PhD thesis, University of Manchester

89 Quinnel R C, Stockdale H R, Willis D S 1983 Observations of pressures within normal discs in the lumbar spine. Spine 8: 166–169

90 Hickey D S, Hukins D W L 1980 Relationship between the structure of the annulus fibrosus and the function and failure of the intervertebral disc. Spine 5: 106–116

91 Klein J A, Hickey D S, Hukins D W L 1982 Computer graphics illustration of the operation of the intervertebral disc. Engng in Med. 11: 11–15

92 Klein J A, Hukins D W L 1982 X-ray diffraction demonstrates reorientation of collagen fibres in the annulus fibrosus during compression of the intervertebral disc. Biochim. Biophys. Acta 717: 61–64

93 Klein J A, Hickey D S, Hukins D W L 1983 Radial bulging of the annulus fibrosus during compression of the intervertebral disc. J. Biomech. 16: 211–217

94 Klein J A, Hukins D W L 1983 Functional differentiation in the spinal column. Engng in Med. 12: 83–85

95 Roaf R 1960 A study of the mechanics of spinal injuries. J. Bone Jt Surg. 42B: 810–823

96 Reuber M, Schultz A, Denis F, Spencer D 1982 Bulging of lumbar intervertebral discs. J. Biomech. Engng 104: 187–192

97 Kazarian L E 1975 Creep characteristics of the human spinal column. Orth. Clin. N. Am. 6: 3–18

98 Smeathers J E 1984 Some time-dependent properties of the intervertebral joint when under compression. Engng in Med. 13: 83–87

99 Farfan H F 1977 A reorientation in the surgical approach to degenerative disc disease. Orth. Clin. N. Am. 8: 9–21

100 Jayson M I V, Herbert C M, Barks J S 1973 Intervertebral discs: nuclear morphology and bursting pressure. Ann. Rheum. Dis. 32: 308–315

101 Markolf K, Morris J M 1974 The structural components of the intervertebral disc. A study of their contributions of the ability of the disc to withstand compressive forces. J. Bone Jt Surg. 56A: 675–687

102 Klein J A, Hukins D W L 1982 Collagen fibre orientation in the annulus fibrosus of intervertebral disc during bending and torsion measured by X-ray diffraction. Biochim. Biophys. Acta 719: 98–101

103 Cossette J W, Farfarn H F, Robertson G H, Wells R V 1971 The instantaneous centre of rotation of the third lumbar intervertebral joint. J. Biomech. 4: 149–153

104 Panjabi MM, Brand R A, White A A 1976 Three-dimensional flexibility and stiffness properties of the human thoracic spine. J. Biomech. 9: 185–192

105 Farfan H F, Huberdeau R M, Dubow H I 1972 The influence of geometric features on the pattern of disc degeneration — a post mortem study. J. Bone Jt Surg. 54A: 492–510

106 Adams M A, Hutton W C 1981 The relevance of torsion to the mechanical derangement of the lumbar spine. Spine 6: 241–248

107 Klein J A, Hukins D W L 1983 Relocation of the bending axis during flexion-extension of lumbar intervertebral discs and its implications for prolapse. Spine 8: 659–664

108 Rolander S D 1966 Motion of the lumbar spine with special reference to the stabilising effect of posterior fusion. An experimental study on autopsy specimens. Acta Orth. Scand. Suppl 90

109 Adams M A, Hutton W C 1982 Prolapsed intervertebral disc: a hyperflexion injury. Spine 7: 184–191

110   Katz J L 1980 The structure and biomechanics of bone. Symp. Soc. Exp. Biol. 34: 137–168

111   Schmorl G, Junghanns H 1971 The human spine in health and disease 2nd Am edn. (Beseman, E F (ed) Grune & Stratton, New York, p 262–265

112   Vernon-Roberts B, Pirie C J 1973 Healing trabecular microfractures. Ann. Rheum. Dis. 32: 406–412

113   Sims-Williams H, Jayson M I V, Baddely H 1978 Small spinal fractures in back pain patients. Ann. Rheum. Dis. 37: 262–265

114   Hansson T, Roos B 1983 The amount of bone mineral and Schmorl's nodes in lumbar vertebrae. Spine 8: 266–271

115   Ball J 1971 Enthesopathy of rheumatoid and ankylosing spondylitis. Ann. Rheum. Dis. 30: 231–223

116   Shah J S, Jayson M I V, Hampson W G J 1979 Mechanical implications of crimping in collagen fibres of human spinal ligaments. Engng in Med. 8: 95–102

117   Tkaczuk H 1968 Tensile properties of human lumbar longitudinal ligaments. Acta Orth. Scand. suppl 115

118   Waters R L, Morris J M 1973 An in vitro study of normal and scoliotic interspinous ligaments. J. Biomech. 6: 343–348

119   Nachemson A L, Evans J H 1968 Some mechanical properties of the third human lumbar interlaminar ligament (ligamentum flavum). J. Biomech. 1: 211–220

120   Adams M A, Hutton W C 1980 The role of the apophyseal joints in resisting intervertebral compressive force. J. Bone Jt Surg. 62B: 358–363

121   Maroudas A 1979 Physicochemical properties of articular cartilage. In: Freeman M A R (ed) Adult articular cartilage, 2nd edn. Pitman Medical, Tunbridge Wells, p 215–290

122   Aspden R M, Hukins D W L 1981 Collagen organisation in articular cartilage determined by X-ray diffraction and its relationship to tissue function. Proc. Roy. Soc. B212: 299–304

123   Cyron B M, Hutton W C 1980 Articular tropism and stability of the lumbar spine. Spine 6: 168–172

124   Farfan H F 1975 Muscular mechanism of the lumbar spine and the position of power and efficiency. Orth. Clin. N. Am. 6: 135–144

125   Borg T K, Caulfield J B 1980 Morphology of connective tissue in skeletal muscle. Tissue and Cell 12: 197–207

126   Katz B 1966 Nerve, muscle and synapse. McGraw-Hill, New York

127   Rowe R W D 1981 Morphology of perimysial and endomysial connective tissue in skeletal muscle. Tissue and Cell 13: 681–690

128   Rowe R W D 1974 Collagen fibre arrangement in intramuscular connective tissue. Changes associated with muscle shortening and their possible relevance to raw meat toughness measurements. J. Food Tech. 9: 501–505

129   Brieg A 1970 Overstretching of and circumscribed pathological tension in the spinal cord — a basic cause of symptoms in cord disorders. J. Biomech. 3: 7–9

130   Panjabi M M, Dicker D B, Dohrmann G J 1977 Biomechanical quantification of experimental spinal cord trauma. J. Biomech. 10: 681–687

131   Wennerstrand J, Jonsson A, Arvebo E 1978 Mechanical and histological effects of transverse impact on the canine spinal cord. J. Biomech. 11: 315–331

132   Hung T-K, Chang G-L 1981 Biomechanical and neurological response of the spinal cord of a puppy to uniaxial tension. J. Biomech. Engng 103: 43–56

133   Hung T-K, Chang G-L, Lin H-S, Walter F R, Busegin L 1981 Stress-strain relationship of the spinal cord of anaesthetised cats. J. Biomech. 14: 269–276

134   Farfan H F, Cossette J W, Robertson G H, Wells R V, Kraus H 1970 The effects of torsion on the lumbar intervertebral joints: the role of torsion in the production of disc degeneration. J. Bone Jt Surg. 52A: 468–497

135   O'Brien J P 1983 The role of fusion for chronic low back pain. Orth. Clin. N. Am. 14: 639–647

136   Paris S V 1983 Spinal manipulative therapy. Clin. Orth. Rel. Res. 179: 55–61

137   Kenedi R M, Gibson T, Evans J H, Barbenel J C 1975 Tissue mechanics. Phys. Med. Biol. 20: 699–717

Biomechanical studies in cadaveric spines

INTRODUCTION

'I often say when you can measure what you are speaking about and express it in numbers, then you know something about it; but when you cannot measure it, when you cannot express it in numbers, your knowledge is of a meagre and unsatisfactory kind.' So said Lord Kelvin in 1891. The numbers concerning the physical properties of the spine and its kinematic behaviour are necessary not for their own sake, but to provide basic understanding and to help clinicians in their work. Diseases and degeneration affect the physical properties of the spinal components: ligaments, discs, facet joints and vertebral bodies, which in turn alter the overall spinal behaviour. An indication of onset and severity of the disease/degeneration may be obtained from the study of the spinal behaviour, especially its physical properties or characteristic movements.

Another important problem concerns injuries. What forces can the spine sustain in different directions? This type of information is necessary, for example, to the designer of restraining systems for cars and the catapult escape seats in high-speed aircraft. Diseases, degeneration and injuries may lead to instability of the spine and low back pain. The physical properties of the spine are helpful in understanding the present treatment modalities as well as in developing new procedures for the future. Finally, mathematical models of the spine are valuable tools for predicting the behaviour of the spine in situations where direct human experiments may not be possible. However, in order for these models to be valid and provide insight, they must incorporate physical properties of the spine that have been obtained by experiments using fresh cadaveric spine specimens.

This chapter is a survey of biomechanics data available to date for the lumbar functional spinal unit (lumbar FSU). The FSU, or motion segment, consists of two adjacent vertebrae and connecting ligamentous tissue. It is the basis for the study of biomechanical properties of the spine, and many phenomena occurring at the FSU level can be directly transferred to gross spinal behaviour. The data presented here are therefore fundamental for any analysis or modelling of the spine.

The chapter starts with a short presentation of the mechanical and mathematical terminology and notation used throughout the presentation. After this comes a part dealing with the anatomy of the FSU, seen from a biomechanical point of view. The biomechanics of the lumbar motion segment is divided into two sections. The first deals with the intact structure and the second with the degenerated or traumatized segment, including fracture. The final part discusses some of the presented data from a functional point of view.

Throughout the chapter, the discussion of the lumbar motion segment will be organized according to its three building blocks: 1. the vertebra, 2. the intervertebral disc, and 3. the ligaments.

TERMINOLOGY AND NOTATION

Anatomical coordinate system

The anatomical coordinate system (Fig. 7.1) is introduced in order to simplify the discussion of three-dimensional phenomena in the spine.[1] It is a right-hand Cartesian coordinate system fixed in space, with the origin at the centre of the upper vertebral body of a motion segment. With this as a basis, all loads on and displacements of the motion

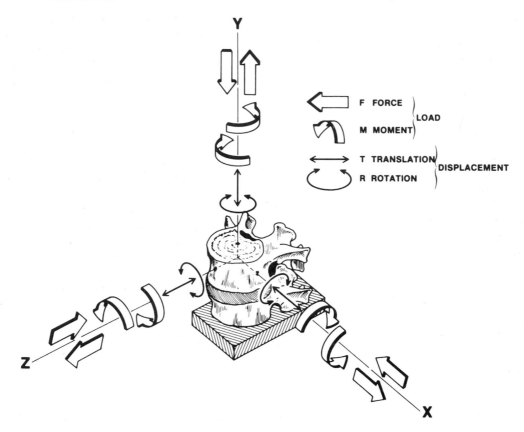

Fig. 7.1 The anatomical coordinate system

segment can be described in a mathematical, unambiguous way.

Kinematics

Kinematics is the study of rigid body motion, with no consideration of the forces involved. Some of the key terms pertaining to spine kinematics are:

Translation

A body is said to be in translation when movement is such that all particles in the body at a given time have the same direction of motion relative to a fixed point.

Rotation

A body is said to be in rotation when movement is such that all particles along some straight line in the body (or a hypothetical extension of it) have zero velocity relative to a fixed point. Rotation is a spinning or angular displacement of a body around some axis. The axis may be located outside the rotating body or inside it.

Degrees of freedom

One degree of freedom is motion in which a rigid body may translate along a straight line or rotate about an axis. Vertebrae have six degrees of freedom, translation along and rotation about each of three orthogonal axes (see Figure 7.1).

Range of motion

The difference between the two points of physiological extremes of movement is the range of motion. Translation is expressed in metres or inches, and rotation in degrees. The range of motion can be expressed for each of the six degrees of freedom.

Coupling

Coupling refers to motion in which rotation or translation of a body about or along one axis is consistently associated with simultaneous rotation or translation about another axis.

Instantaneous axis of rotation (IAR)

For a rigid body in plane motion, there is at every instant a line in the body (or in a hypothetical extension of the body) which does not move. This line is called the instantaneous axis of rotation (IAR) or sometimes the centre of rotation. Plane motion is fully defined by the position of the IAR and the magnitude of the rotation about it.

Helical axis of motion (HAM)

The instantaneous motion of a body in three-dimensional space can be analysed by regarding it as a simple screw motion. The screw motion is a superimposition of rotation and translation about and along the same axis. This axis has the same direction as the resultant of the three rotations about the x, y, and z axes. For a given moving rigid body in space at an instant, the location and direction of this axis and the designation of numerical values for rotation and translation constitute a complete, three-dimensional description of the motion.

Elasticity

Elasticity is the property of a material or a structure to return to its original form following the removal of the deforming load. Energy is stored during loading and released completely during unloading. Thus, no energy is lost in the process, and there is no permanent deformation. Stress–strain curves of an elastic material may be linear or non-linear, but the loading and unloading curves are always the same.

Viscoelasticity

Viscoelasticity is the property of a material to show sensitivity to rate of loading or deformation. This can also be characterized as time-dependent load-deformation behaviour of a material. As the name suggests, the behaviour has two basic components,

viscosity and elasticity. Creep and relaxation are two phenomenological characteristics of viscoelastic materials and are used to document their behaviour quantitatively. During creep tests, the load is suddenly applied and is kept constant thereafter. The resulting displacement is recorded against time. In relaxation tests, a deformation is produced and then fixed; the resulting decrease in load is recorded as a function of time.

There are two other phenomena that are typical of viscoelastic materials. A load-deformation curve of a viscoelastic material is dependent upon the rate of loading. The higher the rate, the steeper the curve. The other phenomenon involves the loading–unloading cycle. A viscoelastic material shows hysteresis (loss of energy in the form of heat during each cycle).

It has been experimentally determined that bone, ligaments, tendons and passive muscles are viscoelastic, and their behaviour can be readily simulated with models for viscoelastic materials.

Fracture criteria

When discussing the strength of materials, one can formulate various theoretical criteria for when a given material will rupture. For metals, the most common parameter is the ultimate stress, which means that if the material is subjected to stresses higher than this value, it will fracture. This criterion has proved to depict reality very well for a large number of construction materials. For many polymers, however, such as plastics and a large group of biomaterials including collagen, other fracture criteria work better. In many cases the ultimate strain is used, meaning that the material will fracture when extended past a certain point. This criterion does not involve any stress considerations whatsoever; it simply states that when the strain is, say, 14%, fracture will occur. More elaborate fracture formulas have also been proposed, especially for high-speed loading (impact fracture) and fatigue fracture.

Units

Two different systems of units are widely used in the biomechanical literature. The standard system for the US is still the traditional one with displacement measured in inches, force in pounds and stress in pounds per square inch (psi). The SI system (Systèm International d'Unités), proposed as a world standard, is gaining recognition throughout the world, and more and more articles will use metres (m) for displacement, newtons (N) for force and newtons per square metre or Pascals (Pa) for stress.

ANATOMY RELATED TO BIOMECHANICS

Anatomy of the vertebra

A vertebra consists of an anterior block of bone, the body, and a posterior bony ring, the neural arch, containing articular, transverse and spinous processes. The vertebral body is a roughly cylindrical mass of cancellous bone contained in a thin shell of cortical bone. Its superior and inferior surfaces, slightly concave, are called the vertebral end-plates. The neural arch consists of two pedicles and two laminae, from which arise the seven processes: the spinous process, the two transverse processes and the four facets.

The basic design of the vertebrae is the same throughout the entire spine, but their size and mass increase continually from the third cervical to the last lumbar vertebra. This is a mechanical adaptation to the increasing loads to which the spine is subjected in its lower regions. The upper two cervical vertebrae, called the atlas and axis, are of special design to allow large rotations of the head.

The pattern of movements of the spine is to a large degree dependent on the shape and orientation of the articulating processes of the diathrodial joints. The facets of the lumbar spine have curved mating surfaces, the inferior facets are convex and the superior concave. Average spatial orientation of the surfaces is depicted in Figure 7.2.

Anatomy of the disc

The intervertebral disc constitutes 20–33% of the entire height of the spinal column. It is comprised of three distinct parts: the nucleus pulposus, the annulus fibrosus and the cartilaginous end-plates.

The nucleus pulposus is a centrally located mass of fine collagenous strands in a very loose and translucent network. The fibres are embedded in a mucoprotein gel matrix containing various mucopolysaccharides. The water content ranges from 70 to 90%. It has its maximum at birth and tends to

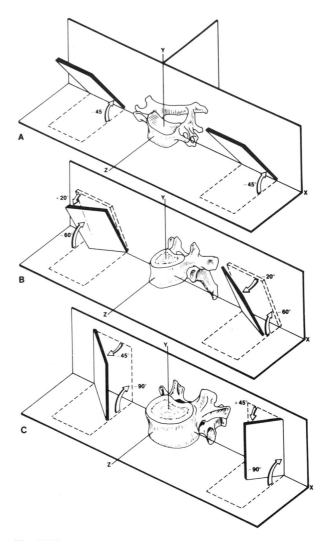

Fig. 7.2 Facet orientation

decrease with age. In the lumbar region, the nucleus fills 30–50% of the total disc area in cross-section. In the low back, the nucleus is usually positioned slightly towards the posterior part of the vertebral body.

The annulus fibrosus is a portion of the intervertebral disc which gradually becomes differentiated from the periphery of the nucleus and forms the outer boundary of the disc. This structure is composed of fibrous tissue in concentric bands. The fibres within each band are arranged in a helicoid manner. In a given band, they run in the same direction, at 30° to the disc plane. In any two adjacent bands, they run in opposite directions. In the inner zone, the annulus fibres attach to the cartilaginous end-plates, while in the outer region they are connected directly to the osseous tissue of the vertebral body. These fibres are called Sharpey's fibres.

The cartilaginous end-plates are composed of hyaline cartilage that separates the other two components of the disc from the vertebral body. Comparatively little is known about this structure.

Anatomy of the ligaments

There are six ligaments of the lumbar spine (Fig. 7.3). A short description of the ligaments arranged from anterior to posterior follows:

The anterior longitudinal ligament (ALL)

This is a fibrous tissue structure which arises from the anterior aspect of the basi-occipital and is attached to the atals and the anterior surfaces of all vertebrae, down to and including a part of the sacrum. It attaches firmly to the edges of the vertebral bodies but is more loosely affixed to the annular fibres of the intervertebral disc. The width of the anterior longitudinal ligament is diminished at the level of the disc.

The posterior longitudinal ligament (PLL)

This arises from the posterior aspect of the basi-occipital, covers the dens and the transverse liga-ment and runs over the posterior surfaces of all the vertebral bodies down to the coccyx. The ligament has an interwoven connection with the disc. In contradiction to the ALL, it is wider at the disc level and narrower at the vertebral body level.

The capsular ligaments (CL)

These are attached just beyond the margins of the adjacent articular processes. The fibres are generally oriented in a direction perpendicular to the plane of the facet joint.

The ligamenta flava (LF)

These extend from the anterior inferior border of the laminae above to the posterior superior border of the laminae below. Although they seem to be paired due to a midline cleavage, each is rather like a single structure that extends from the roots of the articular process on one side to the corresponding process on the other. The ligament is composed of a large amount of elastic fibres and is the most purely elastic tissue in the human body. With ageing there is an increase in the relative amount of fibrous tissue.

The interspinous ligament (ISL)

This connects adjacent spinous processes, and their insertion area extends from the root to the apex of each process.

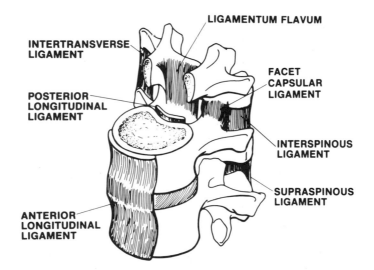

Fig. 7.3 Lumbar ligaments

The supraspinous ligament (SSL)

This originates in the ligamentum nuchae and continues along the tips of the spinous processes as a round, slender strand down to the sacrum.

In a recent project, Panjabi et al[2] measured the spatial orientation, length and cross-sectional area of the lumbar ligaments.

BIOMECHANICAL PROPERTIES OF THE LUMBAR SPINE

Kinematics of the lumbar functional spinal unit

Range of motion

The representative rotations in flexion/extension, lateral bending and axial rotation are shown in Table 7.1.[1] The flexion/extension motion range usually increases from L1 to L5. The lumbosacral joint offers more sagittal-plane motion than do the other lumbar joints. For lateral bending, each level shows about the same range, except for L5–S1, which has little motion. The situation is the same for axial rotation, except for L5–S1, which in this case shows a greater range.

Coupling characteristics

There are several coupling patterns that have been observed in the lumbar spine. Rolander[3] observed an interesting coupling of y-axis rotation (axial) with y-axis translation. There is also a coupling pattern described by Miles & Sullivan[4] in which axial rotation is combined with lateral bending, such that the spinous processes point in the same direction as the lateral bending. This pattern is the opposite of that in the cervical and upper thoracic spine. Although these coupling patterns comprise fundamental and essential elements in the understanding of lumbar spine kinematics, investigators have not been able to attach any clinical significance to them.

Instantaneous axes of rotation (IAR)

The rotation axes for the sagittal plane of the lumbar spine have been described in several reports. Calve & Galland[5] suggested that for flexion/extension the axis is located in the centre of the intervertebral disc. Rolander[3] showed that when flexion is simulated starting from a neutral position, the axis is located in the anterior portion of the disc. Reichmann and colleagues[6] reported that the IAR is occasionally in the region of the disc, but in most cases it is outside the disc and at a considerable distance from it. In lateral bending (frontal plane rotation), the axis falls in the region of the right side of the disc with left lateral bending and in the region of the left side of the disc with right lateral bending. For axial (y-axis) rotation, the IAR is located in the region of the posterior nucleus and annulus.[7]

Helical axes of motion

There is relatively little information available on the HAM parameters for the lumbar spine.[3,8,9] Goel & Panjabi[10] made a study of motion segment kinematics in response to lateral bending and shear loads, in which they measured HAM parameters. They also related HAM data to disc degeneration.

Table 7.1 Representative values of the range of rotation of the lumbar spine

Interspace	Flexion/extension (x-axis rotation)		Lateral bending (z-axis rotation)		Axial rotation (y-axis rotation)	
	Limits of ranges (degrees)	Representative angle (degrees)	Limits of ranges (degrees)	Representative angle (degrees)	Limits of ranges (degrees)	Representative angle (degrees)
L1–L2	9–16	12	3–8	6	1–3	2
L2–L3	11–18	14	3–9	6	1–3	2
L3–L4	12–18	15	5–10	8	1–3	2
L5–S1	14–21	17	5–7	6	1–3	2
	18–22	20	2–3	3	3–6	5

Elastic and viscoelastic properties of the disc

The simple compression test of the disc has been one of the most popular experiments in biomechanics; this is naturally due to the importance of the disc as a major load-carrying element in the spine.[11-16]

Typically, the load-displacement curve of a disc subjected to compressive loading shows three phases. For small loads, the disc displays very low stiffness. This gradually increases with higher loads, and in a fairly wide load range the load-displacement curve is linear. Just prior to failure, the stiffness decreases. Thus, the disc can provide flexibility at low loads and stability at high loads.

Markolf[17] has also studied the load-displacement relation in discs subjected to tensile loads. He found the structure to be less stiff in tension than in compression; this he believes is due to build-up of fluid pressure within the nucleus under compression.

Farfan et al[18] studied the torsional stiffness characteristics of the disc. The torque-rotation curves obtained from the testing had the same triphasic characteristics as those obtained for compression. Markolf[17] has reported stiffness for the disc subjected to shear loading. Numerical values for stiffness properties of the disc are collectively presented in Table 7.2.[1]

The intervertebral disc shows viscoelastic, i.e time-dependent, load-displacement behaviour. Markolf & Morris[19] studied creep under the appli-cation of three different loads and made observations up to 70 minutes. The higher loads produced larger deformation and faster rates of creep. Kazarian[20] performed creep tests on spine motion segments and classified the discs into four grades, from 0 to 3, according to their degree of degeneration (same system as used by Rolander[3]). He observed that the creep characteristics of the disc and its degeneration grade are related. The non-degenerated discs creep slowly and reach their final deformation after considerable time, as compared to the degenerated discs. Thus, the process of degeneration makes the disc less viscoelastic. This implies that, as the disc degenerates, it loses the capacity to attenuate shocks and to distribute the load uniformly over the entire end-plate. Hysteresis, another viscoelastic pheno-menon closely related to energy absorption, has been studied by Virgin.[11] It seems to vary with the load applied, as well as with the disc age and the spine level. It is largest in very young people and the middle-aged. Virgin also reported that the hysteresis decreased when the same disc was loaded a second time. This may imply that we are less protected against repetititve loads.

Elastic and viscoelastic properties of the ligaments

Tkaczuk[21] did an extensive study of the tensile characteristics of the anterior and posterior longi-tudinal ligaments with the purpose of examining the

Table 7.2 Stiffness coefficients of the intervertebral disc (average values)

Authors	Stiffness coefficient*	Maximum load*	Spine region
Compression (−Fy)			
Virgin[11]	2.5 MN/m	4500 N	Lumbar
Hirsch & Nachemson[12]	0.7 MN/m	1000 N	Lumbar
Brown et al[14]	2.3 MN/m	5300 N	Lumbar
Markolf[17]	1.8 MN/m	1800 N	Thoracic and lumbar
Tension (+Fy)			
Markolf[17]	1.0 MN/m	1800 N	Thoracic and lumbar
Shear (Fx, Fz)			
Markolf[17]	0.26 MN/m	150 N	Thoracic and lumbar
Axial rotation (My)			
Farfan[18]	2.0 N m/deg	31 N m	Lumbar

* N = newton, kN = 1000 newton, MN = 1 000 000 newton

influence on the biomechanical properties of these tissues due to degeneration and age. In one set of experiments, specimens of a standard size were used. The samples were loaded up to one-third of the failure load, and the load-deformation curves were recorded. Three parameters were recorded: the maximum deformation, the residual or permanent deformation, and the energy loss due to hysteresis. All these factors were found to decrease with age. The greatest decrease was found in the energy absorption values, documenting the decrease of shock-absorption capabilities in ligaments with age. Tkaczuk also reported that the maximum and residual deformations were lower for specimens with degenerated discs.

Panjabi et al[2] studied the load-strain characteristics of the separate ligaments in the lumbar spine. Their technique allowed recording of axial as well as transverse strain along the ligaments. The stiffest ligament proved to be the posterior, and the superspinous the most flexible.

The function and importance of the ligamentum flavum has been a matter of discussion from the beginning of this century.[22,23] Some biomechanical studies of this important ligament have been reported.[24,25] A report of great interest is that by Nachemson & Evans.[26] Ten specimens of ligamentum flavum and attached laminae, from the L3–L4 segment, were loaded at slow speed along the spine axis. While separating the vertebral laminae from the bodies, Nachemson & Evans found the ligamentum flavum to have pre-tension (tension present in situ when the spine is in its neutral position). This 'resting' tension in the ligament produces resting compression of the disc. Histologically, the ligamentum flavum has the highest percentage of elastic fibres of any tissue in the body. This allows a large amount of extension of the ligament without residual deformation.

Elastic and viscoelastic properties of the lumbar functional spinal unit

Compressive loading, again because of its assumed clinical importance and simplicity of testing, has dominated the studies of stiffness of the spine.[3,12,16,27,28,29] Tension and shear, on the other hand, are probably the least studied.[30]

Experiments have shown that the lumbar FSU is stiffer in compression than in tension. This is probably due to the hydrostatic pressure within the disc. The spine becomes stiffer at higher loads, shown by studies of Hirsch & Nachemson[12] and Rolander.[3]

Liu et al[30] have reported that the shear stiffness in the lumbar region is about twice as high in the lateral as compared to the anteroposterior direction. Lin et al[31] and Berkson et al[32] have, however, come to the conclusion that the difference is not that large. The latter study found the lumbar motion segment to be stiffest in posterior shear. There is no consistent pattern of change with spine level. In general, the spine was found to be much more flexible in shear as compared to compression, the shear stiffness being 15% of the compressive value.[33]

Panjabi et al[29] have reported extensive work on the three-dimensional behaviour of the lumbar spine. For each FSU tested, they recorded 72 load-displacement curves, representing the complete flexibility characteristics of the specimen. The study also investigated the effect of a compressive preload on the spine behaviour (Fig. 7.4). They found that the spine became more flexible in the presence of preload with the physiological forces directed laterally or anteriorly. The preloaded spine was less flexible when subjected to axial tension or axial torsion. No appreciable change due to preload was noticed when axial compression, posteriorly directed force, or extension moment was applied.

Lin and co-workers[34] tested lumbar specimens in complex modes, including eccentric compression and combined compression, bending and shear. The data were used with an optimization routine in order to determine the orthotropic elastic properties of the intervertebral disc.

In a project reported by Schultz et al[35] and Berkson et al,[32] the three-dimensional load-displacement behaviour of 24 lumbar FSUs was measured. Intradiscal pressure was also recorded. The study compared intact specimens with FSUs in which the posterior elements had been removed. Tencer et al[36] reported a study in which 14 lumbar FSUs were tested, with and without preload. An interpretation of the results in terms of relative load-bearing roles of the different parts of the FSU was also presented. The results indicated that the disc is the major load-bearing element in lateral and posterior shear, axial compression and flexion, while

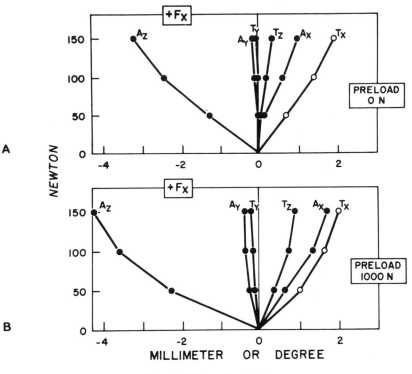

Fig. 7.4 Effects of preload

the facets play an important role in anterior shear and axial torque.

Many papers have reported the spine stiffness behaviour in bending.[37,29] The spine seems to be more flexible in flexion than in extension. The increased flexibility is about 25–30%. On removal of the posterior elements, the extension flexibility increased so that there was no more difference between flexion and extension. The flexion flexibility did not change when the posterior elements were removed.[37]

THE BIOMECHANICS OF DISEASE AND TRAUMA

Failure loads of the vertebra

The ultimate strength of vertebral bodies has been of interest to scientists for a long time, the first study having been done over 100 years ago.[27] In recent times, many of the investigations of this problem have been related to the problem of pilot ejection injuries.[38–40] The experiments show the same general results: the ultimate compressive strength of the

vertebrae is highly dependent on the spine level (Fig. 7.5). With values of about 1.6 kN (340 lbf) in the upper cervical spine, the failure load of the lumbar spine can be as high as 8 kN (1760 lbf). This tendency is of course quite logical: the lower the spine level, the more load must the segment be able to carry. The increase in strength is mainly caused by increased vertebral cross-sectional area.[41]

In general, the strength of the vertebrae decreases with age. Bell et al[39] have shown a definite relationship between vertebral strength and relative ash content of osseous tissue. Studying the lumbar spine, Hansson et al[42] have shown that there is a highly significant correlation between mechanical strength and bone mineral content. Bell et al[39] have also shown that a small loss of bone tissue can produce a large reduction of vertebral strength. The phenomena can be explained in terms of mechanics by a close study of the spongy structure of the vertebra (Fig. 7.6).

This can be seen as a network of vertical columns and horizontal ties, together carrying load from the end-plates.[43–45] According to classical mechanics, the buckling strength of a column is proportional to the

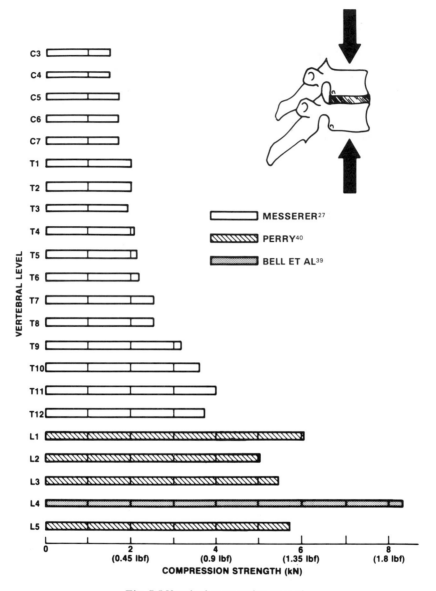

Fig. 7.5 Vertebral compression strength

square of its cross-sectional area, and inversely proportional to the square of its free length. It can hence be seen that a reduction in bone tissue mass, either in the form of reduced cross-sectional area of the vertical columns or as fewer horizontal ties, could drastically reduce the ultimate strength of the vertebral body.

The major part of the compressive load on the spine is carried by the vertebral body; only about 18% of the total load is transferred by the facets.[46] King et al[47] on the other hand, have stated that the neural arch structure under various dynamic conditions can carry anywhere between zero and 33% of the total motion segment load.

Little information is available on the ultimate strength of the neural arch and the facets.

Failure loads of the disc

Compression

Although it is the cause of many problems, the intervertebral disc is a surprisingly tough structure.

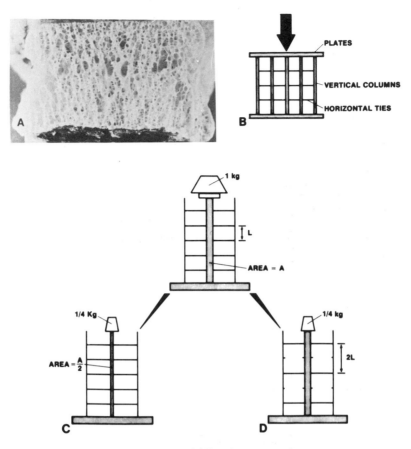

Fig. 7.6 Vertebral failure in osteoporosis

Virgin[11] observed that, although discs were subjected to very high loads and showed permanent deformation on removal of the load, there was no herniation of the nucleus due to the compressive load. Even when a longitudinal incision was made in the posterolateral part of the annulus all the way to the centre and the specimen was loaded in compression, there was no disc herniation. This has been substantiated by several researchers.[13,14,16,19,40]

To compare the relative strength of the disc to that of the vertebral body in supporting compressive loads, static tests were conducted by Brown and colleagues[14] on motion segments (without posterior elements) of the lumbar region. They found that the first component to fail in such a construct was the vertebra, due to fracture of the end-plates. No failure of the disc ever took place. The mode of failure was solely dependent on the condition of the vertebral body. Osteoporotic vertebrae showed extensive collapse of the end-plate and the underlying bone at relatively low loads. Brown and colleagues also observed that there were no differences between the vertebrae with 'normal' and degenerated discs.

Farfan[16] on the contrary, proved by his large number of tests that the degenerated disc was actually stronger than the normal disc when subjected to compression. Experiments were conducted on lumbar spine specimens using discography to demonstrate the movements of the nucleus pulposus under compressive loading. After the first cracks were heard, indicating fracture of the vertebral endplates, the nucleus was found to migrate into the bodies, resembling Schmorl's nodes. The observations suggest that disc herniation is not caused by excessive compressive loading.

With central compressive loading, the disc was observed to bulge in the horizontal plane, but not in any particular direction.[14] This implies that the tendency for the disc to herniate posterolaterally, as seen in the clinical situation, is not inherent in the structure of the disc, but must depend upon certain loading conditions other than compression.

Bending

Bending and torsional loads are of particular interest, since experimental findings suggest that these and not the compression loads are the most damaging to the disc.[16]

Bending of the disc of 6–8° in the sagittal, frontal and other vertical planes did not result in failure of the lumbar disc. However, after removal of the posterior elements and with 15° of bending (anterior flexion), failure did occur.[14] A triangular piece of bone was avulsed from the postero-inferior aspect of the superior vertebra in this experiment. Other interesting findings concerned the bulging of the disc during normal physiological motions. The disc bulged anteriorly during flexion, posteriorly during extension, and toward the concavity of the spinal curve during lateral bending. The disc contracted on the opposite sides (on the convexity of the curve). Very little motion took place in a direction perpendicular to the plane of motion.

Torsion

The hypothesis that torsion may be the major injury-causing load was put forward by Farfan[16] in 1973. In his experiment FSUs were subjected to torsional loading around an axis passing through the posterior aspect of the disc. Torque-angle curves were recorded to failure. About 20° of rotation was generally required to produce failure. Sharp, cracking sounds emanating from the specimen were noted before rupture occurred. No fracture of the endplates was found. The average failure torque for normal discs was about 25% higher than that for degenerated discs.

Fatigue tolerance

As the biological capacity for repair and regeneration of the disc is thought to be low, its fatigue properties are important. Unfortunately, very little is known about this subject. Brown and colleagues[14] performed a single fatigue test on the disc by applying a small constant axial load and a repetitive forward bending motion of 5°. The disc showed signs of failure after only 200 cycles, and it completely failed after 1000 cycles. This indicates that the fatigue tolerance is low, at least under in vitro conditions.

Failure loads of the ligaments

Myklebust and colleagues[48] reported a study in which spinal ligaments (anterior and posterior longitudinal ligaments, joint capsules, interspinous ligaments and ligamentum flavum) were tested to failure. The anterior longitudinal ligaments and the joint capsules were consistently the strongest, and the interspinous and posterior longitudinal ligaments the weakest. The failure loads ranged from 30 to 500 N, with the highest values observed in the lumbar spine.

Panjabi et al[2] tested the ligaments of 17 lumbar FSUs, recording the load-deformation curves as well as the failure loads (Fig. 7.7). The stiffest structure was the posterior longitudinal ligament, while the anterior longitudinal ligament was the strongest. the supraspinous ligament showed the highest failure deformation, and the anterior and posterior longitudinal ligaments the least.

Effects of disc degeneration

It is somtimes assumed that with age the disc space narrows and the disc becomes stiffer; it is also assumed that a herniated disc is biomechanically unsound.[49] In a carefully conducted study of lumbar cadaveric FSUs, Nachemson et al[50] made the following observations. The disc height was found to be about the same in the degenerated and non-degenerated spine specimens. The age and disc level also did not affect the mechanical properties of the functional spinal unit. The most interesting finding concerned disc degeneration: no consistent correlation was observed between disc degeneration and mechanical behaviour. In this study, however, only the elastic behaviour was measured. Kazarian[20] found the viscoelastic behaviour to be significantly altered due to disc degeneration. There was less creep (deformation with time under constant load) in functional spinal units that had degenerated discs as compared to the ones with non-degenerated discs.

In a recent study, Panjabi et al[51] studied the three-dimensional behaviour of the functional spinal units

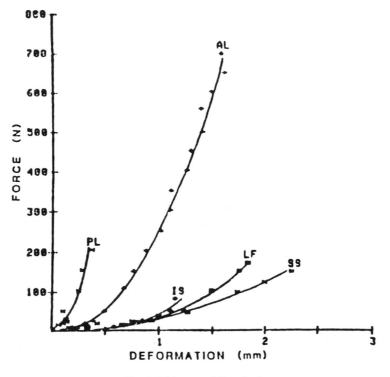

Fig. 7.7 Ligament failure loads

of the lumbar spine subjected to forces and moments in different directions, with special reference to disc degeneration grades. Two parameters were studied: the total ranges of motion and 'neutral zone'. The latter is defined as the amount of motion present in the functional spinal unit due to the application of only a small force. In general, ROMs for different loads did not change with disc degeneration, with one exception. It increased significantly for axial torsion. For this loading, the 'neutral zone' was also found to be significantly related to disc degeneration with a positive correlation coefficient of 0.76. For the load types that produced motions in the plane of the disc, the 'neutral zone' increased significantly with disc degeneration, although the corresponding ROMs did not. Thus, although the range of motion may not be directly related to disc degeneration, yet the 'neutral zone', especially in the horizontal plane, seems to be related to the degeneration of the disc. This may have significance for chronic spinal instability or the mechanics of low back pain.

Effects of disc injury

Some experimental evidence suggest that the construction of the disc is such that, when an intact disc is injured, some type of 'self-sealing' mechanism takes place. Markolf & Morris [19] reported the results of an experiment with compression loading of injured discs. Their basic specimen consisted of a motion segment which had been modified by sawing off the posterior elements at the pedicles. Three models of injury were studied: a radial hole through the annulus, discectomy and an axial hole through the entire construct, removing the central portion of the end-plates and the nucleus. Each specimen was tested before and after injury. The test after injury involved three load/unload cycles. The mechanical characteristics recorded were the load-displacement curve, the creep behaviour and relaxation, all under compressive loading. With the first loading cycle and with subsequent injury, results showed that there were definite changes in the mechanical characteristics of the specimen. But a remarkable 'self-sealing' process came into play when the specimen was loaded for a second and third time. During the third loading cycle, the FSU showed near-'intact behavr.

Panjabi et al[52] came to quite different conclusions in their study. Eight lumbar FSUs were tested three-dimensionally. Three states of the disc were studied: intact structure, lateral annular injury and discectomy. Elastic behaviour as well as creep response were recorded. They found that the injuries significantly altered the mechanical properties of the spinal unit, main motions as well as coupled, but no self-sealing effect was observed (Fig. 7.8).

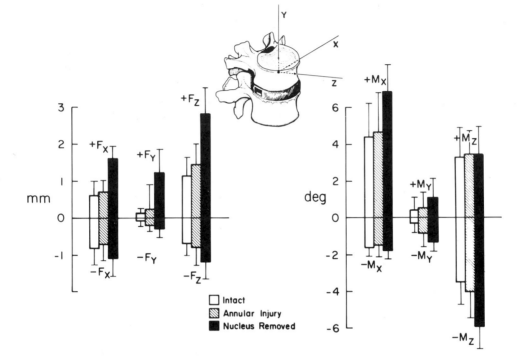

Fig. 7.8 Flexibility response as a function of disc injury

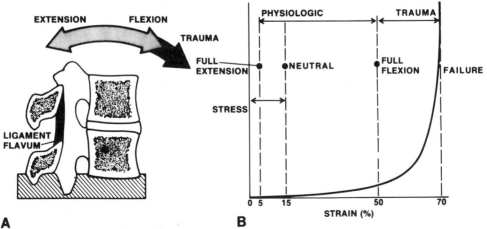

Fig. 7.9 Ligament behaviour

FUNCTIONAL BIOMECHANICS

Function of the facets

The lumbar intervertebral joints are thought to be anatomically designed to limit anterior translation and permit considerable sagittal and frontal plane rotation.[53] The intervertebral joints are aligned to resist axial rotation. In general, these joints are thought to serve as a guide for the displacement patterns of the motion segments.[54,55]

Function of the ligaments

The ligaments are uni-axial structures, acting rather like rubber bands. They readily resist tensile forces but buckle under compressive loads. When a spine motion segment is subjected to different forces and moments, various groups of ligaments are subjected to tension and thus stabilize the segment (Fig. 7.9).

The spinal ligaments have many functions. First, they must allow adequate physiological motion and fixed postural attitudes between vertebrae, with minimum muscle energy expenditure. Second, they must protect the spinal cord by restricting the motion within well-defined physiological limits. Finally, they must protect the spinal cord in traumatic situations where high loads are applied at fast speeds. In these highly dynamic situations, not only is the displacement to be restricted within safe limits, but large amounts of energy suddenly applied to the spine have to be absorbed.

REFERENCES

1 White A A, Panjabi M M 1978 Clinical biomechanics of the spine. Lippincott, Philadelphia
2 Panjabi M M, Jorneus L, Greenstein G 1984 Lumbar spine ligaments: an in vitro biomechanical study. ORS Transactions
3 Rolander S D 1966 Motion of the lumbar spine with special reference to the stabilizing effect of posterior fusion. Thesis, Department of Orthopaedic Surgery, University of Gothenburg, Sweden
4 Miles M, Sullivan W E 1961 Lateral bending at the lumbar and lumbosacral joints. Anat. Rec. 139: 387
5 Calve J, Galland M 1930 Physiologie pathologique du mal de Pott. Rev. Orthop. 1: 5
6 Reichmann S, Berglund E, Lundgren K 1972 Das Bewegungszentrum in der Lendenwirbelsaule bei Flexion und Extension. Z. Anat. Entwicklungsgesch. 138: 283
7 Cossette J W, Farfan H F, Robertson G H, Wells R V 1971 The instantaneous center of rotation of the third lumbar intervertebral joint. J. Biomech. 4: 149
8 White A A 1969 Analysis of the mechanics of the thoracic spine in man. Acta Orthop. Scand. 127 (Suppl)
9 Lysell E 1969 Motion of the cervical spine. Acta Orthop. Scand. 123 (Suppl)
10 Goel V K, Panjabi M M 1984 Motion segment kinematics in response to lateral bending and shear loads. Presented at ISSLS, Montreal
11 Virgin W 1951 Experimental investigations into physical properties of intervertebral discs. J. Bone Joint Surg. 33B: 607
12 Hirsch C, Nachemson A 1954 A new observation on the mechanical behavior of lumbar discs. Acta Orthop. Scand. 23: 254
13 Hirsch C 1955 The reaction of intervertebral discs to compression forces. J. Bone Joint Surg. 37A: 1188
14 Brown T, Hanson R, Yorra A 1957 Some mechanical tests on the lumbo-sacral spine with particular reference to the intervertebral discs. J. Bone Joint Surg. 39A: 1135
15 Roaf R 1960 A study of the mechanics of spinal injuries. J. Bone Joint Surg. 42B: 810
16 Farfan H F 1973 Mechanical disorders of the low back. Lea & Febiger, Philadelphia
17 Markolf K L 1970 Stiffness and damping characteristics of the thoracic-lumbar spine. Proceedings of Workshop on Bioengineering Approaches to the Problems of the Spine, NIH, Septemebr
18 Farfan H F, Cossette J W, Robertson G H, Wells R V, Kraus H 1970 The effects of torsion on the lumbar intervertebral joints: the role of torsion in the production of disc degeneration. J. Bone Joint Surg. 52A: 468
19 Markolf K L, Morris J M 1974 The structural components of the intervertebral disc. J. Bone Joint Surg. 56A: 675
20 Kazarian L E 1975 Creep characteristics of the human spinal column. Orthop. Clin. North Am. 6: 3
21 Tkaczuk H 1968 Tensile properties of human lumbar longitudinal ligaments. Acta Orthop. Scand. 115 (Suppl)
22 Fick R 1904 Handbook der Anatomie and Mechanik der Gelenke. Fischer, Jena
23 Strasser H 1908 Lehrbuch der Musker und Gelenkmechanik. Springer, Berlin
24 Akerblom B 1948 Standing and sitting posture (thesis). A/B Nordiska Bokhandels, Stockholm
25 Nunley R L 1958 The ligamenta flava of the dog: a study of tensile and physical properties. Am. J. Phys. Med. 37: 256
26 Nachemson A, Evans J 1968 Some mechanical properties of the third lumbar inter-laminar ligament (ligamentum flavum). J. Biomech. 1: 211
27 Messerer O 1880 Uber Elastität und Festigkeit der Menschlichen Knochen. Cottaschen, Stuttgart
28 Perry O 1957 Fracture of the vertebral end-plate in the lumbar spine. Acta Orthop. Scand. 25 (Suppl)
29 Panjabi M M, Krag M H, White A A, Southwick W O 1977 Effects of preload on load displacement curves of the lumbar spine. Orthop. Clin. North Am. 88: 181
30 Liu K Y, Ray G, Hirsch C 1975 The resistance of the lumbar spine to direct shear. Orthop. Clin. North Am. 6: 33
31 Lin H S, Liu Y K, Ray G, Nikravesh P 1978 Systems identification for material properties of the intervertebral joint. J. Biomech. 11: 1
32 Berkson M H, Nachemson A, Schultz A B 1979

Mechanical properties of human lumbar spine motion segments. Part II: Responses in compression and shear; influence of gross morphology. J. Biomech. Eng. 101: 53

33   Belytschko T, Andriacchi T, Schultz A, Galante J 1973 Analog studies of forces in human spine: computational techniques. J. Biomech. 6: 361

34   Lin H S, Liu Y K, Adams K H 1978 Mechanical response of the lumbar intervertebral joint under physiological (complex) loading. J. Bone Joint Surg. 60A: 41

35   Schultz A B, Warwick D N, Berkson M H, Nachemson A L 1979 Mechanical properties of human lumbar spine motion segments — Part I: Responses in flexion, extension, lateral bending and torsion. J. Biomech. Eng. 101: 46

36   Tencer A F, Ahmed A M, Burke D L 1982 Some static mechanical properties of the lumbar intervertebral joint, intact and injured. J. Biomech. Eng. 104: 193

37   Markolf K L 1972 Deformation of the thoracolumbar intervertebral joint in response to external loads: a biomechanical study using autopsy material. J. Bone Joint Surg. 54A: 511

38   Ruff S 1950 Brief acceleration: less than one second. In: German aviation medicine in World War II, vol 1. US Government Printing Office, Washington DC

39   Bell G H, Dunbar O, Beck J S, Gibb A 1967 Variation in strength of vertebrae with age and their relation to osteoporosis. Calcif. Tissue Res. 1: 75

40   Perry O 1974 Resistance and compression of the lumbar vertebrae. In: Encyclopedia of medical radiology. Springer, New York

41   Weaver J K 1966 Bone: its strength and changes with aging and an evaluation of some methods for measuring its mineral content. J. Bone Joint Surg. 41A: 935

42   Hansson T H, Ross B O, Nachemson A L 1978 The bone mineral content and biomechanical properties of lumbar vertebrae. Presented at the 24th annual meeting of the Orthopaedic Research Society, Dallas

43   Casuccio C 1962 An introduction to the study of osteoporosis. Proc. R. Soc. Med. 55: 663

44   Atkinson P J 1967 Variation in trabecular structure of vertebrae with age. Calcif. Tissue Res. 1: 24

45   Amstutz H C, Sissons H A 1969 The structure of the vertebral spongiosa. J. Bone Joint Surg. 51B: 540

46   Nachemson A 1960 Lumbar intradiscal pressure. Acta Orthop. Scand. 43 (Suppl)

47   King A I, Prasad P, Ewing C L 1975 Mechanism of spinal injury due to caudocephalad acceleration. Orthop. Clin. North Am. 6: 19

48   Myklebust J B, Pintar F, Maiman D, Sances Jr A 1983 The strength of spinal ligaments.

49   Harris R I, Macnab I 1954 Structural changes in the lumbar intervertebral discs. Their relationship to low back pain sciatica. J. Bone Joint Surg. 36B: 304

50   Nachemson A, Schultz A B, Berkson M H 1979 Mechanical properties of human lumbar spine motion segments. Influences of age, sex, disc level and degeneration. Spine 4: 1

51   Panjabi M M, Goel V K, Summers D J 1983 Effects of disc degeneration on the instability of a motion segment. Orth. Res. Soc. Trans.

52   Panjabi M M, Krag M H, Chung T Q 1984 Effects of disc injury on mechanical behaviour of the human spine. Spine 9: 707

53   Lewin T 1964 Osteoarthritis in lumbar synovial joints. A morphological study. Acta Orthop. Scand. 73 (Suppl)

54   Armstrong J R 1958 Lumbar disc lesions. Livingstone, Edinburgh

55   Nachemson A 1963 The influence of spinal movements on the lumbar intradiscal pressure and on the tensile stresses in the annulus fibrosus. Acta Orthop. Scand. 33: 183

Mathematical models of the spine and their experimental validation

INTRODUCTION

Much evidence, anecdotal and otherwise, exists to show that low back pain is often associated with mechanical loading. The axiskeleton and soft tissues of the lumbar spine deform under applied loads. If these deformations exceed certain limits, nociceptors are activated, which the brain perceives as pain. Within the intervertebral joint complex, nociceptors are located in both cortical and cancellous bone, outer layers of the annulus fibrosus, facet capsules, ligaments and cartilaginous endplates. The present chapter is concerned principally with the mathematical modelling and experimental validation of the vertebral column in general and the lumbar spine in particular. The approach is from the point of view of structural mechanics. The implicit assumption is that the nociceptors are embedded within the structure and are activated by some 'excessive' strain, although no experimental data exist on the threshold values needed to trigger nociception.

ADVANTAGES OF USING MODELS

Mathematical models of a spinal segment or whole spine are significant for the same reasons that models are valuable in other branches of engineering and science: 1. they systematize thinking; 2. they provide a framework for the evaluation of existing evidence; and 3. they show some types of evidence to be more important than others. Furthermore, models enable predictions to be made, and therefore suggest experiments which otherwise might not have come to mind.

Computer models, if viewed as surrogate experiments, offer the ideal opportunity from the point of view of control. They are, if done correctly, characterized by absolute repeatability, with the additional advantage of the user being able to vary any parameter in the most minute degree and observe what effect the change of that particular parameter might have on the final outcome. Once developed, these are perhaps the most compact and economical of all research methodologies available.

Sometimes certain parameters cannot be measured experimentally and one has to resort to mathematical models to find an answer. For example, a knowledge of the state of stress and strain and the forces acting throughout the lumbosacral joint may be helpful to a proper understanding of some of the mechanical causes of low back pain. Technical difficulties preclude direct measurements of these causes in all relevant components of the spine, and a mathematical model may be one of the alternative approaches to overcome these hurdles. The unusual complexity of the spinal structure, however, demands a stepwise approach, i.e. at each step of model development, its predictions should be validated in terms of those parameters amenable to experimental measurement.

A number of analytical models simulating the response of the human spine, exhibiting large displacements, rotations and constantly-changing inertial and stiffness properties, have been developed in the past. These models can be categorized according to whether they simulate static or dynamic situations and each category further differentiated according to whether large displacements can be accommodated, whether the vertebral bodies are modelled as rigid or elastic, and finally the techniques used to model the intervertebral disc and ligamentous structures. The accuracy of a mathematical model is in direct proportion to the accuracy with which the input variables are known. Some of these variables are:

1. Nature of loads acting on the spine
2. Kinematically possible modes of body response and their effects on the stress distribution
3. Material behaviour and mechanisms of injury of the individual components of the spinal column.

WHOLE-SPINE MODELS

As a result of spinal injuries suffered by pilots during ejection from high-speed aircraft, much of the early modelling efforts dealt with responses of the spine to impact loads. Any modelling related to the whole spine naturally applies to the lumbar region as well.

A discrete-parametric, two-dimensional, mid-sagittal model of the total spinal column including the head (Fig. 8.1) was developed by Orne & Liu[1] based on the experimental data available then. The unshaded and shaded areas in the figure represent the vertebrae and intervertebral discs respectively. The orientation of the lowest disc with respect to the spinal axis was determined by the angle ψ. The external forces, $F(t)$, experienced by the pilot during

ejection, were represented by the angle η, as shown in Figure 8.1. The following constitutive equation was used to model the intersegmental behaviour of the 'generalized disc', i.e., all the soft tissues and facet joint interactions between the vertebrae, under axial compressive loads:

$$\sigma + p_1\dot{\sigma} = q_0\epsilon + q_1\dot{\epsilon} \qquad (1)$$

where σ and ϵ denote the axial stress and strain in the disc with respect to local coordinate system and p_1, q_0 and q_1 are material constants. Since the intersegmental 'disc' under the influence of external loads would experience shear, axial plus bending loads, the following three equations, based on equation (1), expressed the relationship between the forces experienced by the disc and the resulting motions with respect to the coordinate system (Fig. 8.2).

$$F_1 = (GA/kl)\,\delta_s$$

$$F_2 = (12EI/l^3)\,\delta_b + (6EI/l^2)\,\delta_3$$

$$F_3 = (6EI/l^2)\,\delta_b + (4EI/l)\,\delta_3$$

and $F_2 + p_1F_2 = (A/l)\,(q_0\delta_2 + q_1\dot{\delta}_2),$

where $\sigma = F_2/A$ and $\epsilon = \delta_2/l$, and k, E, G, A and l denote the shape factor for the cross-section of the disc, the Young's modulus, shear modulus, area of cross-section and disc thickness respectively. The term (GA/kl) represents the shear stiffness of the disc.

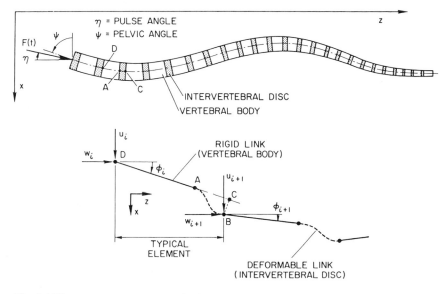

Fig. 8.1 Discrete parameter model of spinal column.

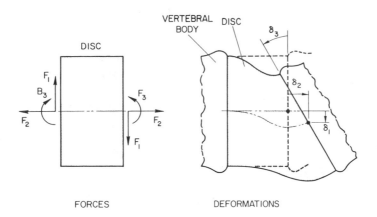

VERTEBRAL BODY   DISC

DISC

FORCES

DEFORMATIONS

Fig. 8.2 Intervertebral disc forces and deformation.

Each vertebra, considered massless, was assumed to support a distributed slice of mass m_i acting at some eccentricity, e_i, as shown in Figure 8.3. The rotational mass moment of inertia, J_i, about an axis passing through the centre of the mass and perpendicular to X–Z plane was also included in the model. The generalized forces, B_i, Q_i and P_i, are the reactions offered by the adjacent disc. Thus, the differential equations of motion for the intervertebral segments were obtained. These solutions of differential equations, using numerical integration techniques, needed some boundary conditions: forces acting at the superior aspect of the head were assumed zero and a known acceleration pulse was applied at the pelvis. Numerical integration determined the distribution of forces (axial as well as shear) and bending moment as a function of time and

at each location of the vertebra within the spinal column. An example of these induced forces and moments at L1–L2 spinal level is shown in Figure 8.4.

It is possible to predict stress and strains within the 'disc' once the forces and moments are known and constitutive equations assumed. This passive model, besides providing the likely cause of fracture during pilot ejection and the spinal region most likely to sustain these fractures, showed an urgent need to determine the following:

1. Variation of material properties along spine under the combined action of axial, shear and bending loads
2. Mechanisms of failure of vertebra subjected to complex loads
3. Variations of rotatory inertia and mass eccentricity along the spinal column.

HEAD AND NECK MODELS

A number of researchers have improved upon the model. McKenzie & Williams,[2] using the model of Orne & Liu,[1] predicted the dynamic response of head and neck during hyperextension and hyperflexion (whiplash). Parsad & King[3] extended the Orne and Liu model by considering the facets as separate entities instead of lumping these with the 'discs'. The more recent lumped-parameter models of Huston et al[4] and Reber & Goldsmith[5] have included the effects of facets, discs, muscles and ligaments for the head and neck. The models

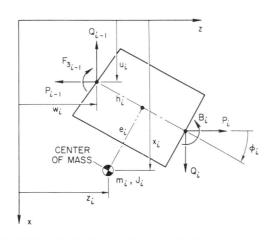

Fig. 8.3 Free-body diagram of vertebral body.

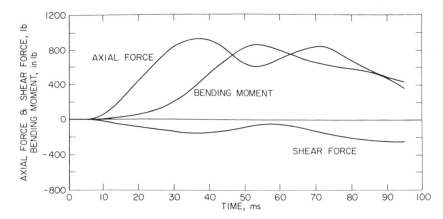

Fig. 8.4 Time history of axial force, shear force and bending movement at disc between vertebrae L1 and L2.

predicted the kinematic response to the frontal acceleration quite well.

The next pioneering work was that of Williams & Belytschko.[6] They proposed a three-dimensional analytical model to predict the kinematic response of the head and neck (including muscles) subjected to impact loads. The cervical vertebrae and head were treated as rigid bodies, and deformable elements were located between adjacent vertebrae representing the intervertebral discs and ligaments (Fig. 8.5). Spring elements were used to model ligaments and beam elements (possessing axial, bending and torsional stiffnesses) for the disc. A special type of spring element in which the axial force may be activated independently of the elongation was used to mimic muscle contraction. In lateral and/or frontal plane accelerations, it was very difficult to ensure the stability of the cervical spine model with facets represented by springs. To overcome this deficiency, a special type of pentahedral continuum element was developed to model the facet interaction. The initial orientation of muscles, ligaments and spinal components was taken from standard anatomical texts. The stiffness values for the elements were also derived from literature. The loads obtained from their hybrid model (combination of lumped-parameter and finite elements) were used as input for the finite element programs for transient analysis.[7-9]

The model was employed to predict the response of the human head and neck under a variety of head impact conditions. The model was validated by comparing the computed time-history of vertical

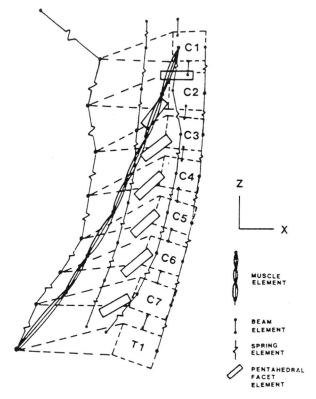

Fig. 8.5 Major muscle and ligament elements in model.

displacement Z of the head in response to $-G_x$ (frontal) acceleration with the results of Ewing et al[10] (Fig. 8.6). The graph shows good agreement with the experimental results up to 200 ms for the model in which muscles were treated as active elements. The results of passive muscle model and ligamentous

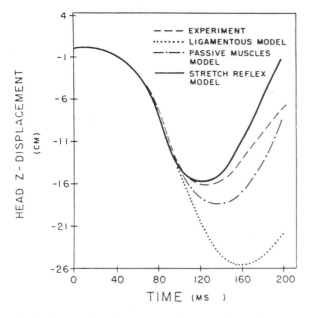

Fig. 8.6 Vertical (z) displacement of head relative to T1 compared to $-G_x$ (experiment of Ewing et al[10]).

model were in agreement with the experiment during the first 90–100 ms. A reasonable agreement was also found between the predictions of the active muscles model with the experimental data of Ewing et al[10] in other acceleration modes.

The effect of muscular activity on forces in the spine was also examined. The axial force in the disc was characterized by an initial tensile peak, followed by a much larger compressive peak. In the active muscle model the peak axial compressive force increased by 20–50% compared to the passive muscle model. The peak shear forces also increased by 25–80% as a result of muscular contraction, while the peak tensile forces remained approximately the same. It is interesting to note that the authors found a decrease in bending moments and ligamentous forces with the use of active muscles in the model.

Belytschko et al[7,8] and Schultz et al[11] developed 3-D structural models of the isolated thoracolumbar spinal motion segment. As a matter of fact, these were the forerunners of their later work on head and neck models. In these models, vertebrae were simulated as rigid bodies and discs and ligaments as deformable elements (springs and beam elements). Geometric and material non-linearities were incorporated within the models, and the stiffness method of structure analysis was employed to compute

forces and displacements of the vertebrae. In this method, the external load was applied in increments [δQ^{ext}], and for each load increment the stiffness equations were iteratively solved until the external forces were balanced by the internal forces [Q^{int}] within a reasonable tolerance limit on the stiffness matrix K. This iterative procedure was achieved by varying the stiffness properties of the deformable elements.

Good agreement between the computed and experimental results was found. For example, a comparison of the computed frontal plane motion, in response to a 3 kg lateral force applied at T1 with the sacrum fixed, was made with the experimental results of Lucas & Bresler.[12] Having established the validity of the model, these authors studied the behaviour of scoliotic spine subjected to a traction/compressive load of 3 kg at T1. The results clearly showed that a scoliotic spine behaved differently compared to the normal spine. The main drawback of the study was inherent in its lumped-parameter representation, i.e. no direct stress analysis of the joint was possible. Thus, important phenomena such as changes in spinal stress or strain distribution with age, arthrodesis, disc degeneration and corrective surgery, can not be investigated through such models. Panjabi[13] proposed a general 3-D discrete-parameter model of the spine with the capability of simulating the spine's response to both static and dynamic loading. The formulation was general and no specific model (or example) related to spine was proposed.

The dynamic aspects of the lumbar spinal segment, using the finite element technique, have been investigated by Koogle et al.[14] The vertebra was considered as a three-dimensional elastic structure, with the ligaments and disc between any two vertebrae modelled as springs possessing non-linear spring force-deflection characteristics. These characteristics were determined experimentally. For numerous loading conditions, excellent results were obtained, although no specific results were reported in the paper.

LOWER-BACK MODELS

The amount of modelling effort in the lower back, in comparison to head and neck models, is relatively small. This is partly due to lack of necessary input data needed for the model and partly to the fact that efforts in attempting to gain a better biomechanical understanding of low back pain have come to the forefront only relatively recently.

Belytschko et al[15] were probably the first to attempt a stress analysis of disc using the well-known finite element technique or method (FEM). They idealized the intervertebral disc and adjacent vertebral bodies as a three-dimensional structure that was rotationally symmetrical with respect to the vertical centre line (axisymmetrical model), as shown in Figure 8.7. The behaviour of the disc subjected to small axial deflections was investigated. The vertebral core (region 1 in Fig. 8.7(b)) and thin outer shell (region 3) were assumed to be isotropic and homogeneous materials with moduli of elasticity equal to 33.4×10^3 MPa (7.5 kp/mm²) and 7.1×10^3 MPa (1.6 kp/mm²) respectively. A Poisson's ratio of 0.25 was assumed. The nucleus pulposus (region 4) was assumed incompressible and in a hydrostatic state of stress. The annulus was subdivided into a number of subregions, and each subregion was modelled as a single homogeneous orthotropic

material. The properties were obtained by averaging the properties of individual lamellae. This approach accounted for the inhomogeneity of the annulus. The cartilaginous end-plate (region 6) was also assumed to be an isotropic and homogeneous material with a modulus of elasticity and Poisson's ratio of 10.8×10^3 MPa (2.43 kp/mm²) and 0.4 respectively. A load of 48.9 kN (11 kp) was applied at the top surface such that it resulted in a uniform axial displacement. An axisymmetrical linear finite element technique, with triangular linear displacement elements, was used to determine the state of stress, strain and deflections within the disc. The orthotropic material constants for the annulus were derived by adjusting the material constants[16] iteratively to match the overall disc behaviour (axial compressive load-deflection curves) to the one measured experimentally by Rolander.[17] Good agreement with the experimental results of Markolf[18] and Brown et al[19] was found with these same constants in the model.

The normal, tangential, axial and radial stress distribution within the annulus were studied, since these quantities cannot be measured experimentally. The maximum tangential stress occurred along the outer periphery (3.35 times the applied pressure). The axial stress was compressive at the inner wall of the annulus, while at the outer wall it became tensile. The fibre stresses, along the fibre direction, were tensile. The effect of disc degeneration on the overall disc behaviour (in terms of disc bulge, ratio of nucleus pressure, p_i, and externally applied pressure, p_e, and stresses) was investigated by varying (decreasing) the Young's modulus of the annulus. The ability of the nucleus to generate hydrostatic pressures was not altered. The reduction in the modulus (1:3) resulted in lower intradiscal pressures, a greater compression and bulging of the annulus (Fig. 8.8). The stresses within fibre also showed a decrease.

This pioneering study, even though burdened with a number of simplifying assumptions, revealed the usefulness of the FEM in computing parameters, which are difficult to quantify experimentally. Furthermore, a knowledge of the state of stress and strain within the disc and body can point to those regions most susceptible to failure. Kulak et al[20] extended this study by incorporating non-linear material properties for the disc and using a non-

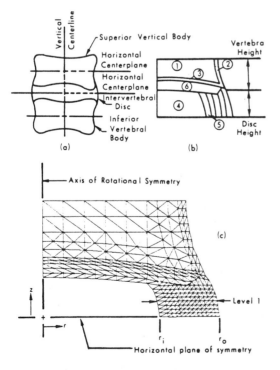

Fig. 8.7 Finite element model of the disc.

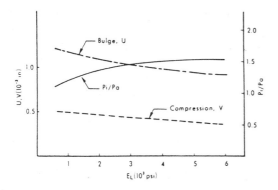

Fig. 8.8 Effect of longitudinal modulus, E_L, on disc bulge, disc compression and nucleus pressure.

linear FEM. The other variables, such as symmetry about the vertical axis and small axial loading, were kept the same.

DISC-BODY UNIT MODELS

The work of Lin et al[21] integrated the FEM with an optimization algorithm to determine the 'disc' material properties so as to match the computed behaviour with the experimental data. It was the beginning of three-dimensional FEM analysis of the disc-body unit of the spine without the posterior elements. Hakim & King[22] and Balasubramanium et al[23] investigated the effect of dynamic loads on the whole vertebra (separated from the rest of the spine) and the effect of laminectomy on the stresses within the vertebral pedicles and pars interarticularis regions respectively.

More recently Spilker et al[24,25] adopted a semi-analytical scheme for axisymmetrical structure subjected to non-axisymmetrical loading and a hybrid stress model to determine the mechanical response of the two vertebral segments with the posterior elements removed. A number of different loading situations: axial compression, shear, bending and torsion, were included in the analysis and the computer results were in agreement with the published experimental data of Berkson et al[26] and Reuber et al[27] The main conclusions of the study are described below:

1. Model intradiscal pressure increases occurred only in response to compression. This is consistent with experimental observations that intradiscal pressure changes are small in other modes of loading compared to those that occur in compression.

2. Model displacements and strains varied inversely with the elastic modulus of the annulus. Stresses and intradiscal pressure increases were independent of this modulus.

3. An elastic modulus of 14 MPa for the annulus produced mean model predictions which were in reasonable agreement with mean experimental measurements of gross disc behaviour under compression, shear and bending. For torsion, a 100 MPa elastic modulus of the annulus was needed to obtain reasonable model–experimental correlations.

4. In general, disc radius and disc height were major determinants of disc displacements. Typically, displacements at a given load increased with increasing disc height and decreased with increasing disc radius.

5. In response to compression, disc enucleation produced a relatively small increase in vertical displacement, but a significant decrease in disc bulge.

The main drawback of the finite element studies reported above is the modelling of the annulus fibrosus as a continuum, whether linear or non-linear and homogeneous or inhomogeneous. This approach has failed to recognize that the annulus fibrosus consists of a number of fibre layers and that the space between the layers is filled by ground substance.[28]

Model used by Shirazi-Adl et al

The pioneering work of Shirazi-Adl et al[29] modelled the disc-body unit, using the finite element technique, with the annulus treated as a composite of fibres and ground substance. Figure 8.9 shows the sections of the finite element grid used in modelling the disc-body unit. The model employed 264 eight-node solid elements, 283 two-node axial elements with a total of 562 nodal points. In axial loading, deformations remain symmetrical about both the mid-sagittal and mid-horizontal planes (through the disc). Only a quarter of the disc-body unit was needed for modelling purposes.

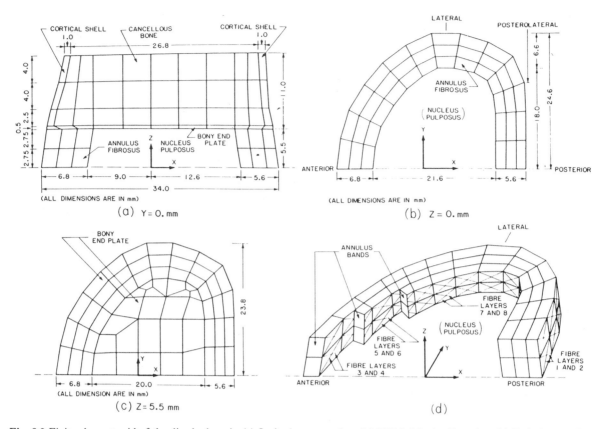

Fig. 8.9 Finite element grid of the disc-body unit: (a) Sagittal cross-section; (b) Mid-height ($z=0$) section; (c) End-plate section; (d) Annulus bands and fibre orientation.

Axial elements were used to model annular fibres. The fibres were arranged in eight layers, in a criss-cross pattern, making an angle of about 29° with the horizontal plane of the disc. The fibre layers were taken as 19% of the annulus and were embedded into the ground substance. The nucleus was modelled as an incompressible material. The effect of cartilaginous end-plate was not included in the model. The material properties taken from the literature are given in Tables 8.1 and 8.2. It may be noted that these non-linear material properties of the components of the composite annular material were not altered during the analysis. This is unlike the earlier finite element studies (e.g., Kulak et al[20]) in which the non-linear orthotropic material constants for the annulus were found by matching the results of the FEM analysis with the experimental axial load-displacement data. The model behaviour for the disc material exhibiting both the geometric and material

non-linearities was predicted for a uniform axial displacement field of the superior vertebra with respect to the inferior. The maximum value of corresponding axial compressive load acting on the vertebra was about 3000 N. The effect of a number

Table 8.1 Material properties of the bulk material. Taken from Shirazi-Adl et al.[29]

Material	Young's modulus E (MPa)	Shear modulus G (MPa)	Poisson's ratio ν
Cortical bone	12 000.0	4615.0	0.3
Cancellous bone	100.0	41.7	0.2
Annulus ground substance	4.2	1.6	0.45

Table 8.2 Material properties of their distribution assumed for the collagenous fibres of the annulus.

	Layers 1 and 2	Layers 3 and 4	Layers 5 and 6	Layers 7 and 8
Ratio of cross-sectional area	1.0	0.78	0.62	0.47
Ratio of elastic constant ($\sigma = 23\,000\ \epsilon^{1.9}$)	1.0	0.90	0.75	0.65

of variables: variation in intradiscal pressure, nucleus removal, disc degeneration, variation of fibre angles and shape variations of the disc on its posterior aspect was investigated.

The output of the model in terms of axial compressive displacement, disc bulge, end-plate bulge in vertical direction (along the z-axis, Fig. 8.9) and intradiscal pressure as a function of axial compressive loads were all compared to experimental and theoretical results of earlier finite element studies. Keeping in mind the wide scatter within the published results, a good comparison was found (Fig. 8.10). Since it is not possible to describe

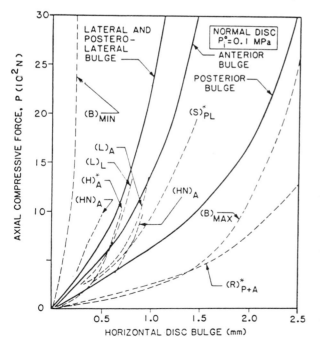

Fig. 8.10 Comparison between predicted and experimental results of disc bulge under axial compressive force.

the findings of their work in detail in a review and expository paper, the following paragraphs summarize their findings and are taken from their paper.

Axial displacement

The disc-body unit exhibited a stiffening effect with increasing compressive load. A decrease in the initial nucleus pressure reduced the axial stiffness. In the case when the disc was considered void of the nucleus, the stiffness was found to be reduced by as much as half from the value computed for the normal disc. A decrease in annulus fibre angle from 29° to 24° and 19° (with respect to the horizontal plane) increased the axial stiffness, while variation in posterior geometry of the annulus had relatively minor effect.

Disc bulge

Similar to axial displacement, the bulge stiffness increased with compressive load and decreased with a reduction in the initial intradiscal pressure. The effect of the removal of the nucleus appeared quite marked in terms of both the magnitude and the relative variation of the bulge around the annulus. For example, in the normal disc the maximum bulge occurred at the posterior location, while in the disc void of the nucleus it occurred at the anterior site. Also, for an identical magnitude of the compressive load, the bulge in a normal disc was predicted to be less than that following nucleotomy at all locations around the annulus except at the posterior aspect. A decrease in the annulus fibre angle increased slightly the posterior bulge, while the bulge at the other locations decreased considerably. Alteration of flat posterior geometry to a re-entrant one increased the bulge.

End-plate bulge

In the normal disc, the vertical end-plate deformation was outward, with the maximum deflection in the centre and uniformly decreasing to zero at its edges. For the disc void of the nucleus, the central portion of the end-plate also bulged outwards, and its maximum magnitude was less than that in the normal disc.

Intradiscal pressure

The intradiscal pressure increased nearly linearly with increasing compressive load. The slope of the variation remained almost identical regardless of the magnitude of the initial intradiscal pressure, but exhibited a slight increase with a reduction in the fibre angle.

Stresses in the vertebral body

In the cancellous bone of the vertebra with a normal disc, the maximum compressive stress occurred at the regions adjacent to the nucleus space, while in the disc void of the nucleus this stress occurred adjacent to the annular attachment region. Also, for an identical compressive load, the maximum compressive stress in the cancellous bone was reduced by one-half when the nucleus was removed. However, the stress increased by 35% in the cortical bone upon nucleus removal. In the end-plate of the normal disc, maximum tensile stresses occurred adjacent to the nucleus space in the fibres close to the cancellous bone, while in the end-plate of the disc without the nucleus this stress occurred at the same location but in the fibres adjacent to the nucleus space. For an identical compressive load, the maximum tensile stress in the end-plate was reduced by 35% when the nucleus was removed. In the cortical shell, for the same external load, the maximum compressive stress increased by 50% if the nucleus was removed.

Stress and strains in the annulus

For a compressive load of 3000 N, the strains in the annulus fibres of the normal disc were always tensile and exhibited a continuous decrease from the inner layers to the outer one. For the disc void of the nucleus, only the fibres located at the outer layers experienced tensile strain when subjected to an axial compressive load of 1750 N. For an identical compressive load, the maximum fibre tensile strain for the normal disc was greater than for the disc without nucleus.

The strains in the annulus ground substance in the horizontal plane were tensile at almost all locations, both for normal disc and the disc void of the nucleus. The stresses, however, were mostly compressive in the normal disc and nearly so for the disc without the nucleus. For the disc void of the nucleus, large tensile strains were predicted, namely 30% in the radial direction for a compressive load of 1750 N.

Vulnerable points in the disc-body unit

Comparison of the predicted stresses and strains in the various materials of the disc-body unit, with the reported ultimate stresses and strains of the materials, indicated that under compressive load the most vulnerable elements in a normal disc were the cancellous bone and the end-plate adjacent to the nucleus space. This prediction appears to correlate with the frequent occurrence of Schmorl's nodes in non-degenerated discs.

For the disc void of the nucleus, however, the most vulnerable element appeared to be the annulus ground subtance that was predicted to undergo large radial tensile strain. This result correlates with the occurrence of circumferential clefts in degenerated discs. Also, the stresses in the cancellous bone and the end-plate, although markedly reduced, still remained sufficiently high to cause failure in regions adjacent to the annulus attachment zone. The annular fibres of the disc did not appear to be particularly susceptible to rupture under compressive load.

In conclusion, this study reinforces the concept of earlier investigators that stress analysis, concurrent with experimental measurements, is an appropriate approach towards the elucidation of the mechanical causes of the disorders affecting the human lumbosacral spine.

Extension of the model

Shirazi-Adl et al[30] have recently extended the disc-body unit model to include the posterior elements: ligaments and facets. Each ligament was represented by a collection of uni-axial elements, oriented along the fibre direction with non-linear stress–strain relations. The facet joints were taken into account by a constant examination of the location of the articulating surfaces of the superior facet (represented by 28 points) with respect to that of the inferior one. In this manner, a relatively rigid connection, normal to the inferior surface, was generated when a region of the superior facet was computed to be in contact with the inferior facet.

The formulation of the rest of the problem was identical to the one described earlier.

The predicted variations of angular displacement and intradiscal pressure with flexion moment were in good agreement with the experimental results. The main results for 60 Nm of flexion moment were as follows:

1. The supraspinous and medial fibres of the interspinous ligaments were subjected to maximum tensile strains of 29.3% and 25.3% respectively. These values compared well with the elastic limit of 18–32% for the interspinous ligament.

2. The cancellous bone of the intervertebral body was subjected to a tensile stress of 0.60 MPa and a compressive stress of 1.75 MPa adjacent to the end-plate at the posterior and the anterior regions respectively. These predictions compared nicely with the ultimate strength of the cancellous bone of 1.18 MPa in tension and 1.37–3.10 MPa in compression.

3. The annular bulk material underwent a maximum tensile strains of 25.1% axially in the posterolateral region and 30.9% radially in the anterior region of the disc. These results compare favourably with the failure strain of 12–35% for this material.

4. The inner layer of the collagenous fibres of the annulus was subjected to a maximum strain of 7.3% at the posterolateral and posterior locations. The elastic limit of this fibre is in the range 3–7%.

5. The bony posterior elements were under maximum stresses of about 18.2 MPa in compression, 18.7 MPa in tension and 10.7 MPa in shear.

Model used by Ueno and Liu

Ueno[31] re-examined the finite element formulation of the intervertebral disc in general and the annulus in particular. Based on a careful examination of the composite, i.e. a collagen-fibre reinforced ground substance, he came to the conclusion that the entire spectrum of the hardening non-linear axial load-deformation curves found experimentally can be simulated by *linear* material properties for both the fibre and ground substance. Stated another way, the non-linear load-displacement curves for axial compression are primarily a geometric non-linearity, and material non-linearities are negligible, if any. The collagen fibres were modelled by axial elements with a wrinkling option, i.e. it carried load only in tension but not in compression. A fully three-dimensional finite element model of the L4–L5 intervertebral joint, including the ligaments, posterior elements, vertebral body end-plates, incompressible nucleus pulposus and composite annulus fibrosus, was constructed using a general-purpose finite-element program, ANSYS. Its simulations were in good agreement with the available experimental data on compression, flexion and extension. In the above sense, Ueno's construction provided additional support to the essential validity of the quarter and half disc-body models of Shirazi-Adl et al[29,30] without invoking the need for the complications of non-linear material properties. Its truly three dimensional nature was exploited to study the axial torsion of the pre-compressed lumbar L4-L5 joint by Ueno and Liu.[32]

The essential asymmetry of the response of the L4–L5 joint to axial torsion begins with facet contact, which theoretically can take place either with the compressive preload as shown by Yang & King[33] or with one of the facet pairs coming into contact as a result of the applied torque shown experimentally by Adams & Hutton.[34] In either mode of torsion, it is clear from the finite-element analysis that the following conclusions can be drawn:

1. The finite element model, constructed by using the general-purpose program, ANSYS, which simulated well the experimental database in compression, flexion and extension, also provided good agreement with the experimental torque-angular displacement data for both the intact and facetectomized joint as shown in Figure 8.11.

2. The facets carried from 10 to 40% of the torque depending on the gap of the facet joint and the load level as shown in Figure 8.12.

3. Facet contact relieved the stresses in the fibres of the posterior margin of the disc.

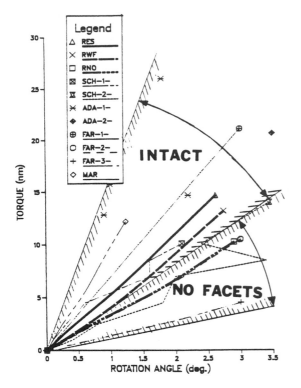

Fig. 8.11 Comparison between predicted and experimental results of applied torque vs angular displacement.

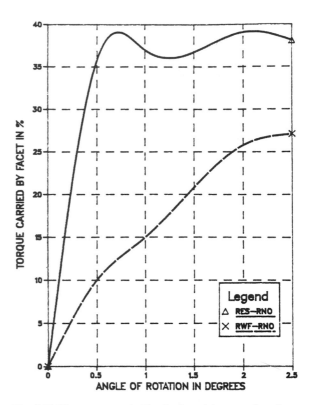

Fig. 8.12 The torque carried by the facet joints as a function of angular displacement in axial torsion. These were obtained by subtracting the torque for the facetectomized case from the intact case. Solid line corresponds to both facets in contact. Dotted line corresponds to only one facet in contact.

There was a corresponding shift of the neutral axis posteriorly as a result of facet contact.

4. Only half of the annular fibres were active in resisting torsion. Thus, the role of annular fibres in resisting torsion is reduced when compared to compression.

5. The pressure rise in the nucleus due to torsion in the physiological range of angular displacement ($<3°$) is minimal compared to that of axial compression.

6. The fibre stresses in the disc were the highest at the lateral margin of the outer layer of the annulus in axial torsion. The corresponding stresses in the ground substance were nearly hydrostatic and the shear stress intensity was negligible there. Therefore, torsion is an unlikely cause for posterior or postero-lateral disc rupture in the absence of facet fracture. Should the disc fail in torsion, the FEM

analysis indicated that the lateral aspect is more vulnerable.

7. The role of ligaments in torsion with a compressive preload was minimal for torsional angular displacement of less than $3°$.

8. Most of the torsional load was transmitted through the cortical shell rather than the cancellous core of the vertebral body. Thus, the cortical shell is more vulnerable to shear failure in torsion.

9. Shear stress intensity is high at the anterior and posterior margins of the vertebral body in contrast to its distribution in the disc. High levels of shear stress intensity and principal stresses were found at the junction of the pedicle and vertebral body for the intact intervertebral joint.

CONCLUSION

In principle, at least, we should be able to extend the intervertebral joint models delineated above to include regions of the spine, e.g. the lumbar vertebral column. In practice, however, such simulations are restrained by computational storage and time. Although the costs have decreased and the capability of digital computers has increased dramatically, it will probably be another five years before it becomes possible to simulate numerically the entire lumbar spine.

ACKNOWLEDGEMENTS

The generous support provided by Grants No. GM 26608 (National Institute of General Medical Sciences), AM 32954 (National Institute of Arthritis, Diabetes, Digestive and Kidney Diseases), and Grant No. 23-P-59176 of the National Institute of Handicapped Research, Department of Education, is gratefully acknowledged.

Tables 8.1, 8.2 and Figs 8.9 and 8.10 are reproduced with the kind permission of Dr A. M. Ahmed and the Editor of *Spine*. Figs 8.1–8.4 are reproduced with the kind permission of the senior author and the Editor of *Journal of Biomechanics*. Figs 8.5 and 8.6 are reproduced with the kind permission of Dr Ted Belytschko and the Editor of the *Journal of Biomechanical Engineering*. Figs 8.7 and 8.8 are reproduced with the kind permission of Dr T. Belytschko and the Editor of *Journal of Biomechanics*. Figs 8.11 and 8.12 are reproduced with kind permission of Drs Ueno and Liu.

REFERENCES

1 Orne D, Liu Y K 1971 A mathematical model of the spinal response to impact. J. Biomech. 4: 49–71

2 McKenzie J A, Williams J F 1971 The dynamic behavior of the head and cervical spine during whiplash. J. Biomech. 4: 546–550

3 Prasad P, King A I 1974 An experimentally validated dynamic model of the spine. ASME J. Appl. Mech. 546–550

4 Huston R L, Huston J C, Harlow M W 1978 Comprehensive three-dimensional head-neck model for impact and high acceleration studies. Avia. Space Envir. Med. 49: 205–210

5 Reber J A, Goldsmith W 1979 Analysis of large heads neck motion. J. Biomech. 12: 211–222

6 Williams J L, Belytschko T B 1983 A three-dimensional model of the human cervical spine for impact simulation. J. Biomech. Engng 105: 321–331

7 Belytschko T, Schwer L, Schultz A 1976 A model for analytic investigation of three-dimensional head-spine dynamics. Aerospace Medical Research Laboratory, WPAFB, Ohio (AMRL-TR-76-10)

8 Belytschko T, Schwer L, Klein M J 1977 Large displacement transient analysis of space frames. Int'l J. Num. Methods 11: 65–84

9 Privitzer E, Belytschko T 1980 Impedence of a three-dimensional head-spine model. Mathematical Modelling 1: 189–209

10 Ewing C L, Thomas D J, Lustik L, Muzzy III W H, Williams G C, Majewski P 1977 Dynamic response of the human head and neck to +Gy impact acceleration. Proceedings of the 21st Stapp Car Crash Conference, SAE paper no. 770928: 549–586

11 Schultz A B, Belytschko T B, Andriacchi T P, Galante J O 1973 Analog studies of forces in the human spine: mechanical properties and motion segment behavior. J. Biomech. 6: 373–383

12 Lucas D B, Bresler B 1961 Stability of the ligamentous spine. Biomechanics Lab, University of California, Berkeley, Report No. 40

13 Panjabi M M 1973 Three-dimensional mathematical model of the human spine structure. J. Biomech. 6: 671–680

14 Koogle T A, Swenson Jr L W, Piziali R L 1979 Dynamic three-dimensional modelling of the human lumbar spine. Advances in Bioengineering, ASME, 65–68

15 Belytschko T, Kulak R F, Schultz A B 1974 Finite element stress analysis of an intervertebral disc. J. Biomech. 7: 277–285

16 Galante J O 1967 Tensile properties of the human lumbar annulus fibrosus. Acta Orthop. Scand. Suppl. 100

17 Rolander S D 1966 Motion of the lumbar spine with special reference to the stabilizing effect of posterior fusion. Acta Orthop. Scand. Suppl. 25

18 Markolf K L 1972 Deformation of the thoracolumbar intervertebral joints in response to external loads. J. Bone Jnt Surg. 54A: 511–533

19 Brown T, Hansen R J, Yorra A J 1957 Some mechanical tests on the lumbosacral spine with particular reference to the intervertebral disc. J. Bone Jnt Surg. 39A: 1135–1164

20 Kulak R F, Belytschko T B, Schultz A B, Galante J O 1976 Nonlinear behavior of the human intervertebral disc under axial load. J. Biomech. 9: 377–386

21 Lin H S, Liu Y K, Ray G, Nikravesh P 1978 System identification for material properties of the intervertebral joint. J. Biomech. 11: 1–14

22 Hakim N S, King A I 1979 A three-dimensional finite element dynamic response analysis of a vertebra with experimental verification. J. Biomech. 12: 277–292

23 Balasubramanium K, Ranu H S, King A I 1979 Veterbral response to laminectomy. J. Biomech. 12: 813–823

24 Spilker R 1980 Mechanical behavior of a simple model of an intervertebral disk under compressive loading. J. Biomech. 13: 895–901

25 Spilker R, Daugirda D M, Schultz A B 1984 Mechanical response of a simple finite element model of the

intervertebral disc under complex loading. J. Biomech. 17: 103–112

26 Berkson M, Nachemson A, Schultz A 1979 Mechanical properties of human lumbar spine motion segment. Part II: Responses in compression and shear influence of gross morphology. J. Biomech. Engng 101: 53–57

27 Reuber M, Schultz A, Kirkhope J, Dennis F 1982 Bulging of intervertebral discs. J. Biomech. Engng 104: 187–192

28 Broberg K, von Essen H 1980 Modelling of intervertebral discs. Spine 5: 155–167

29 Shirazi-Adl S A, Shirvasta S C, Ahmed A M 1984 Stress analysis of the lumbar disc-body unit in compression. Spine 9: 2, 120–134

30 Shirazi-Adl S A, Shrivasta S C, Ahmed A M 1984 Mechanical response of the lumbar intervertebral joint in flexion: a 3-D nonlinear finite element model study. 30th Proc. ORS, Atlanta, Georgia, 204, Feb. 6–9

31 Ueno K 1984 A three-dimensional nonlinear finite element model of the lumbar intervertebral joint. PhD dissertation, University of Iowa, Iowa City

32 Ueno K, Liu Y K 1985 A three-dimensional nonlinear finite element model of the lumbar intervertebral joint in torsion. J. Biomech. Engng (submitted)

33 Yang K H, King A I 1984 Mechanism of facet load transmission as a hypothesis for low back pain. Spine 9/6: 557–565

34 Adams M A, Hutton W C 1981 The relevance of torsion to the mechanical derangement of the lumbar spine. Spine 6/3: 241–248

Lumbar intradiscal pressure

INTRODUCTION

It is obvious to all those suffering from low back pain that the symptoms worsen when the lumbar spine is subjected to increased mechanical load. Patients with low back disorders limit their physical activities, which also indicates that loading of the spine must be a factor in these disorders. It is not definitely known, however, how important mechanical factors are for producing the low back pain symptoms, but it is likely that both biomechanical and chemical/biological factors play a role in disc degeneration and ageing per se. The degenerative process, either directly or indirectly, through chemical reactions and mechanical deficiencies of the motion segment, can play a role in producing pain.

In this chapter I shall present some of the results derived from more than 30 years of research into the normal and pathological mechanics of lumbar discs. I will also correlate the mechanical factors with some of the clinical and biological facts of this disease. Much of the knowledge forming the basis for the low back schools currently in use (Chapter 15) is based on the disc pressure measurements reported here.

INVESTIGATIONS

It has long been said that low back pain was the price humans paid for assuming an erect stance. Many veterinarians, however, have been able to demonstrate that quadrupeds also suffer from back pain syndromes.[1-6] The common denominator in the investigations of all sorts of animals presented so far is that, in general, disc hernias — a definite pain-producing pathological entity — develop in those areas of the spine that are subjected to the heaviest

mechanical stresses.[5,6] In this context, mechanical stresses include not only vertical forces or forces along the spine but also rotational, bending and shearing stresses.

Calculations of loads

Early theoretical calculations of the load on the lumbar spine were often too high; they suggested that, when a person is lifting only 200 N, the forces are above the known fracture load of cadaver spines.[7-10] Clinical observations have shown that normal lumbar spines can withstand around 10 kN of vertical load before fracturing.[10-12] Many authors have been able to demonstrate the theoretical load-relieving effect of intra-abdominal and intrathoracic pressure, although this load-relieving effect, except in a symmetrical position, has been questioned recently.[13-17] In most instances previously theoretically calculated loads exceeded 5–10 kN, which in our present knowledge represents the strength of vertebral bodies.[10,11] (See also Chapter 10).

Experimental disc rupture

Most investigators have been unable to produce true disc herniations by mere compression of specimens composed of an intervertebral disc and two adjacent vertebrae.[10,18-22] Although they were able to show that on pure vertical compression the vertebral endplates will be the first structures to fracture, with a resulting herniation of the nucleus pulposus into the vertebral body, they were unable to produce the sort of disc hernias that we see in our patients. In none of these previously mentioned papers, however, was any attention given to the varying shapes of the nucleus pulposus in relation to the loads producing such fractures.[23] Recently Brinckmann et al[24] demonstrated that on pure compression the end-plate is the weakest part and fractures at a compressive load of 7500 N after a deflection of 0.5 mm. If the disc is degenerated or enucleated, a less compressive force can fracture the end-plate.[25]

Jayson et al[23] have shown that most discs subjected to high vertical loads burst into the vertebral body. This happens with discographically normal as well as with irregular nuclei pulposi. These authors also showed that the pressure necessary to fracture osteoporotic spines could be low — approaching figures, as will be demonstrated later in this chapter, that can be recorded during disc pressure measurements in life.

In some discs, however, where the preceding discography demonstrated a posterolateral extension of the nucleus reaching the border of the vertebra, there occurred a true posterior bursting of the annulus at loads of around 3–6 kN. This was also true in a few discs with a central posterior weakening.

It was obvious from these reports, as well as from the experimental findings of Markolf[26] and Farfan et al,[27,28] on the mechanism for posterior annulus weakening, that we needed to investigate the mechanical background for disc hernia. Earlier writers, as well as myself, have mostly held the opinion that a rather marked weakening of the annulus due to biological reasons has to precede a true disc herniation. Recently-performed biomechanical investigations have, however, again emphasized a possible mechanical background for disc herniation. Adams & Hutton[29] studied cadaver specimens that were laminectomized and then somewhat hyperflexed and could produce disc hernias by not too excessive compression loads.

The nutrition of the intervertebral disc in adults is a mostly passive process which, however, can be positively influenced by motion and negatively by immobilization.[30-32] The area between the nucleus and annulus is fairly poorly nourished by the necessary ion complexes, and the first signs of disc degeneration actually occur in this zone, starting the weakening process of the otherwise mechanically very competent disc. This weakening occurs at an age when the nucleus, and hence the disc pressure from a mechanical point of view, is fairly normal.

Measurements of disc pressure

It has been suggested that the nucleus pulposus, the gelatinous centre of the disc, acts hydrostatically.[33] Although it seems reasonable to assume this from its high water content — 85%[34,35] — it was not proven until 1960.[36] I punctured the nucleus pulposus with a specially constructed hollow needle covered by an elastic polyethylene tubing (Fig. 9.1) and connected it to an electromanometer. By turning the needle in the three directions of principal stress in the loaded disc I was able to show that the nuclei of normal and also of slightly degenerated discs behave hydrostatically.[36-38] Pressures in normal discs were around 1.5 times the vertical load applied per unit area and there was a linear increase in pressure for external loads up to 2000 N.[36]

It was also possible to relate the forces acting in the nucleus to the forces acting in the annulus — the fibrous structure surrounding it.[39] The vertical stress in this structure is about 50% of the applied external load per unit of area while the tangential, tensile strain is four to five times the applied external load, at least in the outer parts (Fig. 9.2). Also, both experiments on cadavers as well in living anaesthetized subjects seem to verify an intrinsic pressure of about 0.1 MPa. This has been noted by Virgin[33] in 1951. It was later demonstrated that the ligamentum flavum, situated between the posterior arches and facets, prestresses the disc by a force of around 0.15 MPa.[40] Because the ligament is at a distance from the motion centre of the disc,[41] it creates an intradiscal pressure of about 0.1 MPa. In this manner some intrinsic stability of the spine is provided — the spine is slightly prestressed.[42]

In vivo studies

The in vitro experiments provided a basis for intravital disc pressure studies[43-44] (Fig. 9.3). In the first series of experiments in 20 subjects we used a needle built on the principles already described and studied different static positions of the body. Figure 9.4 presents a summary of the pressure changes that we observed in the third lumbar disc in a 70 kg subject during different static positions, expressed as a percentage of the pressure in upright standing. (In absolute values, the load on the L3 disc in the upright position is about 500 N (Table 9.3).

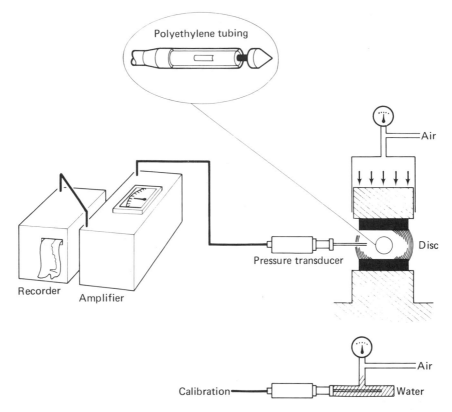

Fig. 9.1 Schematic drawing of a method for measuring intravital pressure in vitro.

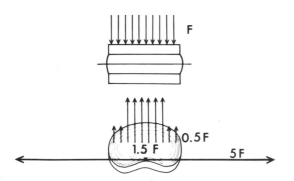

Fig. 9.2 Approximate relationship between vertical stress and mechanical strain in different parts of normal lumbar discs.

The system that we used did not allow for any dynamic measurements because of the poor dynamic characteristics of the polyethylene membrane. Now, with the help of the Toyota Research and Development Company, Nagoya, Japan, we have developed a new pressure gauge.[44] Semiconductor strain gauges embedded in epoxy resin of the tip of a needle, 0.8 mm wide, transmit pressure on the basis of piezoresistive effects (Fig. 9.5). The frequency response of the pressure needle allows measurements of pressure changes up to at least 5000 Hz. The frequency limit of the system is thus set by the recorder, the upper frequency limit of which is about 500 Hz. The calibration of the transducer is always performed before and after each experiment, and on no occasion has any difference been noted.[34-36] Lately, we have observed a slight difference in balance when the bridge was balanced with the needle in air compared with the needle in the disc tissue. This we have found to be due to self-heating of the transducer. In order to reach a temperature equilibrium state during measurements, the needle has to be zero-balanced in the subject's body.[45-47] The results obtained in the earlier investigations show a disc pressure that is 0.2–0.3 MPa in excess of the true value.

It has become evident that the zero position of the pressure transducer must be checked regularly after the study of each particular task. Only minute changes in zero-balance corresponding to less than

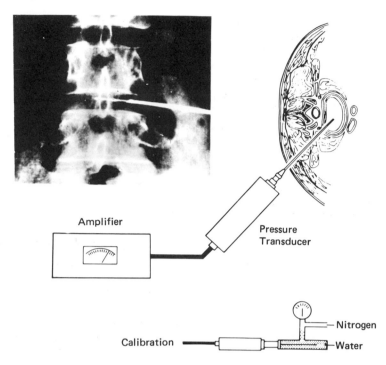

Fig. 9.3 Method for measuring intravital pressure in vivo.

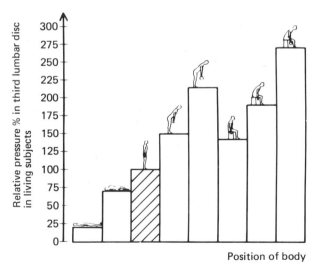

Fig. 9.4 Relative increase and decrease in intradiscal pressure in different supine, standing and sitting postures compared to the pressure in upright standing (100%).

0.05 MPa are then noticed. These changes are probably due to a slight bending of the tip of the needle as the muscles move in relation to the disc, but a slight zero-shift is also caused by the recorder.[48]

Results

With our miniaturized pressure transducer it has been possible to measure the pressure in the disc and calculate the approximate loads on the lower lumbar spine not only in some common static positions, but also when the subject is performing various types of movements, manoeuvres and physical exercises or work tasks. A summary of the results in the supine, sitting and standing positions respectively is shown in Tables 9.1, 9.2 and 9.3. More attention should be paid to the relationship between the different movements etc. than to the absolute values. In these tables the loads have been corrected, taking into consideration the zero-balance error that I previously described and which occurred in the papers published on the subject up to the early 1970s.

We have also recorded the forces to which the lumbar spine is subjected in different work situations. In the sitting position, for example, the importance of a good lumbar support and an armrest for relief of the load on the lumbar spine is clearly seen in Table 9.2. The pressure in the unsupported sitting position is actually 40% higher than that in the standing-at-ease position, probably

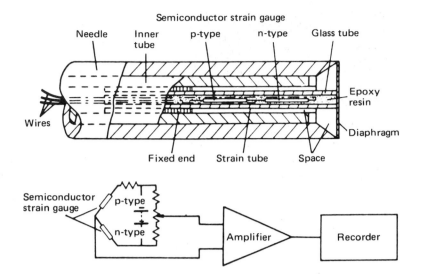

Fig. 9.5 The sub-miniature pressure transducer and the principles of the pressure-measuring system.

Table 9.1 Approximate load on L3 disc in a 700 N (70 kg) individual in different supine postures, activities and exercises.

	N
Supine, awake	250
Supine, semi-Fowler position	100
Supine, anesthetized or paraplegic	80
Supine, traction, passive 30 s*	250
Supine, traction 300N, passive 3 min*	< 100
Supine, active own traction (autotraction)*	500
Supine, arm activities with 20N weight*	600
Sit-up exercises, full movement*	1200
Bilateral leg lifts*	800
Sit-up exercises, isometric, little motion*	600
Tilt-table 80°	300

*Maximum value recorded during dynamic activity.

Table 9.2 Approximate load on L3 disc in a 700 N (70 kg) individual in different sitting postures and activities.

	N
Sitting upright, unsupported	700
Sitting, 100°, seat incl., 4 cm lumbar support	450
Sitting, 100°, seat incl. + armrests	400
Sitting, 100°, seat incl., depressing clutch	500
Sitting, office chair	500
Raising, without armrest max. value*	1000
Raising, with armrest max. value*	700
Sitting, office chair, 20 N arms extended	700
Sitting, forward bent 20°, 100 N each hand	1400
Lifting 50 N, arms extended*	1400

*Maximum value recorded during dynamic activity.

Table 9.3 Approximate load on L3 disc in a 700 N (70 kg) individual in different standing postures and activities.

	N
Standing at ease*	500
Standing, laterally flexed 20°*	600
Standing, coughing*	700
Standing, straining, laughing*	700
Standing, jumping in place*	700
Standing, forward bent 20°	700
Standing, forward bent 40°	1000
Standing, forward bent 20°, 100 N each hand	1200
Standing, forward bent 20°, rotated 20°, 50 N each hand	2100
Lifting 100 N, back straight, knees bent*	1700
Lifting 100 N, back bent, knees straight*	1900
Standing upright, lifting 50 N, arms extended horizontally*	1900
Standing forward bent 30°, 40 N each hand, arms extended	1700
Standing, with corset/brace, forward bent 30°, 40 N each hand, arms extended	1200

* Maximum value recorded during dynamic activity.

due to the vector caused by the line of gravity falling in front of the L3 disc in this latter position. In the studies of the sitting position we also found that the disc pressure was considerably influenced by several of the support parameters, i.e. further inclining the backrest decreased the disc pressure, as did an increase in lumbar support.[46] The less the backrest inclination, the more important was the lumbar support (Fig. 9.6). The use of the thoracic support increased the disc pressure (Fig. 9.7).

When the subject was driving a car, the disc pressure increased by 0.05 MPa when the gear was shifted and still more when the clutch pedal was depressed (about 0.1 MPa).

In general, we conclude that the lumbar support should distribute the pressure over the largest

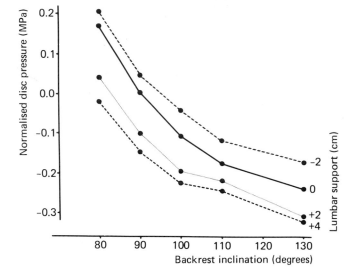

Fig. 9.6 Mean values of normalized disc pressures in MPa. Thoracic support and seat inclination 0°. At each backrest, inclination values are given for −2, 0, +2 and +4 of lumbar support.

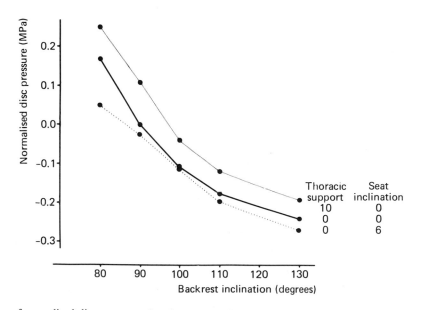

Fig. 9.7 Mean values of normalized disc pressures. Lumbar support 0 cm. The decrease obtained by increased seat inclination as well as the increase obtained by increased thoracic support are demonstrated.

possible area. Within the limits of the investigation, we detected less disc pressure the more the lumbar spine was moved towards lordosis. The level of the back at which the support was placed was of importance. When the support was placed in the upper lumbar region, the effect was less than when it was placed in the lower lumbar region. Too low a position of the support, however, had only limited influence on posture of the spine, as the seated subject was pushed forwards on the seat surface. In order to obtain the best effect in all individuals, a lumbar support should be capable of variation in both size and height above the seat.[45] A radiographic study demonstrated, however, that the lumbar support at L2, L3 or L4 gave the same radiographic picture.[48]

The importance of lever arms for increased disc pressure is most clearly depicted in Table 9.2, which shows that extension of an arm, holding 20 N increases the disc pressure by 40% while bending forwards with 100 N in each hand triples the pressure. Dynamic registration perhaps are even more striking: the lifting of 50 N with arms extended also triples the disc pressure in the sitting position. Also in paraplegic patients, lever arms are important.[49]

Regarding the measurements in the supine position in the awake state, the semi-Fowler position shows the lowest pressure, corresponding to a load of 100 N. We must emphasize the uncertainty with our various traction experiments due to their necessary shortness (experiments on living people). We have never measured an excessive diminution of the pressure. Indeed, in so-called autotraction it increased, as did the electromyography recordings.[47] Other studies using only electromyography as the reference have also demonstrated that only in long-term passive traction do the muscles relax. In the beginning of passive traction there is always an increase in the myoelectric signal.[50]

Various types of exercise are usually performed in the supine position. They produce a substantial increase in disc pressure unless they are performed isometrically.[43]

Japanese,[51-53] Russian,[54] German[55] and South African[56] investigators measured intravital disc pressure by the method I have described, and in essence all verified our findings. It must be pointed out, however, that because the hydrostatic prop-erties of the nucleus are lost when the disc becomes severely degenerated, disc pressure measurements can be performed satisfactorily only in subjects with normal or nearly normal discs.

Technical problems

The calculation of the total force on the disc is subject to some error because, as we found in autopsy material, the obtained pressure must be divided by a factor, 1.5, and then multiplied by the surface area of the disc.[36,42] The division factor varied in autopsy discs from 1.3 to 1.6, showing a tendency to diminish with increasing load, also verified by other authors.[55,56] In life this divisor can only be approximated. The surface area of the disc of the subject must be calculated from special radiographs and is also subject to measurement error.

The systematic error because of temperature drift has already been mentioned. Despite these technical problems, disc pressure measurements are still the only direct way to obtain information on the load of the lumbar spine in various positions etc., and they are now extensively used in spine modelling as well as for patient information in back schools (c.f. Chapter 15).

Aetiology of back pain

It is arguable whether the data obtained can help to clarify the aetiology of back pain. From the knowledge we gained by the autopsy experiments, the tensile stresses in the posterior part of the annulus fibrosus can be calculated. They are three to four times the measured pressure. Galante[57] has shown the strength of these posterior fibres to be as low as 10 MPa. Lifting a weight in the forward bent twisted position with only 100 N in the hand will easily increase the pressure to more than 2 MPa, which will produce a tensile strain in the posterior part of the annulus approaching 8 MPa. At present we cannot say whether such ruptures, which obviously may occur in tasks performed in everyday life, in themselves cause pain, or if they allow chemically irritating substances to leak from inside the disc.[58-64]

Some of our recent studies[17,46,65-67] have concentrated on the measurement of work postures, and again the results can be seen in Tables 9.1–9.3. The often-quoted difference between proper lifting with the knees bent and back straight versus the back bent, knee straight position has not been found so important when the distance between the load and the L3 disc was kept constant, i.e., it is the lever arm that is more important than the way of lifting. This of course has great clinical implications and again has been re-emphasized by measurements of the effect of only 50 N on an outstretched arm (Fig. 9.8 (a)–(c)). Flexion and rotation, i.e. twisting, also subjects the lumbar spine to considerable load (Table 9.2, Fig. 9.9).

Electromyography

Direct intravital measurement of intradiscal pressure is not practical, except under certain well-controlled laboratory conditions.

With the advancement of medical electronics and signal treatment in the field of electromyography (e.m.g.), it is nowadays also possible to express the magnitude of the myoelectric signal, as obtained by both needle and surface electrodes in microvolts (μV).[66-69] The theoretical background and practical modes of application of these systems have been

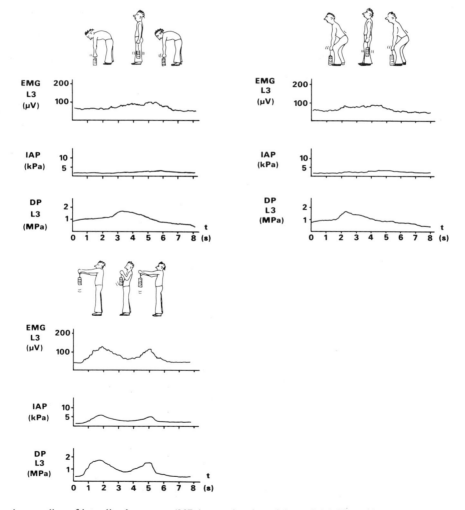

Fig. 9.8 Dynamic recording of intradiscal pressure (MPa), myoelectric activity at L3 (μV) and intra-abdominal pressure (kPa) in back lift (a), and leg lift (b). In these recordings the distance between the body and the load was equal from the beginning. The load was 100 N (10 kg). In (c) the load is only 50 N (5 kg) and the effect of the distance from the body to the load is obvious, both from the disc pressure measurement (the myoelectric activity at L3) and the intra-abdominal pressure.

demonstrated by Örtengren.[69] Bipolar surface electrodes can be utilized for measurements under more rugged conditions, such as a factory floor.

Recently, in both static and dynamic experiments in living humans,[17,65-70] we have been able to demonstrate a definite statistically significant relationship between discometry — the direct measurement of load on the lumbar spine — and the e.m.g. signal. Schematically, some of these results are depicted in Figure 9.9 and Figure 9.10 (a)–(c). It is obvious that the lumbar spine is mechanically stressed, particularly in positions involving both forward bending and twisting.

In numerous papers we have thus correlated the intradiscal pressure obtained in various positions with the results of electromyography, and good correlations have been found with coefficients usually approaching 0.9. On the other hand, intra-abdominal pressure measurements have been found to correlate rather poorly with the other two means of examining the load on the back, even to the point that the importance of intra-abdominal pressure as a force-relieving mechanism per se, except in some very symmetric lifting positions, must be seriously questioned.[17,65,67] In some positions we noted, however, the load-reducing effects of wearing a brace or a corset.[70]

Finally, all these measurements have been used to verify various mathematical models of the spine which are further delineated in Chapters 8 and 10.

The measurements are performed in discs with normal nuclei, since the L3 discs of young healthy volunteers have been chosen. The disc pressure is a direct reflection of the load to which this motion segment of the spine is subjected. Cadaver experiments have demonstrated that compression is the major determinant for disc pressure,[71] not only for L3 but also for L4 and L5 discs. This means that, relatively speaking, the results obtained from the L3 disc can, with an addition of a few per cent of load per segment below, hold for the whole lumbar spine.[11] This is particularly important when relating different postures, positions, manoeuvres and working tasks to each other.

Again, as stated before, only young healthy volunteers with normal discs have been measured. The total load on a degenerate motion segment must be approximately the same as that on a non-degenerate segment. Only the internal stress distribution is likely to be different, i.e. more load is supported by the facet joints and the internal stress distribution in the disc proper also changes with degeneration. In extended positions also the facet joints will support proportionately increased amounts

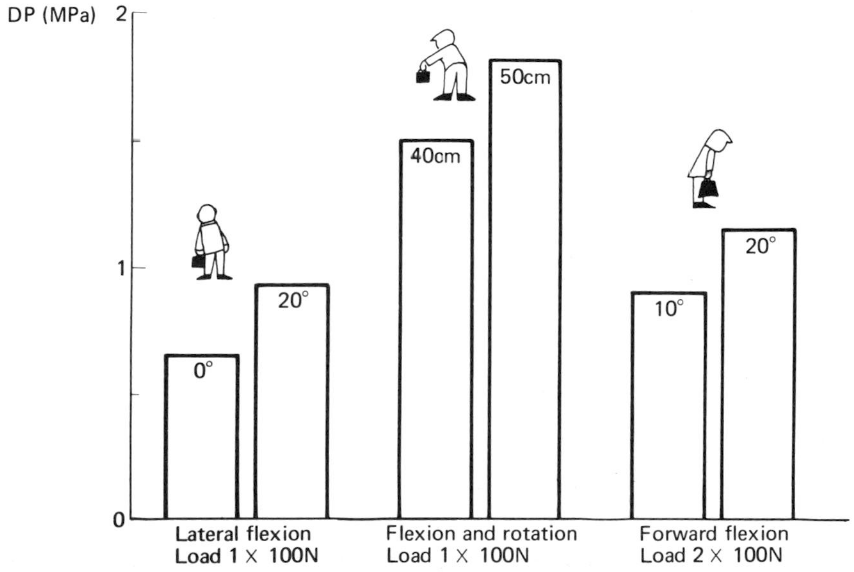

Fig. 9.9 Intravital disc pressures (MPa) during static loading in left lateral flexion with a load of 100 N (10 kg) in the left hand; with a combination of flexion and rotation and a load at a distance of 40 and 50 centimetres from the centre of the body respectively; and, finally, in forward flexion with 100 N (10 kg) in each hand at 10° and 20° respectively.

of load, but very few of the measurements in Tables 9.1–9.3 actually have been performed in any type of extended position. Without doubt and even with due consideration for all the technical and methodological errors that are inherent in the method, we can certainly now say which particular work positions are more taxing for the spine than others.

So far in the various series of experiments over the last 20 years performed on nearly 100 living volunteers, we have met only one complication. This was a 24-year-old woman who was known to have had attacks of headache in the past and had another after discometry that made hospitalization necessary for six days. We cannot exclude the possibility that a root sleeve was inadvertently pierced, even from the posterolateral approach always used since 1962, and caused some leakage of cerebrospinal fluid. The headache disappeared completely after one week, however. There have been no known further complications. Eight subjects have participated twice, and one even three times!

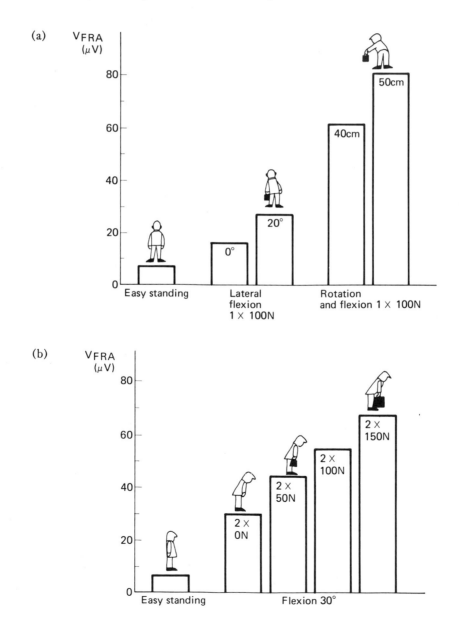

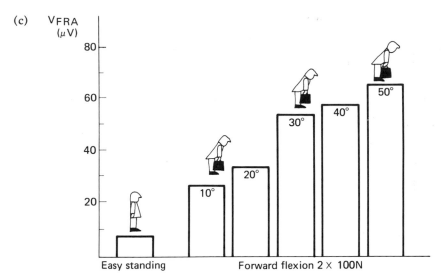

Fig. 9.10 Myoelectric signals (μV) at the L3 level right, at (a) in lateral flexion and in rotation and flexion with 1×100 N (10 kg) load, at (b), in flexion of 30° with increasing loads held by the hand, at (c) in increasing angle of forward flexion with 2×100 N (20 kg) load.

Practical implications of disc pressure measurements

Even if the pressure measurements can only be used hypothetically to explain the aetiology of low back pain, the information obtained is of direct value for treating patients with such pain, because we know more about the forces to which the patients' discs are subjected when they perform various tasks and exercises. Some of this information has served as a basis for the Swedish Back School.[72] In patients with acute low back pain, this mode of treatment has stood the test of a controlled randomized study, resulting in one week's earlier return to work, compared to general physical therapy or placebo treatment.[73]

Epidemiological studies[74-81] have verified the importance of mechanical stresses and strains for the low back problem,[74] and Kelsey[82] recently demonstrated a high over-morbidity in disc prolapse syndromes in those lifting high loads in twisted positions. Also, the importance of proper car seating

was delineated in another similar study.[83] Those driving regularly several hours a week using the Volvo car had significantly less attacks of sciatic syndromes. The seat used in these cars was constructed following the sitting experiments reported.[46]

Thus, it has been demonstrated that the knowledge obtained from disc pressure measurements can be successfully used in treating patients with acute low back pain. It can be used for ergonomic design of work-places, helping the industrial engineers to avoid positions etc. that induce heavy mechanical load on the back. The information also can be used in the creation and design of different types of rehabilitation programs, aimed at the earliest possible return to work. These can usually be performed even if the patient has some pain, if the most strenuous tasks of which we now are aware through these measurements can be avoided. Such programs are now being tested successfully in many parts of the world.[84]

REFERENCES

1 Olsson S-E 1951 On disc protrusion in the dog. Acta Orthop. Scand. suppl. 8
2 Hansen H-J 1959 Comparative views on the pathology of disc degeneration in animals. Lab. Invest. 8: 1242
3 Butler W F 1967 Age changes in the nucleus pulposus of the non-ruptured intervertebral disc of the cat. Res. Vet. Sci. 8: 151
4 Butler W F 1968 Histological changes in the ruptured intervertebral disc of the cat. Res. Vet. Sci. 9: 130
5 Hansen H J, Olsson S-E 1954 The effect of single violent trauma on the spine of the dog. Acta Orthop. Scand. 24: 1

6   Jeffcott L B, Dalin G 1983 Bibliography of thoracolumbar conditions in the horse. Equine Vet. J. 15: 155–57

7   Armstrong J R 1952 Lumbar disc lesions. Livingstone, Edinburgh

8   Bayer H 1954 Mit welchen Kraften wirken die Ruckenstrecker auf die Lendenwirbelsaule ein? Z. Orthop. 84: 607

9   Mattiash H-H 1956 Arbeitshaltung und Bandscheibenbelastung. Arch. Orthop Unfallchir. 48: 147

10   Perey O 1957 Fracture of the vertebral endplates in the lumbar spine. An experimental biomechanical investigation. Acta Orthop. Scand. Suppl. 25

11   Ruff S 1950 Brief acceleration: less than one second. In: German Aviation Medicine, World War II, vol 1. US Government Printing Office, Washington, p 584

12   Hirsch C, Nachemson A 1961 Clinical observations on the spine in ejected pilots. Acta Orthop. Scand. 31: 135

13   Bartelink D L 1957 The role of abdominal pressure in relieving the pressure on the lumbar intervertebral discs. J. Bone Joint Surg. 39B: 718

14   Morris J M, Lucas D B, Bressler B 1961 Role of the trunk in stability of the spine. J. Bone Joint Surg. 43A: 327

15   Eie N 1966 Load capacity of the low back. J. Oslo City Hosp. 16: 73

16   Hemborg B 1983 Intraabdominal pressure and trunk muscle activity during lifting. Thesis, Department of Physical Therapy, University of Lund, Sweden

17   Schultz A, Andersson G, Örtengren R, Haderspeck K, Nachemson A 1982 Loads on the lumbar spine. Validation of a biomechanical analysis by measurements of intradiscal pressures and myoelectric signals. J. Bone Joint Surg. 64A: 713–720

18   Jayson M I V, Herbert C M, Barks J S 1973 Intervertebral discs: nuclear morphology and bursing pressures. Ann. Rheum. Dis. 32: 308

19   Evans F G, Lissner H R 1954 Strength of intervertebral discs. J. Bone Joint Surg. 39A: 185

20   Brown T, Hansen R J, Yorra A J 1957 Some mechanical tests on the lumbosacral spine with particular reference to the intervertebral discs. J. Bone Joint Surg. 39A: 1135

21   Roaf R 1960 A study of the mechanisms of spinal injuries. J. Bone Joint Surg. 42B: 810

22   Smith F P 1969 Experimental biomechanics of intervertebral disc rupture through a vertebral body. J. Neurosurg. 30: 134

23   Jayson M I V, Barks J S 1973 Structural changes in the intervertebral discs. Ann. Rheum. Dis. 32: 10

24   Brinckmann P, Frobin W, Hierholzer E, Horst M 1983 Deformation of the vertebral end-plate under axial loading of the spine. Spine 8: 851–856

25   Horst M, Brinckmann P 1981 Measurement of the distribution of axial stress on the end-plate of the vertebral body. Spine 6: 217–232

26   Markolf K L 1972 Deformation of the thoracolumbar intervertebral joints in response to external loads. J. Bone Joint Surg. 54A: 511

27   Farfan H F, Huberdau R M, Dubow H I 1972 Lumbar intervertebral disc degeneration. J. Bone Joint Surg. 54A: 492

28   Farfan H F 1973 Mechanical disorders of the low back. Lea & Febiger, Philadelphia

29   Adams M A, Hutton W C 1982 Prolapsed intervertebral disc. A hyperflexion injury. Spine 7: 184–191

30   Urban J, Holm S, Maroudas A, Nachemson A 1977 Nutrition of the intervertebral disc: An in vivo study of solute transport. J. Clin. Orthop. 129: 101–114

31   Holm S, Nachemson A 1982 Nutritional changes in the canine intervertebral disc after spinal fusion. J. Clin. Orthop. 169: 243–258

32   Holm S, Nachemson A 1983 Variations in the nutrition of the canine intervertebral disc induced by motion. Spine 8: 866–874

33   Virgin W J 1951 Experimental investigations into the physical properties of the intervertebral disc. J. Bone Joint Surg. 33B: 607

34   Pusshel J 1930 Der Wassergehalt normaler und degenerierter Zwischenwirbelscheiben. Beitr. Path. Anatom. 84: 123

35   Hirsch C, Paulson S, Sylven B, Snellman O 1952 Biophysical and physiological investigations on cartilage and other mesenchymal tissues. VI. Characteristics of human nuclei pulposi during ageing. Acta Orthop. Scand. 22: 175

36   Nachemson A 1960 Lumbar intradiscal pressure. Acta Orthop. Scand. Suppl. 43

37   Nachemson A 1962 Some mechanical properties of the lumbar intervertebral discs. Bull. Hosp. Joint Dis. (New York) 23: 130

38   Nachemson A 1963 The influence of spinal movements on the lumbar intradiscal pressure and on the tensile stresses in the annulus fibrosus. Acta Orthop. Scand. 33: 183

39   Nachemson A 1965 In vivo discometry in lumbar discs with irregular nucleograms. Acta Orthop. Scand. 36: 418–434

40   Nachemson A, Evans J 1968 Some mechanical properties of the third human lumbar interlaminar ligament (ligamentum flavum). J. Biomech. 1: 211

41   Rolander S D 1966 Motion of the lumbar spine with special reference to the stabilizing effect of posterior fusion. Acta Orthop. Scand. Suppl. 90

42   Lucas D B, Bressler B 1960 Stability of the ligamentous spine. Biomechanics Laboratory, Technical Report No. 40, University of California, San Francisco

43   Nachemson A, Morris J M 1964 In vivo measurements of intradiscal pressure. Discometry, a method for the determination of pressure in the lower lumbar discs. J. Bone Joint Surg. 46A: 1077

44   Nachemson A, Elfström G 1970 Intravital dynamic pressure measurement in lumbar discs: a study of common movements, manoeuvres and exercises. Almqvist & Wiksell, Stockholm

45   Andersson B J G, Örtengren R, Nachemson A, Elfström G 1974 Lumbar disc pressure and myoelectric back muscle activity during sitting. I. Studies on an experimental chair. Scand. J. Rehab. Med. 6: 104

46   Andersson B J G, Örtengren R, Nachemson A, Elfström G 1974 Lumbar disc pressure and myoelectric back muscle activity during sitting. IV. Studies on a car driver's seat. Scand. J. Rehab. Med. 6: 128

47   Andersson G B J, Schultz A B, Nachemson A L 1983 Intervertebral disc pressures during traction. Scand. J. Rehab. Med. 9: 88–91

48   Andersson G B J, Murphy R W, Örtengren R, Nachemson A L 1979 The influence of backrest inclination and lumbar supports on lumbar lordosis. Spine 4: 52–58

49   Hein-Sørensen O, Elfström G, Nachemson A 1979 Disc

pressure measurements in para- and tetraplegic patients. Scand. J. Rehab. Med. 11: 1–11

50 Hood J C, Hart D L, Smith H G, Davis H 1981 Comparison of electromyographic activity in normal lumbar sacrospinalis musculature during continuous and intermittent pelvic traction. J. Orthop. Sports Phys. Therapy 2: 137–141

51 Kanematsu H 1970 An experimental study of intradiscal pressure. J. Jap. Orthop. Assoc. 44: 589

52 Okushima H 1970 Study on hydrodynamic pressure of lumbar intervertebral disc. Arch. Jap. Chir. 39: 45

53 Umezawa F 1971 The study of comfortable sitting postures. J. Jap. Orthop. Assoc. 45: 1015

54 Tzivian I L, Rayhinstein V H, Motov V F, Ovseychik J G 1971 Results of clinical study of pressure within the intervertebral lumbar discs. Orthop. Travmatol. Protez. 6: 31

55 Horst M 1980 Messung der Verteilung der Normalspannung an der Grenzfläche Bandscheibe-Wirbelkörper. Thesis, Westfälische Wilhelms-Universität, Münster, West Germany

56 van Dellen J R 1979 Comparative studies of mechanical properties of intervertebral discs from black and white individuals. Thesis, University of the Witwatersrand, Johannesburg, South Africa

57 Galante J O 1967 Tensile properties of the human lumbar annulus fibrosus. Acta Orthop. Scand. Suppl. 100

58 Naylor A 1962 The biophysical and biochemical aspects of intervertebral disc herniation and degeneration. Ann. Roy. Coll. Surg. Eng. 31: 91

59 Feffer H L 1963 A physiological approach to lumbar intervertebral disc derangement. In: Adams J P (ed) Current Practice in Orthopaedic Surgery, vol 1. Mosby, St Louis

60 Hirsch C, Ingelmark B-E, Miller M 1963 The anatomical basis for low back pain. Acta Orthop. Scand. 33: 1

61 Peyron J-G 1967 Biologie du disque intervertébral. Sem. Hop. Paris 43: 3318

62 Nachemson A, Diamant B, Karlsson J 1968 Correlation between lactate levels and pH in discs of patients with lumbar rhizopathies. Experientia 24: 1195

63 Nachemson A 1969 Intradiscal measurements of pH in patients with lumbar rhizopathies. Acta Orthop. Scand. 40: 23

64 Nachemson A 1976 The lumbar spine, an orthopaedic challenge. Spine 1: 59

65 Andersson G B J, Ortengren R, Nachemson A 1977 Intradiscal pressure, intraabdominal pressure and myoelectric back muscle activity related to posture and loading. Clin. Orthop. 129: 156–164

66 Andersson G, Örtengren R, Nachemson A 1978 Quantitative studies of the back in different working postures. Scand. J. Rehab. Med. Suppl. 6: 173

67 Örtgren R, Andersson G, Nachemson A 1978 Lumbar back loads in fixed working postures during flexion and rotation. In: Asmussen E, Jörgenssen K (eds) Biomechanics VI-B. University Park Press, Baltimore, p 159

68 Andersson G B J, Örtengren R, Herberts P 1977 Quantitative electromyographic studies of back muscle activity related to posture and loading. Orthop. Clin. N. Amer. 8: 85

69 Örtengren R 1974 On multichannel acquisition of biomedical data, with special reference to the recording and analysis of myoelectric signals. Thesis, Department of Applied Electronics, Chalmers University of Technology and the Departments of Clinical Neurophysiology and Orthopaedic Surgery I, University of Göteborg, Sweden

70 Nachemson A, Schultz A, Andersson G 1983 Mechanical effectiveness studies of lumbar spine orthoses. Scand. J. Rehab. Med. Suppl. 9: 139–149

71 Berkson M H, Nachemson A, Schultz A B 1979 Mechanical properties of human lumbar motion segments. Part II: Responses in compression and shear; influence of gross morphology. ASME J. Biomech. Eng. 101: 53–57

72 Zachrisson-Forssell M 1981 The back school. Spine 6: 104–106

73 Bergquist-Ullman M, Larsson U 1970 Acute low back pain in industry. Acta Orthop. Scand. Suppl. 170

74 Chaffin D B 1974 Human strength capability and low back pain. J. Occup. Medicine 16: 248

75 Davis P R, Stubbs D A 1977 Safe levels of manual forces for young males. Applied Ergonomics 8: 141

76 Snook S H, Ciriello V M 1972 Low back pain in industry. Am. Soc. Safety Eng. J. 17: 17

77 Magora A 1970 Investigation of the relation between low back pain and occupation. Indust. Med. Surg. 30: 504

78 Magora A 1972 Investigation of the relation between low back pain and occupation. 3. Physical requirements: sitting, standing and weight lifting. Industr. Med. Surg. 41: 5

79 Magora A 1973 Investigation of the relation between low back pain and occupation. 4. Physical requirements: bending, rotation, reaching and sudden maximal effort. Scand. J. Rehab. Med. 5: 191

80 Westrin C-G 1973 Low back sick-listing. A nosological and medical insurance investigation. Scand. J. Soc. Med. Suppl. 7

81 Svensson H-O 1981 Low back pain in forty to forty-seven year old men: a retrospective cross-sectional study. Thesis, University of Göteborg, Sweden

82 Kelsey J L, Githens P B, White A A, et al 1984 An epidemiologic study of lifting and twisting on the job and risk for acute prolapsed lumbar intervertebral disc. J. Orthop. Res. 2: 61–66

83 Kelsey J L, Githens P B, O'Connor T, et al 1984 Acute, prolapsed, lumbar, intervertebral disc. An epidemiologic study with special reference to driving automobiles and cigarette smoking. Spine (In print)

84 Nachemson A 1983 Work for all. For those with low back pain as well. Clin. Orthop. Rel. Res. 179: 77–85

Loads on the lumbar spine

INTRODUCTION

Impairments of the back and spine are the most prevalent cause of chronic disability in the United States in persons younger than 45, and the third most prevalent cause of chronic disability in persons of ages 45–64 years. At least eight million US residents have such impairments.[1] Equally disturbing statistics are available from around the world.

Many of these spine impairments result from low back pain. While some cases of low back pain are accompanied by a clearly observable organic pathology, such as a herniated disc, the vast majority of cases should be classified as idiopathic. This statement sometimes generates controversy. Low back pain is often said to arise from 'instability' or 'degenerative disc disease' or the like. In fact, such conditions are often defined imprecisely, and few controlled, objective studies are available to show that these conditions are primarily responsible for the pain.

Indirect evidence suggests that large mechanical loads on the lumbar trunk structures are linked into the aetiology of idiopathic and other kinds of low back pain. Workers whose jobs are physically strenuous, compared to workers whose jobs are light, seem to have a higher incidence of low back pain.[2,3] Kelsey et al[4] showed that workers performing frequent heavy lifts were three times more likely, and workers performing frequent heavy lifts from twisted positions were six times more likely to experience an acute lumbar disc prolapse, compared to those with lighter work. The role of mechanical loads is also suggested strongly by the fact that patients with low back pain limit their physical activities: they do not move as fast or push as hard as they did before that pain arose.

Thus, an approach likely to bear fruit in scientific studies of low back pain is to determine quantitatively how a given physical exertion loads the structures of the lumbar trunk. This chapter will review advances made in this area of research over the past few years. It will concentrate on how to calculate, using biomechanical models, what loads are imposed on the major structural elements of the lumbar spine, the lumbar spine motion segments and the major muscle groups crossing the lumbar region. Sample results of calculations will be given, to provide a sense of typical load magnitudes. Extensions of the basic concepts, which apply to slow (quasi-static) performances of tasks, to rapid (dynamic) performances will also be discussed.

The chapter will in addition outline how spine loads can be measured in vivo, at least indirectly. It will review a series of studies that have validated the calculations by showing good agreement between indirect experimental measurements and biomechanical model predictions of internal loads.

CALCULATION OF TRUNK LOADS

It is faster, easier, cheaper and safer to calculate lumbar trunk internal loads using biomechanical models than to determine them through experimental measurements. Moreover, model calculations more readily provide insights into the major determinants of those loads than do experimental measurements.

There are two main steps in a biomechanical model calculation of trunk loads: the calculation of the net reaction and the calculation of internal loads.

Calculation of the net reaction

(This and the following subsections are adapted from Schultz & Andersson[5] and Schultz et al[6].)

The net reaction consists of the three components of the force and the three components of the moment that are provided by the lower part of the body to act on the upper part of the body across an imaginary transverse cutting plane passed through the spine level of interest for example at the L3 level. This net reaction needs to be provided in order to keep the body segments above the cutting plane in mechanical equilibrium during a quasi-static task performance. Since in a quasi-static performance the upper part of the body must be in equilibrium, there is little question about the nature of this net reaction. It is determined from the six requirements for equilibrium that result from Newton's Laws; the sums of all the net reaction and external forces acting on the upper body along each, and the sums of all the net reaction and external moments about each of the coordinate axes must be zero. These requirements provide six equations that are solved to find the six components of the net reaction.

There are two types of external loads: loads applied in order to perform the task, and loads from body segment weights. The applied loads are the forces needed to manoeuvre (lift, push, etc.) any object being handled. They are usually applied to the hands and can be measured directly or estimated. The weight loads act at the centres of mass of the upper body segments. The weights of different body segments can be found in the literature (Clauser et al,[7] for example). Mass-centre locations can be estimated by using scaled cross-sectional anatomy drawings (Eycleshymer & Schoemaker,[8] for example) and assuming that the body parts have uniform densities.

The net reaction is not affected directly by anything occurring in the parts of the body below the imaginary cutting plane, nor is it affected by the material properties of any of the hard and soft tissues of the body. Anatomical variables affect the net reaction only in so far as they influence mass distributions and moment arms. The major difficulty in the determination of a net reaction is to gather the data configuration needed to locate the various mass centres. However, it is seldom necessary to locate these with great accuracy; approximate data are usually sufficient.

Sample calculations of the net reaction

These ideas will be illustrated by three examples. First, consider a subject holding weights of magnitude Q in his hands in a sagittally symmetrical upright configuration (Fig. 10.1(a)). Locate a co-ordinate system centred in the L3 inter-vertebral disc, and suppose that the x, y and z directions are to the left, anterior, and superior respectively. Suppose also that the weight of the upper body is divided into the weight of the head and upper neck, W_h; the weights of the left and right upper limbs, W_a; and the weight of the remainder of the trunk above the cutting plane, W_t.

Based upon the body segment weight data cited, assume that W_t is 36% of total body weight when the cutting plane is passed through the L3 level, W_h is 5% of body weight, and W_a is 9% of body weight. Place W_t in the middle of the trunk cross-section at the T9 level, W_h in the middle of a line joining the centres of the left and right ears, and W_a at the mass centre of the limbs, which can be estimated by visual observation of limb configuration. The coordinates of the mass centre locations are specified as (x_t, y_t, z_t), etc.

The net reaction consists of the forces and moments F_x, F_y, F_z, M_x, M_y, and M_z (Fig. 10.1(a) and 10.2). It can be computed from the six equations that must be satisfied for the upper body to be in equilibrium. That is, each component of the net reaction must equal the sum of the corresponding components of the external forces or moments. In this example, four of those requirements are trivially satisfied, since there are no x-direction or y-direction external forces and no external moments about either the y-axis or the z-axis. So, $F_x = F_y = M_y = M_z = 0$. The two non-trivially-satisfied equations of equilibrium are

$$F_z = Q + W_h + W_t$$
$$M_x = y_a W_a + y_h W_h + y_t W_t$$

where F_z and M_x are the two non-zero components of the net reaction. Assume the following representative data:

Q	=	40 N	y_q	=	40 cm
W_a	=	63 N	y_a	=	20 cm
W_h	=	35 N	y_h	=	7 cm
W_t	=	252 N	y_t	=	1 cm

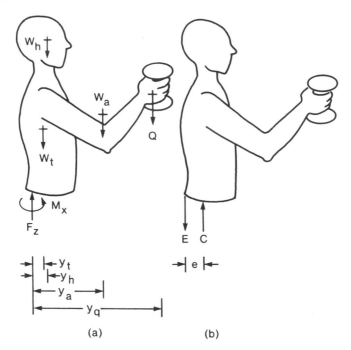

Fig. 10.1 Data for analysis of a sagittally symmetrical weight-holding task

The non-zero components of the net reaction, from the two equations, are

$$F_z = 390 \text{ N}$$
$$M_x = 33.6 \text{ Nm}$$

For a second example, consider the external loads acting on the upper body when a weight of magnitude Q is held in the right hand, and the trunk is upright (Fig. 10.2). In this example, the weight of each limb must be considered separately. Let W^1 and W_r denote these limb weights, and assume they are each 4.5% of body weight. Compute the net reaction components from the requirements for equilibrium of forces in the

x direction: $F_x = 0$
y direction: $F_y = 0$
z direction: $F_z = Q + W_h + W_1 + W_r + W_t$

and for equilibrium of moments about the

x-axis: $M_x = y_q Q + y_h W_h + y_1 W_1 + y_r W_r + y_t W_t$
y-axis: $M_y = x_r W_r - x_1 W_1$
z-axis: $M_z = 0$

In this example, there are again no external forces in the x or y directions, and no force has a moment about the z-axis, so $F_x = F_y = M_z = 0$. In addition, none of W_h, Q or W_t has a moment about the y-axis. If representative numerical values are assumed:

Q	= 40 N	x_q	= 0	y_q	= 40 cm
W_h	= 35 N	x_h	= 0	y_h	= 7 cm
W_1	= 32 N	x_1	= 20 cm	y_1	= 1 cm
W_r	= 32 N	x_r	= 10 cm	y_r	= 26 cm
W_t	= 252 N	x_t	= 0	y_t	= 1 cm

the three non-zero components of the net reaction are

$$F_z = 391 \text{ N} \quad M_x = 23.2 \text{ Nm} \quad M_y = 3.2 \text{ Nm}$$

For a third example (not pictured), consider a subject standing upright while resisting a pull to the right on his chest of 10 kg (98 N). The net reaction that must be supplied across the L3 section in this situation consists of two non-zero forces, a 98 N force to the side (F_x) to equilibrate the right pull, and a net longitudinal force (F_z) equal to the weight of the upper body segments; and two non-zero moments, a flexion moment (M_x) of 1.5 Nm due to the small

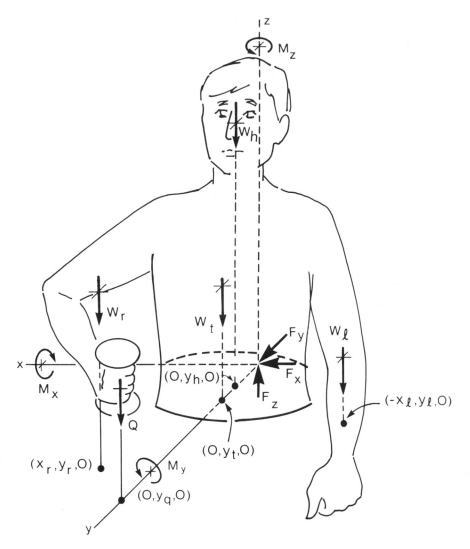

Fig. 10.2 Holding a weight in the right hand: external forces and net reaction components

anterior overhand of the upper body segment weights, and, if that pull acts 33 cm superior to L3, a lateral bending moment (M_y) of 32.5 Nm. F_y and M_z are, once again, zero.

The net reaction computation scheme illustrated by these three examples can readily be generalized to handle more complicated situations.

Calculation of the internal loads

The net reaction needed to equilibrate the upper part of the body is supplied in the lumbar trunk by muscle contractions, connective tissue tensions,

intra-abdominal pressure and the reactions or resistances supplied by the spine motion segments. These are forces internal to the trunk. The most common problem is to determine the motion segment reactions or, in other words, the loads on the spine. But in the course of calculating these loads, the other internal loads will need to be calculated as well.

Lumbar motion segments do not supply significant reaction moments in activities involving upright or near-upright positions of the trunk. A 5 Nm moment causes a lumbar motion segment to rotate from approximately 1° to 5° in bending or torsion.[9]

In physical performances in which the trunk is not substantially bent, net reaction moments of 100 Nm or more are frequently developed, while the motion segments each rotate a few degrees at most. So it will be assumed in the analyses to follow, in which the trunk is not substantially bent, that the motion segments provide zero resistance to bending. On the other hand, lumbar motion segments can resist significant shear and compression forces with only small linear motions,[10] so the analyses will account for that. In performances involving substantial trunk bending, the motion segments do provide significant bending resistances. In those cases, resistances can be estimated from the amount of relative bending between adjacent motion segments and mechanical property data on motion segment stiffnesses. The resistances can then be taken into account in the internal load calculations.

Sample calculation of internal loads

To show how internal loads can be calculated in a mechanically simple situation, consider again the first net reaction calculation example (Fig. 10.1(a)). To calculate a set of internal loads that can provide the required net reaction, assume that there are only two internal forces that supply this: a compressive force C on the lumbar motion segment and a tension E in a single equivalent of the back muscles (Fig. 10.1(b)). These are the assumptions used by Morris et al.[11] These two z-direction forces must provide the net reaction, which consists of non-zero components F_z and M_x. So,

$$F_z = C - E$$
$$M_x = eE$$

Assume $e = 5$ cm, and solve these equations to obtain

$$E = 3360 \text{ Ncm} / 5 \text{ cm} = 672 \text{ N}$$
$$C = 390 \text{ N} + 672 \text{ N} = 1062 \text{ N}$$

The required net reaction can be supplied by these two forces. The simplicity of this calculation resulted from the assumption that the required net reaction was supplied by only two internal forces.

As to the values calculated, the value of the compression force C is considerably larger than the value of the net reaction component in the same direction, F_z. Some thought will show that in this example it is mainly the magnitude of the moments of the external forces about the spine that cause C to be as large as it is, rather than the external force magnitudes themselves. In general, the magnitudes of the external moments will be found to be the major determinants of the internal load magnitudes.

A more general model for calculation of internal loads

Now consider the more-widely applicable model of the trunk shown in Figure 10.3. This model can be used to estimate trunk internal loads in a variety of circumstances. Its use is not restricted to sagittally-symmetrical tasks, for example. It incorporates ten muscle equivalents, five per side, to represent major muscle groups spanning the lumbar region: the rectus abdominus muscles (R); the external oblique abdominal muscles (X); the internal oblique abdominal muscles (I); the lumbar slips of the latissimus dorsi (L); and the erector spinae muscles (E).

Again, in this model, the L3 spine motion segment is assumed to resist compression, lateral shear and anteroposterior shear, but to have no significant moment resistance, for reasons already given. Abdominal cavity pressure resultant force (P) can be accounted for, but will be assumed to be zero in the examples presented here. This assumption is made because in many quasi-static task performances intra-abdominal pressure does not show a consistent relationship with the loads imposed on the spine by task performance, and provides in the mean a spine compression relief of only approximately 15%.[12]

The spine motion segment resistances consist of a compression C, a right-lateral shear S_r, and an anterior shear S_a. The requirement that these three resistances and the ten muscle contraction forces provide the six components of the net reaction that are needed for equilibrium is expressed by the six equations of equilibrium. Since there are 13 unknown internal forces, and only six equations are available to calculate them, the use of this model leads to a 'statically indeterminate' problem. That is, there are more unknowns than there are equations of equilibrium to solve for them.

A good way to solve this statically indeterminate problem is through use of optimization techniques, as proposed, for example, by Seireg & Arvikar.[13] Linear programming (Dantzig,[14] for example) is

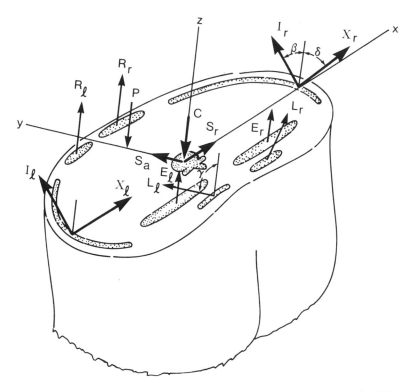

Fig. 10.3 Schematic representation of an L3 cross-sectional model with ten single equivalent muscles. The muscle equivalents represent the rectus abdominus (R); the internal (I) and the external (X) oblique abdominal muscles; the erector spinae (E); and the latissimus doris (L) muscles. The cross-sectional area of each muscle equivalent relative to the product of trunk width times trunk depth, and the location of the muscle equivalent centroids are given in Table 10.1

probably the simplest of these techniques. The major question that arises when linear programming or similar procedures are used for solution is the choice of the 'objective function' or the quantity to be optimized.

An optimization scheme we have used to calculate internal forces minimizes approximately the maximum required muscle contraction force per unit area of muscle cross-section (stress). To achieve this, the maximum allowed contraction stress is set to 10 kPa, and a solution is sought by linear programming so as to minimize the compression force on the spine. If no solution is available, the allowed stress is incremented by 10 kPa, and a solution is again sought. This stress incrementation procedure is iterated until a solution is found. Use of this optimization scheme keeps antagonistic muscle activity to a minimum, while it calls on nearly every muscle that can contribute to an activity to do so at nearly equal contraction stresses. Details of the cross-section model are given in Table 10.1, and details of how this calculation scheme is

implemented are given in the Appendix. Analogous 14 and 22 muscle cross-section models are described by Schultz et al.[6]

Additional sample calculations of internal loads

Calculation of internal loads using the ten-muscle model just described, or more complicated models, cannot readily be done manually. The calculations can readily be done by a computer, using software available for solving linear programming problems. We will consider only the results of such calculations.

For the sample problem of holding a weight in the right hand, when the previously calculated net reaction components and the data in Table 10.1 are utilized, the following are the resulting muscle contraction forces:

E_l = 201 N E_r = 264 N
L_l = 33 N L_r = 33 N

Table 10.1 Data incorporated into the ten single equivalent muscle L3 cross-sectional model

Muscle	Symbol	Line of action	Area ratio per side[a]	Location of centroid Anteroposterior offset ratio[b]	Lateral offset ratio[c]
Rectus abdominus	R	Longitudinal	0.0060	0.540	0.121
Oblique abdominals		Inclined 45° to longitudinal, in sagittal plane			
Internal	I		0.0168	0.189	0.453
External	X		0.0148	0.189	0.453
Erector spinae	E	Longitudinal	0.0390	0.220	0.179
Latissimus dorsi	L	Inclined 45° to longitudinal, in frontal plane	0.0037	0.276	0.211

The vertebral body centre lies in the mid-sagittal plane at 0.66 times the trunk depth from the anterior-most edge of the cross section.

[a] In ratio to trunk width times trunk depth.
[b] From vertebral body centre, in ratio to trunk depth.
[c] From vertebral body centre, in ratio to trunk width.

These forces equilibrate the two net reaction moment components, and no other muscles are required to contract. The right side erector muscles contract somewhat more than the left, in order to equilibrate the net lateral bending moment. The largest muscle contraction stress that results is 140 kPa. Motion segment compression is 865 N, and no shear resistances are called upon.

For the sample problem of resisting the pull to the right, the results of the internal muscle contraction force calculation are:

$$R_l = 40N \quad R_r = 15N$$
$$I_l = 91N \quad I_r = 5N$$
$$X_l = 86N$$
$$E_l = 282N$$

All other muscle contraction forces are found to be zero. The two right-side muscles contract a small amount, but some thought shows that these contractors are not truly antagonistic. They are needed both to balance the net flexion moment, and to counteract the twisting moment produced by the difference in the left internal and the left external oblique muscle contraction forces. The larges muscle contraction stress used to resist the pull is 130 kPa. Motion segment reactions consist of an 812 N compression, an 8 N anterior shear and a 98 N lateral shear.

The calculation schemes outlined provide a complete description, within the assumptions of the model, of what internal forces need to be developed to perform a given physical task.

Calculations of maximum voluntary trunk strengths

The foregoing ideas can be used to predict what the maximum voluntary strengths of the lumbar trunk muscles should be, under the assumptions incorporated into the biomechanical model. Ikai & Fukunaga,[15] for example, reported that human voluntary muscle can contract with a maximum stress of 400–1000 kPa. If, in a reversal of the calculation procedures described, the maximum allowed stress is set to 1000 kPa, the largest net reaction then sustainable can be calculated. The results of this calculation (Table 10.2) suggest what the bounds are on heavy exertions from upright positions. They indicate what moments the lumbar trunk muscles can develop and how large lumbar muscle contraction forces and lumbar spine compressions might become. In fact, the table shows that in an upright maximum voluntary flexion resist-task spine compression might be 4900 N, or more than twelve times the mean weight of the body segments above that level.

Table 10.2 Prediction from ten-muscle model of maximum voluntary trunk strengths and corresponding internal forces. Predictions are for a subject with a lumbar (L3) trunk depth of 20 cm and a trunk width of 30 cm, contracting his muscles at a maximum intensity of approximately 1000 kPa.

Muscle contraction forces (N)		Resist flexion	Resist extension	Resist lateral bend	Resist right twist	Resist
Muscle group						
Internal obliques,	left		1000	890		1000
	right		1000	250		
External obliques,	left		640	640		
	right		640			640
Rectus abdominus,	left		360	360		
	right		360	140		
Erector spinae,	left	2300		2310		
	right	2300				810
Latissimus dorsi,	left	220				210
	right	220				
Spine compression force (N)		4920	3030	4070	2120	
Moment developed (Nm)		220	160	250	160	

VALIDATION OF INTERNAL LOAD CALCULATIONS

While there is little question about the nature of the net reaction, major assumptions are used in the calculation of the internal forces. Before any proposed calculation scheme can be used with confidence, the assumptions it incorporates need to be validated by experimental measurement.

Direct measurement of trunk internal forces in vivo is impractical, but there are at least two means to determine internal forces indirectly in the laboratory: by measurement of intradiscal pressures and by measurement of myoelectric activity. Nachemson[16] reviews the evidence showing that intradiscal pressure measures are indicative of compression loads on the spine, and Ortengren & Andersson[17] review the evidence showing that myoelectric activity in the back muscles relates monotonically to muscle contraction forces. Rectified and integrated myoelectric activity signal levels can essentially be directly related to muscle contraction force magnitudes, by making the myoelectric measurements under nearly identical conditions over periods of 5–15 s in a series of different isometric exertions. Use of mean values over populations of perhaps ten subjects further compensates for individual variations in activity levels. Under those circumstances, myoelectric activity measurements have been shown to be good quantitative measures of muscle contraction force magnitudes.

A series of studies using these two measurement techniques has amply validated the spine load calculation schemes presented here over a range of circumstances. Good agreement between computed tensions and measured myoelectric activities in the erector spinae muscles in many weight-holding tasks performed while the subject is sitting at a table is reported by Andersson et al,[18] and over a range of sagitally symmetrical standing work tasks is reported by Schultz et al.[19] Schultz et al[12] report good agreement in both kinds of tasks between predicted spine compressions and measured spine intradiscal pressures. Good agreement between computed tensions and measured myoelectric activities in several lumbar muscle groups, in tasks involving lateral bending and twisting, is reported by Schultz & Andersson[20] and Schultz et al.[6] So, some confidence can be placed in the results of the trunk load calculations outlined here.

Other evidence suggesting the validity of the calculation schemes comes from measurements in vivo of lumbar trunk maximum voluntary strengths. McNeill et al[21] measured maximum voluntary trunk strengths at the L5 level in 27 healthy men. They found those strengths to be in the mean 210 Nm in tests equivalent to flexion resists, 149 Nm in extension resists, and 148 Nm in lateral bending resists. The ten-muscle model described predicts maximum voluntary trunk strengths at the L3 level in an average-sized adult of 230 Nm in flexion resists, 160 Nm in extension resists, and 250 Nm in lateral bending resist. These compare well with the measured values. The larger predicted lateral bending strength may indicate that the 1000 kPa maximum stress level used to make the predictions is too high, or that factors other than those accounted for in the calculations limit strengths in lateral bending in vivo.

TYPICAL MAGNITUDES OF INTERNAL LOADS

Use of the calculation schemes outlined show that the compression forces on lumbar vertebrae in an adult male of average size range from approximately 400 N, which is roughly the weight of the body segments superior to the lumbar region, when standing or sitting relaxed, to ten or more times that value in slowly-performed heavy physical exertions (Table 10.3). Merely bending the trunk forward 30° triples the relaxed standing compression value, because of the need to equilibrate the flexion moment produced by the anterior overhang of the weights of the upper body segments.

In isometric maximum voluntary exertions in positions of upright standing, the shear forces imposed on the lumbar vertebra may be on the order of 500 N. Correspondingly, the contraction forces in the major trunk muscle groups may be of the order of 2300 N per side in the erector spinae group, and of the order of 400–1000 N in the other muscle groups (Table 10.2).

THE MAJOR DETERMINANTS OF INTERNAL LOADS

The major determinants of the loads that must be resisted by the lumbar spine motion segments and of the contraction forces that must be developed by the lumbar trunk muscles are the moments about the spine of the loads applied to the upper body and of the weights of the upper body segments. The moment of a force about a point is the magnitude of the force times its perpendicular distance to that point (that is, the lever arm over which the force acts on the spine). If a 100N weight is held close to the chest, or about 20 cm anterior to L3, it imposes a moment tending to flex the spine of 100N × 0.2 m = 20 Nm on the trunk. If it is held at arm's length, or about 70 cm anterior to L3, it imposes a flexion moment of 70 Nm anterior on the trunk. Holding the weight at arm's length will impose an increase in lumbar trunk internal loads that is more than three times as large as the increase imposed by holding it close to the chest, although in both cases the weight held is the same. To keep lumbar trunk loads light, it is important to keep the applied loads small, but it is even more important to keep the lever arms over which they act small. When lifting, keep the load lifted as close in to the body as possible.

EXTENSION TO DYNAMIC PROBLEMS

Performance of a physical activity is sometimes called dynamic if it is accompanied by body motion of any kind. However, many activities involving body motion can be analysed without significant error as if they were static. Dynamic considerations are important mechanically only when a motion involves significant linear or angular accelerations. The product of a mass and its linear acceleration is called an inertial force; the product of a moment of inertia and its angular acceleration is called an inertial moment. In a biomechanical analysis, body dynamics need to be considered only when the inertial forces and the inertial moments produced are

Table 10.3 Typical magnitudes of calculated L3 motion segment compression forces imposed by some physical tasks (N). The studies from which these magnitudes were tabulated are reported in the papers cited in the section on validation of internal load calculations

Sitting	
Upright, relaxed	380
arms forward, hold 4 kg	750
Standing	
Upright, relaxed	440
arms forward, hold 8 kg	1170
resist 60 Nm twisting moment	1170
maximum attempted extension	5050
Trunk flexed 30°, relaxed	1400
30°, hold 8 kg	2350
40°, maximum upward pull	4360

of magnitudes that are at least of the same order as the forces and moments needed for equilibrium. If the inertial forces and moments are small when compared with the forces and moments that would be required for static equilibrium, an activity involving body motion is called quasi-static, and can safely be analysed as a static activity.

In truly dynamic activities in which significant inertial forces and moments do arise, these forces and moments can be accounted for easily enough. First, the inertial forces and moments need to be computed. This can be done through measurement or estimation of the appropriate linear and angular accelerations and use of anthropometric data on body segment masses, mass centres and moments of inertia. Once the inertial forces and moments are determined, they are applied at the body segment mass centres as if they were additional external loads. The remaining procedures outlined here are then executed without alteration. In other words, the inertial forces and moments will directly enter the procedures used to calculate the net reaction, but not those used to estimate the internal loads, under almost all circumstances of practical interest.

APPENDIX: DETAILS OF MODEL INTERNAL LOAD COMPUTATIONS

The internal load computations involve six equations which ensure that these internal forces equilibrate the portion of the body above the transverse cutting plane at the L3 level. F_x, F_y, F_z, M_x, M_y and M_z are the six components of the net reaction; their values will have already been computed as outlined. The unknown muscle forces are denoted E_l, E_r, I_l, I_r, L_l, L_r, R_l, R_r, X_l and X_r. Centroidal location data (x_e, x_0, x_l, x_r and corresponding ys) and muscle fibre angles (β, γ, δ) are known from the Table 10.1 data.

If spine compression C is to be minimized, the equation for z-direction equilibrium is used as the objective function:

$$C = F_z + (E_l + E_r) + (R_l + R_r) + (I_l + I_r) \cos\beta + (L_l + L_r) \cos\gamma + (X_l + X_r) \cos\delta \quad (1)$$

Minimization of C is constrained by the requirements that moments about the x, y and z axis be equilibrated:

$$y_e(E_l + E_r) - y_r(R_l + R_r) + y_l(L_l + L_r) \cos\gamma - y_0[(I_l + I_r) \cos\beta + (X_l + X_r) \cos\delta] - M_x = 0 \quad (2)$$

$$x_e(E_r - E_l) + x_r(R_r - R_l) + x_l(L_r - L_l) \cos\gamma + x_0[(I_r - I_l) \cos\beta + (X_r - X_l) \cos\delta] - M_y = 0 \quad (3)$$

$$y_l(L_r - L_l \sin\gamma + x_0[(I_r - I_l) \sin\beta (X_r - X_l) \sin\delta] - M_z = 0 \quad (4)$$

Minimization of C is further constrained by the value of the upper limit on muscle contraction intensities during iteration i, σ_i:

$$\frac{E_l}{A_E} \leqslant \sigma_i \quad (5)$$

for example, where A_E is the cross-sectional area of the erector spinae on one side (Table 10.1 data). Constraints similar to equation 5 must be satisfied for the other nine muscle contraction forces as well.

σ_i is given an initial value, and a solution for the unknowns is sought by linear programming. After each unsuccessful attempt to minimize C while satisfying all constraints, the value of σ_i is increased and another solution is attempted. The process is repeated until a solution is found.

Optimization techniques such as this one may result in non-unique solutions. Despite that, experimental results suggest that this model internal force computation scheme predicts the actual internal forces adequately, under the circumstances considered here.

Once a solution has been found, the remaining two equations of equilibrium are used to calculate the right and anterior shear resistances that must be supplied by the L3 motion segment:

$$S_r = F_x - (L_l - L_r) \sin\gamma \quad (6)$$

$$S_a = F_y - (I_l + I_r) \sin\beta + (X_l + X_r) \sin\delta \quad (7)$$

Internal force computations using more complicated muscle models are similar to those for the ten-muscle model. The equations used in those cases differ from the present equations only in the addition of more unknown muscle forces and their accompanying cross-sectional geometry data.

REFERENCES

1. National Health Survey 1973 Impairments due to injury, United States — 1971. National Center for Health Statistics, Rockville MD, Series 10, Number 87
2. Andersson G B J 1981 Epidemiologic aspects of low back pain in industry. Spine 6: 53–60
3. Damkot D K, Pope M H, Lord J, Frymoyer J W 1984 The relationship between work history, work environment and low back pain in men. Spine 9: 395–399
4. Kelsey J L, Githens P B, White III A A, Holford T R, Walter S D, O'Connor T et al 1984 An epidemiologic study of lifting and twisting on the job and risk for acute prolapsed lumbar intervertebral disc. J. Ortho. Res. 2: 61–66
5. Schultz A B, Andersson G B J 1981 Analysis of loads on the lumbar spine. Spine 6: 76–84
6. Schultz A, Haderspeck K, Warwick D, Portillo D 1983 Use of lumbar trunk muscles in isometric performance of mechanically complex standing tasks: J. Orth. Res. 1: 77–91
7. Clauser C, McConville J, Young J 1969 Weight volume and center of mass of segments of the human body. AMRL-TR-69-70, Wright-Patterson Air Force Base, Ohio
8. Eycleshymer A C, Schoemaker D M 1911 A cross-section anatomy. Appleton-Century-Crofts, New York
9. Schultz A B, Warwick D N, Berkson M H, Nachemson A L 1979 Mechanical properties of human spine motion segments. Part I: Responses in flexion, extension, lateral bending and torsion. ASME J. Biomech. Eng. 101: 46–52
10. Berkson M H, Nachemson A, Schultz A B 1979 Mechanical properties of human lumbar spine motion segments. Part II: Responses in compression and shear; influence of gross morphology. J. Biomech. Eng. 101: 53–57
11. Morris J M, Lucas D B, Bresler R 1961 Role of the trunk in stability of the spine. J. Bone Joint Surg. 43A: 327–351
12. Schultz A, Andersson G, Ortengren R, Haderspeck K, Nachemson A 1982 Loads on the lumbar spine. J. Bone Joint Surg. 64A: 713–720
13. Seireg A, Arvikar R J 1973 A mathematical model for evaluation of forces in lower extremities of the musculo-skeletal system. J. Biochem. 6: 313–316
14. Dantzig G B 1968 Linear programming. McGraw-Hill, New York
15. Ikai M, Fukunaga T 1968 Calculation of muscle strength per unit cross-sectional area of human muscle by means of ultrasonic measurement. Int Z Angew Physiol 26: 26–32
16. Nachemson A L 1981 Disc pressure measurements. Spine 6: 93–97
17. Ortengren R, Andersson G B J 1977 Electromyographic studies of trunk muscles, with special reference to the lumbar spine. Spine 2: 44–52
18. Andersson G B J, Ortengren R, Schultz A 1980 Analysis and measurement of the loads of the lumbar spine during work at a table. J. Biomech. 13: 513–520
19. Schultz A, Andersson G B J, Ortengren R, Bjork R, Nordin M 1982 Analysis and quantitative myoelectric measurements of loads on the lumbar spine with holding weights in standing postures. Spine 7: 390–397
20. Schultz A B, Andersson G B J, Haderspeck K, Ortengren R, Nordin M, Bjork R 1982 Analysis and measurement of lumbar trunk loads in tasks involving bends and twists. J. Biomech. 15: 669–675
21. McNeill T, Warwick D, Andersson G, Schultz A 1980 Trunk strengths in attempted flexion, extension and lateral bending in healthy subjects and patients with low-back disorders. Spine 5: 529–538

Measurement of spinal movement

INTRODUCTION

The measurement of spinal motion is one of the routine methods of examining patients suspected to have disorders of the locomotor system or disorders of other systems known to interfere with spinal movement. In a rheumatological context, the principal disorders in which measurement of spinal movement may be useful are ankylosing spondylitis and disorders of the lumbar disc. The importance of these measurements lies in their value not only in diagnosis but also as means to assess therapy.

Considering the well-established use of measurement of spinal movement in clinical diagnosis, it is surprising that *objective* methods to make these estimations have only been delineated in the last 15 years. A further anomaly stems from the lack, until the 1970s, of normal ranges for spinal movement: these are clearly necessary in order to judge whether measurements from patients are abnormal or not.

In this chapter, spinal mobility measurements will include not only movements of the thoracolumbar spine but also those of the cervical spine. We shall also include a short note on costovertebral motion because of the central importance of limitation of chest expansion in the diagnosis of ankylosing spondylitis. For the most part, comments will be restricted to measurements in clinical practice. However, sections on recent experimental work have been included, since they are important in throwing further light on our understanding of complicated biomechanics of the spine.

RELEVANT ANATOMY

The structure of the human spinal column not only allows flexibility of the trunk but also helps the body to retain an upright posture by means of coordinated action between muscles, ligaments and bones.

The structure of the vertebrae determines to a large extent the mechanics of the spinal column. A particularly important anatomical variation which modifies the type and extent of spinal movement at any one level is the structure of adjacent articular processes of the apophyseal joints. The contact established between the superior articular processes of one vertebra and inferior articular processes of the next restrains vertebral movement and in particular prevents forward displacement of one vertebra on another. The angle of the articular surfaces of the apophyseal joints in relation to the horizontal plane of the vertebral bodies varies at different levels and largely determines the type as well as the amount of movement occurring at various levels of the spine. The vertebral bodies also articulate with each other at the intervertebral disc. The elasticity of this fibrocartilaginous cushion permits sagittal compression of one edge of the disc with compensatory expansion of the other edge as well as some upward, downward and rotary movement between adjacent vertebral bodies. Movement between adjacent vertebrae is maximal at spinal levels where the disc is thickest, such as in the cervical and lumbar regions, and least where the disc is thinnest, as in the thoracic region. The vertebral bodies are bound together by anterior and posterior longitudinal ligaments which extend from the sacrum to the base of the occiput. The dense anterior ligament is stronger than the posterior ligament and limits extension of the vertebral column. The space between the laminae of adjacent vertebrae is occupied by the ligamenta flava, which help to restore the vertebral column to its original position after bending movements. The spinous processes are connected by the supraspinous and interspinous ligaments, which partially limit flexion and lateral bending.

The intrinsic muscles of the back function as an extensor group, and also control or counteract spinal flexion. The erector spinae are particularly important in this respect, and extend from the sacrum to the upper cervical vertebrae and base of the skull. These muscles are the longest in the back and are particularly well developed and prominent in the lumbar region. Flexor muscles of importance include the quadratus lumborum, psoas major and psoas minor, and also the muscles of the abdominal wall (external oblique, internal oblique and rectus abdominis). Abduction (lateral bending) and rotation of the spinal column are performed by contraction of abdominal and intrinsic back muscles on one side, with simultaneous relaxation of comparable muscles on the opposite side.

Recently, a computer analysis of the complex musculature controlling the lumbar spine has been carried out using muscle areas seen on serial cross sections through fresh human cadaver trunks. Rab et al[1] concluded that the total extensor moment only slightly exceeds the total flexor moment. The rectus abdominis, internal oblique and external oblique contribute about one-third towards total flexor moment. The erector spinae group contribute about one-half towards total extensor moment. In rotation, the large abdominal oblique muscles dominate over small 'rotator' muscles of the spine.

The vertebral column permits extension, flexion, lateral flexion and rotation. The extent of these movements varies in different segments of the spine. Movement of the spine is greatest in the cervical region, is more restricted in the lumbar and thoracic regions and is not present in the sacral region. *Flexion* occurs primarily in the cervical, low thoracic and lumbar regions. *Extension* takes place mainly in the cervical and lumbar regions. *Lateral flexion* occurs mostly in the cervical, low thoracic and lumbar regions. *Rotation* is most marked in the cervical region and is relatively restricted in the lumbar and thoracic regions.

MEASURING THORACOLUMBAR SPINE MOBILITY

The widespread traditional practice of assessing spinal mobility subjectively is gradually becoming replaced by an awareness of the importance of objective methods. In the past, it has been popular to judge the degree of spinal movement entirely by eye without assigning to it any numerical value. A slightly more sophisticated approach[2,3] has involved semi-objective techniques based on estimating the amount of spinal deviation fowards, backwards or sideways from a vertical neutral (zero) line using a standard goniometer (Fig. 11.1). This system is still in widespread use, but we believe that it should be

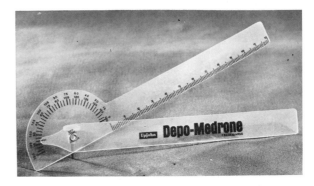

Fig. 11.1 Standard goniometer

abandoned in view of the high degree of inaccuracy involved in assessing angles of movement from an imaginary zero reference point: purely subjective assessment by eye is probably only slightly less accurate. It is possible that increased accuracy may be introduced by using the 'Universal' goniometer (Fig. 11.2) devised by Scott[4] rather than the standard goniometer. Certain further methods, developed to introduce objectivity, possess at least one major disadvantage. Such methods include:

1. Serial radiography of the spine. This has the disadvantage of radiation exposure, expense, and is also time-consuming.[5-7]

2. Serial photography. This has the disadvantage of inaccuracy[8] and is also expensive and time-consuming, as with radiography.

3. Protractor methods. Troup and his colleagues[9] have devised a method to measure sagittal mobility of the spine using a simple protractor, but the extreme postures patients are expected to adopt while measurements are taken by this technique preclude its use in the aged or infirm. (The subjects used in the study of Troup et al were physically active young adults — either physical education

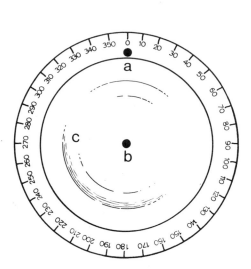

Fig. 11.2 Universal goniometer

Sagittal mobility

Most of the previous work in the field of measuring spinal movement objectively has concerned movement in the sagittal plane alone, lateral flexion and rotation having been relatively neglected. In the measurement of sagittal mobility, thoracic and lumbar movement have been considered together by most investigators; because of this we have used the term 'thoracolumbar' mobility throughout this account. Previous studies have usually considered measurement of the two components of sagittal mobility (*flexion* and *extension*) separately. However, one study has been concerned with considering sagittal movement as a whole.[20] This was based on the following index:

$$\frac{\text{length of fully flexed back}-\text{length of fully extended back}}{\text{length of back in relaxed upright posture}}$$

The main value of this approach lies in the fact that an allowance can be made for the effect of height on spinal mobility.

Thoracolumbar anterior flexion

Most of the movement involved in thoracolumbar forward flexion occurs in the lumbar vertebrae, but a small amount of movement also takes place in the thoracic spine.

Traditionally, an objective method to measure forward bending of the spine has involved recording the distance between fingertips and floor. The popularity of this method is reflected by the commercial production of an instrument to measure this distance (Fig. 11.3). However, as a measure of spinal mobility alone, this technique is notoriously misleading as it includes a contribution from hip movement as well as from spinal movement, and is also governed by other factors such as the degree of tightness of posterior leg muscles and ligaments.

A better clinical technique, not involving any instrumentation, involves simply the placing of two fingers of one hand over adjacent spinous processes and observing the degree of spread of the fingers as the subject bends forward (Fig. 11.4). A more sophisticated application of this technique was first published in the German literature in 1937 by Schober[21] and has recently been modified by Macrae

students or student teachers regularly engaging in sport or athletics.)

Simpler and more suitable methods include:

(a) The 'spondylometer' of Dunham[10] and Goff & Rose.[11] This is essentially a protractor with a long angled extension for measuring 'total' spinal mobility in the sagittal plane.

(b) Another useful instrument is the 'inclinometer' which works on the pendulum principle.[12]

(c) Simpler objective clinical methods requiring no more than a tape measure.[13–18]

Reynolds[19] has done a comparative study of inclinometer and tape measure methods in the measurement of spinal mobility and found the inclinometer to be the most versatile and accurate of the three methods.

Advantages of tape measure methods lie in their inherent simplicity, their low inter- and intra-observer error, and the absence of discomfort or hazard to the patient. A useful offshoot of these methods is that they have been published together with a series of normal values against which the significance of measurements in patients can be assessed.[15]

We shall consider the measurement of thoracolumbar mobility under three heads: (a) sagittal mobility (flexion and extension); (b) lateral flexion; (c) rotation.

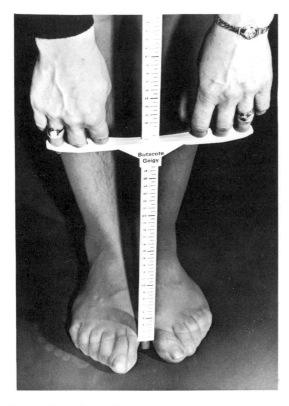

Fig. 11.3 Fingertips-to-floor gauge

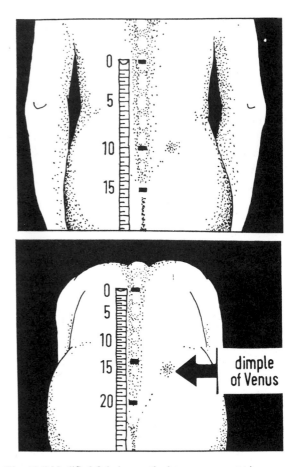

Fig. 11.5 Modified Schober method to measure anterior flexion.[13] (a) Postition 1 to show placing of skin marks; (b) position 2 to show distraction of upper and lower marks on anterior flexion.

& Wright.[13] This is a simple method using a linen or plastic tape measure in which three marks are inked on the skin overlying the lumbosacral spine with the subject standing erect (Fig. 11.5(a)). The first mark is placed at the lumbosacral junction which is represented by the spinal intersection of a line

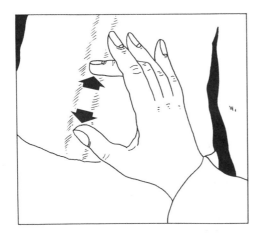

Fig. 11.4 Finger separation test to measure anterior flexion

joining the dimples of Venus. Further marks are inked 5 cm below and 10 cm above the lumbosacral junction. The subject is then asked to touch his or her toes, and the new distance between the upper and lower marks is measured (Fig. 11.5(b)). The *distraction* between these two marks has been found to correlate closely ($r = +0.97$) with anterior flexion measured radiologically. Van Adrichem & van der Korst[18] have reported a similar technique using a steel tape measure to study forward flexion of the spine in children and adolescents. However, in this study both the lower and the upper marks were placed higher up the spine than in our own study. Although the higher placing of the upper mark is doubtless of value because it includes the whole length of the lumbar spine, the higher placing of the lower mark is probably not helpful as the skin is only tethered at the base of the spine, and without tethering of the lower mark the method becomes inaccurate.

Another useful objective clinical method involves the pendulum principle. Asmussen & Heebøll-Nielsen[22] were the first to devise an inclinometric method using this principle. The instrument (Fig. 11.6) allows a numerical value to be ascribed to both posture and movement. This method has been modified by Loebl.[12] Loebl's inclinometer consists of a dial divided into degrees and fixed to two plastic buttons about 9 cm apart. When the buttons are held against the spine, the weighted needle remains vertical and indicates the angle of spinal incline.

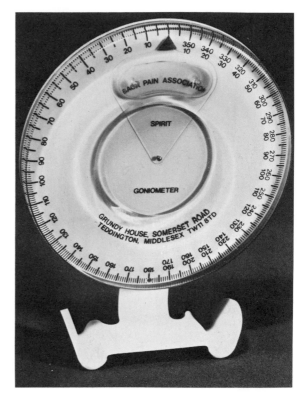

Fig. 11.7 Improved inclinometer of Loebl & Troup[3] (suspension fluid — alcohol in water)

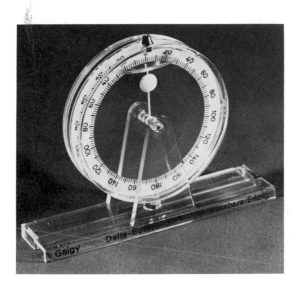

Fig. 11.6 Standard inclinometer (suspension fluid — water)

Loebl & Troup[23] have prepared an improved inclinometer (Fig. 11.7) for commercial production. (The earliest inclinometers were hampered by the use of water as the needle suspension fluid. The damping time of this medium was reduced by using paraffin in Loebl's first inclinometer, and has been further reduced (damping time > 2 s) in Loebl and Troup's commercial production by using alcohol in water as the suspension fluid. However, this can cause the plastic to craze and eventually crack, causing fluid loss. A more versatile design is now available from MIE Medical Research Ltd (Fig. 11.8). Their clinical goniometer is cheap, compact, robust and has the added advantage that is does not

have to be held exactly in a vertical plane, as do pendulum-type goniometers.

Anterior flexion may also be measured by means of the spondylometer (Fig. 11.9). This instrument was first used to measure spinal mobility in the sagittal plane by Dunham in 1949. Since this original report, spondylometry has been used in other centres, and Hart[8] and Sturrock et al[24] have reported their experience with this instrument. The two rubber cushions of the spondylometer protractor are placed over the sacrum and the free end is placed on the vertebra prominens. Readings on the protractor are taken with the patient in the erect and in the fully flexed position. It should be emphasized that the measurement obtained with this instrument does not represent the sum of the angles of movement at each lumbothoracic intervertebral joint. Also, movements at lower intervertebral joints have more effect on the readings than movements at higher levels, so that readings are 'weighted' in favour of the more clinically important movements of the lower spine.

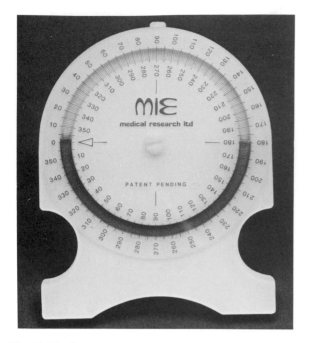

Fig. 11.8 Inclinometer based on the spirit level principle

Thoracolumbar extension

It is only within the last 15 years that objective methods have been developed to measure spinal extension. In the past this movement was assessed subjectively or semi-objectively by asking the patient to bend backwards — the degree of backward bending being gauged by eye or, alternatively, recorded as an angle from an imaginary vertical zero line. Often, measurements of spinal extension were

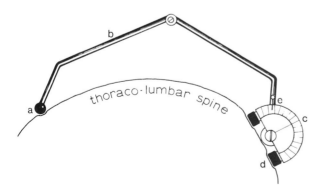

Fig. 11.9 Spondylometer[9] (a) Terminal knob; (b) 'distal' brass rod 40.6 cm long and bend 12.6 cm from the free end through an angle of 35°; (c) protractor; (d) rubber cushion of protractor; (e) pointer attached to 'proximal' brass rod.

incorporated in measurements of total thoracolumbar sagittal mobility. An objective method has been devised by Moll et al.[17] This involves measurement of the distance traversed by a plumb-line pointer held at the side of the trunk (Fig. 11.10). Separate studies using a spinal model have shown that this distance represents a close geometrical function of thoracolumbar extension. The validity of this method has been confirmed by checking the clinical movements against radiological measurements ($r = +0.75$; $p < 0.01$). Satisfactory values have also been obtained in studies to evaluate intra-observer error (coefficient of variation 4.7%), and inter-observer error (the correlation coefficient between measurements taken by two observers (r) was $+0.93$; $p < 0.001$).

However, the method has certain disadvantages, one of which includes the difficulty of making measurements on the lateral trunk in *obese* individuals. Also, difficulties are involved in measuring subjects with hypermobility of the spine. In these subjects, extreme arching of the back causes the plumbline to leave its position against the lateral

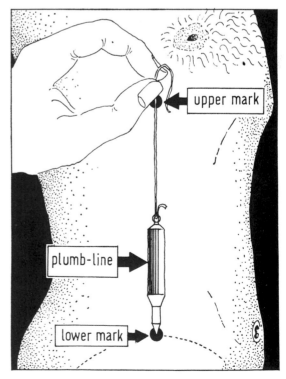

Fig. 11.10 Method of measuring thoracolumbar extension.[17]

trunk. In order to find a more satisfactory method of measuring spinal extension we have recently measured the *attraction* rather than the *distraction* between the landmarks used in measuring anterior flexion by Schober's modified method. The results obtained by this method[25] are reasonably reproducible, but it is not always easy to keep the tape measure close to the skin of the spine while the patient is in a position of extreme extension. In addition to their use in measuring anterior flexion, inclinometry and spondylometry may also be used to measure spinal extension.

Lateral flexion

Traditionally, lateral flexion is assessed by eye by noting how far the fingers can reach down the homolateral thigh. Some observers have introduced objectivity into this method by measuring the distance between the fingers and knee, or between the fingers and floor. Apart from radiographic methods[6,7] and the relatively crude goniometric technique recommended by the American Academy of Orthopaedic Surgeons,[3] until relatively recently there were few other published data on objective methods of measuring this movement. It was with this deficiency in mind that we devised a simple tape measure method to measure spinal movement in this plane.[16] The method involves placing two ink marks on the skin of the lateral trunk with the patient in the 'fundamental' position,[26] as shown in Figure 11.11. The upper mark is placed at a point where a horizontal line through the xiphisternum crosses the coronal line. The lower mark is drawn where a horizontal line through the highest point on the iliac crest crosses the coronal line. The distance between the two marks is measured in centimetres using a tape measure with the patient standing erect, and again after full lateral flexion. The new distance between the two marks is measured and subtracted from the first measurement. The remainder is taken as an index of lateral spinal mobility. In obese subjects, fat folds developing in the lateral trunk sometimes complicate measurement. This source of error may be obviated by measuring the *distraction* of skin marks on the *contralateral* trunk, rather than the *approximation* of marks on the *homolateral* trunk.

Radiological evaluation has shown good correlation between clinical and radiological measurements ($r =$

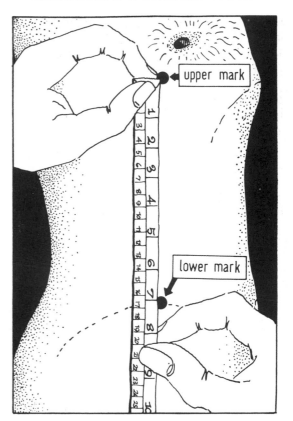

Fig. 11.11 Method of measuring thoracolumbar lateral flexion.[16]

$+0.79$; $p < 0.001$). Evaluation of observer error has also shown the technique to be satisfactory. The coefficient of variation for intra-observer error was 6% to the right and 6.6% to the left. Inter-observer error, represented by the correlation coefficient (r) between measurements taken by two observers, was $+0.68$ ($p < 0.001$). Lateral spinal movement may also be measured using an inclinometer.[12]

Rotation

Few objective clinical studies of thoracolumbar rotation have been done, possibly because of its exclusion as an essential sign in the New York criteria for diagnosing ankylosing spondylitis.[27] Pavelka[14] was one of the first to publish a simple objective clinical method. Marks are made over the spinous process of L5 and over the jugular notch. Using a tape measure, the measurement between these two points is recorded before and after full truncal rotation. The difference between these measurements is taken to represent the degree of rotation. In order to separate lumbar from thoracic movement, the author claimed to be able to measure lumbar rotation separately by estimating the distance between the spinous process of L5 and the xiphisternum before and after truncal rotation. Pavelka made no allowance for the effects of age and sex, although he did recognize the importance of weight and height in modifying these movements.

Franke and his associates[28] have published another study on measurement of spinal rotation, but their data were entirely subjective. So far as we are aware, the only other objective study of spinal rotation is that of Loebl.[29] Using an inclinometer, he measured subjects lying on one side with hips and knees flexed to 90°. The shoulders were rotated to the prone position and the head was rotated further to face in the opposite direction. Maximal passive rotation was achieve to the right and the left. The goniometer was placed on the forehead and on T1, T12 and the sacrum in order to record the surface inclination to the vertical at these points. Regional spinal rotation was calculated from the difference between adjacent inclinations.

MEASURING CERVICAL SPINE MOBILITY

The atlanto-occipital joint allows most of flexion and extension, and the atlanto-axial joint permits rotation. Lateral movement of the neck occurs primarily below the atlas from the mobility of the second to seventh cervical vertebra. Thus the pattern of limitation of neck movement usually indicates the part of the cervical spine involved.[30] Traditionally, cervical spine mobility is assessed subjectively. The patient is asked to tip the head forward for flexion, backward for extension, and for rotation to turn the head to each side as if looking over each shoulder. Lateral mobility is assessed by asking the patient to touch the ear to the shoulder without raising the shoulder girdle.

A useful and simple method to measure cervical spine motion objectively has been reported by Newell[8] and Nichols,[31] who demonstrated how these measurements could be made by placing a conventional patellar hammer on various parts of the head.

Thus, to measure the range of sagittal movement, the base of the hammer is placed on the vertex and the pointed end of the instrument used to indicate the degree of movement. Movement in a lateral plane can also be assessed with the hammer in this position. For assessing the degree of rotation, the hammer is placed with its base on the patient's forehead.

A more complicated method of measuring cervical spine motion has been reported by Soria-Herrera,[32] who used an inclinometer of the type developed by Loebl. When the subject wears the instrument over the ears in the headphones position, the inclinometer needle indicates the degree of movement on full flexion and full extension of the head. To measure rotation, the inclinometer is placed flat on the vertex. To measure lateral flexion, the instrument is placed with its base on the vertex and its dial lying in the coronal plane. It is difficult to assess the accuracy and reproducibility of this technique, as numerical data on these points have not yet been published. It has, of course, the usual disadvantage of involving special and possibly expensive instrumentation. So far as accuracy is concerned, it is probably not significantly better than the much simpler patellar hammer technique of Newell & Nichols.[31]

In Leeds, Murray-Leslie[33] investigated this method further. The accuracy of the technique was improved by using a large protractor and a spirit level, but he was unable to achieve satisfactory inter- and intra-observer concordance. Calcraft and his co-workers[34] used a similar method to measure cervical spine rotation in a study of patients with ankylosing spondylitis.

Another method studied by Murray-Leslie employed a rig with a pointer attached to a head clamp which rotated on fixed bearings and to which was attached a circular scale marked in degrees. An attempt was made to prevent trunk and shoulder movements by asking the subject to clasp her hands behind her chair. With unversity academic and technical staff, reproducibility of the method was satisfactory, but in patients reproducibility was poor. This was in part due to the patients' inability to limit neck movement to pure rotation.

Murray-Leslie also measured, chin-to-suprasternal notch and vertebra prominens-to-occipital protuberance distances to study sagittal motion of the cervical spine. He found some correlation between clinical and radiological measurements, but concluded that the method was not accurate enough.

MEASURING COSTOVERTEBRAL MOTION

Chest expansion may be regarded as a composite movement due to mobility at the costovertebral joints. Rigidity of the thoracic cage is a characteristic feature of ankylosing spondylitis, and has been recognized as a classical feature of this disease since the celebrated description by Bernard Connor in 1691.[35] It is because of the inseparability between chest and spinal involvement in this important rheumatic disorder that chest expansion has been included in this chapter. The generally accepted importance of this sign is evidenced by its inclusion, together with limitation of back movement, by two international symposia as a major criterion for the diagnosis of ankylosing spondylitis.[27,36] Considering the significance of chest expansion as a measure of disease not only in ankylosing spondylitis but also in chest disorders, it is surprising that so little objective work has been done in this area. Traditional methods to assess chest expansion have involved either an assessment of thoracic cage movement by eye, or, semi-objectively, by measuring the degree of separation of the thumbs with the hands placed around the front or the back of the chest.

We have undertaken an objective clinical study of chest expansion, and have used both a tape measure and a modified caliper to measure chest movement.[37] Circumferential mobility was assessed by means of a conventional tape measure at the level of the fourth intercostal space as recommended by the New York symposium.[27] Measurements were taken at the height of maximal inspiration and expiration, and considerable care was taken not to pull the tape too tightly while taking measurements. As subjects vary immensely in their interpretation of the meaning of deep breathing, observations were always preceded by detailed instructions, and, more importantly, by a personal demonstration of what was required. We ensured that measurements were made on subjects standing with *hands on head* and arms flexed in the frontal plane. The advantages of this arm-elevated posture are as follows:

1. Maximal contraction of the main shoulder adductors is prevented, thus obviating a frequent tendency, often observed in young males, to exaggerate expansion by strong voluntary contraction of these muscles, particularly the latissimus dorsi.
2. The scapula and breast are lifted clear of the line of measurement.
3. The field of measurement is more readily observed.
4. Application of the tape measure is considerably easier in this position. A later study[38] at Leeds clearly revealed that female modesty may inhibit chest expansion. It is possible therefore that chest movements in females may be improved by examining patients fully clad: unless thick woollen clothes are worn, clothing should not significantly affect measurement.

Earlier studies of chest expansion had the disadvantage that they involved highly selected populations so far as age and sex distributions were concerned. Such populations have included schoolboys,[39] male and female physical education students,[40] and male medical students.[41] Furthermore, the surface markings used to identify the level of measurement have varied in these and other reports from nipple level[42,43] to the level of the fourth intercostal space,[27,40] and frequently no specific level of measurement was reported.[39,41,44] Broadly speaking, however, numerical data on both circumferential[39,40,42–44] and diametric expansion[40,41] compare reasonably well with the results obtained from the Leeds study.[37]

NORMAL RANGES OF MOBILITY

Spinal mobility

In view of the difficulty in assessing whether individual spinal movements are normal or not, we have delineated normal ranges for several types of spinal movement.[15] This we did on a control population using the objective clinical techniques already described. A normal range of values for spinal movements in anterior flexion, extension and lateral flexion was established. In view of the absence of spinal rotation from international criteria for ankylosing spondylitis we did not study this plane of mobility. Figure 11.12 provides a diagrammatic summary of normal values for each of these directions of spinal movement. The following important features emerged:

1. An initial increase in mean spinal mobility from the 15–24 decade to the 25–34 decade was followed by a *progressive decrease with advancing age*. We calculated that age alone may reduce spinal mobility by as much as 50%.
2. The scatter (mean ± 2 S.D.) of spinal mobility varied between decades, but in each group it was considerable. The wide range of normal mobility was observed in flexion, extension and lateral flexion.
3. A sex difference was observed at each decade in all three planes of movement. In anterior flexion and extension, male mobility exceeded female mobility, whereas in lateral flexion the converse was observed. The predominance of female over male lateral flexion in this study has been supported by a study of spinal mobility in adolescents.[45] Spinal mobility differed by 7–11% between the sexes, and this we found to be statistically significant.

Other workers have found different patterns of spinal mobility between the sexes. Isdale[46] found all spinal movements to be greater in the female. A different pattern was obtained by Sturrock et al,[24] who found female anterior flexion to exceed that in males, although male extension was greater than female extension. The discrepancy between these results has yet to be explained. The striking decrease in spinal mobility with advancing age has both diagnostic and prognostic significance. Although the majority of patients with ankylosing spondylitis present before the age of 30 years, a number experience their first symptom in middle age, or even later.[47] It is important therefore, when considering this disease in the elderly, to allow for the effect of age in order to avoid false positive diagnosis. Prognostically, if the progressive diminution of mobility with increasing age is not considered, the effect due to this in a spondylitic subject may be ascribed to the progress of the disease rather than to the progress of nature.

Another age-dependent feature of diagnostic significance is the delay in peak spinal mobility until the decade following that in which spondylitis most frequently presents, i.e. between the age of 15 and 24 years.[48] As non-spondylitic back pain and radiological changes mimicking sacroiliitis[49] are relatively common at this decade, awareness of this phenomenon is clearly important in order to avoid diagnostic error.

Normal values for thoracolumbar rotation have yet to be delineated. Loebl,[29] however, has reported

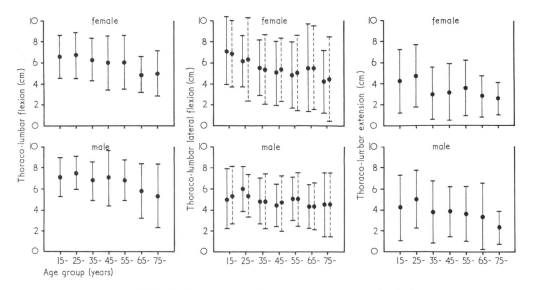

Fig. 11.12 Normal range (mean ± 2 S.D.) of spinal movement.[15] (a) Thoracolumbar anterior flexion; (b) thoracolumbar lateral flexion; (c) thoracolumbar extension

mean figures: 67° in the thoracic spine and 25° in the lumbar spine. These correlate well with traditional figures quoted in textbooks of orthopaedics. For example, Beetham and his associates[30] in their book on physical examination of joints quote figures of 90° of rotation to either side for the 'trunk' and 30° to either side for the 'lower thoracic and lumbar segments'.

The Manchester group,[50] using a spirit inclinometer, have done careful measurements of neck movement and subjected them to rigorous statistical analysis. There was a strong relationship between age and range of movement. More recently Jayson and his colleagues[51] have described instrumentation for the analysis of continuous neck rotation.

Usual textbook *mean* figures for cervical spine movement are as follows: anterior flexion 45°; extention 50–60°; rotation 60–80°; lateral flexion 40°. Clearly, *mean* figures as opposed to a *range* of figures are of very limited value in diagnosis.[50]

Chest expansion

We have reported numerical data (Fig. 11.13) for normal chest expansion obtained using both a traditional tape measure and also a specially adapted caliper.[37] Measurements gained using both techniques have shown patterns similar to those found in the spinal mobility study with respect to the effects of age, sex and scatter. In other words, chest expansion decreases with age, is greater in males and shows a considerable scatter of normal values (mean ± 2 S.D.). The most important observation stemming from this study concerns the way in which the normal scatter of circumferential expansion measurements in both sexes extends well below the 2.5 cm normal/abnormal borderline stipulated by the New York symposium. The danger of false positive diagnosis of ankylosing spondylitis which may arise from using such an arbitrary borderline is self-evident.

DISORDERS WITH LIMITED SPINAL MOBILITY

The principal disorders that may be confused with radiologically borderline or atypical cases of ankylosing spondylitis are shown in Table 11.1. These disorders have in common: (a) spinal pain; (b) restricted chest and/or spinal mobility; and (c) defects of posture.

Ankylosing hyperostosis

Ankylosing hyperostosis is usually clinically distinguishable in view of the following characteristics:

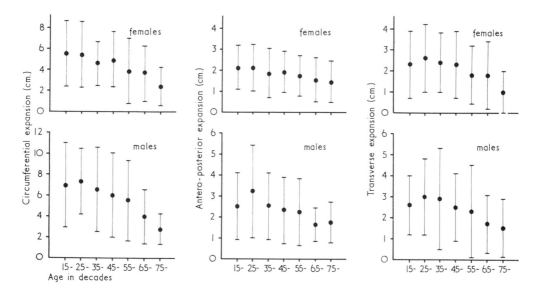

Fig. 11.13 Normal range (mean ± 2 S.D.) of chest expansion.[37] (a) Circumferential expansion; (b) anteroposterior expansion; (c) transverse expansion.

Table 11.1 Disorders clinically resembling ankylosing spondylitis.

Disease	Spinal pain	Reduction of chest expansion	Reduction of spinal mobility			Posture	
			Anterior flexion	Lateral flexion	Extension tension	Thoracic kyphosis	Lumbar flattening
Ankylosing spondylitis	++	++	++	++	++	++	++
Ankylosing hyperostosis	+	0	+	+	+	+	+
Prolapsed lumbar disc	++	0	++	0	++	0	++
Senile osteoporosis	++	0	++	++	++	++	+

0 = absent.
+ = slight.
++ = moderate-severe.

mild pain, normal chest expansion, slight limitation of spinal mobility (apophyseal joints not involved) and slight change of posture.[52]

Prolapsed lumbar disc

Patients with a prolapsed lumbar disc have normal chest expansion (unless concomitant emphysema or other chest disease is present) and normal lateral flexion, in contrast to sagittal mobility which is often severely limited, particularly in the acute phase.[53,54]

Senile osteoporosis

In senile osteoporosis, chest expansion has been reported to be limited.[55] However, in our experience, even in severe cases, this is not so if measurements are corrected for age and sex. Spinal mobility, including lateral flexion,[56,57] may be restricted, but in early cases this is usually to avoid pain rather than due to any real loss of joint movement.

Ankylosing spondylitis

We have undertaken an objective study of movement of the spine and chest in 106 patients with ankylosing spondylitis.[58] Traditional subjective observations that chest and spinal mobility are limited in ankylosing spondylitis were confirmed objectively after correcting the data for age and sex. No difference in the pattern of chest and spinal mobility was noted between patients with uncomplicated spondylitis and those with spondylitis associated with psoriasis, ulcerative colitis, Crohn's disease, and Reiter's disease. On a clinical basis, four patterns of spondylitis were delineated: (1) patients who were

pain-free and had normal chest and spinal mobility (8.6%); (2) patients with painful but normal mobility (14.1%); (3) patients with painful and restricted mobility (66.3%); and (4) patients who were relatively pain-free, but who had completely limited mobility (10.8%). An important observation arising from this survey concerns the marked scatter of spondylitic chest and spinal mobility, and the extensive overlap of these measurements into the normal range. The degree of overlap between normal and spondylitic measurements inevitably increases the yield of false negative results, and therefore weakens the value of these clinical attributes as accurate diagnostic indices of the disease. It is likely that a more realistic diagnostic approach for the future will involve using a *range of abnormality* rather than a range of normality in order to assess the significance of clinical measurements.

DISORDERS WITH SPINAL HYPERMOBILITY

Spinal hypermobility is a manifestation of the hypermobility syndrome, which is inherited as an autosomal dominant.[59] Other disorders associated with hypermobility include Marfan's syndrome, Ehlers-Danlos syndrome, osteogenesis imperfecta, Bonnevie-Ullrich-Turner syndrome (a variant of Turner's syndrome), homocystinuria, Achard syndrome and hyperlysinaemia.

MEASUREMENTS AS DIAGNOSTIC AIDS

At Leeds we have examined 412 subjects (38 with sacroiliitis and 374 controls) to study the value of clinical criteria (pain, limitation of spinal movement and limitation of chest expansion) for ankylosing spondylitis.[60] This was done on the principle that it is not sufficient that criteria be universally agreed, but, more importantly, that they should also be critically and objectively tested. In this investigation the New York clinical criteria for ankylosing spondylitis were studied. Sacroiliitis was assumed to represent the criterion of 'diagnostic truth', as has been adopted in other studies.[61] Particular care was taken in the radiological assessment of sacroiliac joint abnormality, which was made independently by two observers, as we have recommended previously.[62]

Surprisingly, virtually the same evaluation resulted from objective and subjective methodology. This suggests that objective methodology in a diagnostic context is not of such central importance in contributing value to these criteria as was previously thought. Moreover, the comparability between subjective and objective results was consistent with the general observation that an experienced clinician often seems to arrive intuitively at the correct diagnosis, rather in the manner that a familiar face or place is recognized. As yet, however, the actual subjective processes involved in making such decisions are still unknown.[63]

However, despite our inability to demonstrate any clear advantage of objectivity over subjectivity, the considerable value of making objective measurements in clinical rheumatology remains undisputed. The value of objectivity depends not only on the obvious direct advantage based on increased accuracy of the assessment, but also on the indirect advantage of enabling individual correction to be made for age and sex. It was on account of the latter property that we were able to demonstrate the importance of allowing for the effect of age and sex. The value of objectivity is also relevant in therapeutic assessment. Moreover, it may give valuable information concerning the rate of progress, and perhaps also the ultimate prognosis of the disease.

So far as diagnosis is concerned, the following points emerged from our investigation: calculated in terms of frequency of *positive tests, false negative tests, sensitivity*, and the *Youden index* (sensitivity + specificity — 100), criteria were listed in the following order of value: (1) thoracolumbar pain, (2) limited chest expansion, (3) limited back movement. However, in terms of *false positive tests* and

specificity, the reverse order was obtained. It was concluded that individual criteria in their present form failed to provide a satisfactory diagnostic index of ankylosing spondylitis. Thoracolumbar pain is too sensitive and too non-specific, and limited chest and spinal mobility are too insensitive and too specific. In order to obviate this problem it was suggested that the principle of criterion weighting should be adopted, as has been done in other diseases such as thyrotoxicosis.[64]

RECENT EXPERIMENTAL WORK

Kulak and co-workers[65] use the term 'vertebral motion segments'. A motion segment consists of an intervertebral disc, its two adjacent vertebrae and all intervening ligamentous tissues including the facet joints. The total spine can be thought of as a collection of motion segments.

Vertebral motion segments are often capable of reasonably large amounts of motion. Lumbar segments can extend about 20° and can bend laterally about 8°.[66] Farfan et al[67] showed that cadaver motion segments are capable of some 23° of twist in a horizontal plane.

Schultz and his associates,[68] using mathematically modelled motion segments, have shown that even if all deformable elements of a motion segment are assumed to exhibit linear elastic behaviour, changes in geometry that occur when rotations are of the order of 10° produce significant non-linearity of overall response. These geometrical non-linearities often caused model motion segment stiffness to increase by about 50%. These studies also showed that the various ligaments contribute significantly to the rotational stiffness.

Pope and co-workers[69] have developed equipment to study spinal motion of cadavers and live subjects using biplanar radiography. A principal finding was that the lumbar spine exhibits 'coupled motion'. In other words, motion in one direction is dependent on that in another direction. For example, axial rotation is uniformly associated with lateral bending. This work confirms similar observations by Panjabi & White.[70] Another interesting observation of Pope et al concerned the hysteretic behaviour of spinal motion in the cadaver. Movements of spines, transfixed with rods and moved at a rate of 2.5° per second from a neutral starting position to extension and back through flexion, described a hysteresis curve with its centre almost overlying the intersection of the torque vertical axis and the flexion-extension horizontal axis.

In a more recent study Panjabi[71] re-emphasized the complexity of the motion segment in that its mechanical behaviour is a function of ligaments, the disc, the facet joints and the applied load. From studies on cadavers the following conclusions were made:

1. The mechancial behaviour of the spinal motion segment can be expressed by the application of 12 different physiological loads (6 forces and 6 moments (Fig. 11.14)) to the upper vertebrae and measuring the resulting 6 components of three-dimensional motion (3 translations in millimetres + 3 angulations).
2. Each physiological load produces 1 main motion and 5 coupled subsidiary motions.
3. As many as 72 separate load displacement curves are necessary to describe completely the elastic behaviour of a single motion segment.

A further study, by Panjabi & White,[72] used 'pre-loads' of 0, 400 and 1000 newtons as well as 12 physiological loads (Fig. 11.15). The nature of the physiological loads is shown in Figures 11.14 and

11.15. The results of these experiments revealed the following:

1. The spine becomes more flexible in the presence of increasing pre-loads plus physiological forces directed *laterally* or *anteriorly*.
2. The spine becomes less flexible in the presence of increasing pre-loads plus physiological forces producing *axial tension* or *axial torsion*.
3. No appreciable change in flexibility was observed with increasing pre-loads when physiological forces were *axial compression*, a *posteriorly directed* force or an *extension moment*.

RECENT CLINICAL ADVANCES AND POTENTIALS

This section is intended to represent an update in the field of spinal measurement since the last edition of this book. In general, advances have been minimal

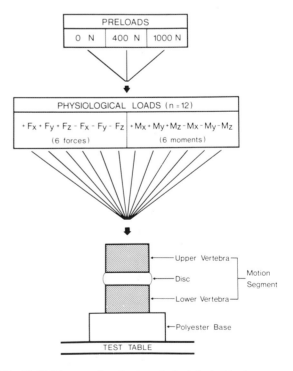

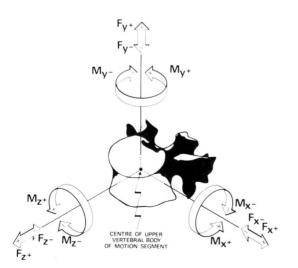

Fig. 11.14 Diagram of forces and moments applied to an experimental spinal motion segment (modified from Panjabi[71]). F = forces (6); M = moments (6).

Fig. 11.15 Diagram of preloads and physiological loads applied to an experimental spinal motion segment (modified from Panjabi[72]).

over the last five years or so, but a number of recent developments deserve mention:

Increased sophistication of existing methods

Flexirule/hydrogoniometry

Previous methods employing the Schober principle and the inclinometer have been combined by Anderson & Sweetman[73] who have studied back movements using a 'flexirule/hydrogoniometer'. With this instrument (Fig. 11.16) the point of anchorage is at the level of the dimples of Venus. The lower inclinometer is placed 5 cm below the anchorage point and measures hip flexion. This measurement is deducted from that recorded by the upper inclinometer (placed 15 cm above the anchorage point) to provide the net movement of the lumbar spine. The flexirule is semi-stiff and only moves in the A–P axis. This allows it to mould into the lordotic profile of the lumbar spine. (Indeed, it has been used by Sweetman to provide a trace of lumbar lordosis in a separate study.)

The flexirule/hydrogoniometer can also be used for measuring lateral flexion using the iliac crest as the reference point. It has at least a theoretical advantage over the tape-measure method[16] in that the measuring device can follow the bulging contours in obese patients.

A further development of hydrogoniometry is the clinical goniometer (Fig. 11.8) by MIE Medical Research Ltd. This device is based on the spirit level principle, thus obviating many of the problems inherent in the pendulum type goniometer.

Cinematography

Mention has already been made of the use of serial photography as a means of providing a permanent record of lateral spinal movement in terms of difference between the resting position and the position at the extreme of movement.[8] Davis, cited by Anderson,[74] has developed this idea by using cinematography either with or without superimposition on a grid. If a grid is used, a pointer can be attached to the dorsal spine and a photographic record made of a subject undertaking a specific task. As with still photography, this method is more applicable to 'laboratory' usage than to clinical practice.

New methods

Long-term electrical recording devices

Various systems have been developed to enable measurements of spinal posture and movement during the act of working. For example, Sweetman et al[75] have used a portable miniature analogue tape recorder with non-invasive monitoring inputs.

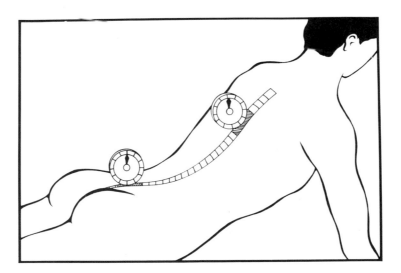

Fig. 11.16 Essential features of, and landmarks used in, flexirule hydrogoniometry (after Anderson & Sweetman[73])

EMG electrodes are placed over the muscles on each side of the lower back, 5 cm below the vertebra prominens (Fig. 11.17). This is damped electronically to act as an inclinometer to record sagittal movement of the upper back. The posture recorded by this device does not distinguish back movement from hip gait movement, but a subsequent development by Kiernan,[76] using more than one electronic inclinometer, provides a more accurate profile of thoracolumbar sagittal motion, as well as simultaneous recording. A further modification by Jackson, cited by Anderson,[74] involved the use of a transducer system designed to record three-dimensional magnetic fields by sensor coils. The magnetic fields are produced in three planes by solenoids (with currents flowing at a frequency on 1 MHz). Continuous recording is made by remote control.

A new 8-channel telemetry system has now been developed that can be of much greater value to back movement research. This system from MIE Medical Research Ltd will allow any combination of EMGs inclinometers, goniometers, or any other trans-ducers to be monitored. The advantages are considerable, especially if real-time computer analysis is required. As the 8-channel system transmits the data by a miniature radiotelemetry device, the subject is free of trailing wires and is therefore able to move freely.

Another device from this company is a computerized gait analysis system. The equipment is designed primarily for clinical use, when objective data on gait patterns are required. The system is based on their radiotelemetry system, with the incorporation of a computer for easy analysis of the data. Patients can have electrogoniometers attached to measure spinal movement, and analysis can be done in 15 minutes. This can monitor the progress of disease and the response to treatment in patients such as those with ankylosing spondylitis and other back disorders.

Potential methods

Williams[77-79] has recently developed a light-sectioning monophotogrammatic method which could be applied to measuring spinal movement in any plane. The method consists of measuring subjects in three dimensions by means of contouring the object optically by a series of light slits of equal size and frequency. The contour plot (Fig. 11.18) is recorded

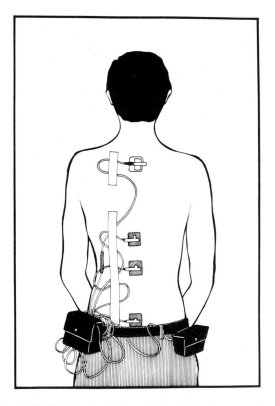

Fig. 11.17 Multiple electrical recording device for measuring spinal posture and movement (after Kiernan[76])

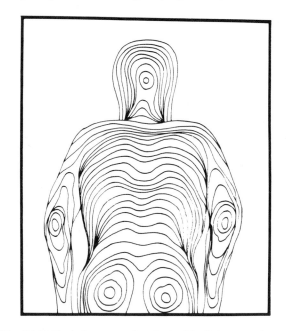

Fig. 11.18 Typical contour plot obtained by light-scattering monophotogrammetry that could be used to measure spinal motion (Williams[79])

photgraphically at 90° to the projection axis. Williams has developed a double-sided system for medical application that is free from geometrical distortion caused by the conical shape of the projection and recording beams. The advantages of such a system are that it is non-contact, instantaneous, simple and relatively inexpensive to operate. Furthermore, it requires only a minimum of special equipment and technique.

So far, the technique has been used clinically largely for volume studies (e.g. measurement of leg oedema, the pregnant abdomen, facial contours in jaw sarcomata, degree of glaucomatous cupping of the fundus). In the field of rheumatology/orthopaedics it has been used to assess spinal deformity. This approach could be extended by 'before-and-after' motion mapping, and any such studies will be awaited with interest.

SUMMARY, CONCLUSIONS AND FUTURE PROSPECTS

This chapter has examined clinical and research techniques to measure spinal movement on a vertebral-segment basis, as well as in different planes of movement.

Accuracy of measurement is not sufficient in itself, and stress has been placed on the importance of knowing normal and disease ranges against which individual measurements can realistically be interpreted. Factors such as age and sex (and race) differences can result in significant variations in normal subjects, and these have to be taken into account when assessing variations due to spinal diseases and other disorders affecting vertebral dynamics. The armamentarium of the 'spinal metrologist' continues to widen, and methods (not necessarily evaluated) so far include: traditional assessment by eye and hand, and various devices incorporating principles of geometry, goniometry, photography, radiography, electronics, electromagnetics and monophotogrammetry.

The choice of methodology must include a consideration of clinical *versus* research usage, as well as the individual balance between advantages and disadvantages. The latter consideration includes: facility and speed of usage, economy and,

not least, the potentially harmful effects (psychological as well as physical) of intrusive techniques. In this regard, mention can be made of a recent study to compare clinical and radiological techniques.[80] It was concluded that the clinical techniques were liable to large errors and that the radiological techniques (biplanar radiography, superimposition of radiographs, vector stereography) gave indices that more truly reflected intervertebral movement. Despite the fact that these criticisms of the clinical techniques were not convincingly supported by a review of the correlation data,[81] the point should be reiterated that 'accuracy' and exact biological representation in measurement, although perhaps of interest in the laboratory, are not always preferable in a clinical context.

For simple routine clinical usage, assessment by eye and hand (e.g. finger separation test) continues to have its merits, although many clinicians are now using more objective methods — particularly the inclinometer (hydrogoniometer), now the standard spinal measuring device used by the Society for Back Pain Research.

In this age of the microchip and the development of sophisticated 'peripheral' electronic devices, we are probably not far from simple, inexpensive extensions of the microcomputer industry to measure musculoskeletal movement. For example, in the future it should be possible to record from patients with disorders of spinal mobility a static or motion print-out (numerical and graphic) of their vertebral movement profile (Fig. 11.19). Such print-outs (which might be termed 'spondylographs') could be taken, read and stored in a comparable way to the present-day ECG, EMG or EEG.

ACKNOWLEDGEMENTS

We thank the Editor of the *Annals of the Rheumatic Diseases* for permission to publish Figs 11.5 and 11.9–11.13 and the Editor of *Rheumatology and Rehabilitation* for permission to publish Table 11.1. We also thank Mrs Edna Dawson, Mrs Pat Drake and Mrs Pat Large for their help in the preparation of this manuscript.

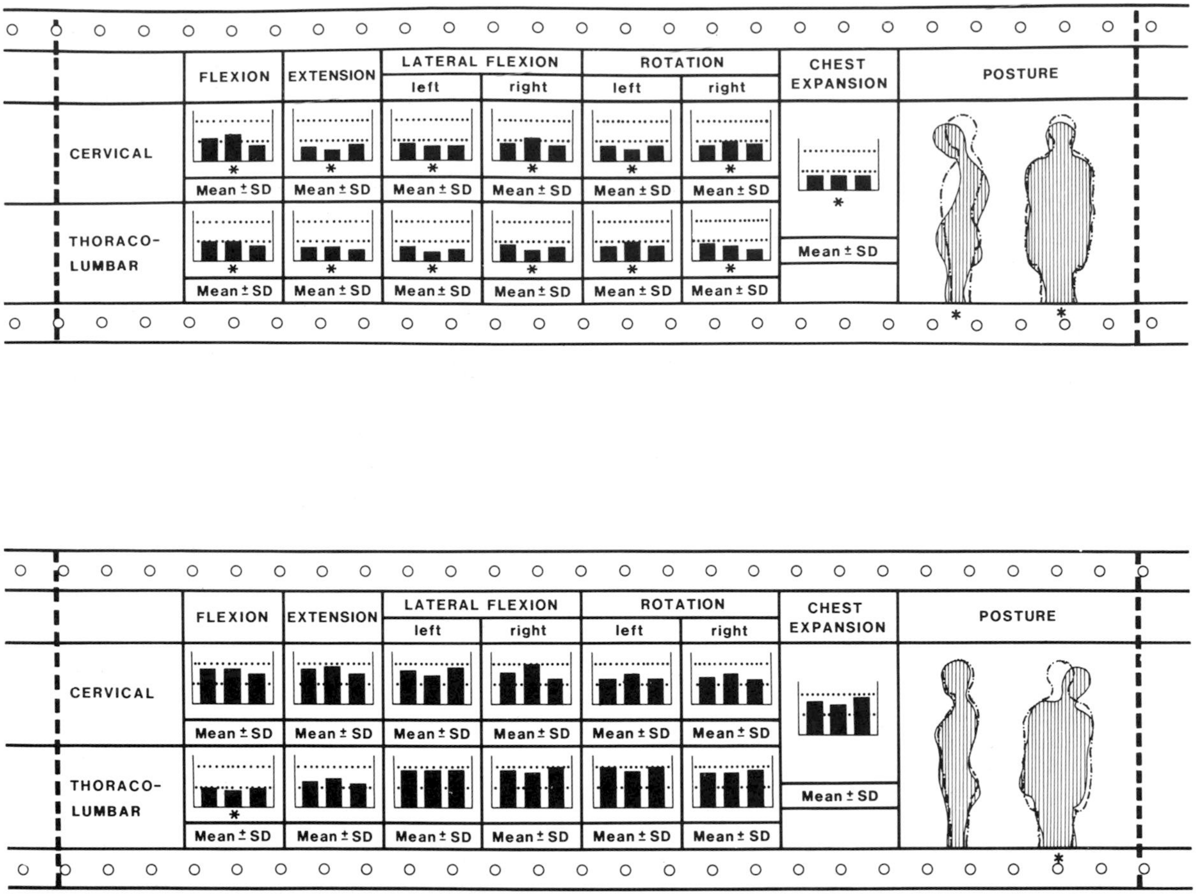

	FLEXION	EXTENSION	LATERAL FLEXION		ROTATION		CHEST EXPANSION	POSTURE
			left	right	left	right		
CERVICAL	Mean ± SD	Mean ± SD	Mean ± SD	Mean ± SD	Mean ± SD	Mean ± SD	Mean ± SD	
THORACO-LUMBAR	Mean ± SD	Mean ± SD	Mean ± SD	Mean ± SD	Mean ± SD	Mean ± SD	Mean ± SD	

	FLEXION	EXTENSION	LATERAL FLEXION		ROTATION		CHEST EXPANSION	POSTURE
			left	right	left	right		
CERVICAL	Mean ± SD	Mean ± SD	Mean ± SD	Mean ± SD	Mean ± SD	Mean ± SD	Mean ± SD	
THORACO-LUMBAR	Mean ± SD	Mean ± SD	Mean ± SD	Mean ± SD	Mean ± SD	Mean ± SD	Mean ± SD	

Fig. 11.19 'Spondylographic' recordings in two contrasting disorders: a proposal for future measurement and documentation of vertebral motion profiles employing microchip technology.
Top: Advanced ankylosing spondylitis — note the limitation of all spinal movements (cervical and thoracolumbar in all directions) and chest expansion; stooped posture. *Bottom*: Lumbar disc protrusion — note the limitation largely confined to forward thoracolumbar flexion; scoliotic posture.

REFERENCES

1 Rab G T, Chao E Y S, Stauffer R N 1977 Muscle force analysis of the lumbar spine. Orth. Clin. N. Am. 8: 193
2 Cave E F, Roberts S M 1936 A method of measuring and recording joint function. J. Bone Jt Surg. 18(2): 455
3 American Academcy of Orthopaedic Surgeons 1966 Joint motion: method of measuring and recording. Livingstone, Edinburgh, p 50
4 Scott B O 1965 A universal goniometer. Ann. Phys. Med. 8: 138
5 Wiles P 1935 Movements of the lumbar vertebrae during flexion and extension. Proc. Roy. Soc. Med. 26: 647
6 Tanz S S 1953 Motion of the lumbar spine: a roentgenological study. Amer. J. Roentgenol. 69: 399
7 Jonck L M, van Niekerk J M 1961 A roentgenological study of the motion of the lumbar spine of the Bantu. S. Afr. J. Lab. Clin. Med. 7: 67
8 Hart F D 1956 Measurement of thoracic and spinal movement in ankylosing spondylitis. In: Goslings J, van Swaay H (eds) Contemporary rheumatology. Elsevier, Amsterdam , p 562
9 Troup J D G, Hood C A, Chapman A E 1968 Measurements of the sagittal mobility of the lumbar spine and hips. Ann. Phys. Med. 9: 308
10 Dunham W F 1949 Ankylosing spondylitis: measurement of hip and spinal movements. Brit. J. Phys. Med. 12: 126
11 Goff B, Rose G K 1964 The use of a modified spondylometer in the treatment of ankylosing spondylitis. Rheumatism 20: 63
12 Loebl W Y 1967 Measurements of spinal posture and range of spinal movement. Ann. Phys. Med. 9: 103
13 Macrae I F, Wright V 1969 Measurement of back movement. Ann. Rheum. Dis. 28: 584
14 von Pavelka K 1970 Rotationsmessung der Wirbelsäule. Z. Rheumaforschg. 29: 366
15 Moll J M H, Wright V 1971 Normal range of spinal mobility: an objective clinical study. Ann. Rheum. Dis. 30: 381
16 Moll J M H, Liyanage S P, Wright V 1972 An objective

clinical method to measure lateral spinal flexion. Rheum. Phys. Med. 11: 255

17 Moll J M H, Liyanage S P, Wright V 1972 An objective clinical method to measure spinal extension. Rheum. Phys. Med. 11: 293

18 van Adrichem J A M, van der Korst J K 1973 Assessment of the flexibility of the lumbar spine. A pilot study in children and adolescents. Scand. J. Rheumatol. 2: 87

19 Reynolds P M G 1975 Measurement of spinal mobility — a comparison of three methods. Scand. J. Rheum. 4(Suppl. 8), (Abstract 20): 16

20 Howes R G, Isdale I C 1971 The loose back: an unrecognised syndrome. Rheum. Phys. Med. 11: 72

21 Schober P 1937 Lendenwirbelsäule und Kreuzschmerzen (The lumbar vertebral column and backache). Münch. Med. Wschr. 84: 336

22 Asmussen E, Heebøll-Nielsen K 1959 Posture, mobility and strength of the back in boys, 7 to 16 years old. Acta Orthop. Scand. 28: 174

23 Loebl W Y, Troup J D G 1974, personal communication

24 Sturrock R D, Wojtulewski J A, Hart F D 1973 Spondylometry in a normal population and in ankylosing spondylitis. Rheumatol. Rehab. 12: 135

25 Moll J M H, Wright V 1974 unpublished data

26 Wells K F 1950 Kinesiology. Saunders, Philadelphia, p 7

27 Bennett P H, Wood P H N (ed) 1968 Population studies of the rheumatic diseases. Proc. Third Intern. Symp., New York, 1966. Intern. Cong. Ser., Series 148. Excerpta Medica Foundation, Amsterdam, p 4–6

28 von Franke J, Wanka C, Salevski H, Runge R 1972 Die Rotationseinschränkung des Rumpfes — ein einfaches klinisches Frühzeichen der Spondylarthritis ankylopoetica (Strumpell-Bechterew-Marie). Dtsch. Gesundh.-Wes. 27: 1326

29 Loebl W Y 1973 Regional rotation of the spine. Rheumatol. Rehab. 12: 223

30 Beetham W P, Polley H F, Slocumb C H, Weaver W F 1966 Physical examination of the Joints. Saunders, Philadelphia, p 98

31 Newell D J, Nichols P J R 1965 The accuracy of estimating neck movements. Ann. Phys. Med. 8: 120

32 Soria-Herrera C 1973 A simple apparatus for measurement of neck movement. Paper presented to a Comb. Prov. Meet. Brit. Assoc. Rheum. and Rehabil. and Roy. Soc. Med. — Phys. Med. Sec., University Hospital of Wales, Cardiff

33 Moll J M H, Wright V 1976 Measurement of joint motion. Clincis in Rheumatic Diseases: Diagnosis and Assessment 2.1: 3–26

34 Calcraft B, Tildesley G, Evans K T, Gravelle H, Hole D, Lloyd K N 1974 Azapropazone in the treatment of ankylosing spondylitis: a controlled clinical trial. Rheum. Rehab. 13: 23

35 Hartung E F 1954 Bett W R (ed) The history and conquest of common diseases. University of Oklahoma Press, Norman, p 133

36 Kellgren J H, Jeffrey M R, Ball J 1963 The epidemiology of chronic rheumatism, vol 1. Blackwell, Oxford, p 326

37 Moll J M H, Wright V 1972 An objective clinical study of chest expansion. Ann. Rheum. Dis. 31: 1

38 Archer I A, Moll J M H, Wright V 1974 Chest and spinal mobility in physiotherapists: an objective clinical study. Physiotherapy 60: 37

39 Wood A G 1970 Rugger team analysed. Brit. J. Phys. Educ. 1: 70

40 Bradbury I, Brooke J D, Maclock M 1969 A comparison of the Rees-Eysenck index of male body shape in males and females. Phys. Educ. 61: 64

41 Malone F F 1904 Relation of chest contour to lung capacity. J. Amer. Med. Ass. 43: 783

42 Hart F D, Maclagan N F 1953 Ankylosing spondylitis: a review of 184 cases. Ann. Rheum. Dis. 14: 77

43 Hunter D, Bomford R R 1963 Hutchinson's clinical methods, 14th edn. Cassell, London, p 186

44 Durrigl T, Mezulic L, Androic S, Vitaus M 1965 Ankylosing spondylitis — clinical examination. Rheumatism 21: 79

45 Moran H M, Hall M A, Barr A, Ansell B M 1978 Personal communication

46 Isdale I C 1973 Personal communication

47 Sharp J 1965 Ankylosing spondylitis. In: Dixon A St J (ed) Progress in clinical rheumatology. Churchill, London, p 189

48 Mason R M 1969 Ankylosing spondylitis. In: Copeman W S C (ed) Textbook of the rheumatic diseases, 4th edn. Livingstone, Edinburgh, p 347

49 Rogers M H, Cleaves E N 1935 The adolescent sacro-iliac joint syndrome. J. Bone Jt Surg. 17: 759

50 O'Driscoll S L, Tomlinson J 1982 The cervical spine. In: Wright V (ed) Clinics in rheumatic diseases: measurement of joint movement. Saunders, London, p 617

51 Rankin I R, Murphy C, Jones B E, Jayson M I V 1983 Instrumentation for continuous analysis of cervical rotation. Eng. Med. 12: 91

52 Forestier J, Lagier R 1971 Ankylosing hyperostosis of the spine. Clin. Orthop. 74: 65

53 Armstrong J R 1965 Lumbar disc lesions. Livingstone, Edinburgh, p 98

54 de Palma A F, Rothman R H 1970 The intervertebral disc. Saunders, Philadelphia, p 210

55 Dent C E, Watson L 1966 Osteoporosis. Postgrad. Med. J. 42: 583

56 Cyriax J 1969 Textbook of orthpaedic medicine. 1. Diagnosis of soft tissue lesions, 5th edn. Baillière Tindall, London, p 447

57 Jesserer H, Kirchnayr W 1961 Presenile and senile osteoporosis: clinical aspects, pathogenesis, diagnosis and treatment. Acta Rheum. 8: 14

58 Moll J M H, Wright V 1973 The pattern of chest and spinal mobility in ankylosing spondylitis. Rheumatol. Rehab. 12: 115

59 Beighton P, Grahame R, Bird H A 1983 Hypermobility of joints. Springer Verlag, Berlin, pp 43–60

60 Moll J M H, Wright V 1973 New York clinical criteria for ankylosing spondylitis: a statistical evaluation. Ann. Rheum. Dis. 32: 354

61 Bennett P H, Burch T A 1968 Bennett P H, Wood P H N (eds) Population studies of the rheumatic diseases. Excerpta Medica Foundation, Amsterdam, Int. Congr. Ser. No. 148, p 305

62 Macrae I F, Haslock D I, Wright V 1971 Grading of films for sacro-iliitis in population studies. Ann. Rheum. Dis. 30: 58

63 McGirr E M 1969 Computers in medicine. In: Rose J (ed) Proc. Symp. Computers in Medicine, Blackburn Coll. Tech. and Design, 1968. Churchill, London, p 19

64 Crookes J, Murray I P C, Wayne E J 1959 Statistical

methods applied to the clinical diagnosis of thyrotoxicosis. Quart. J. Med. 28: 211

65 Kulak R F, Schultz A B, Belytschko T, Galante J 1975 Biomechanical characteristics of vertebral motion segments and intervertebral discs. Orth. Clin. N. Am. 6: 121

66 Bakke S 1931 Roentgenologische Beobachtungen über die Bewegungen der Wirbelsaule. Acta Radiol., suppl. 13: 5

67 Farfan H, Cossette J, Robertson G, Wells R, Kraus H 1970 The effects of torsion on the lumbar intervertebral joint: the role of torsion in the production of disc degeneration. J. Bone Jt Surg. 52A: 468

68 Schultz A, Belytschko T, Andriacchi T, Galante J 1973 Analog studies of forces in the human spine: mechanical properties and motion segment behaviour. J. Biomech. 6: 373

69 Pope M H, Wilder D G, Matteri R E, Frymoyer J W 1977 Experimental measurements of vertebral motion under load. Orth. Clin. N. Am. 8: 155

70 Panjabi M, White A A 1971 A mathematical approach for three-dimensional analysis of the mechanics of the spine. J. Biomech. 4: 203

71 Panjabi M M 1977 Experimental determination of spinal motion segment behavior. Orth. Clin. N. Am. 8: 169

72 Panjabi M M, White A A 1977 Effect of preload on load displacement curves of the lumbar spine. Orth. Clin. N. Am. 8: 181

73 Anderson J A D, Sweetman B J 1975 A combined flexirule/hydrogoniometer for measurement of lumbar spine and its sagittal movement. Rheum. Rehab. 14: 173

74 Anderson J A D 1982 The thoraco-lumbar spine. In: Wright V (ed) Clinics in rheumatic diseases, vol 8. No 3. Measurement of joint movement. Saunders, London, p 631–653

75 Sweetman B J, Moore C S, Jayasinghe W J, Anderson J A D 1976 Monitoring work factors relating to back pain. Postgrad. Med. J. 52 (Supp 7): 151

76 Kiernan P J 1981 Monitoring spinal movements using more than one inclinometer. Proc. Soc. Back Pain Res. unpublished

77 Williams A R 1975 Light-sectioning method — the B M J Award. Medical and Biological Illustration 25: 178

78 Williams A R 1977 Light sectioning as a three-dimensional measurement system in medicine. J. Photogr. Sci. 25: 85

79 Williams A R 1984 Personal communication

80 Portek I, Pearcy M J, Reader G P, Mowat A G 1983 Correlation between radiographic and clinical measurement of lumbar spine movement. Br. J. Rheum. 22: 197

81 Wright V 1983 Editorial. Br. J. Rheum. 22: 193

Radiological investigation of the intervertebral disc

INTRODUCTION

Purpose of radiology

The intervertebral disc undoubtedly represents the major pivotal element of the spine, but it would be wrong to consider it purely in isolation. Schmorl & Junghanns[1] used the term 'motor segment' to embrace such structures as the annulus fibrosus, intervertebral ligaments, apophyseal joints, capsules, dura and paraspinal muscles. The purpose of radiology is to demonstrate in the most definitive manner abnormalities of structure and function in the motor segment with the minimum of radiation and upset to the patient.

From the detailed history and careful clinical examination it may be possible to identify the likely pathological mechanisms of back pain in many patients. The clinician should clearly identify the nature of the problems that require radiological definition. The radiologist should appreciate the clinical dilemma, and be able to offer, in consultation, a logical and appropriate investigative sequence.

In a study from general practice, Dillane and his colleagues[2] observed that 90% of acute back syndromes only needed symptomatic treatment and that 62% of attacks had a duration of two weeks. Only 7.5% of patients had symptoms or clinical signs of a nerve root lesion. Clearly, comprehensive radiological investigation would be inappropriate for the great majority of these patients.

Whenever possible, the clinician should indicate to the radiologist whether the low back or leg pain is likely to be due to an abnormality of movement or to structural damage. The muscle spasm, scoliosis and limitation of straight-leg raising associated with mechanical derangements differ fundamentally from the motor, sensory and reflex loss indicative of nerve root compromise. Ultimately, the accuracy of diagnosis will reflect the frequency of detection of positive clinical signs and radiological findings.

Radiological investigation

There are now an almost bewildering number of methods available to investigate the spine and these are itemised in Table 12.1, but only those relevant to the intervertebral disc and its associated pain syndromes will be considered here.

Although the symptoms of low back pain and sciatica are common to many syndromes, radiological examination should be governed entirely by the particular circumstances of each individual patient. Appropriate procedures should be selected with care to provide the maximum amount of information in the simplest and least harmful way to the patient. The number of examinations should be kept to the minimum necessary to make a firm diagnosis or to assist in the planning of surgical treatment. Routine investigation of symptoms should be avoided for three reasons. First, there is the radiation hazard to be considered. With each lateral radiograph of the lumbar spine, the patient receives a skin dose of 0.02 Gy. This is equivalent to about fifteen times the exposure required for a chest X-ray. Second, comprehensive radiological investigation using contrast medium can be time-consuming to perform and therefore costly in terms of staff time and equipment. Finally, an inappropriate radiological examination will contribute little to the solution of a particular clinical problem and, even worse, may serve to obscure it.

Table 12.1 Radiological methods for investigating the spine

Conventional radiographs
  Biplanar views
  Supplementary views
  Dynamic studies
  Tomography
	Vascular imaging
	  Spinal angiography
	  Ascending lumbosacral venography

Computerized imaging
  Computerized tomography
  Nuclear magnetic resonance
	Provocation radiology
	  Nucleography
	  Facet arthrography

Myelography
  Iodized oil
  Tomopneumomyelography
  Water-soluble myelography
  Epidurography
	Intervention radiology
	  Aspiration needle biopsy
	  Chemonucleolysis
	  Therapeutic angiographic embolization
	
	Ultrasound
	Radio-isotope organ imaging
	  Bone scintigraphy
	  Myeloscintigraphy

CONVENTIONAL RADIOGRAPHY

The lumbar spine is particularly challenging to the radiologist because the shadows cast by the bones form only a proportion of the structures under scrutiny. It must be appreciated that a standard examination only portrays one limited modality of spinal disorder. Soft tissue involvement will usually require additional enhancement techniques.

Standard radiographic examination of the lumbar spine consists of three films taken in the antero-posterior, lateral, lying and coned lumbosacral projections. In view of the high gonadal dose of lumbar radiography, a single well-centred lateral with the beam at the level of the crest may negate the need for the coned lateral.[3]

Oblique views do not significantly enhance the information on the AP and lateral and should not form part of the initial investigation.[4]

The radiographs should be taken with meticulous attention to positioning, collimation and exposure factors and the results viewed with adequate illumination.

The pathological lesions of the common lumbar spine diseases are well known to morbid anatomists. Disc degeneration, spondylolysis, apophyseal joint arthrosis and spinal stenosis can all be demonstrated on these standard views.

Disc degeneration

Signs of disc degeneration are frequently found in the adult population and increase with advancing age. The lumbosacral level is most susceptible.

Gresham & Miller[5] performed discograms on randomly selected cadavers of different age groups and compared the results with histological findings. Between the ages of 14 and 34, they found 90% of all discs were normal. With ageing, the incidence of degenerative changes increased until, at the age of 60, only 5% of discs could be considered normal. Therefore the predictive value of radiographic examinations that show these changes must be limited unless supported by supplementary evidence.

Begg & Falconer[6] reported radiological evidence of degenerative disc spaces at one or more levels in four out of five patients with proven lumbar disc protrusion. In half of these patients, degenerative changes occurred predominantly at the offending level. However, in a larger series, also surgically proven, Epstein[7] found disc narrowing in 16% at the lumbosacral junction and 25% at the L4/5 level. Severe degenerative changes involving several discs are more commonly associated with back pain,[8] but moderate or mild degeneration shows no correlation.[9]

In a population survey of Leigh, Wensleydale, Watford and Rhondda in the UK, Lawrence[10] studied the frequency of disc degeneration and its relationship to back-hip-sciatic pain. In broad terms the results showed that, using conventional criteria for disc degeneration, the sensitivity of radiographic examination was 59% (false negative rate 41%) and the specificity 55% (false positive rate 45%). It was estimated that in 13% of those with disc degeneration the symptoms of pain were due to the disease, and this was more common than prolapsed intervertebral disc, osteoarthrosis, rheumatoid arthritis or ankylosing spondylitis. A history or signs of nerve root involvement was found in 10% of the 224 patients with moderate or severe lumbar disc degeneration.

Early changes

Harris & Macnab[11] have drawn attention to two early features of disc degeneration:

1. Loss of height of the anterior disc space. Normal lumbar lordosis is maintained by the intact intervertebral disc, which assumes a wedge-shaped configuration with the apex directed backwards. Loss of the anterior disc space height in early degeneration causes the adjacent vertebral margins to lie parallel to one another in the neutral position (Fig. 12.1). Measurements of disc height from lateral X-rays can vary considerably,

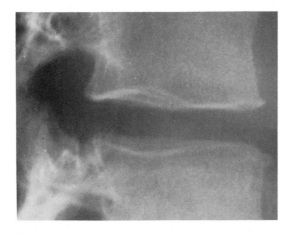

Fig. 12.1 Early disc degeneration. The height of the disc space is reduced anteriorly and the vertebrae pivot to allow the adjacent margins to lie parallel to each other. The posterior apophyseal joints separate slightly to permit this. There are small osteophytes arising from the adjacent vertebral angles (traction spurs).

depending on lateral angulation and rotation. Any judgement that a disc space is narrowed compared to an adjacent disc should be made with care.[12]

2. Anteroposterior intervertebral shift. This is a subtle sign which can be demonstrated using the measuring technique of Knutsson.[13] The natural history of this type of lesion after nineteen years is shown in Figure 12.2.

Late changes

Progressive reduction in the disc space and the presence of intranuclear gas are positive evidence of long-standing disc degeneration. The gas accumulates in spaces created by the deterioration and fissuring of the nucleus and annulus (Fig. 12.3). Visualization on the plain films may be difficult, particularly in the presence of overlying abdominal viscera and is only seen in 12% of cases. The use of CT scanning, however, has shown that it is very common above 40 years of age, with an incidence in the over-70s of 92%.[14]

The accumulation of gas, which is principally nitrogen,[15] is ascribed to a vacuum phenomenon similar to that seen in joints under stress.[16] The gas may be centrally or eccentrically situated, depending on the place of cleavage in the disc and the direction of the distraction forces applied to the vertebra. During flexion the pivoting moment around the nucleus tends to separate and widen the posterior intervertebral disc space. Fissures situated in the posterior half of the disc will be demonstrated best in this position as they become outlined with gas.

The posterior disc space is compressed during extension, and distraction is exerted anteriorly. Intense reactive sclerosis may also be present in the adjacent vertebral end-plates. The presence of the gas, the well-defined vertebral contour and small osteophytes will all aid the differentiation from infection.[17]

Osteophytes

Marginal osteophytes of the vertebral bodies are usually associated with disc degeneration. Macnab[18] separated the osteophytes into two groups, the claw and the traction spurs. The traction spurs develop

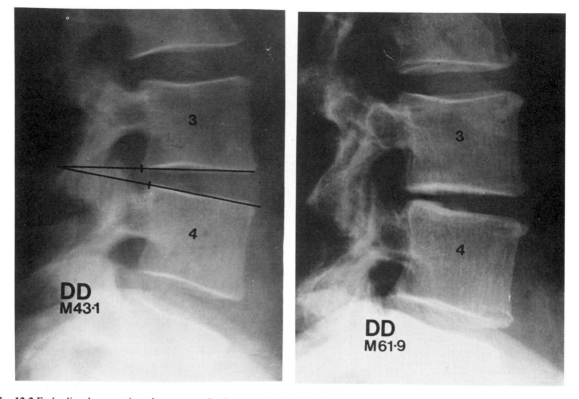

Fig. 12.2 Early disc degeneration. Anteroposterior intervertebral shift (left). There is 4 mm posterior displacement between the 3rd and 4th lumbar vertebrae. Nineteen years later the disc degeneration between these two vertebrae is now clearly established (right).

with a definite gap between the end-plate and the osteophyte. These are due to elevation of the periosteum from the vertebral margin by the bulging annulus provoking the formation of new bone in a beak-line protruberance (Fig. 12.4(a)). The annular

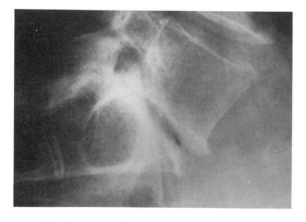

Fig. 12.3 Chronic disc degeneration with intranuclear gas. A localized pocket of intranuclear gas is visualized in the anterior portion of the lumbosacral disc space.

bulging is usually associated with some disc degeneration and penetration and migration of nuclear material outwards through the tears in the inner annulus. In some cases, the appearances may be found with a normal nucleogram, however.[19] In these circumstances, softening and loss of elasticity of the annular fibres may still produce bulging and periosteal elevation.

The claw osteophytes are less common and arise from the vertebral margin without a gap between the end-plate and the osteophyte (Fig. 12.4(b)). These are more commonly associated with normal nucleograms.[19] It should be stressed that at times the differentiation between the two may be impossible. The syndesmophyte of inflammatory spondylitis, which passes vertically across the disc margin, should not be confused with osteophytes.[20]

Apophyseal joint alignment

The apophyseal joints are sagittally orientated in the upper lumbar spine, rotating towards the coronal

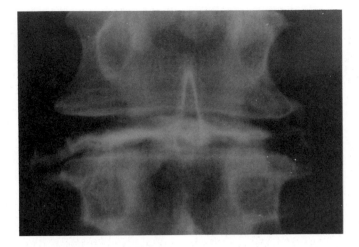

Fig. 12.4(a) The osteophyte forms a beak-like protruberance below the margin of the vertebral end-plate. Contrast within the degenerate disc is seen outlining the inner margin of the osteophyte.

plane at the lumbosacral junction. It has been suggested that impairment of the function of these joints, through malalignment or tropism, may result in a higher degree of disc degeneration.[21] Experiments have shown that these variations impose torsional strains on the intervertebral disc complex, sufficient to produce annular rupture. Other authors, however, suggest that the torsional strains necessary to cause tears in the annulus are considerably greater than physiological levels and would damage the apophyseal joints rather than the annulus.[22]

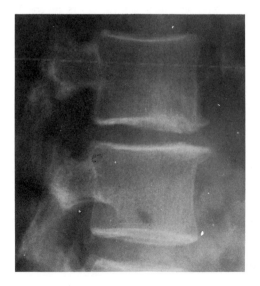

Fig. 12.4(b) The inferior osteophyte is of the claw type from the margin of the end plate.

Malalignment may sometimes be accompanied by subtle vertebral rotation, evident by deviation of the spinous process from the midline. It is difficult to reproduce these effects from standard radiographs, hence a specimen from a cadaver is shown for illustrative purposes (Fig. 12.5). The damage to the disc complex represented an incidental finding in a 32-year-old male in a discographic survey of 'normal' lumbar spines. The intervertebral foramina, infralamina recesses and pars interarticularis are well shown by an oblique projection.

Spondylolysis

Defects in the pars interarticularis affect approximately 6% of the population.[23] They are not seen at birth[24] but are usually present by the age of 6.[25] Inheritance plays a role in the development of the pars interarticularis defect in the form of a hereditary weakness or dysplasia in the cartilaginous model of the arch of the affected vertebra.[26] A further group occur in young adults undergoing severe physical exercise, and these are due to true stress fractures.

Forward displacement may be accentuated by performing a lateral with the patient standing, and further separation of the defect occurs on forward bending (Fig. 12.6).

Spondylolysis may be associated with a forward displacement of the vertebral body. The pars defects will usually be evident on the lateral projection, but

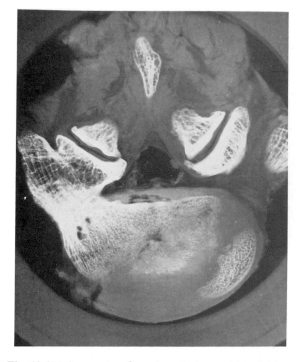

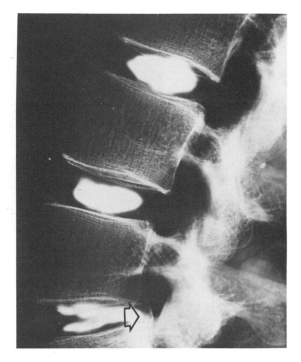

Fig. 12.5(a) Asymmetry of apophyseal joints, axial projection. A transverse horizontal section has been cut through the intervertebral disc and the apophyseal joints at the L4/5 level. The facet joints are clearly asymmetrical. The right side is inclined towards the coronal plane and the left side is more saggital.

Fig. 12.5(b) Radial fissuring of the posterior annulus. The facet joint asymmetry is associated in this instance with posterior disc damage (arrow) not evident at higher levels, where the facet joints are symmetrical.

oblique views (Fig. 12.7) and even lateral tomography may be necessary to confirm the diagnosis. In the adult group, with increased stress, a bone scan may provide the earliest indication of the lesion.

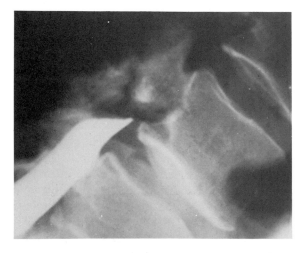

Fig. 12.6 Spondylolisthesis. Lateral flexion myelogram, shows the separation of the defects in the pars interarticularis.

Severe forms of displacement may be associated with deformity of the vertebral body leading to posterior wedging and also a dome effect of the upper end-plate of the S1.[26] A true kyphosis may occur with the slip, which is best measured using the upper end-plate of L5 and the lower end-plate of S1.[27]

There is no clear association between symptoms and the defect, except where a moderate or severe forward slip has occurred. Disc damage may occur at or above the level of a spondylolysis or listhesis, and this may be a source of pain. Facet-induced pain and nerve root compression have also been reported.[23]

Inclined plane radiography

In the sagittal plane, the spine curves throughout its length. In order to delineate clearly individual vertebrae or disc spaces on the AP view, it is necessary to tilt the X-ray tube at varying degrees along the body axis (Fig. 12.8). This facility is

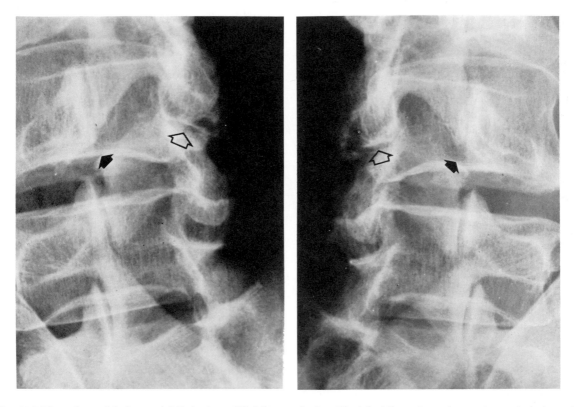

Fig. 12.7 Bilateral spondylotic spondylolisthesis — 45° oblique projection. The left oblique shows the pars interarticularis on the left while the right oblique shows the defect on the right side. The oblique components of the defects are shown in the region of the neck of the Scottie dog (closed arrow). The horizontal component of the defect on the opposite side is shown in the rear of the Scottie dog (open arrow).

particularly valuable at the junctional zone of the cervicodorsal and lumbosacral spine and aids the differentiation of such variations as partial sacralization and the deep-set 5th lumbar vertebra.

Dynamic studies

The normal range of lumbar movement is 70° between flexion and extension, and 40–50° of this occurs in the lower three segments. Many methods have been described for measuring both normal and abnormal displacements.[6,13,28–33] Although the methods of measurement vary, there is general agreement that the characteristic feature of the normal is the regular, sequential rotation of each segment coordinated in a smooth pattern during movement. A recent study comparing discographic appearances of the nucleus with methods of measurement on flexion and extensions films concluded that those methods involving assessment of relative linear interbody displacement[31] most accurately correlated with discogenic damage.[34] This is further supported by experimental studies selectively sectioning the nucleus, posterior annulus fibrosus and posterior longitudinal ligament. Hypermobility of the intervertebral segment was induced which manifested itself in minor horizontal shear motion.[35] The degree of mobility will depend to a certain extent on the state and progress of disc degeneration.

In the early stages of disc damage, there is a tendency to hypermobility.[35] Long-standing disc degeneration with marked narrowing of the intervertebral disc space, on the other hand, tends to reduce mobility. In these circumstances, and in more extreme circumstances, when a fusion is present, additional stress is thrown on the adjacent segments.[36] Less attention has been paid to diagnostic value of dynamic lateral bending procedures. Vernon,[37] however, suggests that isolated segmental pathomechanical behaviour is uncommon and does

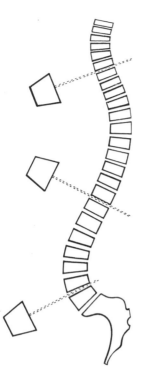

Fig. 12.8 Inclined plane radiography.

not provide adequate discrimination of a specific diseased lumbar segment.

Three-dimensional motion studies are now being performed using computerized biplanar radiographic measurement techniques. Using this technique, a consistent pattern of asymmetric facet motion at levels of proven herniated nucleus pulposus has been shown. Patients clinically suspected of disc herniation, but with normal myelograms, had some asymmetry, but the magnitude was uniformly greater in the myelographically proven lesions.[38] There is little unaniminty regarding the overall correlation between abnormal movement patterns and symptomatology. When, however, there is significant excessive intervertebral tilt or horizontal shear, a higher incidence of symptomatology in the low back has been found.

Post-surgery assessments

Assessment of spinal mobility may be helpful in the assessment of surgical results. Froning & Frohman[39] found that there was generally reduced motion of both the L4/5 and L5/S1 levels after disc removal in patients with good relief of pain and satisfactory results. Those patients with persistence of pain and unsatisfactory results seem to retain almost normal motion at the operated level. The authors found no relationship between the height of the intervertebral disc at the operated level and the degree of intervertebral motion or clinical result.

White & Wiltse[40] found 76% with progressive spondylolisthesis after decompressive laminectomy which included apophyseal process excision and particularly in those under 40 with normal disc height. In contrast, a recent study has indicated that one-level discectomy and unilateral or bilateral apophyseal joint excision will seldom lead to an unstable vertebral segment and will frequently have a satisfactory subjective result.[41]

O'Brien & Evans[42] in a five-year follow-up of patients who underwent laminectomy for disc prolapse, reported abnormal patterns of spinal movement in 75% of patients still suffering pain and disability. Similar patterns were recorded in only 12% of pain-free patients. The poor results also correlated with a history of chronic back pain, multiple total laminectomy procedures and equivocal myelogram findings for disc herniation prior to the laminectomy.

Degenerative spondylolisthesis

Intervertebral subluxation of degenerative spondylolisthesis occurs most frequently between the 4th and 5th lumbar vertebrae, especially when the lumbosacral junction is low-set in the pelvis. Considerable displacement may be found between the flexed and extended positions (Fig. 12.9). In flexion, the upper vertebra glides forwards, attenuating the intervertebral foramen as a result of subluxation of the posterior apophyseal joints. There is an additional displacement in extension. The upper vertebra pivots sharply backwards with overriding of the apophyseal facets. The joint surfaces become damaged following excessive wear and ultimately terminate in severe osteoarthritis. Hypermobility adjacent to a fixed or fused segment may occur and lead to disc damage. This may exert a profound effect on the dural tube because it lies within the spinal canal, even though the amount of displacement on the radiograph may appear to be minor in degree (Fig. 12.10). The epidural space is

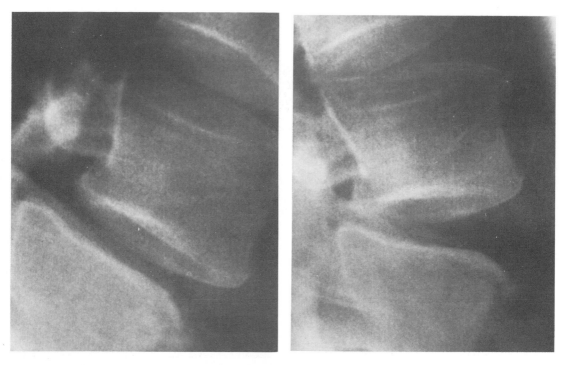

Fig. 12.9 Degenerative spondylolisthesis. Flexion (left). The 4th lumbar vertebra glides forwards accompanied by subluxion of the posterior joints and oblique elongation of the intervertebral foramen. Extension (right). The upper vertebra pivots backwards reducing the vertical height of the intervertebral foramen.

adversely affected by the shape of the bony canal — particularly narrowing of the lateral recesses — by loss of disc height and osteoarthrosis of the posterior apophyseal joints. Erect myelography, in flexion and extension, may be the only method by which this defect is demonstrable.

A small proportion of patients with a remote or generalized form of spinal deformity may suffer low back and leg pain. The relevance of the lumbar contribution in scoliosis, dorsal kyphosis or lordosis may become apparent only when whole-spine views are taken. Standing radiographs have been found to accentuate the displacement in spondylolisthesis.[43] Where it is necessary to obtain follow-up radiographs of spinal problems, e.g. following surgical fusion, standardization of technique is vital for valid comparison.

Linear tomography

It is occasionally necessary to supplement standard radiographs by linear tomography to demonstrate a particular feature (Fig. 12.11). This form of examin-ation is particularly helpful in demonstrating subtle bone injury, neoplasm, osteomyelitis and post-operative states.

Conclusion

Many causes of back pain may be demonstrated or excluded by standard radiographic examination. Spinal neoplasm, tumours of bone, myeloma, metastasis, as well as Paget's disease and fracture or dislocation, are unlikely to be found in more than 2–3% of patients who are radiographed for backache on a routine basis. Vertebral osteomyelitis, both tuberculous and pyogenic, is being seen a little more frequently in the UK, particularly in the immigrant population, and the condition is always associated with back pain. The clinical presentation of ankylo-sing spondylitis is usually characteristic enough to enable a confident diagnosis to be made. An alert radiologist may occasionally have the satisfaction of detecting unsuspected sacroiliitis or a renal calculus on a lumbar spine examination. Syndromes assoc-iated with narrowing of the lumbar canal are fully

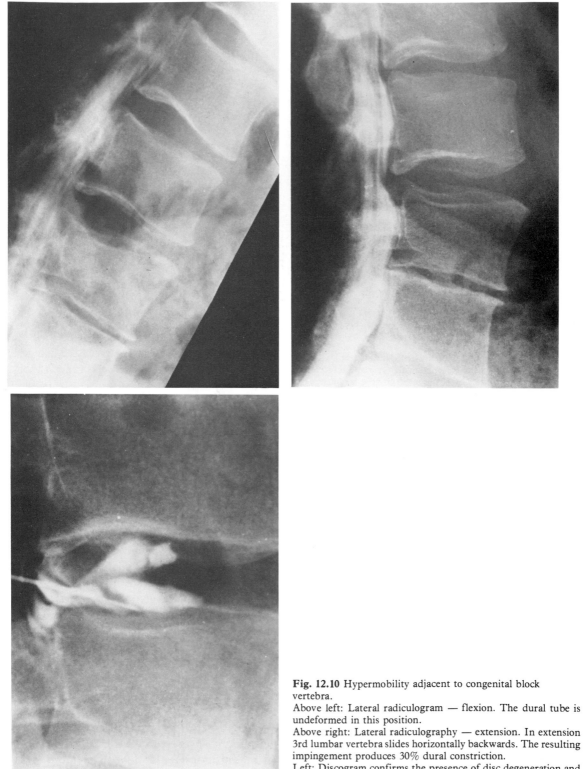

Fig. 12.10 Hypermobility adjacent to congenital block vertebra.

Above left: Lateral radiculogram — flexion. The dural tube is undeformed in this position.

Above right: Lateral radiculography — extension. In extension 3rd lumbar vertebra slides horizontally backwards. The resulting impingement produces 30% dural constriction.

Left: Discogram confirms the presence of disc degeneration and fissuring of the posterior annulus of the L3 disc.

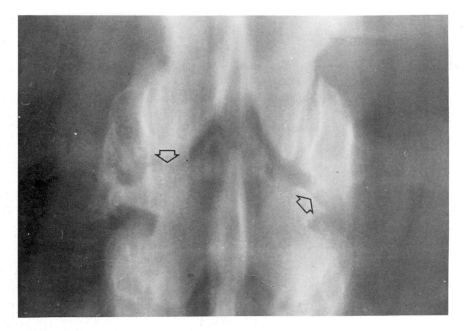

Fig. 12.11 Spondylolytic spondylolisthesis. Anteroposterior tomography reveals the direction of the defects in the pars interarticularis. Florid callus in relation to the pseudoarthrosis may produce entrapment of the emerging spinal nerve below the pedicle.

discussed in Chapter 19. Other forms of advanced imaging, computerized tomography and magnetic resonance, are presented in Chapter 13.

MYELOGRAPHY

For many years, contrast examinations have been used to examine the spinal cord, subarachnoid space and nerve root sleeves. In America and Britain, iodized oil iophendylate (Myodil® or Pantopaque®) used to be the main agent. Unfortunately, the viscosity of iodized oil frequently does not permit the satisfactory filling of the nerve root sheaths, and 30% of lateral protrusions may have been missed.[44] Chronic and sometimes symptomatic arachnoiditis can occur, whether or not the substance has been completely removed from the subarachnoid space. This contrast method has now been superseded by the ready availability of water-soluble media.

Water-soluble myelography

Initial water-soluble contrast agents (Conray 280® and Dimer X®) proved toxic to the cord and also caused arachnoiditis in some cases. Non-ionic agents, the first of which was metrizamide, have proved safe in clinical practice with minimal neurotoxicity, in both the short and long term, and have led to universal acceptance of water-soluble myelography.

Disadvantages of metrizamide, however, are present in the form of high incidence of headache (43%), nausea (14%) and vomiting (12%).[45] Other symptoms, including myoclonic spasms, fever and back pain and occasional psychomotor disturbances, have been reported, and severe e.e.g. disturbances may occur.[46]

The inconvenience of the powdered form and the expense of the media have led to further developments in the form of Iohexol® and Iopamidol®. These substances have chemical and physical properties similar to metrizamide but have a higher osmolality and are stable during autoclaving in solution.

Clinical assessment indicates less excitory or depressive changes in the nervous system, and the incidence and severity of minor adverse reactions is considerably reduced, with an overall incidence of 25%.[47] Most adverse reactions occur within the first 48 hours, but late-onset headache, neck stiffness and photophobia may develop, and post-myelographic chemical and streptococcal meningitis have been reported.[48]

This new generation of water-soluble media also allows the safe examination of the cervical and dorsal spinal canal and cord and has thus replaced oil products for intrathecal investigation.

Prolapsed intervertebral disc

Water-soluble myelography is of maximum value in the diagnosis of root compression by a prolapsed intervertebral disc. Radiologically, there may be an extradural impression of the dural sac. The nerve root sleeve of the affected level usually fails to fill and, in larger lesions, the nerve roots below the affected level will be deviated (Fig. 12.12). More laterally placed lesions may only deviate the root at the affected level or amputate the root sleeve without deviation. In some cases where root filling is incomplete, lateral decubitus films with a horizontal beam may prove valuable to ensure maximal root sleeve filling on the dependent side.

Predictive value of water-soluble myelography

Clinicians vary in their use of the investigation, the presence of a classical history and definite clinical findings being sufficient to proceed directly to surgery. Indeed, Jepson and colleagues[49] have claimed a lower surgical accuracy rate using water-soluble myelography than in those operated upon on purely clinical grounds. However, other authors have indicated the accuracy of clinical assessment alone in determining the exact level of disc disease is unlikely to be much better than 50%.[44] Nachemson has shown that the accuracy of pre-operative diagnosis of a disc rupture at the proper level can be improved to 90% by additional confirmation from a positive straight-leg raising test, e.m.g. studies and radiculography. It has been claimed that the additional sign of cross straight-leg raising increases the accuracy to 97%.[50] Hirsch & Nachemson[51] found a disc lesion in 90% of those patients with neurological disturbances and a positive straight-leg raising. Numerous other series have produced accuracy rates ranging from 90% to 97%.[52-54]

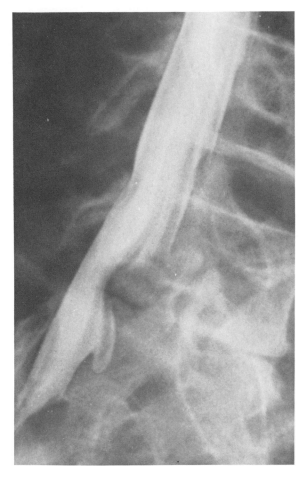

Fig. 12.12 There is a large extradural defect which is compressing the L5 nerve root, leading to failure of filling of the root sleeve. The S1 nerve root is deviated within the dural sac.

False negatives do occur in cases where the prolapse lies very posterolaterally in the foramen and in cases where root sleeves fill poorly. This is particularly the case at the L5/S1 level in the presence of a short dural sac.

Myelography is also helpful in patients who have only mechanical signs, i.e. muscle spasm, scoliosis and some limitation of straight leg-raising. Either a positive or a negative water-soluble myelogram will significantly increase the accuracy of diagnosis. The radiographic features of disc prolapse themselves, however, are no justification for operation, as disc bulges have been shown to be present in a number of examinations performed for other reasons than low back pain or sciatica[55] (Fig. 12.13). In these

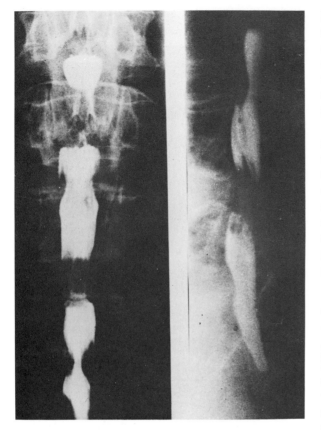

Fig.12.13 Asymptomatic narrowing of the lumbar canal. This was an unexpected finding in a 62-year-old company director who underwent myelography because of neck, shoulder and arm pain associated with cervical spondylosis. There were no symptoms referrable to the lumbar spine.

circumstances, symptoms consistent with disc herniation may develop over the following months or years, and are more likely to produce deficits in sensation than pain.[56] On myelographic evidence alone, it may be difficult for the radiologist to differentiate between a small disc prolapse of intermittent type or diffuse annular bulging associated with more extensive damage and degeneration. This is of diagnostic significance, since these bulges may disappear on forward flexion and, therefore, are not always recognized by the orthopaedic surgeon who operates on a completely relaxed patient, flexed over a prop to facilitate surgical access. In the past, this has undoubtedly been the source of some apparently false negative examinations. The use of erect or semi-erect lateral views on myelography, in both flexion and extension, will differentiate these

lesions (Fig. 12.14). Oblique views in flexion and extension may also identify this type of concealed disc. Operative confirmation may be achieved by means of a hyperextension manoeuvre performed on the operating table. Flexion and extension views may reveal significant spinal canal narrowing which is not solely due to disc damage.

Knuttson[57] described three components of canal narrowing anterior encroachment due to thickening and shortening of the flaval ligaments and lateral encroachment through approximation of the articular facets. All are accentuated by lumbar extension and relieved by flexion. In spinal flexion there is marked elongation of the spinal canal with concomitant stretching of the dural sac and nerve root fibres. Thus lumbar flexion may aggravate symptoms of disc herniation.[58]

Lateral recess stenosis

When significant disc degeneration is present, particularly in the presence of facet hypertrophy, the lateral recess through which the nerve passes may be significantly narrowed and lead to compression of the nerve root within it. Despite the improved filling of the nerve root sleeves with water-soluble contrast media, 50% of these lesions may be missed.[59]

ASCENDING LUMBAR VENOGRAPHY

Contrast visualization of the epidural venous plexus was introduced due to inaccuracies of oil-based myelograms, particularly at the L5/S1 level. It has proved to be a safe procedure of proven value in the diagnosis of lumbar disc herniations.[60-62] Contrast is injected into the lateral ascending lumbar veins or anterior and lateral sacral veins via femoral catheterization. The technique requires some experience to perfect, and variable filling of the epidural plexus may make multiple selective injections of the supplying veins necessary.

The anterior epidural vertebral veins are closely applied to the backs of the intervertebral discs and bodies (Fig. 12.15). At the L3/4 and L4/5 levels they lie laterally, forming a regular hexagonal, whereas at L5/S1 there is a cushion of veins behind the posterior disc surface. Communication with the ascending lumbar veins occurs via radicular veins

Fig. 12.14 Discogram — disc prolapse.

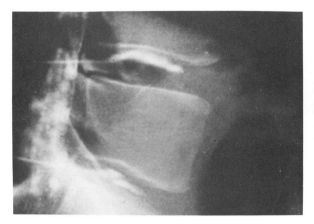

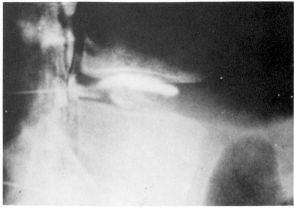

Fig. 12.14(a) Lateral decubitus — flexion. There is a small disc protrusion. Myodil outlines the dural sac, revealing only minor extradural indentation by the disc at L4/5. The epidural space is wide.

Fig. 12.14(b) Lateral decubitus — extension. There is now quite definite indentation of the dural sac by the protrusion.

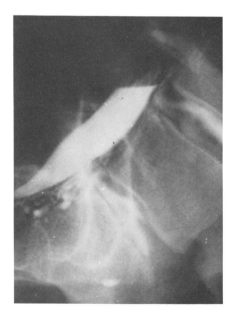

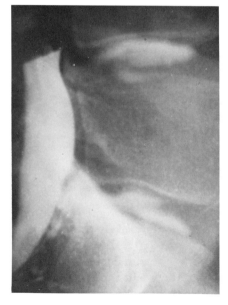

Fig. 12.14(c) Erect lateral — flexion. When the patient bends forward, only minor deformity of the dura is evident. (There is some loss of detail of the discogram because of absorption of contrast medium.)

Fig. 12.14(d) Erect lateral — extension. In this position, there is the most marked deformity of the dural sac. 54-year-old miner with back pain and left sciatica. Back pain reproduced by the L4/5 discogram. Disc protrusion confirmed at operation. Discectomy followed by relief of symptoms.

which pass through the intervertebral foramina above and below the pedicles. Visualization is enhanced by photographic subtraction.

Indication of disc herniation — phlebographic diagnosis is based on demonstrating interruption of an anterior epidural vein. This may be associated with enlargement and increased density of veins above and below the obstruction due to slowing of

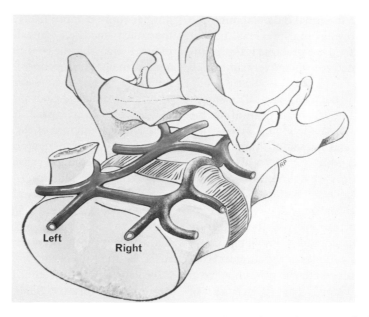

Fig. 12.15 Anterior epidural vertebral veins. These are closely applied to the vertebrae and consequently deform readily with prolapsed disc (right).

venous flow (Fig. 12.16). Interruption of the radicular veins under the pedicle and in the intervertebral foramena may indicate a lateral extrusion of disc material. Partial interruption, deviation or decreased density without complete occlusion indicate a milder degree of venous compression.

Predictive value of epidural venography

Various published works indicate a sensitivity of epidural venography in the diagnosis of disc herniation of between 83% and 99%.[54,60,62] False positives, however, may occur, and these are usually in cases of partial vein compression or deviation. Veins are soft and easily compressed[63] and anatomic variations at L5/S1 may occur.[60] Failure of radicular vein filling is usually accompanied by other changes, and disc herniation is unlikely if this sign is present alone.

A series of patients with suspected disc prolapse has been reviewed[64] in whom the radiculograms were either normal or equivocal. Epidural venography confirmed normality in 16 out of 41 (39%) and indicated a disc lesion in 25 out of 41 (61%). Twenty of these later had the findings confirmed at operation, but two were falsely positive. In the same

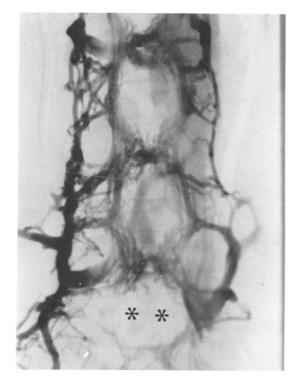

Fig. 12.16 Epidural venogram. The spine has been removed by a photographic subtraction technique to display the internal vertebral veins more clearly. These are occluded at the lumbosacral level (* *) by a large central prolapse of the intervertebral disc.

series, three cases had abnormal radiculograms due to arachnoiditis following the previous use of Myodil® and Dimer X®. Disc prolapse was phlebographically demonstrated and operatively confirmed in two.

Ascending lumbar venography is a safe examination. It has the advantage of not invading the subarachnoid space and, therefore, avoids the consequent headache and nausea of lumbar puncture and injected water-soluble contrast. The theoretical complication of deep-vein thrombosis does not occur in practice. The examination, however, is more time-consuming for the radiologist and requires practice to gain the expertise. The radiation dose is higher than radiculography. Previous surgery will distort the venous complex at the surgical level, but useful diagnostic information may be obtained at the levels above or below. The replacement of Myodil® by water-soluble contrast agents and the advent of CT have substantially curtailed the use of ascending lumbar venography.

Compression of the veins is non-specific and may be due to either disc herniation or bony entrapment. It is, however, a safe procedure and, provided false positive examinations are avoided, an accurate diagnostic tool. It is used, therefore, in most centres as a secondary investigation in cases where the radiculogram is equivocal, due to a short dural sac, poor root sleeve filling or in the presence of arachnoiditis.

EPIDUROGRAPHY

Epidurography outlines the external surface of the dural tube and its extensions along nerve roots. It is, therefore, possible that most deformities may be identified in areas not visualized by intrathecal injection of contrast medium. This is of importance in disc prolapse in very lateral locations not reached by the dural tube. Epidurography, using ionic water-soluble contrast agents, has not been widely accepted because of neurotoxicity and pain.[65] Experimental work on animals and early clinical studies with non-ionic contrast medium suggests that these are more suitable agents.[66]

Contrast may be introduced via the sacral or lumbar route. Transgression of the dural sac in the lumbar route is more likely, due to the presence of the plica mediana dorsalis which substantially reduces the thickness of the posterior epidural compartment.[67] Injection of contrast via needle puncture through the sacral hiatus also provides technical problems. Considerable escape of contrast in the pre-sacral space often takes place, and occasionally puncture of the epidural venous plexus may occur. Also, the presence of the plica can totally separate the epidural space into right and left compartments, hindering opacification of the appropriate side of the epidural space.[68] Technical failure rates range from 7.5%[69] to 15%.[70] Catheterization via a Seldinger technique from the sacral hiatus has recently been advocated, although technical failures still occur.[70]

Prolapsed intervertebral disc produces dural or nerve root deformity. Such defects may be reversible, as shown by Mathews[71] on repeat epidurography, in patients treated conservatively and by traction therapy.

Accuracy levels vary, but a significant number of false negative and false positive examinations have been reported.[72] The misinterpretation of lobulated epidural fat as a disc prolapse is an important cause of a false positive examination. The variable contour of the epidural space and unpredictable filling make interpretation difficult unless the appearances are completely normal. Recurrent disc prolapse and post-laminectomy syndromes are also a limitation for the investigation as adhesions obliterate the epidural space (Fig. 12.17). Epidurogrpahy therefore has no role in the primary evaluation of back pain and should be reserved for those occasions where lateral nerve root compression is suspected and conventional evaluation has failed to answer the clinical question.

PROVOCATION RADIOLOGY

This term defines those circumstances in which radiological interpretation depends not only on the imaging of pathology, but also on the reproduction of clinical symptoms in the patient. Discography and facet arthrography are the two major spinal investigations included in this category. The latter will be discussed in another chapter.

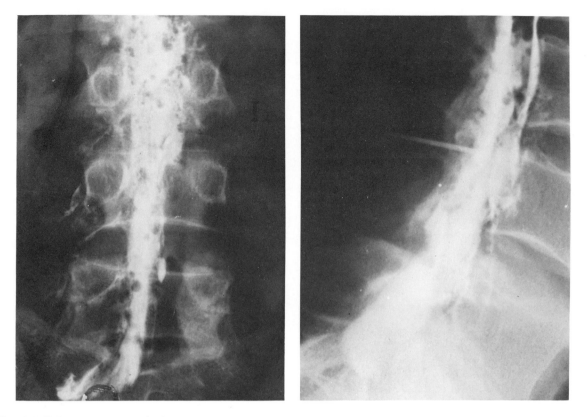

Fig. 12.17 Epidurogram — post-laminectomy. Anteroposterior (left). The epidural space is obliterated on the left side from L4 to the sacrum following L5 hemilaminectomy. Lateral projection (right).

Scientific evidence of the value of this type of procedure is difficult to obtain, since it requires correlation with pathological lesions and largely undefined clinical syndromes. Current experience indicates that these procedures are of some value in patients with genuine atypical pain patterns in whom conventional studies and clinical examination have failed to indicate a specific source of symptomatology.

Discography

The term was first used by Lindblom,[73] who demonstrated the morphology of the intervertebral nucleus by injecting contrast medium. The procedure did not find favour in Great Britain largely because of the neurotoxicity of the contrast media then available and the absence of television image intensification for easy intranuclear placement of the needle. Despite these difficulties, discography was performed by a number of clinicians in the United States and Europe. As with any other complicated investigations, it is becoming increasingly clear that careful selection of the patient maximizes the value of the procedure.

Technique

The examination is best performed on a relaxed, cooperative patient who understands its nature. A careful record of the type and distribution of the patient's pain should be made prior to the examination, preferably by an independent observer. The patient should not be told directly that the discogram might reproduce any previously experienced symptoms, in order to provide a valid objective assessment of the pain response. The pain pattern and character of the induced pain is then compared with the original assessment.

Pre-medication

Most patients do not require pre-medication. Deep sedation or complete analgesia should be avoided, since this will influence the response. Where necessary, diazepam is usually effective in producing relaxation.

Puncture technique

The patient should be positioned on an X-ray table so that anteroposterior and lateral radiographs can be taken. The skin is surgically prepared and draped, with the patient lying on the left side.

There are three approaches to disc puncture (Fig. 12.18). Midline puncture penetrates the subarach-

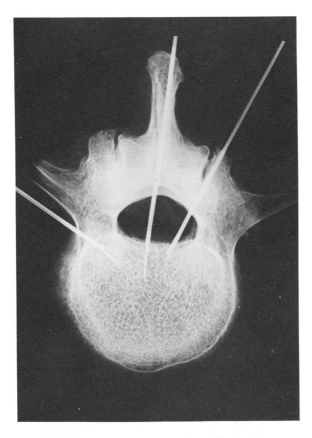

Fig. 12.18 Discogram puncture technique. The dural sac has been outlined in white. Even allowing for post-mortem shrinkage, the dura cannot cover more than half of the posterior aspect of the disc space. The midline puncture approach is transural. The posterolateral and lateral approaches avoid this.

noid space and, therefore, a specimen of cerebral spinal fluid can be collected at the same time. Since this approach involves multiple dural perforation, some examiners choose to perform the procedure under antibiotic cover. For the posterolateral approach, the needle is introduced between the spinous processes, just under 4 cm from the midline and directed 15° downwards to the table top. Finally, the lateral puncture, a point 8–10 cm from the midline and close to the posterior border of the iliac crest is selected. The needle should be inserted separately, for each level where possible, in order that the directional vectors be limited to AP and lateral.

Entry to the lumbosacral space may be difficult when this is deep-set into the pelvis, and more individual manoeuvring may be necessary. The discogram needles are introduced in two stages. A guide needle (21G) is introduced under local anaesthetic and television control until it reaches the outer fibres of the annulus fibrosus. The inner stillette is removed and replaced by a finer needle (26G) which protrudes in beyond the guide. The 26G needle may have to be curved to assist entry into the lumbosacral disc space. Accurate positioning in the centre of the nucleus should be confirmed by direct fluoroscopy before the injection is made. Misplacement of the needle in the annulus may occur. In a normal disc there will be great resistance to the injection, which may even be impossible.

If the annulus is soft due to early degeneration, some contrast may be injected. The appearances are characteristic, with the contrast remaining as a blob or producing a criss-cross pattern of annular fibres (Fig. 12.19). A discogram report and conclusion can be reached only after a combination of the following features has been analysed.

Injection pressure

The normal and intact nucleus pulposus behaves like a ball of fluid within the annular fibrosus. In this state the nucleus resists compressive forces as well as direct introduction of either saline or contrast medium at discography. The injection is usually made with a 1 ml tuberculin syringe to permit efficient application of pressure. Quinnell & Stockdale[74] have, however, recommended a more elabor-

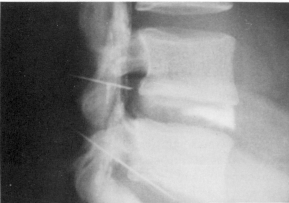

Fig. 12.19(a) Discogram — false injection into annulus fibrosus. Lateral projection. The contrast medium has been introduced into the fibres of the annulus fibrosus giving a characteristic wedge-shaped appearance. (The needle was partly withdrawn following the injection.)

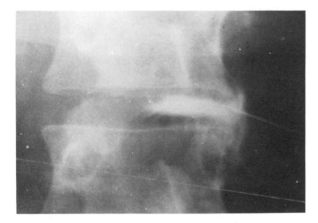

Fig. 12.19(b) Anteroposterior view. This shows the localization of contrast more accurately.

ate pressure-standardized injection technique to monitor the flow of contrast medium into the disc.

The gentle injection of contrast into the normal nucleus will lead to a gradual increase in resistance and in some cases a definite recoil in the syringe with the removal of pressure. The pressure curves delineate this pattern.[74] When the disc undergoes degeneration, the pressure required to fill the disc will be reduced but will still gradually increase as the injection proceeds. If a radial rupture through all levels of the annulus is present, extravasation into the surrounding tissues occurs and the late injection

resistance will be lost. Wiley and his associates[75] have warned than 15% of degenerate discs can have firm resistance to injection pressure. This may represent non-nuclear injection patterns as described by Quinnell & Stockdale.[76]

There is a theoretical possibility of creating planes of cleavage in the nucleus by excessively high injection pressure. This might potentiate subsequent premature degeneration. Injections should not, therefore, be made against significant resistance.

Disc capacity

The volume of contrast fluid accepted by the disc will give a measure of the disc's intrinsic internal elastic properties. The normal disc is limited in its ability to accept fluid by injection, and up to 1 cc will usually be sufficient. Grossly degenerate discs will accept 2–3 cc, but if the outer annulus is ruptured with escape of contrast, there will be no limit to the injectable volume.

Pain

Patients may feel pain during discography for the following reasons:

1. Irritation of lumbar spinal nerves by the close proximity of the needle track
2. Irritation of sensitive nerves in the outer margin of the annulus fibrosus
3. Irritation by the use of an irritant contrast medium
4. Presence of symptomatic disc disease.

It is necessary to distinguish the source of pain because of the difference in significance.

Nerve root irritation. There should be no difficulty recognizing this. A sharp shooting pain occurs down the right leg in a dermatomal distribution, often accompanied by parasthesia. The needle should be withdrawn and a new line to the disc sought. Care must be exercised at the time of disc injection not to confuse residual pain from this source with part of the induced pain pattern due to the injection.

Annular sensitivity. Sometimes the patient experience components of the symptomatic pain when the discogram needle comes in contact with the annulus. This must be clearly distinguished from the nerve root irritation just described. The induced pain may be severe in some cases. The presence of annular sensitivity occurs in approximately 5% of degenerate discs in the lower lumbar spine. It may also occur in a disc which is subsequently shown to have a normal nucleogram. In these circumstances the normal disc is invariably adjacent to a severely symptomatic level. It is possible that this phenomenon may be explained by the intersegmental distribution of nerve supply in this region.

Irritant media. The choice of contrast is of prime importance. It is possible, for example, to provoke bizarre patterns of pain, often severe in intensity, when sodium diatrizoate is used and extravasates outside the nucleus. Symptoms presumably arise from contact with nerve endings in sensitive tissues. This can be alarming and confusing for both the patient and the radiologist. Such was the experience of Holt[77] when he performed a series of discograms on asymptomatic volunteer inmates of a United States penitentiary. The ages ranged in the third and fourth decade. Sodium diatrizoate extravasated into the epidural space from the nucleus in 37% of patients, producing very severe back pain in 15% and combined with sciatica in the other 22%. Experiments have shown that sodium diatrizoate penetrates brain tissue more deeply than meglumine compounds, and this may be an important factor in the neurotoxic action of contrast media on the central nervous system.[78]

There is also evidence that sodium ions increase permeability of capillaries or tissue cells to the anionic component of the contrast media in controlled animal experiments.[79] Recently introduced non-ionic, low osmolar contrast media have very low neurotoxicity and may well prove to be the ideal substances for this investigation, as they increase the specificity of discography with regard to induced pain.

Symptomatic disc disease. In patients with severe low back or leg pain, without conclusive clinical signs, diagnosis of the pain source is difficult, and pre-operative discography in the lumbar region has been found to be a reliable indicator of the symptomatic level.[80] The injection of contrast into the nucleus delineates the morphology and may produce low back pain, leg pain or a combination of both. Symptom provocation is variable, but is commonly present in frank nuclear prolapse. Gardener and co-workers[81] found that the symptoms of sciatica could be well reproduced during discography in two-thirds of patients with proven disc prolapse at surgery. Symptom provocation is less common in the presence of posterior annular tears and disc degeneration. Because symptoms arising from disc degeneration are not usually considered to need surgical treatment, it will always be difficult to obtain convincing proof of a specific lesion or syndrome.

Discography performed in 210 patients with back-hip-leg pain, but without disc prolapse, indicated disc degeneration was more common at the L4/5 and L5/S1 levels. When disc degeneration was present, the lower levels were more commonly symptomatic than the higher lumbar levels but, overall, asymptomatic disc degeneration was more common than symptom-producing changes (Table 12.2).

Fraser et al,[82] in a review of 370 discographically proven degenerate discs, found that symptomatic reproduction occurred most commonly when the contrast bulged into the dural canal in a collar-stud pattern, being contained by the peripheral annular fibres or the posterior longitudinal ligaments (Fig. 12.20(a)). When the contrast was contained, but did not extend beyond the confines of the normal annular margins, symptomatic reproduction was less

Table 12.2 Findings of lumbar discography in 210 patients with back-hip-leg pain without disc prolapse.

Level	L2–3 %	L3–4 %	L4–5 %	L5–S1 %
Normal	45	67	50	26
Symptomatic disc degeneration	10	10	25	24
Asymptomatic disc degeneration	45	23	25	50

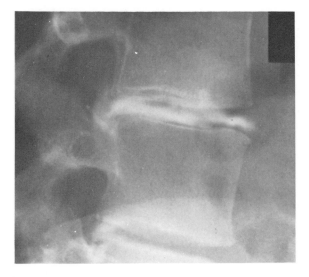

Fig. 12.20(a) The disc space is narrowed. The contrast medium extends throughout the disc and is contained by the outer fibres in a collar-stud fashion beyond the posterior vertebral margin.

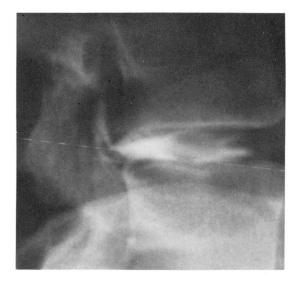

Fig. 12.20(b) Contrast delineates the degenerate disc but escapes posteriorly into the epidural space through a tear in the annulus.

common. If contrast escaped directly into the epidural space on injection, symptomatic reproduction was uncommon (Fig. 12.20(b)). These differences were found to be statistically significant (Table 12.3). It would therefore seem that symp-

Table 12.3 Radiological and symptomatic analysis of 370 proven degenerate discs.

	Symptomatic		Non-symptomatic		P
Contained	29	34%	57	6%	0.051
Herniated	90	76%	29	24%	0.001
Extravasated	35	21%	130	79%	0.001

tomatic pain at discography, and perhaps in the clinical setting, is more likely to occur with intradiscal pressure and tension which produces stretching of the outer annular fibres or the posterior longitudinal ligaments.

Radiological appearances

Contrast medium injected into the nucleus may assume a variety of appearances, depending on the morphology of the nucleus and the volume of injection.

Normal disc. The nucleus should always be clearly identified within the annulus fibrosus on all radiographic projections. A careful radiographic technique is essential, with collimation of the X-ray beam to provide optimum detail. the meglumine range of compounds or non-ionic contrast media provide satisfactory radiographic density of nuclear morphology. After removal of the puncture needle, it is possible to examine the behaviour of the nucleus under the stress of spinal movement (Fig. 12.21). Radiographic extravasation of contrast medium from the nucleus back along the needle track has not been observed following this manoeuvre on conventional radiography, but some contrast has been demonstrated in the needle tracks using CT.[83] An 18 gauge needle was used in these cases, however.

Damaged discs. A variety of different appearances are to be found as the disc becomes damaged. The distribution of the contrast within the nucleus and annulus then depends on the extent of the disruption.

Internal annular disruption. These lesions are characterized by circumferential tears between adjacent rings of the annulus fibrosus or radial tears in these fibres short of complete extension to the outer annular layers (Fig. 12.22).[84] There is no escape of nuclear fragments from the normal

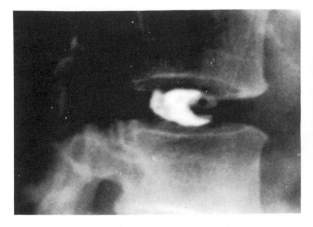

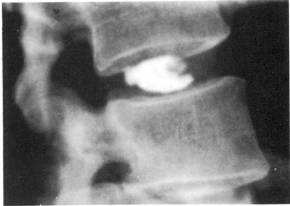

Fig. 12.21a Normal discogram–erect flexion. The nucleus is bilocular and acts as a pivotal moment during vertebral movement.

Fig. 12.21b Normal discogram–erect extension. The vertebra pivots backwards reducing the height of the intervertebral foramen and causing the posterior fibres of the annulus fibrosus to bulge into the spinal canal.

confines of the intervertebral disc space. The exact cause of symptoms is not clear, but may be either mechanical or chemical. The annulus may undergo diffuse bulging secondary to abnormal vertebral movements which stretches the outer innervated fibres of the annulus[85] and posterior longitudinal ligaments. Irritation of the structures adjacent to the affected disc, especially the sympathetic system, may be caused by catabolites diffusing out.[86] The pain in these patients is a deep-seated dull ache in the back, with widespread limb radiation often deep inside it. There is an absence of most physical signs. Flexion, however, particularly sitting up from the lying position, may be severely restricted. Discography is the only means of diagnosis. Concentric bands of contrast will be seen in the posterior annulus which

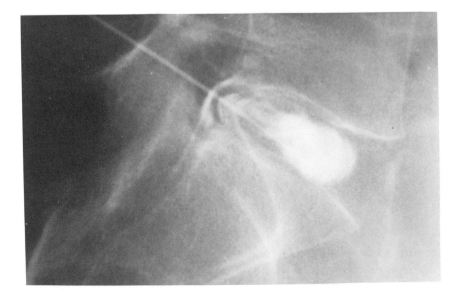

Fig. 12.22 The nucleus is of formal height and shape. Concentric rings of contrast are present in the posterior annulus, indicating disruption between annular fibres. No prolapse is present.

do not extend to the outer margin of the annulus. The disruption may involve one side, both or predominantly the central part of the annulus. When the contrast enters the disrupted disc, the symptomatic pain is reproduced in character and distribution.

Radial annulus rupture. Internal annular disruption may predispose to complete tears in the annulus.[1] Radial annular tears may also occur in previously normal discs in the presence of significant trauma. In these circumstances the clinical picture is often characteristic.[87] The patients are young adults with severe backache over a number of years and an absence of neurological signs or other definite evidence of prolapsed intervertebral disc. There is usually a history of a twisting or lifting injury or a fall at sport. Clinically they have severe disability due to back-hip-leg pain, with only muscle spasm on examination. Plain X-rays are normal and radiculography is usually negative or shows a mild central indentation of the dural sac without nerve root compression. Discography reveals a characteristic 'collar stud' extrusion of contrast extending from the nucleus into the outer fibres of the annulus fibrosus posteriorly (Fig. 12.23). In the small number of patients who have required surgery because of the degree of disability, the operative findings have been consistent. A rent without nuclear herniation has been found in the posterior annular fibres. Varying degrees of rupture are possible, and the natural history may be later nuclear prolapse, disc narrowing and disc degeneration. Inflammatory response is often seen extending into the tear from the outer annular margin. Pathological correlation of the lesion has been observed in the autopsy lumbar spine specimens from an 18-year-old motor cyclist who died in a road traffic accident. The discographic and dissection findings are illustrated in Figure 12.24.

Disc prolapse. There is quite a marked variation in the appearances of disc prolapse found at operation. In some patients there is an obvious localized bulge of the annulus, or when this is incised there may be a spontaneous and explosive extrusion of nuclear material. This is the protruded disc, and the nuclear material is confined solely by a few of the outermost fibres of the annulus. Discography will outline to the margin of the bulging annulus, and extension views will increase the prominence of the hernial sac. Conversely, it will be reduced by flexion. When the

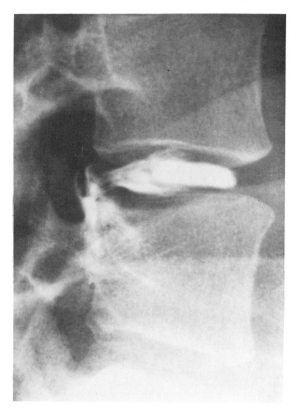

Fig. 12.23 Radial fissure of posterior annulus fibrosus.

nuclear material is extruded through a rent in the posterior annulus, it may be contained by the posterior intervertebral ligament. Contrast injected into the nucleus extrudes from the confines of the annulus fibrosus more than 3 mm beyond the posterior margins of the vertebral body. A radiolucent defect may appear within the pool of contrast, but this is often only seen on the oblique projections and represents the extruded disc fragment.[88] Contrast medium may be seen leaking into the epidural space after delineating the prolapse.

Finally, the nuclear material may be sequestered lying free in the spinal canal. Discography will not demonstrate this lesion, although sequestered tissue may be seen in a filling defect within the extravasated extradural contrast medium.[89]

The extrusions and sequestrations will usually impinge on the dural tube or emerging root sleeves. These types of lesions are, therefore, best demonstrated by water-soluble myelography or epidural

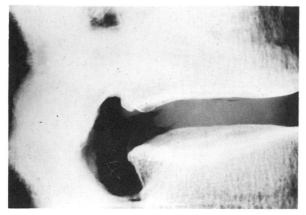

Fig. 12.24a During flexion, the posterior disc space is distracted causing intranuclear fissuring to become outlined by air. The defect in the annulus fibrosus is also revealed in this position.

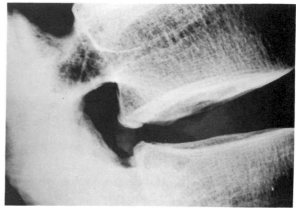

Fig. 12.24b In extension, the posterior disc space is compressed and the air is expelled. Air can now be identified in the anterior disc space within a narrow slit inferiorly. In this specimen, it is also possible to demonstrate the amount of annular bulging which occurs during extension.

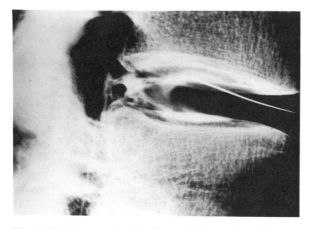

Fig. 12.24c Discography. The fissures have now been filled with contrast medium. In flexion, the contrast extravasates into epidural tissue through the fissure in the annulus fibrosus.

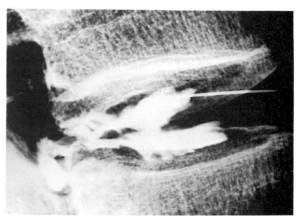

Fig. 12.24d In extension, the epidural extravasation of contrast medium remains localised.

venography. Protrusions, on the other hand, are best demonstrated by discography.

Interosseous extension of nucleus. Central or anterior interosseous disc herniation may occur. the most benign lesion is a small beak of contrast entering a Schmorl's node in the centre of the end-plate from an otherwise normal nucleus (Fig. 12.25). This is the commonest lesion and is not clinically significant. A more severe form of interosseous

herniation exists which is accompanied by considerable back pain. This follows significant compression/flexion stress to the spine in adolescent patients. The interosseous herniation is in the anterior third and is often accompanied by disc narrowing and poor definition of the end-plate defect. The injection often accurately reproduces the distribution of symptomatic pain[90] (Fig. 12.26).

A third form of this lesion is the nuclear extension

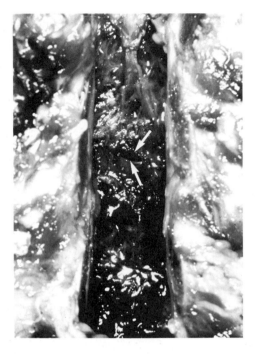

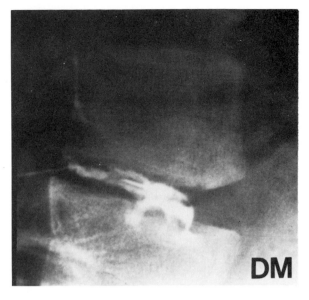

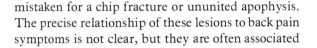

Fig. 12.26 Contrast delineates a partially degenerate disc. The interosseous herniation is outlined by contrast entering from the nucleus.

Fig. 12.24e Operative findings. The laminae and dura have been removed exposing the vertical rent in the posterior fibrosus (arrowed).

into the anterior aspects of the inferior end-plate, which is sclerotic. In some cases a discrete triangular bone fragment may be present which can be mistaken for a chip fracture or ununited apophysis. The precise relationship of these lesions to back pain symptoms is not clear, but they are often associated

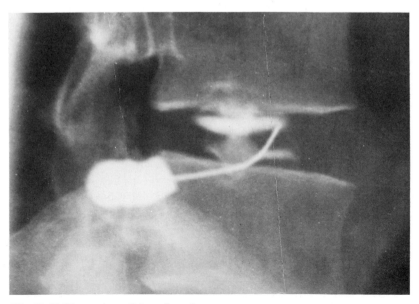

Fig. 12.25 Discogram — Schmorl's node.

with evidence of Scheuermann's disease in the thoracic spine and are likely to be due to the same aetiological mechanism.[91]

Disc degeneration. The nucleus pulposus normally provides the hydrostatic component of the disc, with a high proteoglycan, low collagen content and contains 80–90% water. As age progresses there is a gradual reduction in hydration of both the nucleus and annulus which reduces their capacity to withstand strain. As degeneration progresses, the nucleus becomes desiccated and splits, and clefts occur. Contrast injected into degenerate discs disperses in all directions, extending to the outer margins of the annulus. It is usually possible to inject 2 cc or more into the disc. Extravasation into the epidural space may occur, allowing an indefinite quantity of contrast to be injected. Degenerate discs are commonly asymptomatic, but when contrast is contained by the outer fibres of the annulus and the annulus bulges into the spinal canal, symptomatic pain is often present.[82] The loss of the nuclear cushioning action leads to abnormal movements in flexion and extension. In extension the posterior part of the disc becomes flattened, whereas in flexion the upper vertebra squats squarely on its neighbour due to widening of the posterior disc space (Fig. 12.27).

Post-discectomy syndromes. Patients who complain of persistence of pain following laminectomy or discectomy constitute a group that can be extremely difficult to manage clinically. Post-operative fibrosus and scarring will deform the dural sac and obscure the myelographic interpretation. Discography can be used in these patients to assess the condition of the operated disc and to exclude significant disease at adjacent levels. Occasionally, a post-operative defect of the annulus fibrosus persists and thus permits the free extravasation of contrast into the epidural space. The symptomatic examination is helpful in identifying the offending and significant level.

A negative myelogram provides only indirect evidence that the disc is normal, and discography is the only method that at present can confirm this. If surgical fusion is being considered, it is necessary to anticipate the effect that this will have on the rest of the spine. Additional stress will be imposed on the levels immediately adjacent to the immobilized segment, as the pivotal moment moves upwards. After a time, the disc above the level of fusion can begin to show evidence of damage and abnormal mobility even in quite young patients.[92] This complication is least likely to occur when a normal

Fig. 12.27 Disc degeneration-asymptomatic discogram injection

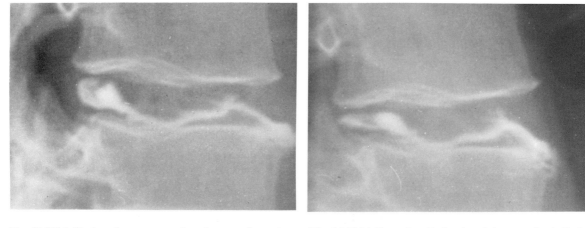

Fig. 12.27(a) Flexion. the upper vertebra sits squarely on the lower one due to widening of the posterior disc space. Note how the intervertebral forament opens out in this position.

Fig. 12.27(b) Extension. Deformity of the posterior half of the disc is marked during extension. No symptoms of pain were invoked during the discogram. There is a small degree of intra-osseous extravasation anteriorly.

disc forms a new fulcrum of movement following intervertebral fusion.[93]

Complications

Discography should be avoided if there is a likelihood of a large disc protrusion being present. In these cases it is possible to convert this into a complete spinal block and cauda equina lesion by injection of contrast medium. Contrast injections should be avoided if there is a convincing history of iodine sensitivity.

Discography is an invasive procedure and therefore carries with it a theoretical possibility of provoking damage or infection in the nucleus. Every precaution should be exercised in the selection of patients and procedural technique to minimize this possibility. In 1952, Cloward & Buziad[94] reported their experience with discography over a ten-year period. They were unable to find a single case where significant damage to a disc had followed the procedure. Collis & Gardner[88] described similar findings in a review of over 4000 injected discs. Nevertheless, occasional and infrequent complications have been reported.

Massie & Stevens[95] reported one disc-space infection in a series of 622 patients after discography. Wiley and associates[75] also found one instance of disc infection from a total of 2500 separate injections. De Haene[96] reported three patients with the same complication in 192 discograms. In every instance there was completely satisfactory recovery with conservative treatment and antibiotics, often leading to spontaneous intervertebral fusion. The examination should not be performed, however, if there is a focus of infection close to the site of puncture, such as pustules, or acne or systemically such as active sinuses, meningitis or vertebral osteomyelitis.

De Sèze and Levernieux[97] carefully followed up 55 patients after discography over a period of 12 months and detected a loss of intervertebral disc space height in 13 patients.

Post-discographic damage has been intensively investigated both by direct examination of nuclear material, removed at operation and by experimental models. In an animal experiment, Garrick & Sullivan[98] could find no gross microscopic, or radiological abnormality in discs that had been subjected to discography. On the other hand, Key & Ford[99] performed needle-puncture experiments on 14 dogs and found one histological example of nuclear material extending through the needle track into the fibres of the annulus fibrosus.

The vulnerability of the intervertebral disc to injury has been assessed in cadaveric experiments. Freiberg[100] subjected spine specimens to passive flexion and extension following puncture of the annulus fibrosus with a wide-bore needle. No extrusion of nuclear material could be demonstrated, even with the largest-calibre needle. The bursting pressure of intervertebral discs in the cadaver has also been studied.[89,101] In the normal disc this is extremely high and certainly far in excess of the injection pressure achieved at discography.

Disc material removed at surgery from patients who have previously undergone discography does not differ histologically from control specimens. Goldie,[102] however, did find that approximately 50% of the specimens showed a number of small droplets refractive to light, which were considered to represent some form of reaction between the contrast medium and the nucleus pulposus. Perey[103] reported no histological evidence of tissue necrosis in the discs of a patient who died of a non-related abdominal condition shortly after discography.

Repeat discography has been performed on a small number of patients with long-standing symptoms and the suspicion of disc disease. Massare[104] noted that a second discogram had been performed in 6 patients in a series of 500. The initial discogram was normal in each patient and in 5 out of the 6 on the second examination. Gresham & Miller[3] reported one patient in whom a second discogram had been performed 7 years after the first. On both occasions the discogram was normal.

Predictive value of discography

It is evident from post-mortem studies that discography demonstrates the morphology of the intervertebral disc very accurately. In 1952 Erlacher[105] reported a study of 200 discograms that had been performed on cadavers. After a mixture of methylene blue and water-soluble contrast had been injected, the dispersal could be accurately determined directly by visualization and indirectly on film. Complete agreement was found between the radiographic distribution of the contrast medium throughout the disc space and the extent of straining by the dye.

The morphological accuracy of discography is most readily translated into the clinical field in the diagnosis of disc prolapse. This is also the anomaly that is most easily correlated, as surgical verification is readily available. Early protagonists of the technique used it to confirm disc prolapse, and most authors considered it an adjunct to myelography. Collis & Gardener,[88] however, claimed its superiority for the method over myelography. Massare[104] and his associates performed discograms on 31 patients clinically suspected of having disc prolapse but with negative or equivocal radiculography. Discography revealed frank disc protrusion in 24 patients and degeneration in the remainder.

Recently, Hudgins[107] has studied the accuracy of lumbar discography in disc herniation, subjecting the data from different centres to predictive value analyses. A positive discogram showed herniation and a normal or degenerative pattern were classified as negative, the latter because surgical treatment was not performed for this condition. It was concluded that lumbar discography has an 83% sensitivity (false negative rate of 17%) and a 78% specificity (false positive rate of 22%). The diagnostic accuracy of discography in patients with back, hip or leg pain without disc herniation is more difficult to assess. The discographic results have to be assessed against the outcome of surgery, but the type of surgical treatment may vary.

Simmons & Segil[80] compared the value of clinical study, myelography and discography in 361 patients. These patients had undergone either discectomy alone, discectomy with fusion, or fusion alone. Analysis was based on relief or significant improvement of pre-operative symptoms by operation at the particular level or levels selected by the pre-operative assessment. Their results indicated that discography was the most accurate method, with an 82.2% accuracy rate, as opposed to 44.2% for clinical examination and 45.6% for myelography.

Brodsky & Binder[105] performed discography on over 1500 patients but reported a detailed series of 199 cases in which they found that in 155 (78%) discography had significantly influenced the operative decisions, 69.4% of positive discograms were

matched by full pain replication and 13.6% had partial pain reproduction. They concluded that lumbar discography is a valuable adjunct in the diagnosis of lumbar disc lesions and as a decision-making tool in the treatment of lumbar discopathy subjects. Milette & Melanson[106] studied 500 patients whose Pantopaque® myelograms were considered negative, dubious or inconclusive. 320 discs were normal, of which 95% were painless and 5% had reproduction of clinical symptoms. These, however, were viewed with scepticism in view of medico-legal implications in most cases. 52% of diseased discs were not associated with pain on injection, and 37% reproduced symptoms. The remaining 11% caused pain which differed from normal symptoms. The examination proved the major determinant factor in the surgeon's decision. 97.3% of those patients submitted to operation, had abnormal discograms and reproduction of symptoms was present in 73%.

SELECTIVE NERVE ROOT INJECTION

Macnab[107] has indicated a number of situations where irrefutable clinical evidence of root irritation may still lead to a negative surgical exploration. Investigation prior to surgery in these cases may have failed to demonstrate an abnormality, although the advent of water-soluble contrast investigations and CT scanning has reduced the number of false negatives.

Even with these sophisticated methods, more than one level of pathology may be demonstrated, and the problems of interpretation are even greater in the post-operative state.[108] In these circumstances, selective nerve root injections may be of diagnostic value.[107,109] Krempen & Smith[110] have also suggested that it is primarily indicated for patients with sciatica and multiple surgical procedures or those patients with sciatica in whom the myelograms, discograms and electromyograms are not diagnostic.

Technique

The lumbar nerve roots are approached just after their passage around the pedicle and under the transverse process of their related vertebral bodies. Needle placement for the sacral nerve roots is via the sacral foramina. The patient lies prone and a needle is inserted for the fifth lumbar root, at an angle of 45° perpendicular to the back, approximately 6cm lateral to the midline. Movement in a cephalad direction with subsequent caudal angulation may be necessary in some instances. To avoid the iliac crest, the needle is advanced down to the emerging nerve root and the patient usually experiences a sharp stab of nerve root pain when the root is found. This pain is evaluated for site and character. 0.2–0.5 ml of a non-ionic water-soluble contrast medium are injected to delineate the nerve root sleeve which has a characteristic linear appearance (Fig. 12.28). Alterations in anatomy may be demonstrated due to disc herniation or pedicle kinking. Roetgenographic interpretation of the pattern of contrast medium may be misleading, especially if fibrosis is present. Finally,

0.5 ml of Bivocaine® (Marcaine® 0.5%) are injected into the sleeve, and relief of pain should be evident within a few minutes.

The S1 nerve root is more difficult to inject. The first sacral foramen is approached to the back — angles varying from perpendicular to 45°. This requires image intensification, and the foramen may be difficult to visualize. The first sacral nerve root lies in the sacral canals, and the anterior primary division exists from the sacral foramen anteriorly. The nerve root must, therefore, be localized by the clinician placing the needle directly into the first sacral foramen.

Krempen & Smith[110] describe the use of nerve sleeve injections in 22 selected patients who had had previous laminectomies and multiple investigations. Four cases had no reproduction of pain on needle

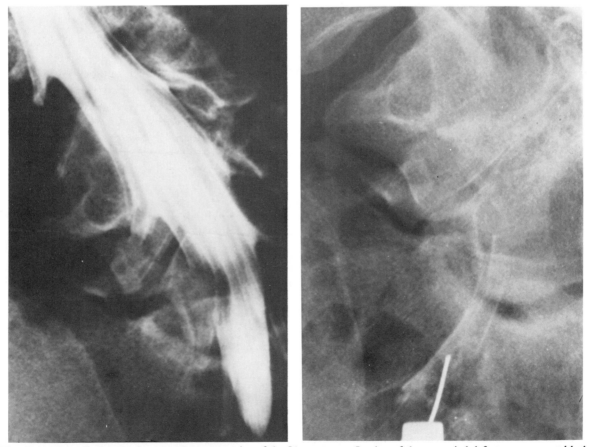

Fig. 12.28 The radiculogram demonstrates compression of the S1 nerve root. In view of the congenital defect, a nerve root block was performed to confirm this as the total source of symptoms. Contrast is demonstrated flowing along the line of the S1 nerve root sleeve.

insertion. The remainder were able to pin-point the level of the lesion to either of two levels. Sixteen of these patients underwent repeat exploration. Two had retained disc material, one had bone entrapment in the lateral recess and the remainder had scar tissue. All patients responded well to surgery.

More recently, Kikuchi et al[111] have reported examinations on 332 patients with radicular pain from a number of causes. They found it very useful in the 19.5% of patients where the clinical neurological findings did not correlate with the affected level on the contrast studies, or regarding which of a number of radiologically abnormal levels was the cause of the symptoms. The study indicated that single nerve root involvement was common in spondylosis or degenerative spondylolisthesis, irrespective of the number of levels involved in contrast studies. These authors also recorded a therapeutic value for these injections, with some cases of long-term pain relief in the disc prolapse group.

The specificity of nerve root blocks is open to question. If the area around the nerve root is injected especially close to the foramen, the sinuvertebral nerve may also be affected, leading to anaesthesia of the dura and posterior longitudinal ligament. If pain originates from these structures, a false assessment of the problem of sciatica may be reached. However, if the needle is in the root sleeve, it is relatively certain that the pain originates from irritation of the root, not the adjacent structure. Therefore, with care in needle placement and limitation in the amount of local anaesthetic injected, nerve root sleeve injections can prove a useful diagnostic adjunct in disc disease.

FACET ARTHROGRAPHY

The spinal apophyseal joints are an integral part of the motor segment and, as such, are directly affected by any change in the status of the intervertebral disc. The facet is no different from any other synovial joint where pain may originate from the synovial capsule, ligaments or surrounding soft tissues. Isolated apophyseal joint disease may follow a traumatic episode, but usually facet arthrosis accompanies disc degeneration. It is therefore important to identify the precise origin of the low back pain. Unfortunately, because of the close proximity of many facet joints and their depth beneath the skin surfaces, it is more difficult for the patient to describe where the pain is felt or for the clinician to elicit physical signs of joint damage.

The use of provocation techniques may also, therefore, be of value in isolating individual painful pathological facet joints. The facet capsule is punctured by a spinal needle under fluoroscopic control. A small quantity of water-soluble contrast medium may be injected to confirm the intracapsular position (Fig. 12.29). The capacity of each joint varies from 0.5 ml in the higher lumbar spine, to 1ml at the lower levels. A small quantity of local anaesthetic may then be injected and the response of symptoms monitored.

A full account of facet arthrography and its place in the facet pain syndrome is found in Chapter 18.

CONCLUSION

The clinical and radiological investigation of patients with back, buttock and leg pain should be entirely influenced by individual circumstances. Fortunately, for most subjects the episode is transient and self-limiting. Symptoms may, however, persist, and plain radiographs are valuable to identify occasionally a specific single-level pathological process. They also have a therapeutic value by reassuring the patient and physician that continued conservative therapy is justified.

If symptoms are severe enough to warrant consideration of surgery, comprehensive radiological investigation is required to assist in planning the most appropriate procedure. If nerve root embarrassment is clinically evident, then investigations such as radiculography or ascending lumbar venography are indicated. On the other hand, if pain of a non-dermatomal nature is experienced, discography with pain assessment is the investigation of choice. By this means, symptomatic and asymptomatic degenerate discs can be identified, normality of discs can be confirmed and the specific discogenic pain syndromes can be identified.

Care should always be taken to avoid the concept of the routine radiological examination, and the number of procedures should be restricted to those providing necessary information for management.

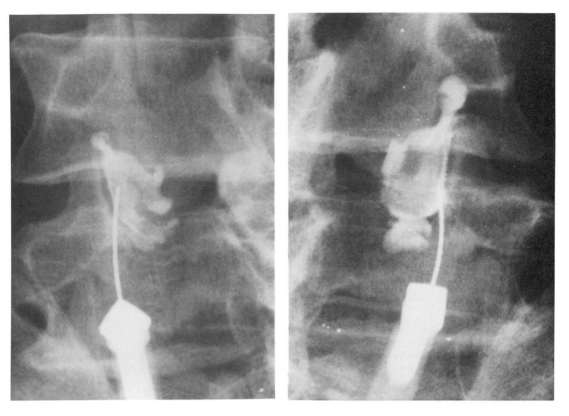

Fig. 12.29 Lumbar facet arthrogram. Oblique projection showing the interarticular joint space (left). Showing the superior and inferior articular recesses (right).

On the other hand, radiologists should not retreat from the use of invasive techniques when value has been substantiated in cases where substantial therapy is being contemplated.

REFERENCES

1   Schmorl G, Junghanns H 1971 The human spine in health and disease, 2nd American edn. Grune & Stratton, New York

2   Dillane J B, Fry J, Kalton G 1966 Acute back syndrome — a study from general practice. Br. Med. J. 2: 82–84

3   Eisenberg R L, Akin J R, Hedgcock M D 1979 Single well-centred lateral view of lumbosacral spine: Is coned view necessary? Am. J. Roentgenol. 133: 711–713

4   Scavone J G, Latshaw R F, Weidner W A 1981 Antero-posterior and lateral radiographs. An adequate lumbar spine examination. Am. J. Roentgenol. 136: 715–717

5   Gresham J L, Miller R 1969 Evaluation of the lumbar spine by discography and its use in selection of proper treatment of the herniated disc syndrome. Clin. Orth. Rel. Res. 67: 29–41

6   Begg C A, Falconer M A 1949 Plain radiography in intraspinal protrusion of lumbar intervertebral discs: a correlation with operative findings. Br. J. Surg. 36 (143): 225–239

7   Epstein B 1969 The spine — a radiological text and atlas, 3rd edn. Lea & Febinger,

8   Magara A, Schwartz A 1976 Relation between low back pain syndrome and X-ray findings. 1. Degenerative osteoarthritis. Scand. J. Rehab. Med. 8: 115–125

9   Splithoff C A 1953 Lumbosacral junction — roentgenographic comparison of patients with and without backache. J. Am. Med. Assn 152: 1610–1613

10 Lawrence J S 1969 Disc degeneration: its frequency and relationship to symptoms. Ann. Rheum. Dis. 28: 121–137

11 Harris R I, Macnab I 1954 Structural changes in the lumbar intervertebral disc. J. Bone Joint Surg. 36B: 304

12 Andersson G B J, Schultz A, Nathan A, Irstam L 1981 Roentgenographic measurement of lumbar intervertebral disc height. Spine 6: 154–158

13 Knutsson F 1944 The instability associated with disc degeneration in the lumbar spine. Acta Radiol. 25: 593–609

14 Larde D, Mathieu D, Frija J, Gaston A, Vasile N 1982

Spinal vacuum phenomenon: CT diagnosis and significance

15 Ford L T, Gilula L A, Murphy W A, Gado M 1977 Analysis of gas in vacuum lumbar disc. Am. J. Roentgenol. 128: 1056–1057

16 Edeiken J, Pitt M J 1971 The radiological diagnosis of disc disease — symposium on disease of the intervertebral disc. Orth. Clin. N. Am. 2: 405

17 Resnick D 1982 Letter to the Editor. Spine 7: 86–88

18 Macnab I 1971 The traction spur. J. Bone Joint Surg. 53A: 663–670

19 Quinnell R C, Stockdale H R 1982 The significance of osteophytes on lumbar vertebral bodies in relation to discographic findings. Clin. Radiol. 33: 197–203

20 Schumachen T M, Genant H K, Kellet M J, Mall J C, Fye K H 1978 HLA-B27 associated arthropathies. Radiology 126: 289–297

21 Farfan H F, Cossette J W, Robertson G H, Wells R V, Kraus H 1970 Effects of torsion on the lumbar intervertebral joints. J. Bone Joint Surg. 52A: 468–497

22 Adams M A, Hutton W C, Stott J R R 1980 The resistance to flexion of the lumbar intervertebral joint. Spine 3: 245–253

23 Frederickson B E, Baker D, McHolick W J, Yuan H A, Lubicky J P 1984 The natural history of spondylosis and spondylolisthesis. J. Bone Joint Surg. 66A: 699–707

24 Hitchcock H H 1940 Spondylolisthesis: observations on its development, progression and genesis. J. Bone Joint Surg. 22: 1–16

25 Wiltse L L 1957 Etiology of spondylolisthesis. Clin. Orth. Rel. Res. 10: 48–59

26 McPhee I B, O'Brien J P, McCall I W, Park W M 1981 Progression of lumbosacral spondylolisthesis. Australasian Radiology 25: 91–95

27 Speck G R, McCall I W, O'Brien J P 1984 Spondylolisthesis. The angle of kyphosis. Spine (In press)

28 Allbrook D 1941 Posterior protrusion of the lumbar intervertebral disc. J. Bone Joint Surg. 23: 444–456

29 Jirout J 1957 The normal mobility of the lumbosacral spine. Acta Radiol. 47: 345

30 Gianturco L 1944 A roentgen analysis of the motion of the lower lumbar vertebrae in normal individuals and in patients with low back pain. Am. J. Roentgenol. 52: 261

31 Morgan F P, King T 1957 Primary instability of lumbar vertebrae as a common cause of low back pain. J. Bone Joint Surg. 39B (1): 6–22

32 Pennal G F, Conn G S, McDonald G, Dale G, Garside H 1972 Motion studies of the lumbar spine. A preliminary report. J. Bone Joint Surg. 54B: (3) 442–452

33 Abel M S 1977 The unstable apophyseal joint: an early sign of lumbar disc disease. Skeletal Radiol. 2: 31–37

34 Quinnell R C, Stockdale H R 1983 Flexion and extension radiography of the lumbar spine: a comparison with lumbar discography. Clin. Radiol. 34: 405–411

35 Akkerveeken P van, O'Brien J P, Park W M 1979 Experimentally induced hypermobility in the lumbar spine. Spine 4: 236–241

36 Pearcy M, Burrough S 1982 Assessment of bony union after interbody fusion of the lumbar spine, using a biplanar radiographic technique. J. Bone Joint Surg. 64B: 228–232

37 Vernon H 1982 Static and dynamic roentgenography in the diagnosis of degenerative disc disease. A review and comparative assessment. J. Manip. Physiol. Therap. 5: 163–169

38 Stokes I A F, Wilder D G, Frymoyer J W, Pope M H 1981 Assessment of patients with low back pain by biplanar radiographic measurement of intervertebral motion. Spine 6: 233–240

39 Froning E C, Frohman B 1968 Motion of the lumbosacral spine after laminectomy and spine fusion. J. Bone Joint Surg. 50A: 897–918

40 White A H, Wiltse L L 1976 Spondylolisthesis after extensive lumbar laminectomy. Proc. Am. Acad. Ortho. Surg.

41 Hazlett J W, Kinnard P 1982 Lumbar apophyseal process excision and spinal instability. Spine 7: 171–176

42 O'Brien J F, Evans G 1978 Pain topics. Surgical removal of ruptured lumbar discs. A five-year follow-up. (7): 5

43 Lowe R W, Hayes T D, Kaye J, Bagg R J, Leukens C A 1976 Standing roentgenograms in spondylolisthesis. Clin. Orth. Rel. Res. 117: 80–84

44 Edgar M A, Park W M 1974 Patterns of induced pain produced on passive straight leg raising — a clinical, myelographic and operative study. J. Bone Joint Surg. 56B (4): 658–667

45 Grainger R G, Kendall B E, Wylie I G 1976 Lumbar myelography with metrizamide — a new non-ionic contrast medium. Br. J. Radiol. 49: 996–1003

46 Irstam L 1978 Lumbar myelography with Amipaque®. Spine 3: 70–82

47 Kendall B, Schneidan A, Stevens J, Harrison M 1983 Clinical trial of Iohexol® for lumbar myelography. Br. J. Radiol. 56: 539–542

48 Schlesinger J J, Salit I E, McCormack G 1982 Streptococcal meningitis after myelography. Arch. Neurol. 39: 576–577

49 Jepson K, Nada A, Rymaszewski L 1982 The role of radiculography in the management of lesions of the lumbar disc. J. Bone Joint Surg. 64B: 405–408

50 Nachemson A 1976 The lumbar spine: an orthopaedic challenge. Spine 1: 59–71

51 Hirsch C, Nachemson A 1963 The reliability of lumbar disc surgery. Clin. Orth. Rel. Res. 29: 189–194

52 Holmes E, Rothman R H 1979 The Pennsylvania plan. An algorithm for the managment of lumbar degenerative disc disease. Spine 4: 156–162

53 Hansen E B, Praestholm J, Fahrenkrug A, Bjeraum J 1976 A clinical trial of Amipaque® for lumbar myelography. Br. J. Radiol. 49: 34–38

54 Herkowitz H N, Wiesel S W, Booth R E, Rothman R H 1982 Metrizamide myelography and epidural venography. Their role in the diagnosis of lumbar disc herniation and spinal stenosis. Spine 7: 55–64

55 Trowbridge W V, French J D 1954 The 'false positive' lumbar myelogram. Neurology (Minneap) 4: 339–344

56 Wilberger J E, Dachling Pang 1983 Syndrome of the incidental herniated lumbar disc. J. Neurosurg. 59: 137–141

57 Knuttson F 1942 Volum- und Formulariationen des Wirbelkanals bei Lordosierung und Kyposierung und ihre Bedeutung für die Myelographische. Acta Radiol. Diagnos. 23: 431–443

58 Breig A 1978 Adverse mechanical tension in the central

nervous system. Stockholm Almqvist and Wiksell International

59 Euinton H A, Locke T J, Barrington N A, Getty C J M, Davies G K 1984 Radiological diagnosis of bony entrapment of lumbar nerve roots using water soluble radiculography. Proc. Intern. Soc. Study Lumbar Spine, Montreal. Orthopaedic Transactions (In press)

60 Gershater R, Holgate R C 1976 Lumbar epidural venography in the diagnosis of disc herniations. Am J. Roentgenol. 126: 992–1008

61 Theron J, Houtteville J P, Ammerich H, Alves de Souza A, Adam H et al 1976 Lumbar phlebography by catheterization of the lateral sacral and ascending lumbar veins with abdominal compression. Neuroradiology 11: 175–182

62 Macnab I, St. Louis E L, Grabias S L, Jacob R 1976 Selective ascending lumbosacral venography in the assessment of lumbar disc herniation. J. Bone Joint Surg. 58A (8): 1093–1098

63 Lepage J R 1974 Transfemoral ascending lumbar catheterization of the epidural veins. Exposition and technique. Radiology 111: 337–339

64 McCall I W, Cosgrove H Unpublished data

65 Nagamine K 1970 Clinical and biochemical study of accidents in periurography. Nagoya J. Med. Sci. 32: 429–444

66 Bromage P R, Bramwell R, Stuart B, Catchlove R F H, Belanger G, Pearce C G A 1978 Radiology 128: 123–126

67 Husemeyer R P 1978 Pain topics. A word of caution regarding injections into the lumbar epidural space

68 Lewitt K 1976 The contribution of peridurography to the anatomy of the lumbosacral canal. Folia Marphol (Praha) 24: 289–295

69 Luyendijk W 1963 Canalography, roentgenological examination of the peridural space in the lumbosacral part of the vertebral column. Belge Radiol. 46: 236–253

70 Roberson G H, Hatten H P, Hesselink J H 1979 Epidurography. Selective catheter technique and review of 53 cases. Am. J. Roentgenol. 132: 787–793

71 Hatten H P 1980 Lumbar epidurography with metrizamide. Radiology 137: 129–136

72 Mathews J A 1976 Epidurography. In: Jayson M I V (ed) The lumbar spine and back pain. Sector, London

73 Lindblom K 1948 Diagnostic puncture of intervertebral discs in sciatica. Acta Orth. Scand. 17: 231

74 Quinnell R C, Stockdale H R 1980 Pressure standardised lumbar discography. Br. J. Radiol. 53: 1031–1036

75 Wiley J J, Macnab I, Wortzman G 1968 Lumbar discography and its clinical applications. Canad. J. Surg. 11: 280

76 Quinnell R C, Stockdale H R 1980 An investigation of artefacts in lumbar discography. Br. J. Radiol. 53: 831–839

77 Holt A P 1968 The question of lumbar discography. J. Bone Joint Surg. 50A: 720–725

78 Tuohimaa P J, Melartin E 1970 Neurotoxicity of iothalamates and diatrizoates. II. Historadioautographic study of rat brains with iodine-tagged contrast media. Invest. Radiol. (Philadelphia) 5: 22

79 Fischer H W, Redman H C 1971 Comparison of a sodium methylgucamine diatrizoate contrast medium of minimal sodium content with a pure methylglucamine diatrizoate preparation. Invest. Radiol. (Philadelphia) 6 (2): 115

80 Simmons E H, Segil C M 1975 An evaluation of discography in the localisation of symptomatic levels in discogenic disease of the spine. Clin. Orth. Rel. Res. 108: 57–69

81 Gardner W J, Wise R E, Hughes C R, O'Connell F B, Weiford E C 1952 The X-ray visualisation of the intervertebral disc with a consideration of the morbidity of disc puncture. Arch. Surg. 64: 355

82 Fraser J, McCall I W, Park W M, O'Brien J P 1983 Discography in degenerating disc disease. Orth. Trans. 7: 466

83 McCutcheon M E, Thompson III W C 1984 CT scanning of lumbar discography: a useful diagnostic adjunct. Proc. Intern. Soc. Study Lumbar Spine, Montreal

84 Crock H V 1970 A reappraisal of intervertebral disc lesions. Med. J. Austr. 1: 983–989

85 Yoshizawa H, O'Brien J P 1980 The neuropathy of intervertebral discs removed for low back pain. J. Path. 132: 95–104

86 Nachemson A 1969 Intradiscal measurements of pH in patients with lumbar rhizopathies. Acta Orth. Scand. 40: 23–42

87 Park W M, McCall I W, O'Brien J P, Webb J K 1979 Fissuring of the posterior annulus fibrosus in the lumbar spine. Br. J. Radiol. 52: 382–387

88 Collis J S, Gardner W J 1962 Lumbar discography — an analysis of 1000 cases. J. Neurosurg. 19: 452

89 Walk L 1953 Diagnostic lumbar disc puncture. Arch. Surg. 66: 232

90 Park W M, Seal P, O'Brien J P, McCall I W 1981 Acute traumatic intraosseous disc herniation. Proc. Intern. Soc. Study Lumbar Spine, Paris

91 Alexander C J 1977 Scheuermann's disease. A traumatic spondylodystrophy? Skeletal Radiology 1: 209–221

92 Calabrese A S, Freiberger R H 1963 Acquired spondylolysis after spinal fusion. Radiology 81: 492

93 Harris R I, Wiley J J 1963 Acquired spondylolysis as a sequel to spinal fusion. J. Bone Joint Surg. 45A: 1159–1170

94 Cloward R B, Buzaid L L 1952 Discography technique — indications and evaluation of normal and abnormal intervertebral disc. Am. J. Roentgenol. 68: 552

95 Massie W K, Stevens D B 1967 A critical evaluation of discography. J. Bone Joint Surg. 49A: 1243

96 De Haene R 1971 La discographie lombaire. J. Belge Radiol. 54 (III): 403

97 De Sèze S, Levernieux J 1952 Accidents in discography. Revue du Rhumatisme 19: 1027

98 Garrick J G, Sullivan C R 1970 Long-term effects of discography in dogs. Minnesota Medicine 53: 1027

99 Key J A, Ford L T 1948 Experimental intervertebral disc lesions. J. Bone Joint Surg. 30A: 621

100 Freiberg S 1941 Low back pain and sciatica by intervertebral disc herniation — anatomical and clinical investigation. Acta Chirurg. Scand. 85: Suppl 64

101 Jayson M I V, Herbert C M, Barks J S 1973 Intervertebral discs: nuclear morphology and bursting pressures. Ann. Rheum. Dis. 32: 308

102 Goldie I 1957 Intervertebral disc changes after discography. Acta Chirurg. Scand. 13: 438

103 Perey O 1950 Contrast medium examination of the intervertebral discs of the lower lumbar spine. Acta Orth. Scand. 20 (4): 327

104 Massare C 1970 Réflexions sur la discographie après 500 cas. J. Radiol. d'Électrol. Méd. Nucléaire (Paris) 51: 571

105 Brodsky A E, Binder W F 1979 Lumbar discography. Its value in diagnosis and treatment of lumbar disc lesions. Spine 4: 110–120

106 Milette P C, Melanson D 1982 A reappraisal of lumbar discography. J. Assoc. Canad. Radiol. 33: 176–182

107 Macnab I 1971 Negative disc exploration. J. Bone Joint Surg. 53A: 891–903

108 Coventry M B, Stauffer R N 1969 The multiple operated back. In: Symposium on the spine. American Academy of Orthopaedic Surgeons. Mosby, St Louis, p 132–142

109 Schultz H, Longheed W M, Wortzman G, Awerbuck B G 1973 Intervertebral nerve root in the investigation of chronic lumbar disc disease. Canad. J. Surg. 16: 217–221

110 Krempen J F, Smith B S 1974 Nerve root injection. J. Bone Joint Surg. 56A: 1435–1444

111 Kikuchi S, Hasue M, Nishiyama K, Ho T 1984 Anatomic and clinical studies of radicular symptoms. Spine 9: 23–30

New investigative techniques
CT scanning in the assessment of lumbar spine problems

INTRODUCTION

Conventional X-ray transmission techniques, despite increasing sophistication of both clinical and radiological procedure, provide only differential 'shadowgrams'. The problems of both imaging the bony spine and its neural content related to the presentation of three-dimensional information on two-dimensional recording media, together with the acquisition of quantitative data concerning both bone and soft tissues.

Computerized transmission tomography (CT) employing X-rays enables a transaxial section of finite thickness, usually 10 mm or less, to be demonstrated without blurring interference from surrounding structures. The cross-sectional reconstruction is based on precise X-ray attenuation characteristics of biological tissue. These digitally-derived data permit quantitative interrogation.

CT, whilst providing a highly efficient system of using X-rays, is neither operator-dependent nor organ-specific. It, therefore, provides much additional information about related organs and structures and their involvement in disease processes. The impact of CT on diagnostic management has been dramatic, first in the investigation of brain disorders and later in the spine and other parts of the body. Success has resulted from the high sensitivity of the method to very small changes in X-ray attenuation occurring in soft tissue and accompanying disease processes.

The radiological armamentarium for the investigation of spinal disorders is now very extensive and some of it potentially hazardous. Computerized tomography is a non-invasive procedure which provides, in the first instance, an axial projection of spinal topographical anatomy against a detailed background of paravertebral muscles, vascular structures and body cavity organs. Further computer processing of the basic digital data enables sagittal, coronal or oblique planes to be re-formated. It enables an assessment of the shape and size of the spinal canal to be made, and in particular presents a more precise location of the apophyseal joint articular surfaces, together with their relationship to the spinal canal and intervertebral foramina. Herniated disc material can be identified on unenhanced scans, but the introduction of a suitable low osmolarity contrast material into the subarachnoid space permits the better study of neural tissue and the pathological processes affecting it.

PHYSICAL BASIS OF COMPUTERIZED TOMOGRAPHY

Computerized tomography was introduced as a diagnostic imaging tool by Hounsfield in 1972.[1,2] The mathematical techniques of image reconstruction had been considered earlier. Computerized tomography employs collimated X-rays directed only at the layer under investigation. Radiographic film is replaced by sensitive scintillation or ionization detectors. If then a sufficient number of projection or views are obtained across this plane of interest, an image can be derived from the measurements of transmitted radiation intensities.

Various types of scanning motion have been employed incorporating different detector systems, from the early rotate and translate machines to rotate-only instruments featuring fixed detector rings. The data acquisition time can now be less than 2 seconds for one section. From the recorded transmission measurements the distribution of attenuation coefficients in the scanned section can be computed as a matrix of numbers, usually 320×320 or 512×512. Each number relates to a volume of tissue (voxel) of which the size is determined by the resolution of the scan and the depth of the section. The numbers are very precisely related to the difference between the attenuation coefficients of the material scanned and water and are termed Hounsfield numbers (H). The scale of numbers usually ranges from –1000 to +1000, i.e. from air to bone, with water as 0. Most biological tissue in the body occupies only a small fraction (3%) of this range, close to water values.

The distribution of attenuation coefficients expressed as Hounsfield numbers may, by digital-to-analogue conversion, be displayed as a grey level picture on a television monitor. High numbers, e.g. bone, are white, and low numbers, e.g. air, are black. The picture so produced from digital information has the unique property that it may be interrogated by the observer. Both the level on the Hounsfield scale, i.e. window level (WL) and the number of Hounsfield units displayed, i.e. window width (WW), may be varied and thus the whole dynamic range of body tissues explored.

Hard copy or film obtained from the television display and selected by the observer represents only a fraction of the information contained within the numerically-derived image. The basic principles of CT and the main methods of computing tomographic cross-sections from transmission measurements have been comprehensively reviewed in the literature.[3,4]

ANATOMY

CT sections of conventional depth, i.e. 10 mm, in 'ideal' position, i.e. without spinal curvature, demonstrate appearances related specifically to the level of the section. The detailed appearances of CT of the lumbar spine have now been well reviewed.[5-9]

Upper segment of vertebral body

The contour of the spinal canal is continuous and formed by a concave posterior margin on the vertebral body, vertically oriented pedicles and the caudally convergent laminae in the base of the spinous process. The spinal canal is triangular, with an interlaminar notch at the apex. The transverse processes are well seen. The cortico-medullary boundary in the vertebral body is indistinct (Fig. 13.1(a)).

Central vertebral body

The intervertebral foramina play an increasingly important part in the lateral margins of the spinal canal. The dorsolateral walls are formed by the posterior articular processes of the pars inter-articularis. The spinal canal is triangular. The corticomedullary boundary zone is clearly identifiable, with a dense cortical anterior margin to the vertebral body (Fig. 13.1(b)).

Lower segment of vertebral body

The bony ring of the spinal canal is discontinuous, due to the intervertebral foramina forming the lateral wall. The superior articular facets of the adjacent caudal segment form the dorsal margins of the intervertebral foramina and are, therefore, centrally situated at the apophyseal joints. The upper aspects of the apophyseal joints are situated at an approximate angle of 50° to the coronal plane; the inferior articular facets and laminae form the dorsal margin of the spinal canal. The canal at its most capacious is clearly influenced by the articular segments. The anterior margin of the vertebral body is ill-defined at the disc margins (Fig. 13.1(c)).

Intervertebral disc level

The intervertebral foramina form the lateral wall of the spinal canal, which therefore appears discontinuous. The apophyseal joints and the laminae form the dorsal margins. A 10 mm section through and in the same plane as the intervertebral disc must incorporate the bony margins of the adjacent vertebral bodies, which therefore appear indistinct, especially anteriorly (Fig. 13.1(d)).

LIMITATIONS

Despite the obvious advantages offered by CT there are significant constraints limiting its full exploitation.

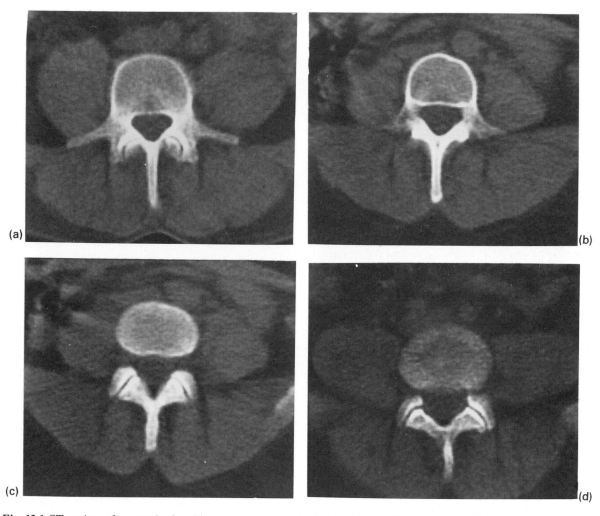

Fig. 13.1 CT sections of a normal spine: (a) upper segment vertebral body; (b) central vertebral body; (c) lower segment of vertebral body; (d) intervertebral disc level.

Physical

There is a fixed and immutable physical relationship between resolution, i.e. picture sharpness or picture element size, sensitivity (i.e. density discrimination or signal-to-noise ratio) and radiation dose. This may be expressed as

$$\frac{\text{dose} \propto (\text{signal-to-noise ratio})^2}{\text{resolution}^3}$$

To improve the information content of an image without incurring a radiation-dose penalty requires a trade-off between density discrimination, i.e. signal-to-noise ratio, and resolution. At a fixed dose, as resolution improves, the signal-to-noise ratio reduces and the ability to see low-contrast objects deteriorates. Optimal conditions depend on the size and contrast of the structure under investigation.

Significant statistical fluctuations occur in the quantitative data relating to the near-isodense spinal canal contents. Identification of neural tissue is therefore particularly unreliable without recourse to contrast material in the subarachnoid space or significant changes in both resolution and density discrimination.

Anatomical

Spinal curvature in either anterosuperior or lateral directions may result in significant variation of the anatomical features displayed in one section (Fig. 13.2). Caution should therefore be exercised in the interpretation of possible bone defects or new growth when displayed in single section.[5]

Radiological

Reproducibility

Precise positioning and accurate reproducibility of a thin body section in all spatial coordinates can present significant problems. Scanned projection radiographic facilities enabling digital AP or lateral images to be obtained are now available on most CT scanners (Fig. 13.11(c)). From these views, with the additional aid of a tilting gantry, reproducibility of transverse sections adequate for practical clinical purposes can be achieved, but detailed comparisons of pixel attenuation values must be made with caution.

Partial volume effect

The computed volume of tissue (voxel) does not contain uniformly homogeneous material. Both high- or low-density material can contribute to the mean attenuation of a voxel. This fact becomes especially important when anatomical interfaces obliquely placed within the scan section are to be evaluated. Structural margins may then be difficult to identify and the accuracy of linear measurement significantly reduced.

Boundary definition

Definition of boundaries is essential in obtaining linear or area measurements, particularly in the

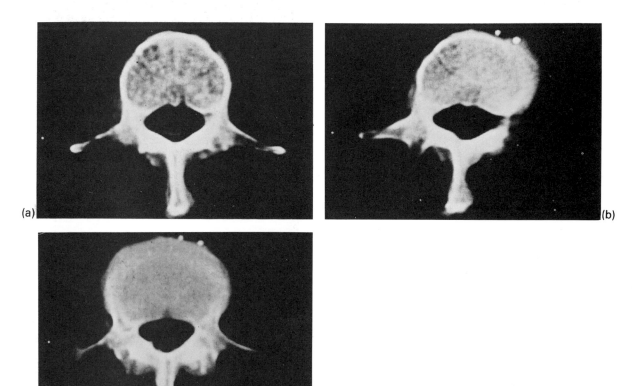

Fig. 13.2 CT sections of a disarticulated spine. (a) mid-vertebral body, no tilt; (b) 10° lateral tilt; (c) 10° upward tilt.

spinal canal. Many features contribute to both systematic and random errors in measurement from CT images. In identifying bony margins it may be necessary, because of the partial volume effect, to define an arbitrary attenuation value which most effectively separates bone from adjacent soft tissue. Higher resolution and reduced section thickness can contribute to a more accurate definition, but increased noise and obliquity of section can result in significant errors. Higher resolution in a limited area of reconstruction may enable density discrimination to be preserved and the dose penalty minimized. The impulse response inherent in the instrument may exert a significant effect on the attenuation values of the 'boundary zone'.[10]

Tissue characterization

Despite the ability of CT to demonstrate certain density differences, simple attenuation value analysis does not permit histological characterization.[11]

Radiation dose

Consideration of radiation dose should relate to information gained per unit of dose.[12] CT provides a highly efficient system for the utilization of X-rays, whereas conventional radiology enables only a small fraction of the incident X-rays to contribute to the final image. The measurement of maximum skin entry dose under similar conditions of resolution, noise, slice thickness, scan field and scan diameter permits some comparison of dose efficiency. Spinal CT scans, in the authors' experience on an IGE 8800 General Purpose Scanner, have resulted in a maximum skin entry radiation dose of 0.01 Gy. Radiation to one section can result in scatter to adjacent tissue, but scan profiles on most scanners are sufficiently good to minimize this risk.

COMPUTER-ASSISTED MYELOGRAPHY

Computer assisted myelography refers to the study of water-soluble contrast medium in the spinal subarachnoid space by computerized tomography[13,14] (Fig. 13.3).

Metrizamide (Amipaque®), the first non-ionic low-osmolality glucose amide with a molecular

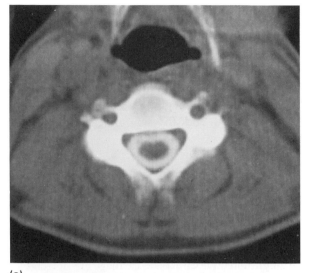

(a)

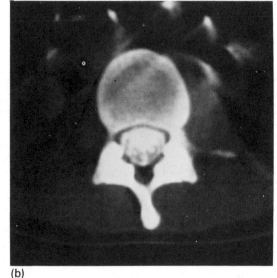

(b)

Fig. 13.3 Computer assisted myelography with contrast medium in the spinal subarachnoid space. (a) Cervical spine demonstrating normal spine cord; (b) lumbar spine demonstrating cauda equina.

weight of 789.1 and containing three iodine atoms, was a major advance over previous contrast media used for myelography.

More recent additions to the non-ionic low osmolality contrast media include Iopamidol® (Niopam®: Merck) and Isohexol® (Omnipaque®: Nyegaard). These contrast media are detectable in much lower concentrations than would be possible by conventional radiology because of the greatly increased sensitivity of CT. When introduced by the lumbar route, such contrast appears in the thoracic spine in one hour and in the cervical and intracerebral subarachnoid spaces at 1–2 hours.[14] The pattern of movement and diffusion of water-soluble contrast medium relates to a number of factors, including gravity, CSF concentration, body cavity pressures and diffusion in neural tissue.[14]

CLINICAL APPLICATIONS

Structural

Intervertebral disc herniation

Schmorl's nodes or herniations of disc material through defective end-plate cartilage are detectable by conventional CT as well-demarcated areas of decreased attenuation value with sclerotic margins and are readily distinguished from intrinsic intra-vertebral bone defects (Fig. 13.4).

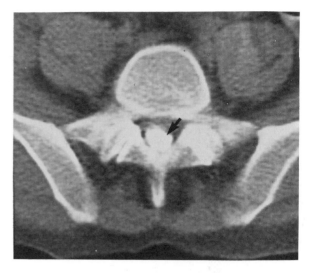

Fig. 13.5 Prolapsed intervertebral disc. Contrast filled subarachnoid space displaced by posterolateral disc herniation (arrow).

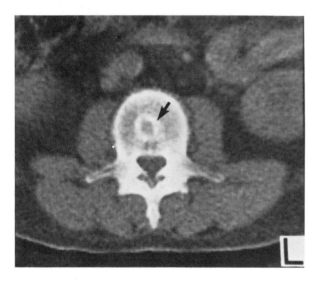

Fig. 13.4 Schmorl's node. Note sclerotic rim (arrow).

Computer-assisted myelography may enable not only the subarachnoid compartment (Fig. 13.5) to be identified but also the contrast-filled root pockets (Fig. 13.6). Either may be displaced in posterior or posterolateral disc herniation.

A number of scanning techniques have been used in the CT investigation of disc disease (Fig. 13.7), including contiguous 5–10mm sections with a vertical gantry, 5mm sections at 3mm intervals with[15] or without re-formating,[16] and 1.5mm contiguous sections with a gantry tilt. This last method is limited by noise and tube loading.

Bulging of the intact annulus is recognized by a convex extension of soft tissue density disc beyond the vertebral body margins. Central protrusion produces deformity or obliteration of the anterior dural margin. The density of such a herniated disc is 80–120 HU unless it is calcified. This value may be higher than fibrosis, but is unreliable in tissue characterization.

Extruded disc material can migrate and thus mimic other pathology, including perineural cysts. If CT is limited to specific disc levels without adequate clinical localization, migration of extruded disc,[17] higher discs or even conus tumours may give rise to false negative results. The sensitivity of CT for identifying disc hernations in 107 patients, 52 of whom went to surgery, has been reported as 96% compared to 93% for myelography.[18]

CT as a primary investigative procedure for suspected disc herniation is only justifiable if the clinical level can be clearly identified. If this is not possible, then myelography followed by CT is preferable. CT is more sensitive in lateral disc herniation or in posterior disc herniation where the epidural space is wide, e.g. L5/S1.[19]

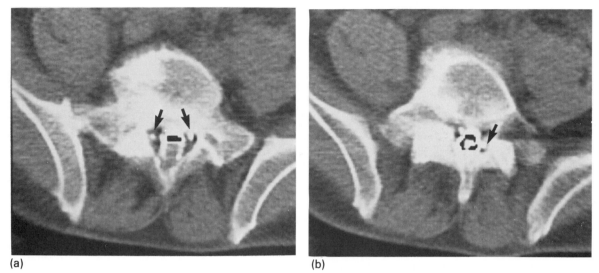

Fig. 13.6 Prolapsed intervertebral disc: normal contrast-filled root pockets (arrows) (left); root pocket displaced by lateral disc herniation (arrow) (right). Note computer artefact (black) within high-density contrast medium (Myodil®) and anterolateral osteophyte formation.

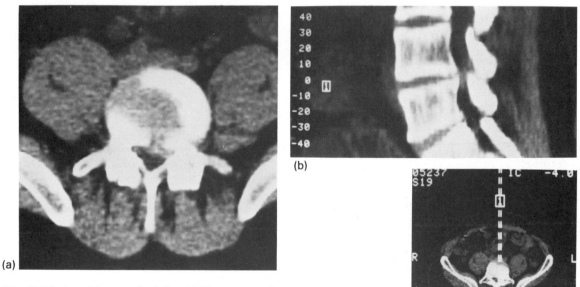

Fig. 13.7 Prolapsed intervertebral disc. (a) Transverse section; (b) reformatted sagittal image; (c) transverse section with cursor in sagittal plane.

The inability of CT to characterize tissue makes post-operative evaluation of recurrent disc herniation, post-operative fibrosis and arachnoiditis difficult. Post-operative fibrosis can be detected in asymptomatic patients.[20]

Spondylolisthesis

Spondylolisthesis is usually detectable on plain lateral radiograms. Narrowing of the spinal canal or the intervertebral foramina and the presence of associated disc herniation may require more specialized procedures. CT may demonstrate not only the shape of the spinal canal and defects of the pars interarticularis,[21] but also subluxation of the apophyseal joints (Figs 13.8 and 13.9).

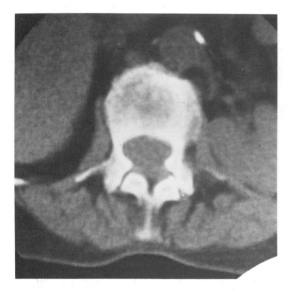

Fig. 13.8 Spondylolisthesis. Note displacement of articular facet.

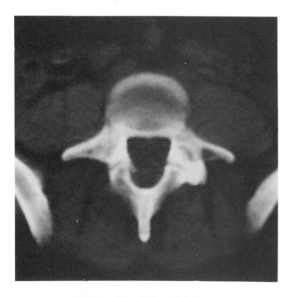

Fig. 13.9 Spondylolysis. Note bilateral defects in the pars interarticularis.

Apophyseal joint disease

The role of apophyseal joint disease in the pathogenesis of back pain remains speculative, but there is little doubt that osteoarthrosic outgrowths from these joints may not only inhibit movement in the lumbar spine but also compromise nerve roots in the intervertebral foramina and spinal canal. The value of computerized tomography in these circumstances lies in its unique ability to display in transverse section the angulation and articular surfaces of the apophyseal joints, the extent and direction of adjacent new bone growth and the shape and size of the spinal canal (Fig. 13.10). In a series of 100 consecutive cases of low back pain and sciatica examined by CT, abnormal facet joints were found in 65 patients.[22]

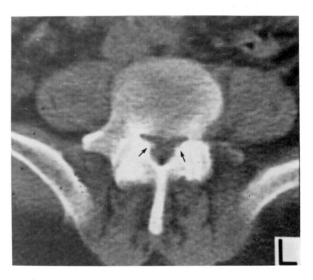

Fig. 13.10 Apophyseal joint disease. Extensive new bone formation encroaching into the spinal canal (arrow).

Trauma

The role of computerized tomography in the assessment of spinal injury is concerned specially with the demonstration of fractures in the transverse axial plane and their effect on neural tissue in the spinal canal (Figs 13.11 and 13.12). Computer-assisted myelography is necessary in the assessment of neural tissue damage, the differentiation between extradural compression and intramedullary swelling and can be influential in the selection and guidance

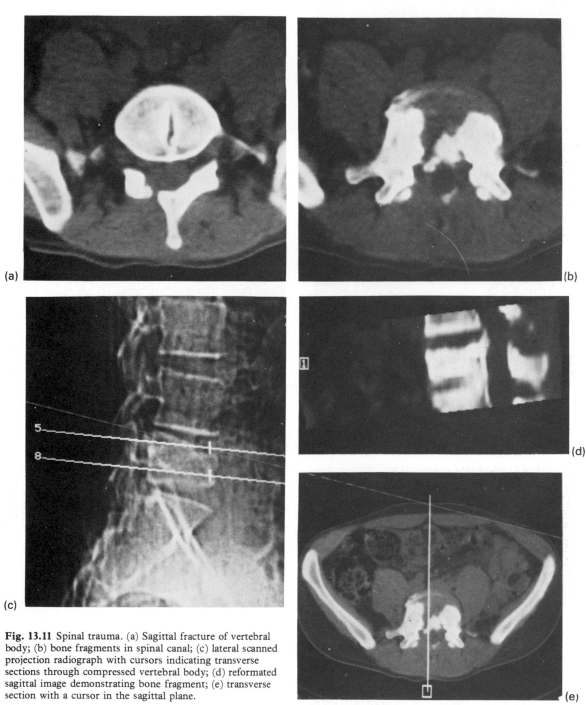

Fig. 13.11 Spinal trauma. (a) Sagittal fracture of vertebral body; (b) bone fragments in spinal canal; (c) lateral scanned projection radiograph with cursors indicating transverse sections through compressed vertebral body; (d) reformatted sagittal image demonstrating bone fragment; (e) transverse section with a cursor in the sagittal plane.

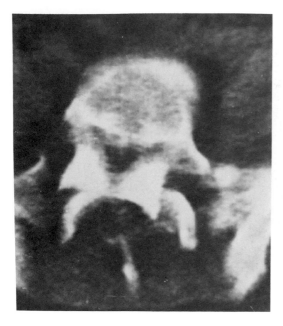

Fig. 13.12 Fracture dislocation of the lumbar spine. Transverse section. Note rotational deformity.

of decompression surgery. Spinal cord[23,24] deformity and distal atrophy may be important prognostic indicators (Fig. 13.13).[25] Acute haemorrhage is detected as a high-attenuation abnormality due to accumulation of haemoglobin or by its mass effect.

Spinal stenosis

The incidence and implications of lumbar spinal stenosis are gaining increasing attention. The varying clinical presentations of this syndrome have been well documented.[26,27]

Alterations in the linear dimensions and cross-sectional area of the spinal canal may sometimes be deduced from careful inspection of plain radiographs obtained under controlled conditions,[28] but no conventional radiographic projections can demonstrate the true shape of the spinal canal. Computerized tomography enables the total cross-sectional area of the bony canal to be explored, together with its shape, and also permits an accurate assessment to be made of the factors contributing to both primary and secondary canal narrowing.

Achondroplasia represents an extreme example of developmental spinal stenosis where the pedicles are abnormally short and the premature fusion of the neural epiphyseal plates leads to considerable narrowing of the entire canal (Fig. 13.14).

Spinal osteophytes arising posteriorly or postero-laterally may be difficult to localize by conventional radiology and yet may compromise the spinal canal or exit foramina (Fig. 13.15).

Spinal stenosis secondary to degenerative disease in the lumbar spine is usually localized or segmental. New bone formation with or without fusion of the

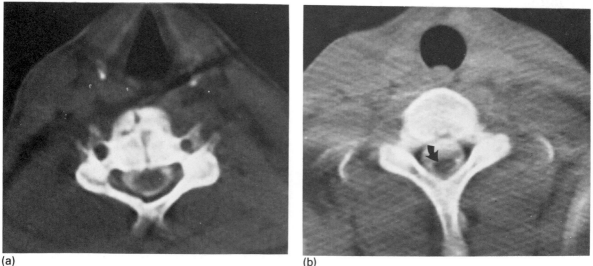

(a)   (b)

Fig. 13.13 Trauma — cervical spine. Sagittal fracture encroaching on anterior aspect of spinal cord (left); distal cord atrophy (arrow) demonstrated by computer-assisted myelography (right).

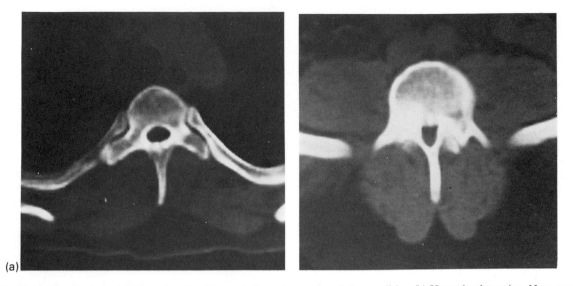

Fig. 13.14 Achodroplasia. (a) Thoracic spine. Note spinal canal stenosis and short pedicles. (b) Upper lumbar spine. Note canal stenosis.

apophyseal joints, as previously discussed, may result in narrowing of the exit intervertebral foramina (Fig. 13.10), sometimes described as lateral canal stenosis. The spinal canal may assume a trifoliate shape as a result of bony changes adjacent to the apophyseal joints (Fig. 13.16).

Intrinsic bone disease may be easily recognized on plain radiographs, but the presence of secondary spinal stenosis is more readily explored by com-

puterized tomography in the transverse axial plane (Fig. 13.17), whilst the configuration of the spinal canal is ideally displayed by conventional computerized tomography.

A number of authors have discussed methods of measuring the spinal canal by CT.[29,30] AP diameters less than 11.5mm, interpedicular distances less than 16mm and cross sectional areas less than 1.45cm^2 have been considered small.[30] Area measurements do not take soft tissue structures, e.g. ligamentum

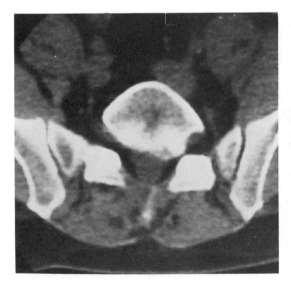

Fig. 13.15 Lateral canal stenosis. Note posterolateral osteophyte obstructing left exit foramen:

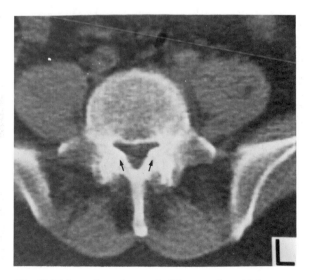

Fig. 13.16 Lateral canal stenosis. Note apophyseal joint sclerosis (arrow) and trifoliate shape of the spinal canal.

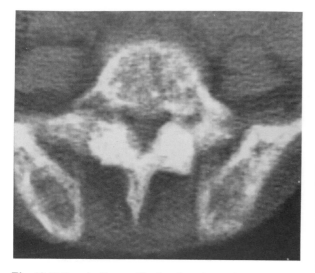

Fig. 13.17 Paget's disease affecting the spine and pelvis. Note secondary spinal canal stenosis.

flavum, into account and are, of course, subject to the constraints relating to boundary definition discussed earlier.

In the presence of lateral stenosis, cross-sectional measurements are insensitive. A lateral recess height of more than 5mm has been used to exclude lateral recess stenosis.[31] Foraminal narrowing can be assessed by CT.

Infection

Involvement of paravertebral structures in spinal infection (Fig. 13.18) is readily displayed by CT in addition to direct bony involvement (Fig. 13.19). A psoas abscess is characterized by an increase in size of the psoas muscle with low attenuation areas within it.[32,33] Contrast enhancement of the abscess margin is confirmatory evidence. Extradural collections and

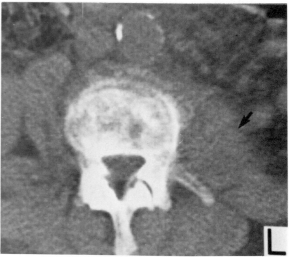

Fig. 13.19 Osteomyelitis. Metastatic abscess due to subacute bacterial endocarditis. Note paravertebral mass (arrow).

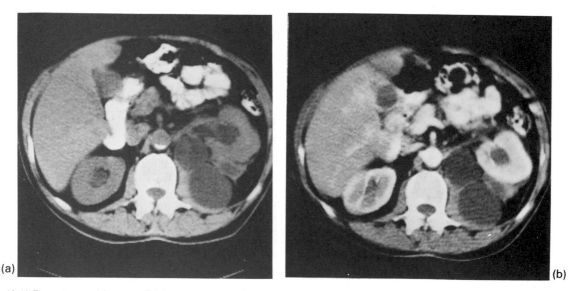

(a)

(b)

Fig. 13.18 Psoas abscess (a) pre- and (b) post-contrast enhancement. Note loculi of pus enlarging the psoas outline with peripheral enhancement.

disc space infections have also been recorded[29] (Fig. 13.20).

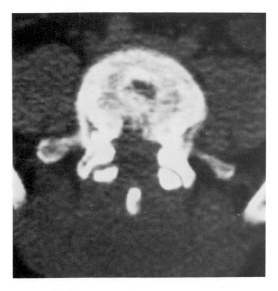

Fig. 13.20 Discitis. Note adjacent bone sclerosis.

Neoplastic disorders

Pain is an almost universal symptom in patients suffering from tumour involvement of the spine, whether primary or secondary. Primary tumours of the bony spine are infrequent but metastatic disease, either by direct or haematogenous spread, is not.

In the early stages of bone destruction, conventional radiology may reveal only minimal trabecular disturbance. Computerized tomography is then often capable of delineating clearly the area of bony abnormality (Fig. 13.21). In those circumstances where a diagnosis is available from conventional films, computerized tomography offers an additional dimension and an analysis of adjacent soft-tissue structures.

The determination of precise anatomical extent of a tumour and its relation to surrounding structures can be of significant diagnostic value but, more importantly, enable either surgical or radiotherapeutic planning to be more precise (Fig. 13.22). Computerized tomography has an obvious role in the non-invasive monitoring of disease and its response to treatment (Fig. 13.23). The restricted sectional thickness (5–13mm) offered by computerized tomography does not, however, permit the method to be employed as a screening technique.

A unique advantage of computerized tomography is its ability to determine the heterogeneity of composition of pathological processes — a quality already so successfully exploited in the brain. This is of particular value in those tumours containing high-density material (calcium) (Fig. 13.23) or low-

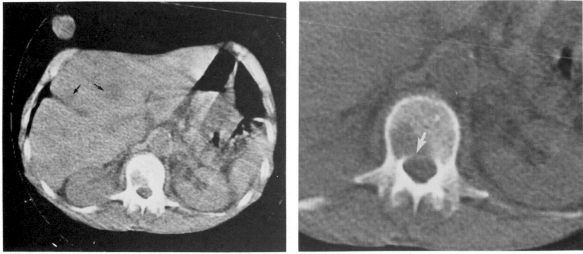

(a)   (b)

Fig. 13.21 Metastatic deposit from carcinoma pancreas. Left: total body section also demonstrating liver metastases (arrow). Right: detailed display of lytic deposit encroaching on spinal canal (arrow). The bone lesion is not detectable on plain radiographs.

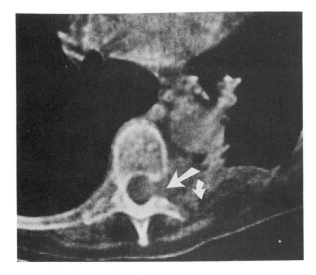

Fig. 13.22 Lymphoma eroding rib and pedicle (arrow) and infiltrating adjacent soft tissue.

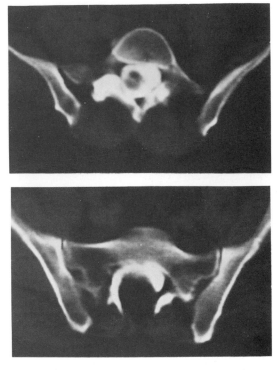

Fig. 13.24 Spinal dysraphism. (a) Lipoma of spinal cord outlined by contrast medium. Note low-density fat. (b) Lipoma outlined by contrast medium extending into sacral spinal canal.

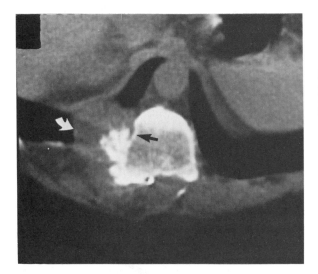

Fig. 13.23 Recurrent chondroma. Calcified mass (arrow) extending retropleurally. Note pressure erosion of vertebral body (arrow) and laminectomy.

tomography at the appropriate anatomical level is then of practical clinical importance in differentiating between metastatic and degenerative joint disease, even when the two are coincident (Fig. 13.25).[34]

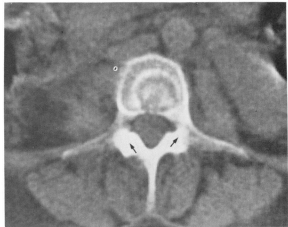

Fig. 13.25 Metastasis carcinoma, breast. Lytic lesion with sclerotic rim. Note apophyseal joint disease (arrow).

density material (fat) (Fig. 13.24). The precise histological nature of disease processes cannot be differentiated, though current research is directed towards the problem of tissue characterization.[11]

The role of isotope bone scanning in the evaluation of metastatic disease is well established. Degenerative joint disease of intervertebral or costovertebral origin may, however, give rise to falsely positive appearances. Plain radiology in these circumstances can be unhelpful. Computerized

Metabolic bone disease

Osteoporosis and osteomalacia may present with back pain due to local bone disease or associated fractures and spinal canal narrowing (Fig. 13.26).

Earlier studies[35] in the appendicular skeleton suggested that the mineral content of trabecular bone could be quantified reproducibly with accuracy and precision by CT. Current studies are directed towards the quantification of bone mass and bone mineral in the axial skeleton.[36]

The presence of fat in trabecular bone may, as a

result of partial volume effect, influence computed attenuation values. In these circumstances separation of elements with differing atomic number may be achieved by scanning the same section at two different beam energies.[37]

Referred back pain

Back pain may be the presenting feature not only in pelvic joint disorders (Fig. 13.27) but also in

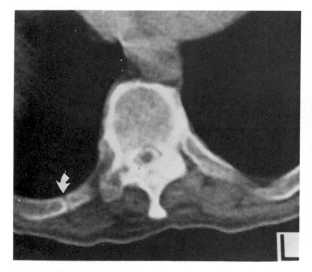

Fig. 13.26 Osteomalacia. Note Looser's zone (arrow) and contrast in spinal subarachnoid space.

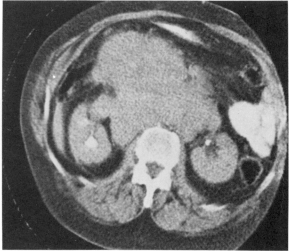

Fig. 13.28 Retroperitoneal sarcoma. Soft-tissue mass obliterating fascial planes and displacing kidneys laterally. Note the contrast medium in pelvicalyceal systems.

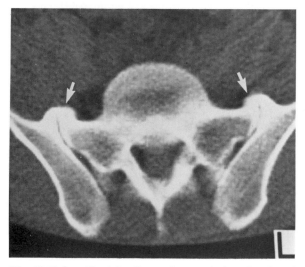

Fig. 13.27 Sacroiliac joint disease. Juxta-articular sclerosis and prominent anterior new bone formation (arrows).

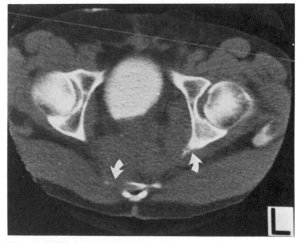

Fig. 13.29 Recurrent carcinoma rectum. Soft-tissue mass occupying ischiorectal fossae and invading left obturator muscle. Contrast-filled bladder displaced to the right. Note sacral erosion (arrow) and ischial spine erosion (arrow). Neither bone lesion was detectable on plain radiographs.

retroperitoneal (Fig. 13.28) and pelvic diseases (Fig. 13.29). CT is not organ-specific and, whilst offering a low disease specificity, has nevertheless considerable potential in the detection and exploration of abdominal soft-tissue disease.

CONCLUSIONS

CT, though employing ionizing radiation, is non-invasive, relatively operator-independent and is not organ-specific. It permits unique visualization of the spine and associated soft tissues in cross-section. While offering low disease specificity, CT is particularly valuable in identifying and localizing spinal stenosis and apophyseal joint disease. The digital derivation of the image allows access to the quantitative study of trabecular bone. Whilst CT is valuable in the study of disc disease, computer-assisted tomography is necessary to demonstrate neural tissue fully. The anatomical configuration of the spine, together with restricted sectional thickness, places significant constraints on the role of CT as a screening procedure in spinal disorders.

REFERENCES

1   Hounsfield G N 1972 Patent specification 1283915. Patent Office, London
2   Hounsfield G N 1973 Computerized transverse axial scanning (tomography). Part 1 — Description of system. Br. J. Radiol. 46: 1016–1022
3   Pullan B R, Rutherford R A, Isherwood I 1976 Computerized transaxial tomography. In: Medical images: formation, perception and measurement. Wiley, New York, p 20–38
4   Brooks R A, De Chiro G 1976 Phys. Med. Biol. 21: 689–000
5   Isherwood I, Antoun N M 1984 In: Textbook of radiological diagnosis. Lewis, London, p 581–601
6   Haughton V M, Williams A L 1982 Computed tomography of the spine. Mosby, St Louis
7   Haughton V M (ed) 1983 Computed tomography of the spine, vol 2. Churchill Livingstone, Edinburgh
8   Teplick J G, Haskin M E (eds) 1983 Radiological Clinics of North America, vol 21. Saunders, Philadelphia
9   Donovan Post J M (ed) 1984 Computed tomography of the spine. Williams & Wilkins, Baltimore
10 Checkley D R, Zhu X P, Antoun N M, Chen S Z, Isherwood I 1984 An investigation into the problems of attenuation and area measurements made from CT images of pulmonary nodules. J.C.A.T. 8: 237–243
11 Isherwood I 1984 Tissue characterization: imaging by numbers. Diagnostic Imaging 6: 44–52
12 Isherwood I, Pullan B R, Ritchings R T 1978 Radiation dose in neurological procedures. Neuroradiology 16: 477–481
13 Di Chiro G, Schellinger D 1976 CT of spinal cord after lumbar intrathecal introduction of metrizamide (computer assisted myelography). Radiology 120: 101–104
14 Isherwood I, Fawcitt R A, Forbes W St C, Nettle J R L, Pullan B R 1977 CT of the spinal canal using metrizamide. Acta Radiol. Supp 355
15 Williams A L, Haughton V M, Syvertsen A 1980 Computed tomography in the diagnosis of herniated nucleus pulposus. Radiology 135: 95
16 Glenn V W Jnr, Rothman S L, Rhodes M L 1982 Computed tomography/multiplanar reformatted (CT/MPR) examinations of the lumbar spine. In: Genant H K, Chafetz N, Helms C A (eds) CT of the lumbar spine. University of California Press
17 Fries J W, Abodeely D A, Vijungco J G, Yeager V L, Gaffey W R 1982 CT of herniated and extruded nucleus pulposus. J.C.A.T. 6: 874–887
18 Haughton V M, Eldevik O P, Magnaes B, Amundson P 1982 A prospective comparison of computed tomography and myelography in the diagnosis of herniated lumbar disks. Radiology 142: 103–110
19 Williams A L, Haughton V M, Daniels D L, Thornton R S 1982 CT recognition of lateral lumbar disc herniation. Am. J. Neuroradiol. 3: 211–213
20 Braun I F, Lin J P, Benjamin M V, Richeff I I 1984 CT of asymptomatic postsurgical lumbar spine. Analysis of the physiological scar. Am. J. Roent. 142: 149
21 Rothman S L G, Glenn W V 1984 In: Donovan Post M J (ed) Computed tomography of the spine. Williams & Wilkins, Baltimore
22 Carrera G F, Haughton V W, Syvertsen A, Williams A L 1980 CT of lumbar facet joints. Radiology 134: 145
23 Brant-Zadawksi M, Miller E M, Federle M P 1981 CT in the evaluation of spine trauma. Am J. Roent. 136: 369–375
24 Brant-Zadawski M, Jeffrey R B Jnr, Minagi H, Pitts L H 1982 High resolution computed tomography of thoracolumbar fractures. Am. J. Neurorad. 3: 69–74
25 Seibert C E, Dreisbach J N, Swanson W B, Edgar R E, Williams P, Hahn H 1981 Progressive post-traumatic cystic myelopathy. Am. J. Neurorad. 2: 115–119
26 Blau J N, Logue V 1961 Intermittent claudication of the cauda equina. An unusual syndrome resulting from central protrusion of lumbar intervertebral disc. Lancet I: 1081–1086
27 Blau J N, Logue V 1978 The natural history of intermittent claudication of the cauda equina. Brain 101: 211–212
28 Roberts G M 1978 MD thesis, London University
29 Lee B C P, Kazam E, Newman A D 1978 CT of spine and spinal cord. Radiology 128: 95
30 Ulrich C G, Binet E F, Sanacki M G, Kieffer S A 1980 Quantitative assessment of lumbar spinal canal by CT. Radiology 134: 137
31 Ciric I, Mikhael M A, Tarkington J A, Vick N A 1980 The lateral recess syndrome. J. Neurosurg. 53: 433–443
32 Jeffrey C D, Callen P W, Federle M P 1980 CT of psoas abscesses. J.C.A.T. 4: 639–641

33 Feldberg M A M, Koehler R, Van Maes F G M 1983
    Psoas compartment disease studied by CT. Radiology
    148: 505–512
34 Best J J K, Adam N M, Isherwood I, Sellwood R A
    1977 The interpretation of radio-isotope bone scans: a
    comparative study. Br. J. Surg. 64: 822
35 Isherwood I, Rutherford R A, Pullan B R 1976 Bone
    mineral estimation by computer assisted transverse axial
    tomography. Lancet II: 712–716

36 Isherwood I, Pullan B R, Rutherford R A, Strang F A
    1977 Electron density and atomic number determination
    by CT. Part I: Methods and limitations. Part II: A study
    of colloid cysts. Br. J. Radiol. 50: 613–619
37 Adams J E, Chen S Z, Adams P H, Isherwood I 1982
    Measurement of trabecular bone mineral by dual energy
    CT. J.C.A.T. 61: 601–607

New investigative techniques
Magnetic resonance imaging of the lumbar spine

INTRODUCTION

Magnetic resonance imaging (MRI) has emerged as a powerful clinical and research tool. Although this technology can be applied usefully to almost any part of the body, examination of the spine is already among the most important applications. The purpose of Part B of this chapter is to introduce the reader to the principles of MRI and to illustrate its role in evaluating the lumbar spine.

PHYSICS[1]

Basic principles

Magnetic resonance (MR) is based on the behaviour of certain nuclei in a strong magnetic field. Any nucleus with an uneven number of protons and neutrons will act as if it has a small magnetic field, and will tend to align itself in the direction of a stronger external field. Hydrogen, which has only one proton, is the nucleus used most often in MRI because it is present in great abundance in biological tissues. Other nuclei which can be used include phosphorus 31, sodium 23 and carbon 13.

When the hydrogen proton is placed in a magnetic field, it will not align directly with the field, but will precess or wobble around the axis of the magnetic field lines (Fig. 13.30). This precession occurs at a fixed frequency (called the Larmor frequency), which is directly proportional to the strength of the magnetic field. At a magnetic field strength of 0.35 tesla (T) (or 3500 times as powerful as the earth's magnetic field), which is the field strength used in our imaging device, hydrogen precesses at 15 mHz. Since many protons are present in the sample and are precessing in random phase relative to one another,

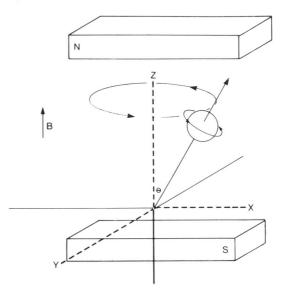

Fig. 13.30 A proton in a magnetic field precesses or 'wobbles' around an axis parallel to the field at a rate proportional to the strength of the magnetic field

the net magnetic orientation of all protons in the sample will be parallel to the magnetic field.

If a radio frequency (RF) pulse is applied at the Larmor frequency, the net magnetic orientation of the sample will be tilted from its alignment with the external field. The degree of tilt is dependent on the strength and duration of the applied RF pulse. The tilted protons will continue to precess, and thus the net magnetic orientation will also precess. The frequency of precession of the net magnetic orientation also occurs at the Larmor frequency.

The tilted net magnetic orientation can be described as having two components with respect to the magnetic field: one component parallel to the magnetic field and another component perpendicular to the field. In an x–y–z coordinate system, the parallel component is along the z-axis, and is called M_z. The component of the net magnetic orientation which is perpendicular to the magnetic field is in the x–y plane, and is called M_x. The perpendicular component, M_x, continues to precess around the z-axis. As long as M_x exists, the hydrogen protons emit a radio frequency signal, which is the magnetic resonance (MR) signal. The frequency of the emitted radio signal is determined by the local magnetic field strength, and the amplitude of the signal is determined by the magnitude of M_x. The net magnetic orientation is usually tilted 90°, since this produces the greatest M_x, which generates the strongest MR signal.

Several factors operate simultaneously to cause M_x to decrease rapidly, which consequently causes the MR signal to decay rapidly. First, the net magnetization vector proceeds to realign with the external magnetic field, i.e. along the z-axis. This realignment results in an increase in M_z. The growth of M_z occurs exponentially with a time constant $T1$ (the 'spin-lattice' relaxation time). $T1$ is a basic property of biological tissue and fluid, and ranges in value from 100 ms to 3.0 s.

Second, each hydrogen proton is exposed to a slightly different magnetic field due to the interaction of other hydrogen protons nearby. Since the frequency of the MR signal is directly proportional to the local magnetic field strength that the proton is in, the protons emit MR signals of slightly different frequencies. This causes the protons to become slightly out of phase with each other, which causes M_x to shrink even more rapidly. This decay is characterized by another exponential decay constant called $T2$ (the 'spin-spin' relaxation time). $T2$ is also a basic property of biological tissue and fluid, and occurs much more rapidly than $T1$. $T2$ values range from 25 to 200 ms.

The final factor which causes M_x to decrease is machine-related non-uniformity of the magnetic field, which also causes proton dephasing. Thus there are two causes of proton dephasing: local proton interaction ($T2$ decay), and magnetic field non-uniformity.

Signal intensity and pulse sequences

The intensity of the MR signal at any point is primarily dependent on hydrogen density, $T1$, $T2$

and flow. The contribution of hydrogen density to signal intensity is fairly obvious: the greater the hydrogen density, the more intense the signal. Thus lung and cortical bone, which have few hydrogen protons, generate a weak MR signal and are dark on the image. Conversely, fat, which has a high hydrogen density, generates a strong signal and is very bright on the image. However, fast-flowing blood generates a weak signal because of the rapid movement through the tissue being imaged.

The contribution of $T1$ and $T2$ to signal intensity is more complicated. First, $T1$ will be considered (Fig. 13.31). When the net magnetic orientation is tilted 90° by a radio frequency pulse, M_z becomes zero. Immediately M_z begins to increase exponentially by the time constant $T1$. The strength of the MR signal that a quantity of protons will emit depends on how large M_z is when the next 90° pulse is applied. If the 90° pulse is applied when M_z is maximal, then the MR signal will be maximal. However, if the 90° pulse is applied before M_z is maximal, then the signal will be less. MRI involves multiple pulsing cycles, and the cycles are usually too short to allow M_z to become maximal for all tissues (in order to keep imaging time reasonably short). Since the strength of M_z is dependent on $T1$, then image intensity is also dependent on $T1$. Consequently, objects with different $T1$s will have different intensities. As is shown in Fig. 13.31, objects with a short $T1$ will be brighter than objects with a long $T1$.

The $T2$ of the object under study also has an important contribution to the signal intensity. If the

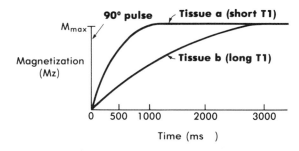

Fig. 13.31 The intensity of the MR signal is determined by the degree of magnetization parallel to the main magnetic field (M_z) when the 90° pulse is applied. M_z recovers exponentially with a time constant $T1$. Substances with a short $T1$ (tissue (a)) recover faster than those with a long $T1$ (tissue (b)). Hence tissue (a) will be brighter than tissue (b) on a $T1$ weighted image

signal is sampled at increasing intervals after the radio pulse, its intensity will be seen to decrease at a rate determined by $T2$ (Fig. 13.32). In contrast to $T1$, objects with a *long* $T2$ will return more signal than those with a short $T2$, and thus the long $T2$ object is brighter on the image.

Now the radio pulse sequence needs to be considered. The spin echo technique (Fig. 13.33) is the pulse sequence most often employed for the spine. The first component of this technique is a 90° pulse. Shortly thereafter a 180° pulse is applied in order to compensate for the proton dephasing due to magnetic field non-uniformity. After the 180° pulse the protons begin to rephase, and the 'spin echo' is then detected. The spin echo is the actual MR signal from which the images are constructed. If desired, several spin echoes can be obtained after each 90° pulse. Each subsequent spin echo is progressively weaker in signal strength; that progressive decline is

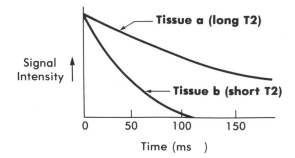

Fig. 13.32 The signal intensity after the RF pulse decays with an exponential time constant $T2$. Substances with a long $T2$ (tissue (a)) will lose signal more slowly than those with a short $T2$ (tissue (b)); hence tissue (a) will be brighter than tissue (b) on a $T2$ weighted image. (This graph ignores the effect of machine-related magnetic field non-uniformity)

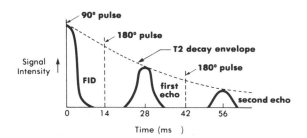

Fig. 13.33 After the 90° pulse the MR signal decays very rapidly due to $T2$ decay and magnetic field non-uniformity. The 180° pulse reverses the dephasing due to magnetic field non-uniformity, and after a delay the spin echo is detected. Multiple spin echoes allow the $T2$ decay constant to be calculated

the $T2$ decay. The time between the 90° pulses is called the repetition time or TR. The time between the 90° pulse and the spin echo is called the echo time or TE. In imaging, the cycle of 90° and 180° pulses is generally repeated; often four averages are obtained in order to increase the signal strength.

The relative contribution of $T1$ and $T2$ to the image intensity and contrast is determined by the TR and TE in the following manner. The time between the 90° pulses determines how much the parallel magnetization, M_z, is allowed to recover. At a short TR (0.5–1.0 s) $T1$ strongly influences image contrast, since M_z has not fully recovered for most tissues. Thus objects with different $T1$s will have different intensities; as noted previously, objects with a short $T1$ are brighter than those with a long $T1$. (When TR is very long, M_z has recovered for most tissues; thus objects with different $T1$s will have the same intensity, assuming $T2$ and hydrogen density are the same.) On the other hand, TE largely determines the contribution of $T2$ to image contrast. As TE is prolonged, the overall signal intensity decreases as a result of proton interaction dephasing ($T2$ decay). Thus images with a long TE have relatively more $T2$ contribution.

In summary, in the spin echo technique varying the TR and TE affects the relative contribution of $T1$ and $T2$ to the image intensity. A short TR, short TE pulse sequence is said to be '$T1$ weighted', while a long TR, long TE sequence is '$T2$ weighted'. The effects of $T2$ and $T2$ on image intensity are different. On a $T1$ weighted image, objects with a short $T1$ are most intense, while on a $T2$ weighted image objects with a long $T2$ are brightest.

Imaging

Imaging entails determining the location of the various tissues which are emitting the MR signal. Imaging is accomplished by using the relationship between magnetic field strength and precessional frequency. The frequency of the applied radio pulse which will tilt the protons and the frequency of the emitted MR signal (both are the same) are directly proportional to the magnetic field strength. That is, a proton in a stronger magnetic field emits an MR signal of higher frequency than a proton in a weaker magnetic field. Thus when a low-strength-gradient magnetic field is introduced along the axis of the larger static magnetic field, the protons emit MR signals of different frequency. Since the gradient field position is known, and since the MR signal frequency is proportional to the gradient field, then the position of the emitting protons can be determined and an image can be generated.

Imaging protocol

A number of options are available when imaging with MR. We have exclusively used the spin echo pulse sequence when examining the spine and other musculoskeletal structures. In our system one can select a TR of 0.5, 1.0, 1.5 or 2.0 seconds. The choice of TR affects the number of slices obtained and the image acquistion time (Table 13.1). Two spin echoes, with TEs of 28 and 56 ms, are routinely obtained. Presently, the sections are 7 mm thick with a 3 mm gap between sections. Five millimetre contiguous sections can be acquired, but require a significantly longer acquisition time. Image resolution is usually 1.7 or 2.0 mm. A higher resolution of 0.8 mm is available, but this also lengthens examination time. Our routine lumbar spine exam generally employs 7 mm sagittal sections with both a short (0.5 s) and long (1.5 or 2.0 s) TR pulse sequence at a resolution of 1.7 mm. More recently surface coils have been employed which increase signal to noise ratio and permit imaging with 5 mm thick sections and high resolution without major time penalty.

Table 13.1 Spin echo imaging sequences

TR (ms)	TE (ms)	No. of sections	Imaging time (min)
500	28, 56	5	4.5
1000	28, 56	10	9
1500	28, 56	15	13.5
2000	28, 56	20	18

ADVANTAGES OF MRI

Magnetic resonance imaging has a number of advantages over computerized tomography. First, MR can directly image in either the transaxial, coronal or sagittal planes. In contrast, CT is generally limited to the transaxial plane. Although computer-generated reformations can give CT images in other planes, these reformations have a limited field of view and reduced resolution.

Another advantage of MR is the absence of beam hardening artefacts. Beam hardening often greatly complicates the interpretation of lumbar spine CT scans. Similarly, MR does not have streak artefacts from surgical clips or other metallic densities.[2] Probably the greatest advantage of MR is the enhanced soft-tissue contrast. Thus structures which are of similar density on CT (e.g. annulus and nucleus pulposus; disc and thecal sac) can have very different intensities on MR. The ability to manipulate soft-tissue contrast with MR by altering the TR and TE allows great flexibility in imaging.

NORMAL ANATOMY

The normal structures of the lumbar spine are well defined by MRI (Fig. 13.34). Subcutaneous and epidural fat are very intense, especially in images with $T1$ weighting. The intensity of fat is in part due to its very short $T1$. Marrow, which contains a significant amount of fat, is also fairly intense. Cortical bone, on the other hand, shows essentially no intensity, since there are very few available hydrogen protons. Yet cortical bone can be seen, since structures which surround it (marrow and soft tissue) do generate a signal. Muscle is generally intermediate in intensity.

The ability of MRI to depict clearly the intervertebral disc heralds an important future role of this technology in the evaluation of back pain. The nucleus pulposus (NP) has an intermediate signal on $T1$ weighted images (short TR, short TE). However, the normal NP becomes relatively more intense as a more $T2$ weighted pulse sequence (long TR, long TE) is employed. The relative increased intensity is due to the high water content of the NP, which results in a long $T2$. (Remember that an object with a long $T2$ will be very bright on a $T2$ weighted image.) The annulus, however, is less well hydrated, and consequently has a lower intensity than the nucleus (especially on a $T2$ weighted image). The outer layers of the annulus, which blend with the anterior and posterior longitudinal ligament complex, generate very little signal and are depicted as black on most images. The ability of MRI to separate NP from annulus is an important advantage over CT.

The thecal sac also shows varying intensity because of a high water content. On a $T1$ weighted image, the thecal sac has an intermediate or low

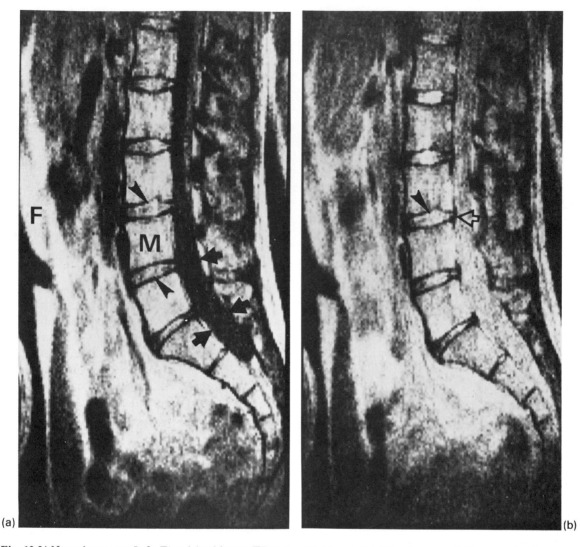

(a)   (b)

Fig. 13.34 Normal anatomy. Left: $T1$ weighted image (TR=1.0 s, TE=28 ms). Fat (F) and marrow (M) are very bright, whereas cortical bone (i.e. vertebral endplates) and air are dark. The inververterbral discs (arrowheads) are intermediate in intensity. CSF (arrows) is dark on this image because of its long $T1$. Right: $T2$ weighted image (TR=2.0 s, TE=56 ms). Fat and marrow remain bright. Note the marked relative increase in intensity of both CSF and the nucleus pulposus (NP), due to their long $T2$. The NP (arrowhead) can be separated from the annulus and longitudinal ligaments (arrow)

intensity. When a more $T2$ weighted image is generated, the relative intensity of the thecal sac increases. On a strongly $T2$ weighted image, the thecal sac can be very bright, almost like a metrizamide myelogram. The nerve roots cannot be seen separately within the thecal sac, although they can be imaged within the neural foramina because of the surrounding epidural fat (Fig. 13.35).

MRI can also image the spinal cord without the use of intrathecal contrast (Fig. 13.36).[3,4] The cord is best seen on a $T1$ weighted image where the intermediate-intensity cord is surrounded by low-intensity CSF. However, on a $T2$ weighted image the CSF becomes more intense and the cord is more difficult to visualize as a separate structure.

DISC DISEASE

MRI is presently the most sensitive imaging modality for detecting degenerative disc disease.[5] Pathologically, disc degeneration begins with the

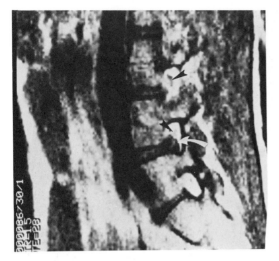

Fig. 13.35(a) Nerve roots in neural foramen. Parasagittal MR section. The nerve roots (arrowheads) are surrounded by high-intensity epidural fat in the neural foramen. At L4-5 on the left there is an osteophyte encroaching the neural foramen (arrow).

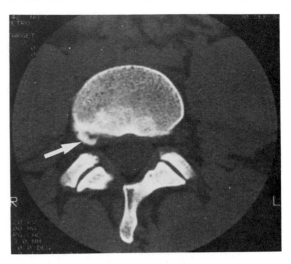

Fig. 13.35(b) CT scan on the same patient shows an osteophyte in the left L4-5 neural foramen (arrow)

breakdown of the proteoglycans in the NP. Consequently, the nucleus is unable to retain as much water as normal, and it begins to dehydrate. This reduction of water content decreases the number of hydrogen protons, which shortens the $T2$; thus the degenerated disc is lower in intensity

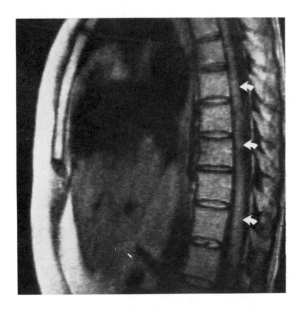

Fig. 13.36 Normal spinal cord. Sagittal MR scan ($T1$ weighted) of the thoracic spine shows the spinal cord (arrows) to be intermediate in intensity. The surrounding CSF is dark

than the normal disc (Fig. 13.37). This difference in intensity is usually best appreciated on strongly $T2$ weighted images. In the early stages of disc degeneration, the plain films and CT are usually normal.

Abnormal encroachment of the intervertebral disc on neural structures is usually well defined by MRI (Figs 13.38, 13.39 and 13.40).[5,6] Bulging of the low-intensity annulus is usually best depicted on a $T2$ weighted image where the CSF is relatively bright. However, sometimes a $T1$ weighted image is useful in showing the intermediate intensity of a herniated disc against the dark thecal sac. The sagittal images demonstrate well the relationship between the disc and the thecal sac. Axial images are frequently helpful in showing encroachment of the nerve roots within the neural foramen.

The ability of MRI to separate the annulus from the NP is important in the evaluation of the abnormal disc (Figs 13.38, 13.39 and 13.40). MRI has the potential to determine whether nuclear material has escaped from the confines of the annulus. Thus it is hoped MR can distinguish between a disc protrusion (nuclear bulge contained within annulus), a disc extrusion (nuclear material beyond confines of annulus but still in contact with nucleus) and a sequestered disc (nuclear material beyond confines of annulus and not in contact with

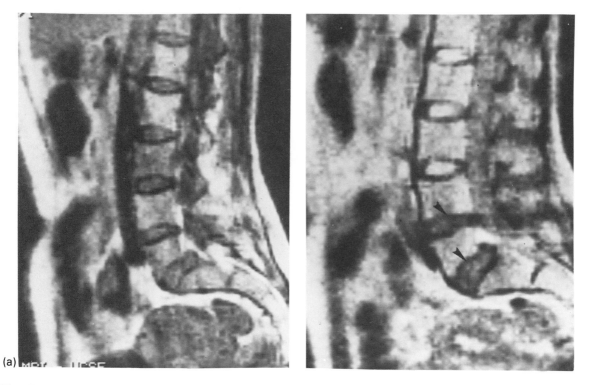

Fig. 13.37 Disc degeneration. (a) $T1$ weighted image. There is little difference in intensity between the intervertebral discs. A grade 1 spondylolisthesis is present at L5-S1. (b) $T2$ weighted image. The L4-5 and L5-S1 discs (arrowheads) are darker than the other normal discs. A degenerating disc dehydrates, which shortens the $T2$ and consequently decreases the signal intensity on a $T2$ weighted image

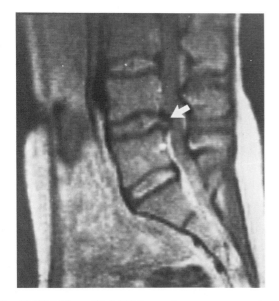

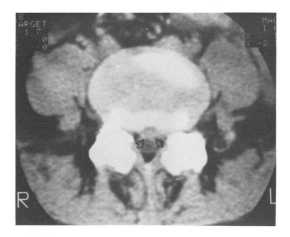

Fig. 13.38(a) The sagittal MR image shows gross protrusion of disc material at L4-5 (arrow) into the thecal sac. There is intermediate intensity within the herniated disc indicating true protrusion of nuclear material

Fig. 13.38(b) Herniated disc. A CT scan (same patient) documents the L4-5 disc herniation (arrows). The NP and annulus have the same density and thus usually cannot be distinguished on CT

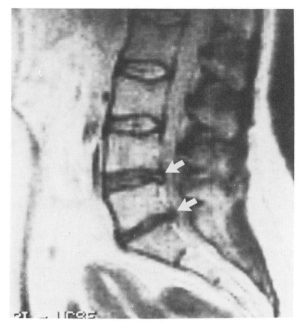

Fig. 13.39 Herniated disc. There is encroachment of the intervertebral disc into the thecal sac at L4-5 (arrows). The intermediate intensity from the herniated disc at L4-5 indicates that there is true protrusion of the nucleus pulposus beyond the confines of the annulus. A purely annular bulge would not have this intermediate intensity

nucleus). CT has particular difficulty in this distinction, since on CT the nucleus and annulus have the same density. The failure of CT to detect a sequestered disc (free fragment) is an important cause of chemonucleolysis failure.

SPINAL STENOSIS

Bony and soft tissue encroachment on the thecal sac and nerve roots can be readily detected by MRI. Central canal stenosis is best seen on $T2$ weighted images, where the high-intensity thecal sac is seen in sharp contrast to the low-intensity region of stenosis (Fig. 13.41). Encroachment on the neural foramen is perhaps best depicted on a $T1$ weighted image where the high-intensity epidural fat surrounds the medium-intensity nerve root and sheath. MRI has been reported to be as accurate as CT and myelography in demonstrating spinal stenosis, although CT was more accurate in distinguishing bony from soft tissue narrowing.[5]

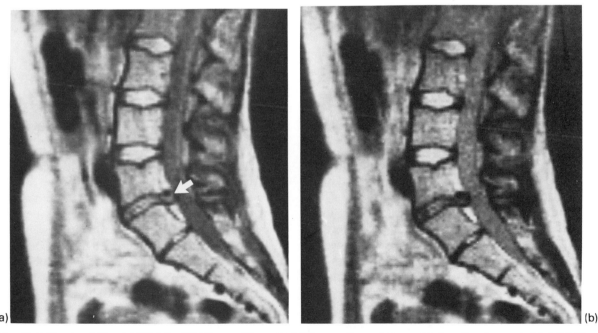

(a)   (b)

Fig. 13.40 Herniated disc. (a) TR 1.5 s, TE 28 msec. The sagittal MR scan shows a large protrusion of nuclear material at L5-S1 (arrow). The L5-S1 disc is slightly lower in intensity than the adjacent normal discs. (a) TR 1.5 s, TE 56 ms. As the TE is prolonged, the image is more $T2$ weighted; hence the difference between abnormal and normal discs is accentuated. Also note the increasing intensity of the CSF, which allows better definition of the posterior extent of the disc protrusion

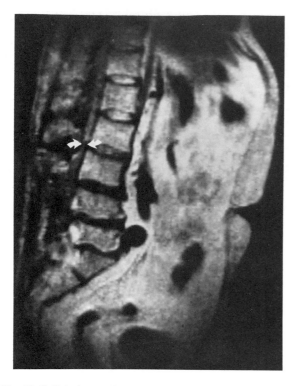

Fig. 13.41 Spinal stenosis. A *T*2 weighted image shows marked posterior narrowing of the spinal canal at L2-3 (arrows). Severe degenerative disc disease is present at L3-4, L4-5 and L5-S1

CHEMONUCLEOLYSIS

Magnetic resonance dramatically documents the effect of chemonucleolysis on the intervertebral disc (Fig. 13.44).[5,6] A decrease in the signal of the nucleus is usually seen. This change is probably due to the dehydration that occurs secondary to the breakdown of collagen in the disc. In addition, the volume of the disc herniation often decreases on the post-injection images. Occasionally a marked increase in signal is seen adjacent to the end-plates on a strongly *T*2 weighted image.[5] This finding is of uncertain significance, but may be related to inflammation and oedema.

MRI may also become important in selecting patients for chemonucleolysis. As noted above, the ability to distinguish annulus from NP may be helpful in detecting the sequestered disc. Just as important, however, is the information about the herniated disc. An acutely herniated disc is still partially hydrated, and thus will show some intensity on a *T*2 weighted image. On the other hand, a chronic disc herniation (sometimes called a 'collagenase disc') may be completely desiccated, and consequently may show no significant intensity on any pulse sequence. Since the collagenase disc does not respond to chemonucleolysis, the absence of signal from a herniated disc is probably a contra-indication to this therapy.

POST-OPERATIVE SPINE

Our initial experience with using magnetic resonance to evaluate the post-operative spine has been promising.[6] MRI will probaby prove to be valuable in distinguishing post-operative fibrosis from recurrent disc herniation. In several cases, surgically-proven post-operative fibrosis showed as an intermediate-intensity material that became brighter on the longer TE image (Fig. 13.42). The appearance of the fibrosis was clearly distinct from the intervertebral disc at that level. On the other hand, in another post-operative case a large recurrent disc herniation was clearly shown (Fig. 13.43). In these cases the CT scan was nonspecific and was consistent with either fibrosis or recurrent disc.

INFECTION

Spinal osteomyelitis has a unique appearance on magnetic resonance.[5] On *T*1 weighted images the intervertebral disc and adjacent vertebral bodies show a decreased signal intensity. The extent of any destructive process and surrounding soft tissue mass is also clearly depicted. On a strongly *T*2 weighted image, however, the image dramatically changes. The intervertebral disc shows a relatively increased intensity, in contrast to the decreased intensity seen with disc degeneration. In addition, the adjacent vertebral end-plates also demonstrate an increased intensity. This appearance — increased intensity of both the disc and end-plate on a *T*2 weighted image — appears to be quite specific for spinal osteomyelitis.

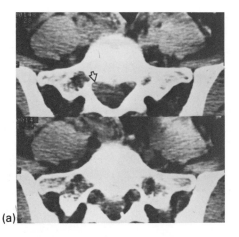

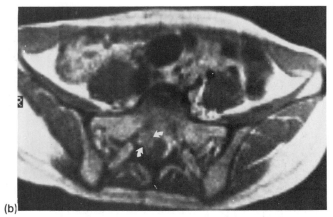

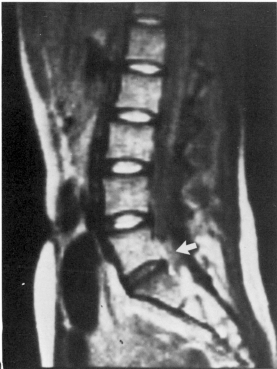

Fig. 13.42 Post-operative fibrosis. (a) CT demonstrates marked asymmetry of the epidural fat in the right S1 lateral recess (arrow). In this post-operative patient, the appearance is consistent with either fibrosis or recurrent disc herniation. (b) The corresponding transaxial MR image (T2 weighted) shows an irregular area of increased intensity around the right S1 root (arrows). (c) The MR sagittal section (T2 weighted) shows an irregular region of increased intensity (arrow) at the L5-S1 level. At surgery this was proven to be post-operative fibrosis. The appearance of the fibrosis is completely different from the abnormal L5-S1 disc

NEOPLASM

MRI clearly defines primary and secondary neoplasms of the vertebral elements, although the appearance is different for blastic and lytic lesions. Blastic tumours show a decreased intensity compared to adjacent marrow on both $T1$ and $T2$ weighted images (Fig. 13.45). This decreased signal is probably due to the reactive bone formation which, like cortical bone, will have few hydrogen protons available for imaging. On the other hand, the appearance of lytic vertebral tumours is often different (Fig. 13.46). On a $T1$ weighted image the intensity of the lesion is decreased, due to a long $T1$. However, on a $T2$ weighted image the intensity of the lytic tumour is increased due to a long $T2$. Prolongation of the $T1$ and $T2$ is characteristic of many musculoskeletal tumours.

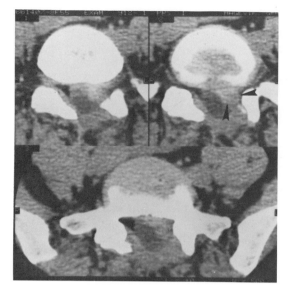

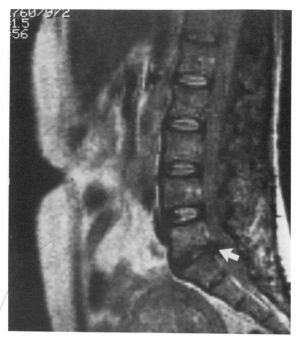

Fig. 13.43(a) Recurrent disc herniation. CT demonstrates a large mass effect at L5-S1 on the left which is displacing the thecal sac (arrowheads). Although the appearance is more suggestive of recurrent disc herniation, post-operative fibrosis can appear similar.

Fig. 13.43(b) Recurrent disc herniation. MR clearly demonstrates protrusion of NP into the thecal sac (arrow). A large recurrent disc herniation was found at surgery. Compare this appearance with Fig. 13.42(c)

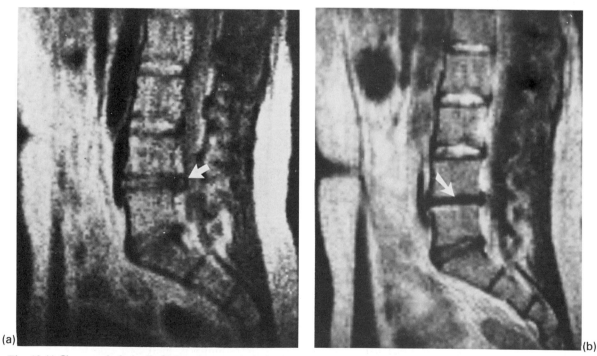

(a)

(b)

Fig. 13.44 Chemonucleolysis. (Left) Pre-chemonucleolysis. An early-generation MR scan shows a large herniated disc at L4-5 (arrow). The intensity of the L4-5 disc is decreased. (Right) Post-chemonucleolysis. There is marked loss of signal intensity from the L4-5 disc (arrow) and loss of disc height. The disc herniation has decreased in size.

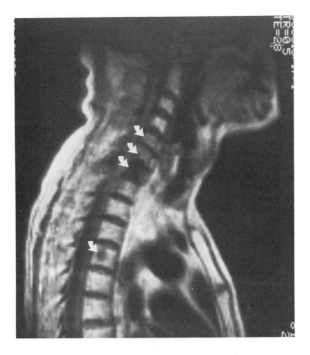

Fig. 13.45 Blastic metastases. Blastic metastases from a prostate primary show decreased intensity in the T5-7 and T11 vertebral bodies (arrows)

The local soft tissue extent of neoplasm is also well defined. Invasion into surrounding muscle is best imaged on a $T2$ weighted image, where the tumour (long $T2$) is brighter than the muscle (shorter $T2$). However, defining the extent of the lesion into fat is often best visualized on a $T1$ weighted image. In this case fat (short $T1$) is brighter than tumour (long $T1$). Tumour encroachment on the thecal sac and spinal cord is also easily demonstrated by MRI, often giving as much information as a myelogram (Fig. 13.46(b)). MRI, because of its superior soft-tissue contrast, is often better than CT in defining soft-tissue extent of neoplasm.

Although not often a problem in the lumbar spine, MRI is superb in defining tumour and tumour-like conditions of the spinal cord.[3,4] Both neoplasms and syringomyelia/hydromyelia are often better depicted by MR than by conventional techniques. In fact, MRI may replace myelography, since the former can directly image the cord without the use of intrathecal contrast or ionizing radiation.

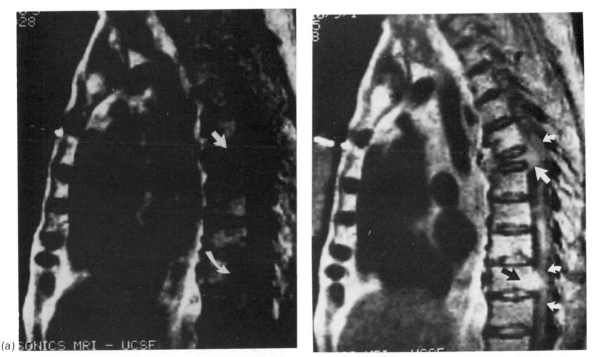

Fig. 13.46 Lytic metastases (lung primary). (a) $T1$ weighted image. There is complete destruction of the T8 vertebral body (straight arrow) with preservation of the adjacent intervertebral discs. Another lesion at T12 (curved arrow) shows loss of signal intensity compared to the adjacent normal marrow. (b) $T2$ weighted image. The lesions at both T8 (white arrow) and T12 (black arrow) show increased intensity. The spinal cord (curved white arrows) is displaced posteriorly at both levels

DISADVANTAGES OF MRI

There are several disadvantages to MRI. Our previous routine utilized 7 mm thick section with a 3 mm gap between sections. Although moderate-to-large disc herniations are readily demonstrated with this technique, small focal bulges can be missed because of partial volume averaging and the non-imaged gap. However, now 5 mm and 4 mm contiguous sections are becoming more widely available,[5] which is comparable to CT. MR also has a lower spatial resolution compared to CT. This lower resolution is partially offset by the greater soft-tissue contrast available with MR. The resolution of MR can be improved by using surface coils, which increase the signal-to-noise ratio. However, fine bony detail is still better defined by CT. Most of the disadvantages of MRI will diminish through continuing advances in instrumentation and imaging techniques.

SUMMARY

Magnetic resonance imaging shows great promise in the evaluation of the lumbar spine. Degenerative disc disease, spinal stenosis and neoplasms are demonstrated as well as or better than CT. Moreover, the ability to distinguish the annulus from the nucleus pulposus and the absence of streak artefacts are important advantages over CT. With the continuing technical advances that are certain in this decade, MRI may supplant CT in the evaluation of the spine during the 1990s.

REFERENCES

1 Moon K L Jr, Genant H K, Davis P L et al 1983 Nuclear magnetic resonance imaging in orthopedics: principles and applications. J. Orthop. Res. 1: 101–114

2 Mechlin M, Thickman D, Kressel H Y, Gefter W, Joseph P 1984 Magnetic resonance imaging of postoperative patients with metallic implants. A J R 143: 1281–1284

3 Modic M T, Weinstein M A, Pavlicek W, Boumphrey F, Starnes D, Duchesneau 1983 Magnetic resonance imaging of the cervical spine: technical and clinical observations. A J R 141: 1129–1136

4 Han J S, Kaufman B, El Yousef S J et al 1983 NMR imaging of the spine. A J R 141: 1137–1145

5 Modic M T, Pavlicek W, Weinstein M A et al 1984 Magnetic resonance imaging of intervertebral disk disease. Radiology 152: 103–111

6 Chafetz N I, Genant H K, Moon K L, Helms C A, Morris J M 1983 Recognition of lumbar disk herniation with NMR. A J R 141: 1153–1156

Conservative treatment of back pain

INTRODUCTION

To utilize *conservative* treatment effectively, one must embrace the *radical* notion that it will prove successful. The emphasis in this chapter is on that majority of low back pain problems wherein non-surgical intervention is not only conservative but effective. The outlook for restoration to an essentially normal lifestyle is excellent for patients with discogenic lumbar pain, provided that litigation, Workman's Compensation issues or other psychosocial stresses do not compromise the patient's motivation to comply with an appropriately structured regimen.[1-6]

What is involved in lumbar pain? Over 90% of lumbar pains can be related to perturbations of functions of the L4–L5 and L5–S1 discs.[7] Trauma to these discs (sprains) with varying amounts of annular ligamentous swelling, discal bulging, herniation and disc fragment extrusion can cause low back pain with or without radiation and with or without sciatic nerve compression. Dysfunction of the adjacent disc-vertebral connected facet joints (and/or possible sacro-iliac involvement) with development or exacerbation of facet osteoarthritis explain most of the remaining symptoms in patients with low back pain. It may seem cavalier to express no greater concern for the patient who also manifests sciatic or femoral radiculopathy, but one anticipates a spontaneous recovery in 80% of these patients, and the outcomes at one year and four years with surgical treatment are no better than after conservative treatment.[3, 5, 8, 9–11]

To undertake a truly conservative course of action in patients presenting with lumbar pain it is necessary to be conversant with the common low back pain problems in order to recognize and diligently pursue the diagnostic considerations of the rare causes. The diagnosis of lumbar pain due to causes other than disc-related usually suggests itself at the time of the initial evaluation or within the next few visits when it is apparent that conservative therapy is failing for reasons other than non-compliance to a well-considered regimen.

If one is to advocate conservative therapy, one has to be able to recognize it when one sees it. By and large, it is not found in a surgical operatory nor even during chemonucleolysis — but it can be! In a patient with relatively progressive paresis and/or bowel and bladder impairment, there is no justification for a wait-and-see approach. By the same token, a patient with acute or subacute leg and low back pain and manifest radiculopathy (positive straight-leg raising or Ely tests; knee jerk, medial hamstring, or achilles reflex impairment; or sensory and minor motor impairment consistent with femoral or sciatic dysfunction) even in the presence of E.M.G. documentation and/or positive CT or myelogram is best conservatively managed.[8, 11] Institution of chonucleolysis or surgery is considered only after conservative treatment has failed to conserve.[6, 11–14]

It should be remembered that surgery best serves those who respond best to conservative treatment — the acute lumbar-pain patient with sciatica. Surgery for low back pain per se, e.g. lumbar facet osteoarthritis or spondylolisthesis with low back strain is less effective and is potentially capable of aggravating rather than relieving the pain.[11, 15, 16] Refractory chronic spinal or root stenosis secondary to discal fragments or bony encroachment are two other difficult problems that may be better served by a more radical (surgical) intervention.[11, 17]

So, what is truly conservative therapy?[18–20] The

question is better stated, 'What is conservative therapy for what condition?' Granted that most causes for low back pain originate in the 4th and 5th lumbar discs and the related facet joints, neural structures and their pain referral patterns, the extent of tissue injury, the duration of its effect, the pain and suffering it causes and its potential for long-term impairment of function determine how each problem is best approached.[15, 21]

PHASES

A hierarchial categorization of lumbar pain by phases (Phase I to Phase IV) provides the physician, the associated health professionals and, above all, the patient with a concrete frame of reference for the severity of the problem, the requisite therapeutic options and the activity (or rest) level that is appropriate.

In establishing the patient's 'phase', it is important to consider the *duration* of symptoms — acute when less than four weeks, subacute when less than 12 weeks, chronic when greater than 12 weeks — as well as the *severity* of the low back pain problems in terms of pain intensity and the status, if present, of disc-related neurological complications. The use of 'acute', defined as duration of symptoms rather than the severity of the problem, helps avoid semantic confusion and inappropriate assessments of the patient's status.

Phase I patients have severe pain and/or an unstable neurological deficit and have acute, or subacute duration of symptoms. This includes patients with a severe exacerbation of previous chronic stable low back pain. Phase II patients have moderate pain and/or a resolving neurological deficit of acute-chronic duration. Phase III patients have mild pain of subacute or chronic duration with occasional moderate exacerbations during stressful activity. Any neurological deficit has now stabilized. Phase IV patients have minimal or no pain and a minimal stable chronic neurological deficit of no functional significance, e.g. a patch of numbness or slight weakness of toe extensors. The initial assignment of the patient to his or her appropriate phase level, with reassignments to higher phases as the patient progresses in his or her recovery, permits a rational ordering of therapies and activities. It also

serves as a reminder of the need for increasing activities and reconditioning through each phase of the recovery process, and it gives a motivating reinforcement to the patient that he or she is indeed progressing in his or her recovery.[22]

PAIN CONTROL MEASURES

In the vast majority of low back pain sufferers, relief of pain is their primary goal. Although many pharmacological agents are now available, it should be emphasized that there are a number of non-pharmacological methods available which are effective and economical and have a low risk of side-effects. It is our experience that, if non-pharmacological modalities are optimized, the need for pharmacological therapy is reduced or obviated entirely.

Heat

Heat (both superficial and deep) is useful because it eases pain, raises the pain threshold, reduces pain and muscle spasm and reduces joint stiffness.[23] Because of its potential for thermal damage, heat should not be used on areas which have impaired sensation, diminished circulation, or in subjects who are sedated or mentally compromised. A worrisome example is the over-sedated patient with acute severe back pain who also has impaired sensation or circulation in the lower extremities.

Superficial heat

Superficial heating modalities (e.g. hot packs, hydrocollator, heating pad) may be effective in relieving pain in deep tissues such as muscle, even though the heat they generate fails to penetrate the superficial subcutaneous tissues, possibly by reflex circulatory changes and by increasing pain threshold.

Deep heat

Diathermy and ultrasound are capable of delivering deep heat (heat which penetrates the superficial subcutaneous tissue). Although diathermy can produce deep heat, it has fallen by the wayside primarily because it has no major advantage over superficial heat in treating low back pain or pain of other musculoskeletal origin. The use of ultrasound, on the other hand, remains well established in clinical usage.[23] Ultrasound is generated by a high-frequency-sound generator which agitates molecules and produces heat. Areas which appropriately can be treated with ultrasound include locally tender areas such as muscle trigger points and tender bursae, entheses and tendon insertions. A typical treatment series might consist of 20-minute sessions 2–3 times per week for 2–3 weeks. A desirable effect is usually evident in the first or second session. Its use is contra-indicated in anaesthetised areas, in infected tissue, around prosthetic joints and over portions of the spinal cord which have been exposed by a laminectomy.

Cold

Efficacy of cold seems to be related to reduction or changes in local metabolic activity, decreased spindle activity and slowing of nerve conduction.[23] Trigger points and other focally tender areas may be treated with a two-minute application of ice massage in the form of an ice cube applied in a slow circular stroking manner over a small circumscribed area. Larger areas may be treated with a cold pack for 10–20 minutes. An improvised bag of ice or a bag of frozen peas or corn can be used in an emergency, but commercially available envelopes filled with pliable silicate gel that can be easily refrozen and can be fitted to areas of treatment are more suitable for use in chronic cases.

Electrical stimulation

Transcutaneous electric nerve stimulation (TENS or TNS) is one of several modalities which modify pain perception through electrical stimulation. The basic TNS unit consists of a small easily portable battery-powered unit the size of a deck of playing cards with two electrodes which can be attached to the skin proximal to or bridging the painful area. Optimization of pain relief usually requires adjustment of pulse frequency (high or low), pulse intensity, pulse duration and length of stimulation. High-frequency stimulation is more often useful for instant pain relief, while low-frequency stimulation is generally believed to give more prolonged pain relief.[24]

TNS may be administered continuously, but is usually delivered in shorter increments interspersed with periods of rest (e.g. two hours of TNS alternating with two hours of rest) for a maximum of 8 to 10 hours per 24-hour period. Complications of TNS include skin irritation from the adhesive, allergic reactions to the electrode gel, and sparking from poor contact causing cutaneous burns. TNS has been shown to decrease the pain of neuropathies and radiculopathies (particularly when applied over the related nerve), and this adjunctive control of sciatic pain makes this complication the main indication for its use in low back pain therapy.[24] Although the efficacy of TNS has not been shown as clearly for low back pain, it also appears occasionally to be a useful modality in patients with low back pain of a variety of causes, even in the absence of radiculopathy.[25, 26]

The Point Finder and Stimulator, an alternative method of electrical stimulation, employs a small battery-powered unit with a metal probe or applicator which can be used for locating and treating focally painful areas such as tender trigger points and tendon insertions, bursitis and focal muscle spasm. When point stimulation is used for treatment, the current is applied to the centre of the painful or tender area. Since each point can adequately be treated with 15–90 seconds of stimulation, multiple areas can be treated at any one session. Its use, as with TNS, is best avoided in subjects who are pregnant or reportedly in subjects who have demand cardiac pacemakers.

If pain relief is not provided by TNS or point stimulator, faradic or high-frequency galvanic muscle stimulation will occasionally afford relief of painful muscle spasm.[23]

Traction

In theory, the idea of distracting lumbar vertebrae by traction and thereby reducing pain emanating from a bulging intervertebral disc with or without nerve entrapment is an attractive one. It has in fact been demonstrated by epidurography that transient vertebral distraction and reduction of disc bulging can occur during traction.[27] A multitude of methods and apparatuses have been devised to administer traction. Unfortunately, their clinical efficacy has not been well substantiated in controlled studies.[28, 29]

The force required to overcome friction and inertia on a horizontal bed and yet provide vertebral distraction has been found to approximate 50% of body weight. On a friction-free table (split traction table) with a mobile lower segment, about one-half of that force would be required to produce vertebral distraction.[30] Inverted traction and hanging traction take advantage of the body's own weight to provide the distracting force. In clinical practice we have found very little value in horizontal traction. Despite the popularity and apparent simplicity of various forms of inverted traction, we have found none to be of particular value in those low back pain patients who were able to tolerate the inverted position. An alternative upright hanging device has recently been advocated.

Despite the popularity of hanging and inverted traction methods, their efficacy has not yet been substantiated and they do not appear to have significant advantages over standard horizontal methods, which themselves have not been shown to be efficacious in controlled series. Users of inverted traction should be aware that retinal detachment, regurgitation of stomach contents and aggravation of hypertension and pulmonary compromise may result from the inverted position.

Hydrotherapy

Heated tubs with or without water agitation have limited use as a heating modality. This is in part due to difficulty for the low back pain patient with getting into or out of the pool. However, swimming can be useful once patients have sufficiently recovered to tolerate pool buoyancy activities. A buoyancy belt or tube around the waist may minimize lumbar hyperextension or serve as an aid to swimming for subjects who are not well-qualified swimmers.

Medications

Several classes of medication have been advocated for the treatment of low back pain: analgesics, non-steroidal anti-inflammatory drugs (NSAIDs), skeletal muscle relaxants and tricyclic antidepressants. Analgesic medications (e.g. codeine, oxycodone plus aspirin) have been shown to reduce pain, but do not speed the period to recovery.[5] Although it is not clear that muscle relaxants are effective by virtue of relaxing skeletal muscle, several (e.g. carisoprodol, cyclobenzaprine) have been shown in placebo-controlled studies to be efficacious in relieving low back pain.[31, 32] Conversely, in the management of low back pain, the NSAIDs have not been shown to speed recovery nor to provide pain relief beyond that provided by bed rest alone.[5] In subjects with a large component of fibromyalgia, low-dose tricyclic antidepressant therapy (e.g. amitriptyline or doxepin, 10–75 mg near bedtime or in divided doses) may provide an additional margin of pain relief and often improve accompanying sleep disorders.[33]

Pain in the acute situation is a useful reminder to reduce or obviate activity which would interfere with the normal healing processes. Thus, to the extent possible, analgesic drugs should not be used in subjects with acute pain or radiculopathy in doses which would permit a level of activity beyond that which would allow natural resolution of the disorder. Conversely, if chronic pain persists (e.g. painful chronic facet osteoarthritis), analgesics may be useful in returning the patient to a higher level of activity.

Local injections

Patients with primary or generalized fibrositis and those with local or regional secondary soft tissue tenderness in muscles or their attachments often benefit from injections of local anaesthetics (2–5 ml of 1% lidocaine and/or depository steroids), seemingly regardless of the primary diagnosis. In patients with low back pain and regional myofascial pain, there are a few specific sites that are apt to be particularly tender and that often respond well to local injections where other pain-control measures have proven unsuccessful. These focal areas of palpable tender muscle induration ('spasm') are: over the sciatic outlet; deep in the gluteus maximus muscle; in the mid-belly of the gluteus medius muscle between the tip of the greater trochanter and the iliac crest; and in the mid-belly of the lateral wall of the quadratus lumborum muscle, halfway between the iliac crest and the lower ribs. These trigger areas closely correspond to established acupuncture points.[34, 35]

Two areas of bony tenderness that may benefit from local injections of steroids (2.5 mg of triamcinolone in 2–4 ml of 1% lidocaine) are: the area of the gluteus submaximus bursa just below the lateral aspect of the greater trochanter, and the medial aspect of the posterior superior iliac spine. Many other trigger areas can be found. One of the above is usually present during symptomatic episodes of low back pain in most patients. Injections of these as well as particularly sensitive, less common 'triggers' can be associated with a lessening of pain and more rapid restoration of function.

Exercises

There are three major schools of exercise therapy for low back pain. In addition to the exercise regimens advocated by these schools, there are a great number of variations of 'standard' exercises, despite the fact that at best the abdominal isometric strengthening exercise has been the exercise most often shown favourably to influence the outcome of patients with low back pain.[36-39]

The best-known school of low back pain is the flexion school most strongly advocated by Williams and Macnab.[40-42] The extension school, proposed by McKenzie, is rapidly gaining in popularity; and the eclectic or the anything-or-nothing school, e.g., 'take it easy', 'walk', 'swim', 'don't do any exercise', 'lift weights', 'hang upside down', etc., accounts for the remaining exercise regimens.[43]

The flexion school stresses avoidance of extension of the lumbar spine and the associated potential problems of compression of bulging posterior annular fibres and/or arthritic facet joints, while emphasizing the stretching of tight posterior muscles and ligaments for pain relief.[41,42] The flexion regimen also presumes that the posterior longitudinal ligament and posterior annular fibres, when made taut by the lumbar kyphotic posturing, help push the bulging posterior annular fibres and adjacent intradiscal contents anteriorly and away from compressed nerve roots and dural structures. it is also assumed to relieve nerve root compression at the posterior aspect of the intervertebral foramina from facet joint encroachment during extension.[41]

The extension school's rationale is based on the concept that, when the lumbar spine is extended, the posterior vertebral end-plates are approximated and

can act as a wedge to pinch and squeeze any posteriorly bulging nuclear material anteriorly and away from the posterior annular fibres and adjacent nerve roots.[43,44]

The *eclectic* approach is just that — do anything that does not hurt too much; do nothing; or do whatever — however arbitrarily. Given no certain outcome for any exercise regimen and the polarization of approaches in the two most widely used regimens, e.g., flexion versus extension, it seems prudent to re-examine the rationale for exercises in low back pain problems.

It is widely accepted that acute–severe (Phase I) low back pain problems respond to bed-rest.[3,10] Even here the flexion and extension advocates argue about the proper rest posture: supine with knees bent and legs propped up (flexion), and prone with a pillow under the chest in the rest position (extension).[41,43] One can assess both options during an examination and essentially take the cue from the patient's response to pain during an extension or flexion manoeuvre. Prone positioning seems to assist back and sciatic pain control for some and clearly exacerbates it for others.

In our experience the flexion regimen for the acute Phase I patient who must take to bed is the easiest to implement, requires less instruction and will allow for re-examination of alternatives after a few days to a week. Even bed-rest requires instructions if it is to prove its worth in proper transferring in and out of bed (or on and off the floor if the mattress is placed there for firmness), rolling from side to side to a side-lying posture with a pillow between the legs to minimize pelvic rotation. Grooming, toileting, eating and car seating for the ride home and the return visit also require careful instruction to a Phase I patient.

EXERCISES TO RELIEVE PAIN

Pain-relieving or 'feel-good' exercises

Teaching exercises, like one's cooking, is better served if first tasted or tried. Therefore it is incumbent on the teacher of exercises to be familiar with the proper performance of the exercise and the problems that can occur if it is performed incorrectly. Like a well-prepared menu, the exercise to be taught should be accompanied with a well-written illustrated handout. Even if the handout is optimal and the exercise instruction is optimal, both are required at least once in a second session and often need to be retaught in order to be properly learnt.

The exercises to relieve pain or 'feel-good' exercises are selected because of their ability to enhance patient comfort and thereby provide the patient with a measure of control over his or her disorder. These exercises are performed as slow stretches; they are not accompanied with jerking or ballistic movements and are typically held for 5–10 seconds at the termination of each gentle stretch.

Phase I patients are on a full bed-rest regimen, up only for lavatory privileges and meals when tolerated. The importance of bed-rest in Phase I and II in expediting recovery cannot be overstressed.[3, 5, 8, 10]

In Phase I, when the patient is able to move without undue distress, a gentle pelvic tilt repeated as often as required for comfort can be instituted. In many patients, further relief of low back pain can be obtained by lying in the supine position, grasping the knees and then squeezing the thighs against the chest for about 5 seconds.[40] For the patient who is more comfortable in extension, prone press-ups in which the head, shoulders and upper trunk *but not the pelvis* are raised and lowered at a slow count (up one and two, down one and two) can be repeated 10 times hourly and before and after each required trip out of bed (e.g. to the lavatory).[45]

In the conventional flexion mode the patient may find that alternating supine single or bilateral 'double' knee-to-chest stretches give relief of lumbar tightness and associated discomfort. For some, Macnab's 'kick-up' exercise is helpful for pain control.[41, 46] The exercise is begun by clutching the hands behind flexed knees and slowly rocking, or by slowly raising the pelvis and thighs, with the knees and hips flexed at 90°. With the knees flexed, a gentle 'kick-up' is performed in which the knees move toward the face. The buttocks are then lowered to the starting position to the bed. The exercise is repeated five times. Another often helpful exercise for reducing pain in the lumbosacral and buttock areas is the 'knee-back' exercise which can be performed in the supine or sitting position (see Figure 14.1).

All of these exercises can be introduced in Phase I and are useful in Phases II and III as well. Even if the patient when first seen is capable of functioning at a Phase II–IV level, it is advisable to begin the exercises with Phase I 'feel-good' and abdominal

isometrics. To further assure proper conditioning and to avoid exercise-related exacerbations, the patients are progressed through a hierarchy of more intensive exercises ('do-good' exercises) until they reach their optimal goal in Phase I–IV.

It is important to bear in mind when prescribing exercise therapy that compliance can be lost by an excessively demanding regimen. We recommend that the total time spent on the exercise program each day be limited to 30–60 minutes during the therapeutic and convalescent phases. The total time can be broken into shorter exercise units (e.g. 15 minutes twice daily). For maintenance exercise, exclusive of recreational athletics, a 5–10 minute regimen should suffice.

Reconditioning or 'do-good' exercises

The patient in Phase I, when no longer in severe discomfort, can usually begin the abdominal isometric exercise.[47] Since most patients in Phases I and II require a corset for pain control at least some of the time, it has been our experience that, when a patient can hold an abdominal isometric contraction in the supine knee-flexed position for 40 seconds, he or she is usually ready to discontiue corset-wearing except for special circumstances — e.g., heavy work.[47, 48]

In Phase II the patient is up and about 10–90% of the time, walking or riding short distances and perhaps has returned to part-time work or light household activity. He or she is ready for additional stretches which are now introduced in a stepwise fashion. The stretches include a hamstring stretch in the supine position (deferred if sciatic symptomatology is aggravated); supine pelvic rotation with both knees flexed and feet on the floor (moving the legs together slowly to the floor from one side and then to the other), and then a standing Achilles tendon stretch.[47] It is notable that even patients with generalized joint laxity seem to be made more comfortable by mild stretches when the stretch commences at or near the end of the limits of their available pain-free range.

More rigorous abdominal isometric strengthening can be achieved through a shift of the centre of gravity by changing the hand placement from initially over the knee to the chest, then behind the

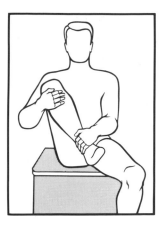

THE KNEE BACK (SITTING)

PURPOSE: TO RELIEVE PAIN RADIATING INTO THE
BUTTOCKS BY S-T-R-E-T-C-H-I-N-G TENSE
BUTTOCK MUSCLES.

1. SIT DOWN.
2. GRASP THE UPPER SIDE OF YOUR RIGHT (OR LEFT —
   CHOOSE MOST PAINFUL SIDE) ANKLE WITH YOUR LEFT (OR
   RIGHT — THE OPPOSITE SIDE) HAND IN AN OVERHAND
   HOLD.
3. PLACE YOUR LEFT (OR RIGHT — MOST PAINFUL SIDE)
   HAND UNDER YOUR LEFT (OR RIGHT) KNEE.
4. GENTLY PRESS YOUR HEEL TOWARD YOUR GROIN AND AT
   THE SAME TIME GENTLY PULL YOUR KNEE TOWARD THE
   PAINFUL SIDE'S SHOULDER.
5. HOLD THIS POSITION AND COUNT: 1001 TO 1010.
   COUNT MAY BE INCREASED TO 1020.
6. REPEAT_____TIMES PER DAY.

PRECAUTION: STOP EXERCISE IF PAIN INCREASES OR
NUMBNESS OR TINGLING OCCURS.

R.L. Swezey, M.D. A. Swezey
M. Deckert. © 1983

Fig. 14.1 The knee-back (sitting) position

neck, and finally with the elbows extended horizontally behind the head (see Figures 14.2 and 14.3).

Strengthening of the quadriceps muscles also commences with a supine back-protective, leg-extended, 'quad-set' isometric exercise. In this exercise the opposite hip is flexed, posteriorly rotating the pelvis to flatten and stabilize the spine. The quadriceps are further strengthened in a standing exercise wherein the back is flattened against a wall and then the body slowly lowered to hold an isometric contraction initially at 30° for 5–10 seconds and ultimately at 60° for 40–60 seconds. The purpose of the quadriceps strenghtening is to facilitate squatting, kneeling and arising in a back-protective manner. The gluteal muscles can be further strengthened (they, like the quadriceps, are essential to accomplish controlled kneeling or squatting for back protection), by a raised pelvic tilt exercise. This is performed from the supine pelvic tilt position, raising and holding the pelvis above the floor in an isometric contraction. All of these exercises are designed so as to avoid a backstrain posture. They are seqentially implemented to permit gradual reconditioning and to help prepare patients for participation in their daily activities with less vulnerability to back strain.

PARTIAL "SIT-UP" (ABDOMINAL ISOMETRIC):
LYING DOWN WITH ARMS STRAIGHT
PURPOSE: TO STRENGTHEN ABDOMINAL MUSCLES IN ORDER TO HELP ALLEVIATE STRESS ON BACK MUSCLES.

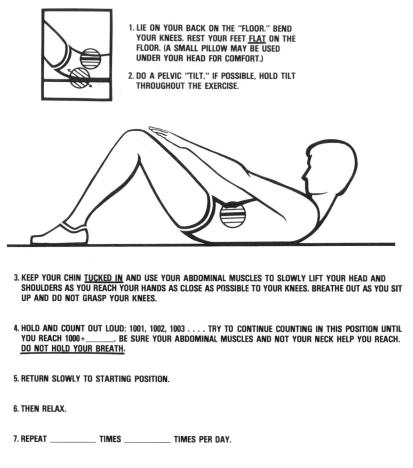

1. LIE ON YOUR BACK ON THE "FLOOR." BEND YOUR KNEES. REST YOUR FEET <u>FLAT</u> ON THE FLOOR. (A SMALL PILLOW MAY BE USED UNDER YOUR HEAD FOR COMFORT.)

2. DO A PELVIC "TILT." IF POSSIBLE, HOLD TILT THROUGHOUT THE EXERCISE.

3. KEEP YOUR CHIN <u>TUCKED IN</u> AND USE YOUR ABDOMINAL MUSCLES TO SLOWLY LIFT YOUR HEAD AND SHOULDERS AS YOU REACH YOUR HANDS AS CLOSE AS POSSIBLE TO YOUR KNEES. BREATHE OUT AS YOU SIT UP AND DO NOT GRASP YOUR KNEES.

4. HOLD AND COUNT OUT LOUD: 1001, 1002, 1003 . . . . TRY TO CONTINUE COUNTING IN THIS POSITION UNTIL YOU REACH 1000+_____. BE SURE YOUR ABDOMINAL MUSCLES AND NOT YOUR NECK HELP YOU REACH. <u>DO NOT HOLD YOUR BREATH.</u>

5. RETURN SLOWLY TO STARTING POSITION.

6. THEN RELAX.

7. REPEAT _____ TIMES _____ TIMES PER DAY.

Fig. 14.2 Partial 'sit-up' (abdominal isometric): lying down with arms straight

Phase III exercises

The Phase III patient is engaging in normal activities and in less vigorous sports with no or only mild restrictions. If his or her condition warrants, he or she is moving into preconditioning for more potentially vigorous activities. Such patients may or may not be resting in the afternoon, walking more vigorously, may be swimming and bicycling (in the upright position), and may even play light doubles tennis or golf. The Phase III exercises provide additional rotary spinal stretches to mobilize both the lumbar spine, hips and gluteal fascial attachments overlying the greater trochanter. These include: advanced pelvic rotations, a seated forward-bending stretch, and the quadruped or hand-and-knees position 'catback' stretch.[47]

It is well to consider that, whereas 'feel-good' exercises can be performed at any time for pain control, further stretching of tight tissues in order to improve mobility is more effectively done when muscles have been warmed by activity, e.g., a walk, swim or bike ride. Progressive back extensor muscle strengthening in the back protective quadruped position can be instituted. These would include the single arm raise, the single leg raise, and the opposite arm and leg raise, all performed with an isometric 5–10 second hold of the raised extremities.

PARTIAL "SIT-UP" (ABDOMINAL ISOMETRIC):
LYING DOWN WITH ARMS EXTENDED ALONG SIDES OF HEAD

PURPOSE: TO STRENGTHEN ABDOMINAL MUSCLES IN ORDER TO HELP ALLEVIATE STRESS ON BACK MUSCLES.

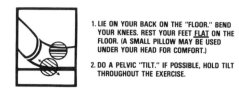

1. LIE ON YOUR BACK ON THE "FLOOR." BEND YOUR KNEES. REST YOUR FEET <u>FLAT</u> ON THE FLOOR. (A SMALL PILLOW MAY BE USED UNDER YOUR HEAD FOR COMFORT.)

2. DO A PELVIC "TILT." IF POSSIBLE, HOLD TILT THROUGHOUT THE EXERCISE.

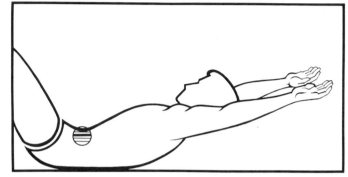

3. EXTEND BOTH ARMS ALONG THE SIDES OF YOUR HEAD.

4. KEEP YOUR CHIN <u>TUCKED IN</u> AND USE YOUR ABDOMINAL MUSCLES TO SLOWLY RAISE YOUR HEAD, SHOULDERS, AND ARMS UNTIL YOUR SHOULDER BLADES NO LONGER TOUCH THE FLOOR. KEEP YOUR LOWER BACK FLAT.

5. BREATHE OUT AS YOU SIT UP.

6. HOLD AND COUNT OUT LOUD: 1001, 1002, 1003 . . . . TRY TO CONTINUE COUNTING IN THIS POSITION UNTIL YOU REACH 1000+_____. <u>DO NOT HOLD YOUR BREATH.</u>

7. RETURN SLOWLY TO STARTING POSITION.

8. THEN, RELAX.

9. REPEAT _____ TIMES _____ TIMES PER DAY.

Fig. 14.3 Partial 'sit-up' (abdominal isometric): lying down with arms extended along the sides of the head

All of the quadruped exercises are best performed with care taken to avoid raising the extremity above the level of the spine in order to minimize strains in an extended lumbar posture. These exercises seem appropriate to recondition the dorsal-lumbar musculature, particularly for osteopenic patients, but they must be carefully instituted, as they can exacerbate symptoms of back pain and strain. Prone extension strengthening, with a pillow under the abdomen raising the abdomen to maintain a protective lumbar flexion posture, can be initiated before attempting exercises in the quadruped position.

Phase IV exercises

The patient in Phase IV is resuming heavy work and/or vigorous athletics. He or she will, like any athlete, benefit from all-round exercise in order to achieve optimal strength, agility, flexibility and endurance. He or she will also require specific conditioning for specific sports as well as appropriate instructions in back-protective measures for each sport (tennis — avoid arching and back extension in the serve and overhead shots; golf — avoid arching in the follow-through, and remember to kneel to tee up).

Formal Phase IV exercises include prone back extension exercises (performed without a pillow) with single arm raises, then opposite arm and leg raises. When each of these exercises can be done without difficulty (three repetitions in each position held as a terminal isometric contraction for 10 seconds), bilateral arm raises, bilateral leg raises and finally simultaneous bilateral arm and leg raises are introduced. These are strenuous exercises and should be used cautiously, particularly in patients with facet syndromes, spinal stenosis, spondylolysthesis or radiculopathy. Further back and upper extremity conditioning is achieved through prone push-ups, starting first with knees bent and pushing off from the knees and hands, progressing to the classic push-up from the toes with the legs extended.

Aerobic conditioning (in patients without knee problems) can be initiated with repetitions of standing wall slides (the patient stands with his or her back against the wall and slides up and down repeatedly), progressing to repeated deep-knee bends, standing behind a counter or a chair for balance. Most patients with low back pain can achieve a satisfying high level of physical exercise by swimming (no diving, no butterfly stroke); walking, gradually increasing the distance and the pace (no hip swinging race walking); or bicycling (preferably seated upright with a short seat to crank distance to minimize lumbopelvic rotation).

In summary, exercise is first initiated to relieve pain and then progressed to assure reasonable flexibility and strength sufficient to engage in daily activities and ultimately to resume, when possible, more vigorous work, recreational and athletic pursuits.

POSTURE

For a back patient, good posture is the posture that minimizes the stresses and strains from gravitational forces. If one views the patient standing in profile, a line ideally should be drawn through the external auditory canal, the point of the shoulder, the vertical trunk, the greater trochanter, the anterior aspect of the knee and the proximal tarsal joints. But our patient also sits, lies, bends, reaches, walks, climbs, shops, plays the piano and rides bicycles, among other activities. He or she does these activities en face as well as in profile and at various angles, with the anatomical defects (short leg or round shoulders) with which he or she was endowed or acquired, and with little conscious awareness of how he or she is actually aligned.

It is the Extension School's advocacy of maintaining lordosis as opposed to the traditional Flexion or Pelvic-Tilt-At-All-Times School that has caused contention.[41, 43] Our experience is that a middle ground can be found wherein the patient is taught to flatten the lumbar curve with a mild gluteal contraction (gluteal pinch) to assure a measure of conscious control over lumbar alignment without stressing either extension or flexion.

Posture, for the patient in bed, means lying supine with the knees supported on a firm pillow, bolster, suitcase, folded blanket, or in a gatched hospital bed with a supportive but not board-like mattress; side-lying with the hips and knees partially flexed (hook-lying) and, for most patients, with a firm pillow between the knees to minimize lumbosacral rotary stresses. To change positions, the patient is taught to squeeze the buttocks in order to flatten and stabilize the lower back and then 'log roll' the shoulders, trunk, pelvis and knees as one unit from side to back or to the opposite side.

When the patient is seated, the back is supported against a firm seat-back by a folded blanket, a flat pillow, purse, briefcase or a folded sweater or coat (a tablecloth in a restaurant will do in an emergency). The hips and knees are flexed and the feet are preferably raised a few inches on a footstool, briefcase, book, etc. Chairs with arms and with firm and relatively high seats are sought for ease of seating and arising.

Standing postures can be taught with these few simple rules: 'back first, back flat, back straight and back last'.

'Back first' means plan ahead and think of back protection first before engaging in any activity.

'Back flat' reminds the patient to perform a mild pelvic tilt in order to flatten the back by pinching the buttocks together and tightening the stomach muscles before engaging in any activity that might stress the back.

'Back straight' reminds the patient to avoid bending over, twisting and reaching.*

'Back last' tells the patient to position himself or herself using the arms and legs first and the back last in lifting, pulling, pushing and other potentially stressful activities.

Ergonomics and kinetics

Although optimal static posture minimizes disc pressure and strain on lumbar structures, it is increasingly important as the patient becomes more active (Phases II–IV) to consider kinetic postural factors. The accumulative stress of a mildly lurching gait on the patient with a functionally short leg may necessitate a corrective heel lift or instruction provided for cane-assisted walking.[48a] Choice of proper supportive shoes, techniques for kneeling and lifting, instruction in pushing vs pulling heavy objects and in the use of a stepstool or ladder rather than overhead reaching all require deliberate patient education and training. The reader is referred to additional resources for specific recommendations in patient instruction guidelines.[41, 49–53]

Corsets and braces

Corsets are important adjuncts to posture and ergonomic methods for stabilizing the lumbar spine. Classic studies on the efficacy of corsets and braces have demonstrated that abdominal compression and not limitation of lumbar motion is the essential ingredient.[54, 55] Indeed, some corsets and braces that give considerable support in static postures may actually increase lumbar motion during ambulation.[54, 56] Aside from the fact that braces are made more sturdily, generally require less surface contact for support and are therefore cooler, there is no particular reason for prescribing a brace over a corset.[57] This is particularly true in view of the customary short-term need for corsets.

Lumbar corsets come in many forms. We have found that most of the patients with Phase I–II low back pain problems get adequate support for pain control with an elastic cinch that utilizes a heat moulded rigid plastic lumbosacral pad.[58] An inexpensive motorcyclist's elastic 'kidney belt' can also serve well. Occasional patients prefer a narrow (5–10 cm) elastic or webbed 'sacroiliac trochanteric belt'. This provides little abdominal support but does restrict lumbosacral and sacroiliac movement sufficiently for pain control in some patients. In pregnancy, where lumbosacral strains are associated with ligamentous laxity, these small 'belts' are easily fitted under the protruberant abdomen and can add to patient comfort. More rigorous support is achieved with a heavy cloth garment employing three anterior straps and buckles to permit firm anchoring and also to create the option for release of the upper belt and snaps for comfort while sitting.[44]

We all come in different sizes and shapes, but most patients can be fitted with 'off-the-shelf' ready-made garments using one of the above alternatives. Needless to say, corseting the extremely obese or very 'hippy' patient, or patients with sensitive skin or ribs or with scoliosis and kyphosis, can become extremely difficult and even futile. It should be remembered that the patient not only needs to be properly fitted, but also requires careful instruction in donning and doffing a corset. The corset is best donned with the patient supine, the knees flexed and the back flat, or when standing, leaning against the wall with the garment between the patient's flattened lumbar spine and the wall. At the very least, back strain is to be avoided during the actual process of applying the therapeutic corset.

Finally, it should be established that the patient has sufficient abdominal muscle strength (e.g. holds an abdominal isometric contraction for 40 seconds) so that when pain control permits, he or she is able to be 'weaned' from the corset. We usually recommend more corset-wearing in the afternoon and evening, when the patient is apt to be fatigued, before finally relinquishing all use of corsets. Even when the corsets are no longer used on a daily basis, we recommend that some patients wear them like 'work gloves' during activities that are particularly stressful.

MANUAL THERAPIES (MASSAGE, MOBILIZATION AND MANIPULATION)

If it can be accepted that some exercises or particular movements performed by patients can relieve low

---

*A supplementary rule in this case is: 'feet first and face it'. This means that, to avoid twisting, the patient should position the body directly over the feet and face the task to be done, rather than twist to do it. This would apply to reaching into a file drawer from a desk seat or preparing to lift an object from the floor or overhead, no matter how light; or the stance that one should take at the moment of racket impact on a tennis ball.

back pain, and that restriction of untoward movement by postural control or corseting can also prevent or relieve pain, then it is possible to consider that there may be specificity in the relationship of certain spinal movements to the treatment of back disorders. McKenzie and Macnab have placed particular emphasis on mobilizing intradiscal or facetal structures by active (patient self-performed) exercises.[40, 45] Cyriax, Macnab and many others also advocate passive movements applied to the patient by the physician or therapist to relieve pain, muscle spasm and/or to restore normal structural relationships and mobility in disc, facet or sacroiliac joints.[40,44,59-63]

The problem of convincing the sceptical that there is specificity to the clinical assessments of manual therapists and therefore to their manipulations is considerable. One has but to reflect on the confusing overlap of innervations in paralumbar structures, or the notable difficulties encountered with correlating CT, E.M.G., myelogram, clinical signs and surgical findings.[11,64-66]

There is inadequate scientific documentation for the efficacy of massage or mobilization of low back pain disorders (the reports on efficacy of manipulation in the treatment of low back pain show either no efficacy or at best a slightly accelerated rate of recovery during the first few weeks). One then has to ask what it is about manual therapy that continues to provide literally millions of patients to those who employ manual therapeutic methods.[64, 67-70]

Massage

Massage, perhaps because it is time-honoured and usually relatively benign, is the least controversial of the various manually-applied therapeutic movements. In various massage techniques soft tissue can be stroked, pounded, kneaded, squeezed or compressed in order to relieve pain, relax focal or diffuse muscle contractions and/or to increase musculoskeletal mobility. Recent advances in neurophysiology suggest that pain control and muscle relaxation may have common pathways.[70a,71,73] Superficial stimulation by vibration, heat or cold, or musculoskeletal movement can inhibit the firing of a muscle spindle directly or stimulate large sensory afferent fibres and thereby inhibit pain centrally by a variety of

mechanisms including the recent observations of endorphin release.[24,70a,71,73-75] It is thought that these mechanisms explain many of the phenomena observed in association with massage therapy.

The introduction of acupuncture and its offshoots, including acupressure and electroacupuncture, and the development of transcutaneous nerve stimulation have dramatically accelerated our appreciation of the importance of peripheral stimulation on pain control.[73-75] The final common path of these peripheral stimulations from the standpoint of manual therapies includes manual stimulation of a variety of muscle and skeletal structures that appear to be highly associated with the sensory pathways extensively studied in connection with acupuncture and transcutaneous nerve stimulation.[74-76]

Mobilization

If massage can be viewed in part as a variety of techniques that serve to inhibit pain through selective passive manual movements, then mobilization can also be considered in that light. Gentle oscillating or rotary movements of lumbar and lumbosacral structures are often accompanied by reduced pain and lessened associated muscle spasm.[62, 73] Whether the more vigorous mobilizations serve to stretch or rupture micro- or macroadhesions in facet joints and paradiscal structures in order to permit further freedom of movement as a means of reducing postural or activity-related strains has not been proved.[77] One can, however, argue from the example of the lessening of pain that so often accompanies restoration of mobility in the 'frozen shoulder' that more vigorous skeletal mobilization may act similarly on contractures of paraspinal ligaments and muscle. Indeed, it is the expectation that more vigorous mobilizations and manipulations do restore more normal skeletal mobility and structural relationships that provides the primary purpose for mobilization.[60, 61, 63, 77-79] It is the same hope, too often unfulfilled, that underlies the persistence of chiropractors and other manual therapists in persevering in manipulating and remanipulating to 'restore normal alignment' that also serves to cast doubt on the efficacy of all manual therapies.

Manipulation

If one can put aside legitimate concerns that harm can be caused by manipulation (indeed, it can, although this is rare when manual therapies are applied for low back pain in the absence of sciatica), one can consider that manipulation may be a potentially useful adjunct to the management of some low back pain disorders.[60, 61, 63, 79–82]

First the distinction must be made between mobilization, a passively-induced controlled movement by the physician or therapist, and manipulation, which also uses a passively-induced but momentarily uncontrolled movement accomplished through a high-velocity purposefully-directed thrusted manoeuvre. It is this brief high-velocity thrust which, once set in motion (and therefore no longer controllable), provides the potentially dangerous but gratifying cracking sound that may be associated with pain reduction and restoration of movement.[61,62,77] It also may be associated with wrenching pain, onset of sciatica or fracture of an overlooked malignant infiltrate or osteopenic bone.[79–82]

It is the sound and fury of manipulation that attracts and repels, and in general has relegated its practices to the lay practitioner or paraprofessional. There its wide acceptance by the public continues to gall the medical profession. The fury is in the uncontrolled thrust, its potential for harm, and in the lack of scientific justification for its use.

Why the thrust? If other more controlled forms of manual therapy can relieve pain and restore mobility, why the thrust? The rationale for the thrust is that the high-velocity movement occurs so rapidly that reflex protective muscle contraction or guarding is momentarily inhibited, allowing for properly-positioned articular structures to be moved or 'adjusted'.[77] The thrust presumably accomplishes for the manipulator what anesthesia does for the surgeon, when, for example, he reduces a subluxation of a shoulder or a torn meniscus. Manipulation is done with the patient fully awake, thereby allowing for immediate assessment of the effort. It is this opportunity to abruptly impact on perceived articular derangements with, hopefully, immediate results that gives manipulation its glamour and staying power. It is the firm conviction of many manual therapists that disc fragments can be replaced, or blocked facet joints can be released by their handiwork. But this is supported only by fragmentary and unconvincing evidence, perhaps indicating as much the inadequacy of our current technology and research as the unwarranted convictions.[64, 67–70, 78]

Unquestionably, many patients with low back pain have 'limped in and danced [or at least walked] out' of the treatment room following a manipulation. This is also true for spray-stretch, acupressure, or local lidocaine injections and for less aggressive massage or mobilization therapies. Obviously, at the time of this writing the need for manipulation as such in the management of low back pain is not great, and the best that can be said for it is that it may play a role in shortening the early weeks of painful disability, and this remains to be proved.[64,67–70,78] It nonetheless seems reasonable to attempt manipulation in selected cases where pain and muscle spasm permit and, more importantly, the risk of fracture or aggravation of disc-related radiculopathy is not likely. Furthermore, even if it is not reasonable, it is sensible to assume that it will probably be done anyway to millions of patients by thousands of practitioners of manipulative therapy.

PRACTICAL CONSIDERATION FOR SPECIFIC SPINAL DISORDERS

The principles of Phase I–IV therapies are generally applicable to the major disorders of the lumbar spine. Exercise and posture emphasizing lumbar extension are contra-indicated in patients with spondylolisthesis, spinal stenosis and facet syndromes. Although manipulation is occasionally dramatically successful in ankylosing spondylitis, skeletal hyperostosis, facet syndrome and in patients with lumbar strains, it should not be risked in patients with radiculopathy, spinal stenosis and obviously not in those patients with severe osteopenia or tumour. Nonetheless, gentle mobilization can be an adjunct for pain relief in many cases, with perhaps a major benefit coming from the support of the 'hands-on' therapist.

Scoliosis

Patients with scoliosis come in three major groupings: those whose scoliosis is secondary to a short leg and thereby correctable with a heel lift (typically a heel or a heel-sole correction of two-thirds of the leg length discrepancy suffices); those whose scoliosis is structural and usually congenital; and those whose scoliosis is secondary to lumbar disc derangements — so-called sciatic scoliosis.

Congenital scoliosis has not been shown to be influenced by exercises, but instruction in ergonomics and emphasis on rotary stretches often provide symptomatic relief.[83–85] These patients are at least as susceptible as the general population to disc-related problems, and therefore management of low back pain in such patients as those with disc-related disorders (Phase I–IV) is frequently successful — particularly if exercises designed to stretch painful dorsal lumbar structures by trunk rotation are emphasized.[86]

The 'sciatic' scoliosis presents a special problem. In the absence of radiculopathy, these patients can sometimes be promptly relieved by manipulation, and certain others do well with an intensive extension regimen.[62, 87]

The majority of patients with sciatic scoliosis will do just as well treated in the Phase I–III manner. By the end of one month there is no detectable difference in the outcomes of these patients treated with or without manipulation.[64, 67–70, 78] There is a small group of patients with resistant discogenic scoliosis (sometimes evident only when the standing patient bends forward) that are often relieved of their scoliosis and associated pain by specific mobilizing exercises described by McKenzie as 'flexion in step standing'.[59]

Ankylosing spondylitis

Ankylosing spondylitis and related spondyloarthropathies primarily require emphasis on erect posture with gentle stretching, deep breathing and back extension strengthening in addition to NSAID drugs.

SUMMARY

The conservative treatment of back pain requires the skill of the practitioner to conserve the potential for the injured tissues to repair themselves. This requires a judicious balance of rest, exercise and activities. It usually demands pain-control measures which can range from household remedies (heat and ice) to more sophisticated pharmacological and physical therapy modalities.

The conservative treatment of low back pain ultimately rests on education. The education of physicians and associated health professionals and their ability to educate the patient as to his or her role, responsibilities and the means to achieve short- and long-term goals often determines the outcome. Conservative treatment often demands psychological support and sometimes psychological, social and vocational counselling. For the low back pain patient, it is not enough to tell him or her to 'live with it'. We have both the opportunity and obligation to teach the patient with low back pain how to live *well* with it.

REFERENCES

1   Cairns D, Mooney V, Crane P 1984. Spinal pain rehabilitation: inpatient and outpatient treatment results and development of predictions for outcome. Spine 9: 91–95

2   Hammonds W H, Brena S F, Unikel I P 1978 Compensation for work-related injuries and rehabilitation of patients with chronic pain. Southern Med. J. 71: 664–666

3   Johnson E W, Fletcher F R 1981 Lumbosacral radiculopathy: review of 100 consecutive cases. Arch. Phys. Med. Rehab. 62: 321–323

4   Quinet R J, Hadler N M 1979 Diagnosis and treatment of backache. Seminars in Arth. Rheum. 8: 261–287

5   Wiesel S W, Cuckler J M, Deluca F, Jones F, Zeide M S, Rothmen R H 1980 Acute low-back pain. An objective analysis of conservative therapy. Spine 5: 324–330

6   Wiltsie L L, Widell E H, Mausen A Y 1975 Chymopapain in lumbar disc disease. JAMA 231: 478–483

7   Grabias S L, Mankin H J (1980) Pain in the lower back. Bull. Rheum. Dis. 30: 1040–1045

8   Bell G, Rothman R H 1984 The conservative treatment of sciatica. Spine 9: 54–56

9   Porter R W, Hibbert C, Evans C 1984 The natural history of root entrapment syndrome. Spine 9: 418–421

10 Pearce J, Moll J M H (1967) Conservative treatment and natural history of acute lumbar disc lesions. J. Neurol. Neurosurg. Psychiat. 30: 13–17

11 Rothman R H, Simeone F A 1975 The spine. Saunders, Philadelphia, p 484–510

12 Benoist M, Deburge A, Heripret G, Busson J, Rigot J, Cauchoix J 1982 Treatment of lumbar disc herniation by chymopapain chemonucleolysis. Spine 7: 613–617

13 Crawshaw C, Frazer A M, Merriam W F, Mulholland R C, Webb J K 1984 A comparison study of surgery and chemonucleolysis in the treatment of sciatica. Spine 9: 195–198

14 Fraser R D 1982 Chymopapain for the treatment of intervertebral disc herniation. Spine 7: 608–612

15 Sprangfort E V 1972 The lumbar disc herniation: a

computer aided analysis of 2504 operations. Acta. Scand. Orth., suppl 142: 1–95

16 Stauffer R N 1977 An approach to failure of lumbar spine operations. In: Ruge D, Wiltsie L L (eds) Spinal disorders diagnosis and treatment. Lea & Febiger, Philadelphia, p 328–333

17 Wiltsie L L, Rocchio P D 1975 Preoperative psychological tests as predictors of success of chemonucleolysis in the treatment of the low back syndrome. J. Bone Joint Surg. 57A: 478–483

18 Dixon A St J 1976 Diagnosis of low back pain — sorting the complainers. In: Jayson M I V The lumbar spine and back pain. Grune & Stratton, New York, p. 77–92

19 Fry J 1972 Back pain and soft tissue rheumatism. Advisory Services Colloquium Proc. Advisory Services (Clinical and General) Ltd, London

20 Godfrey C M, Morgan P P, Schatzker J 1984 A randomized trial of manipulation for low-back pain in a medical setting. Spine 9: 301–304

21 Farfan H F 1973 Mechanical disorders of the low back. Lea & Febiger, Philadelphia, p 138

22 Swezey R L 1980 Low back pain. In: Fries J F, Ehrlich G E (eds) Prognosis. Charles Press, p 360–364

23 Lehman J F, Delateur B J 1982 Diathermy and superficial heat and cold therapy. In: Kottle F J, Stillwell G K, Lehman J F (eds) Krusen's handbook of physical medicine. Saunders, Philadelphia, p 275–350

24 Anderson S A 1979 Pain control by sensory stimulation: In: Bonica J J (ed) Advances in pain research and therapy, vol 3. Raven Press, New York, p 569–585

24a Thorsteinsson G, Stonnington H H, Stillwell G K, Elveback L R 1977 Transcutaneous electric stimulation: a double-blind trial of its efficiency for pain. Arch. Phys. Med. Rehab. 58: 8–13

25 Ersek R A 1976 Low back pain: prompt relief with transcutaneous neuro-stimulation. A report of 35 consecutive patients. Orthop. Rev. 5: 27–31

26 Fried T, Johnson R, McCracken W 1984 Transcutaneous nerve stimulation: its role in the control of chronic pain. Arch. Phys. Med. Rehab. 65: 228–31

27 Mathews J A 1968 Dynamic discography: a study of lumbar traction. Ann. Phys. Med. 9: 275–9

28 Mathews J A, Hickling J 1975 Lumbar traction: a double-blind study for sciatica. Rheumat. Rehab. 14: 222–225

29 Weber H 1973 Traction therapy in sciatica due to disc prolapse. J. Oslo City Hosp. 23: 167–176

30 Judovich B, Nobel G R 1957 Traction therapy: a study of resistance forces. Am. J. Surg. 93: 108–14

31 Baratta R R 1976 A double-blind comparative study of carisoprodol, propoxyphene and placebo in the management of low back syndrome. Curr. Ther. Res. 20: 233–240

32 Brown B R Jr, Womble J 1978 Cyclobenzaprine in intractable pain syndromes with muscle spasma. JAMA 240: 1151–52

33 Smythe H A 1979 Nonarticular rheumatism and psychogenic musculoskeletal syndromes. In: McCarthy D I (ed) Arthritis and allied conditions. Lea & Febiger, Philadelphia, p 881–91

34 The Academy of Traditional Chinese Medicine 1975 An outline of Chinese acupuncture. Foreign Languages Press, Peking, p 140–190

35 Melzack R, Stillwell D M, Fox E V 1977 Trigger points and acupuncture points for pain: correlations and implications. Pain 3: 3–23

36 Davies J E, Gibson T, Tester L 1979 The value of exercises in the treatment of low back pain. Rheumat. Rehab. 18: 243–247

37 Kendall P H, Jenkins J M 1968a) Exercises for back ache: a double-blind controlled trial. Physiotherapy 54: 154–157

38 Kendall P H, Jenkins J M 1968b Lumbar isometric flexion exercises. Physiotherapy 54: 158–163

39 Lidstrom A, Zachrisson M 1970 Physical therapy on low back pain and sciatica. Scand. J. Rehab. Med. 2: 37–42

40 Macnab I 1977 Backache. Waverly Press, p 136–138

41 Williams P C 1953 The conservative management of lesions of the lumbosacral spine. The American Academy of Orthopedic Surgeons Instructional Course Lectures 10: 90–121

42 Williams P C 1955 Examination and conservative treatment for disc lesions of the lower spine. Clin. Orthop. 5: 28–35

43 McKenzie R A 1981 The lumbar spine. Spinal Publications, p 122

44 Cyriax J 1980 Textbook of orthopedic medicine, vol II. Ballière Tindall, London, p 266

45 McKenzie R A 1981 The lumbar spine. Spinal Publications, p 50–62

46 Macnab I 1977 Backache. Waverly Press, p 139–158

47 Swezey R L 1978 Arthritis: rational therapy and rehabilitation. Saunders, Philadelphia, p 65–77

48 Bierins-Sorensen F 1984 Physical measures as risk indicators for low-back trouble over a one-year period. Spine 9: 106–119

48a Friberg O 1983 Clinical symptoms and biomechanics of lumbar spine and hip joint in leg length inequality. Spine 8: 643–651

49 Frederick B B, Clark V L, Brown B E, Nelson-Allen C E, Amble D S 1979 Body mechanics instruction manual. Express, p 3–37

50 Lettvin M 1976 Maggie's back book. Houghton Mifflin, p 6–157

51 Tessman J R 1980 My Back Doesn't Hurt Anymore. Quick Fox pp 23–117

52 White A H 1983 Back school and other conservative approaches to low back pain. Mosby, St Louis, p 43–176

53 Zachrisson F M 1981 The back school. Spine 6: 104–106

54 Lumsden R M, Morris J M 1968 An in vivo study of axial rotation and immobilization at the lumbosacral joint. J. Bone Joint Surg. 50A: 1591–1602

55 Norton P L, Brown T 1957 The immobilizing efficiency of back braces. J. Bone Joint Surg. 39A: 111–139

56 Waters R L, Morris J M 1970 Effect of spinal supports on the electrical activity of muscles of the trunk. J. Bone Joint Surg. 52A: 51–60

57 Perry J 1970 The use of external support in the treatment of low-back pain. J. Bone Joint Surg. 52A: 1440–1442

58 Russek A S 1976 Biomechanical and physiological basis for ambulatory treatment of low back pain. Orthop. Rev. 4: 21–31

59 McKenzie R A 1981 The lumbar spine. Spinal Publications, p 65–80

60 Mennell J Mc M 1960 Back pain. Little Brown, New York, p 38

61 Maigne R 1972a Orthopedic medicine. Thomas, Springfield, p 27–54

62 Maitland G D 1977 Vertebral manipulation. Butterworth, London, p 170–185
63 Stoddard A 1980 Manual of osteopathic practice. Hutchinson Medical, London, p 142–143
64 Eisen A, Hoirch M 1983 The electrodiagnostic evaluation of spinal root lesions. Spine 8: 98–105
65 Macnab I 1977 Backache. Waverly Press, p 184–195
66 Meyer G A, Haughton V M, Williams A L 1979 Diagnosis of herniated lumbar disk with computed tomography. New Eng. Med. J. 301: 1166–1168
67 Doran D M L, Newell D J 1975 Manipulation in treatment of low back pain: a multicentre study. Br. Med. J. 4: 161–164
68 Evans D P, Burke M S, Lloyd K N, Roberts E E, Roberts G M 1978 Lumbar spine manipulation on trial. Part I — clinical assessment. Rheumat. Rehab. 17: 46–53
69 Glover R, Morris J G, Khosla T 1974 Back pain: a randomized clinical trial of rotational manipulation of the trunk. Brit. J. Indust. Med. 31: 59–64
70 Hoehler F K, Tobias J S, Buerger A A 1981 Spinal manipulation for low back pain. JAMA 245: 1835–1838
70a Ottoson D, Ekblom A, Hansson P 1981 Vibratory stimulation for the relief of pain of dental origin. Pain 10: 37–45
71 Wall P D, Cronly-Dillon J R 1960 Pain, itch and vibration. Arch. Neurol. 2: 365–375
73 Wyke B D 1980 Articular neurology and manipulative therapy. In: Idczak R M (ed) Biomechanical aspects of manipulative therapy. Lincoln Institute of Health Sciences, p 67–72
74 Sjolund B, Terenius L, Eriksson M 1977 Increased cerebrospinal fluid levels of endorphine after electro-acupuncture. Acta. Physiol. Scand. 100: 382–384
75 Wolf S L 1978 Perspectives on central nervous system responsiveness to transcutaneous electric nerve stimulation. Phys. Ther. 58: 1443–1449
76 Simons D G 1981 Myofascial trigger points: a need for understanding. Arch. Phys. Med. Rehabil. 62: 97–99
77 Droz-Georget J H 1980 High-velocity thrust and pathophysiology of segmental dysfunction. In: Idczak R M Biomechanical aspects of manipulative therapy. Lincoln Institute of Health Science, p 81–87
78 Chrisman O D, Mittnacht A, Snook G 1964 A study of the results following rotatory manipulation in the lumbr intervertebral-disc syndrome. J. Bone Joint Surg. 4cA: 517–524
79 Livingston M C B 1968 Spinal manipulation in medical practice: a century of ignorance. Med. J. of Australia 2: 552–554
80 Kleynhans A M 1980 Prevention of complications from spinal manipulative therapy. In: Idczak R M (ed) Biomechanical aspects of manipulative therapy. Lincoln Institute of Health Sciences, p 133–141
81 Maitland G D 1961 Lumbar manipulation: does it do harm? A five-year follow-up survey. Med. J. of Australia 9: 546
82 Pratt-Thomas H R, Berger V E 1947 Cerebellar and spinal injuries after chiropractic manipulation. JAMA 133: 600–603
83 Jackson R P, Simmons E H, Stripinis D 1983 Incidence and severity of back pain in adult idiopathic scoliosis. Spine 8: 749–756
84 Rothman R H, Simeone F A 1982 The spine, vol I. Saunders, Philadelphia, p 339
85 Ruge D, Wiltie L L 1977 Spinal disorders. Lea & Febiger, p 185
86 Nachemson A 1979 Adult scoliosis and back pain. Spine 4: 513–517
87 Maigne R 1972 Orthopedic medicine. Thomas, Springfield, p 301

Back schools

INTRODUCTION

Teaching as part of medical care is as old as medical care itself. In a way a physician is a teacher, sometimes of simple concepts such as how to take medication and what to do following surgery, but sometimes teaching involves much more complex concepts requiring audiovisual aids. Pressure of time will then realistically interfere. Group education is an effective means of reducing this problem and, with a formalized curriculum, teaching can often be done by someone other than the physician. With increasing emphasis on prevention in low back pain as the solution to a significant clinical problem, the teaching aspect has become even more important and complex. Gradually a schooling system has emerged, the back school, and has become widely accepted. Education and training in manual material handling has been given widely over many years, as has strength and fitness training.

In this chapter, I will not discuss these types of training, but rather the more general back school concept, which represents a much more comprehensive approach in which all aspects of back care are included. To that purpose I will review the concepts, content and indications for back schools in prevention and treatment. A review of the scientific support of the back schools will also be given, along with some thoughts about future developments and use.

CONCEPT AND DEVELOPMENT OF BACK SCHOOLS

Although back education has been part of reha-bilitation programmes for many years, the first modern back school was developed in 1969 in Sweden.[1,2] While there were several reasons why the school was produced, the aim was to educate the patient to be able to manage his or her own back and back problems. Based on knowledge current at that time, a programme was developed that would help the patient to live well in spite of back pain and understand how to prevent recurrence or aggravation by working as correctly as possible. It is important to realize that the back school was developed for *patients* when considering its content and usefulness in primary prevention. As stated by another early developer of a back school, 'The development of the back school as a conservative treatment for patients who experienced low back pain is a logical step in the evolution of back care.'[3]

Following the 'Swedish Back School', so-called Canadian Back Education Units were developed in 1974 in Toronto,[4] and the concept was popularized in the US by Fahrni[5] and White and Mattmiller.[6,7] Numerous back schools have developed since, all with the same basic concept of patient education but with different emphases.[8] It is established that at present more than 300 back care institutions in Scandinavia provide back schools, and in 1980 there were 11 Toronto-based Canadian units with eight affiliated programmes in other states of Canada and two units in the United States.

While there are differences in content, indications, distribution and methods between the different schools, they all seem to subscribe to the same basic philosophy that education will help patients take responsibility for their own management of their spine problems.

GOALS

The goals of back schools differ with their proposed use. When prevention is the aim, the purpose is to teach the 'student' what to avoid in life and at work so as not to develop back pain. When a change in lifestyle and work method is desired, this requires an understanding of the importance and beneficial effects of such changes.

When back schools are used as part of a treatment programme or in secondary prevention, the immediate goals are often to reduce pain, to stress the importance of rest and to convey the message that the prognosis of most low back pain episodes is good. Long-range goals in that situation are to teach the patient how to use proper body mechanics, how to cope with painful episodes and to convey the message that the responsibility in recovery is shared by the patient and the treatment group. An improved physical condition is also often desired for secondary prevention.

CONTENT

The format and curriculum of back schools differ. Generally one or more of three types of classic learning are involved: cognitive, psychomotor and affective learning.

Cognitive learning is classroom-type presentation of information. Psychomotor learning, on the other hand, involves observation and physical instruction in how to perform work tasks or activities of daily living correctly. As will be seen, this is a strong component of the California back school. Finally, in affective learning motivation is important, which requires that the material presented is relevant to the student. Different proportions of the three types of learning are relevant to different purposes of the back school. This means that flexibility must be maintained, and programmes tailored to meet the specific requirements.

All back schools include sections on anatomy, physiology and function of the spine, on body mechanics and preventive back care, on the natural course of low back pain, on treatment principles and on the importance of personal involvement.

When reviewing the content of the back school, three currently popular ones will be presented: the Swedish Back School, the Canadian Back Education Unit and the California Back School.[1, 2, 4, 7] This is not to advocate these particular schools, but rather to use them as examples and to point out similarities and differences. They are summarized in Tables 15.1 and 15.2.

The Swedish Back School

The Swedish Back School consists of four lessons given over a two-week period. A sound–slide programme is presented by a physiotherapist to groups of 6–8 patients. Each lesson in the slide programme takes about 15 minutes, after which instruction follows for another 30 minutes. The purpose of the school is outlined at the start and a test of comprehension given at the end.

During the *first lesson*, epidemiology, anatomy and function of the back, as well as different treatment methods, are reviewed. Rest positions are taught and some treatment advice is given. The *second lesson* concentrates on the mechanical strain placed on the back from posture, manual handling and similar. Physical training of the abdominal muscles is also taught. The *third lesson* is a practical

Table 15.1 Basic structure and administration system used in the Swedish, Canadian and California back schools

School	Lessons (*n*)	Time lessons (min)	Subjects (*n*)	Instructor
Swedish	4	45	6–8	Physiotherapist
Canadian	4(5)	90	15–20	Orthopaedic surgeon Physiotherapist Psychiatrist Psychologist
California	4	90	4	Physiotherapist (Consulting orthopaedic surgeon)

Table 15.2 Content of Swedish, Canadian and -California back schools

Lesson	Swedish	Canadian	California
1	Epidemiology Anatomy Function Treatment	Anatomy Physiology Pathophysiology	Interview and assessment Obstacle course exercise tolerance test Basic education
2	Body mechanics Abdominal muscle training	Body mechanics Temporary relief exercise	ADL Co-ordination exercises Isometric exercises Back protection at work
3	Practice of 1 and 2 Ergonomics ADL	Chronic pain concepts Muscle tensions	Load handling Sports Activities
4	Physical activity Summary and review	Demonstration of: relaxation exercises, flexion exercises, isometric technique, pelvic tilting	Review and individual problem- solving
(5)		Review	

application of the first two. Ergonomic work methods are illustrated and practised, and the patient learns how to get in and out of beds, chairs, etc. when he or she has pain. In the *fourth lesson*, physical activity is stressed and a summary made. The patient is also given a written summary when leaving the programme.

The Canadian Back Education Unit

The Canadian Back School typically consists of four 90-minute lectures held at weekly intervals. The classes allow 15–20 people. The first lesson is given by an orthopaedic surgeon, the second by a physiotherapist, the third by a pschiatrist, and the fourth by a psychologist and physiotherapist together. A review class follows six months after the basic series. A pre-test, end-of-lecture series test and a final test of the review class are given. Slides are used to illustrate points, but other technical teaching materials are also used.

The *first class* is on anatomy, physiology and pathophysiology of the spine. The patients have considerable time for personal questions. The *second class* concentrates on body mechanics and methods to obtain temporary relief. The role of exercise is also emphasized. In the *third class* the psychiatrist

explains psychiatric aspects of chronic pain, and discusses the influence of emotions on muscle tension and pain. The *fourth class* is held outside the classroom. A psychologist demonstrates relaxation exercises and the physiotherapist supervises a practice of simple flexion exercises, isometric techniques and pelvic tilting.

The California Back School

The California Back School is different because it includes an obstacle course used for assessment and to plan the training, to practise and to coordinate exercise. There are three weekly 90-minute visits, with a fourth follow-up a month later. The patient's case is reviewed by a consulting orthopaedist. Four patients are seen in each class, and patients are divided into groups depending upon symptoms and signs. A sound–slide programme is used as an aid.

The obstacle course is used on *day one* to measure performance objectively, along with an exercise tolerance test. Basic education is given on the natural history of spinal pain, on which activities to avoid, and on the anatomy and ageing of the spine. Advice is given about how pain can be relieved, and about work activities and body mechanics. The *second day*, after a week of rest, concentrates on daily-living body mechanics, coordination exercises and training at the obstacle course. Patients are taught the programme of home exercises, and back protection at work is reviewed. On *day three*, a quiz on the theory is given, along with the final obstacle course to test coordination in theory and practice. Instruction is also given on load-handling and on sports activities. The follow-up visit, on *day four*, is a problem-solving day on which the patient is again tested on individual problems, which are reviewed and discussed.

INDICATIONS

All human beings should have basic knowledge about their backs, which means that back schools would be indicated for everyone, preferably already during the early school years. However, none of the back schools today is suitable to that purpose, nor are they designed for primary prevention, i.e. to prevent back pain from developing in healthy individuals. Rather, they are either useful as part of a treatment programme or in secondary prevention, i.e. to prevent recurrent back pain.

A back programme aimed at primary prevention would have to be entirely different from those illustrated in this chapter. Concepts would have to be simplified and made meaningful to someone who has never had back pain, a much more difficult task than making someone with experience of low back pain interested.

Of the three back schools mentioned, the Swedish one is general and as such useful to patients with acute or chronic pain who need to improve their knowledge as an aid in their treatment regimen. It is also useful to prevent recurrence when the pain episode is over, and for someone who is prone to recurrences.

The Canadian Back School is designed to deal with chronic back pain, and to change the patients' attitudes toward their problem. Fifty per cent of a patient group reviewed had had low back pain for more than three years, 40% for more than five years. The thrust on pain management is obvious from the content and administration.[3]

The California Back School, on the other hand, treats mainly patients with acute back pain, and integrates the schooling in a low back programme for

diagnosis and treatment.[7] Preventive back programmes including schooling have also been developed under the California Back School's direction, and there is a Canadian back education industrial programme.

In general, the back school is not intended to be a treatment by itself. Neither can it be a substitute for physical evaluation and traditional conservative treatment methods. The suitable back school patient, therefore, is the one who is not in need of specific treatment, but needs information to reduce the risk of recurrence. This is important because, as has often been said, the problem is not to treat back pain but to prevent it from recurring. Another suitable group are patients in whom the back school is an adjunct to other treatment modalities.

DISTRIBUTIONS

Any media can be used for teaching, but slide programmes with supplementary review folders are most frequent. There are examples where the back school is illustrated in a book, on flip-overs, on video and on film. All these methods are acceptable, but the cost–benefit of expensive production is doubtful. Most important is the person who does the teaching. Usually a physiotherapist is in charge, but, as discussed previously, there are alternative possibilities. The person delivering the programme must not only be a good teacher, sensitive to individual needs, but also capable of answering any of the many questions usually posed in the session.

The instructors must be able to sell their message and motivate the student, because the student must not only learn a few facts but also be guided to a proper understanding of the problem. Only then will lifestyle changes occur and educational objectives be met. Undoubtedly, adult education is difficult. Reliance on educational material only is bound to result in failure. Instructors must be trained and their basic knowledge about back problems must be highly professional. Only then can the proper atmosphere be ensured. And, whenever possible, the back school should be supplemented with such material that the student identifies as relevant. Also, there is no substitute for guided practical instruction.

EVALUATION

An early evaluation of the effect of the Swedish Back School was made by Zachrisson-Forssell,[1] on about 140 patients who had completed the back school nine months to eight years previously. About 75% were positive, but no attempt was made to determine the outcome, and controls were lacking. The only controlled prospective study of a back school has been made by Bergquist-Ullman & Larsson.[9] Two hundred and seventeen Volvo employees with acute low back pain were randomly divided into three treatment groups: physiotherapy, placebo and back school. The duration of symptoms was significantly less in the physiotherapy, (15.8 days) and back school (14.8 days) groups than for the placebo group (28.7 days). The number of days off work was 20.5 for the back school group, 26.5 for physiotherapy and 26.5 for placebo. The difference was statistically significant. Sickness absence, change of pain and recurrence within the first year were similar in the three groups. The investigators concluded that the back school was at least as effective as physiotherapy and economically preferable, since one therapist could treat several patients at a time.

Hall & Iceton[3] have provided a detailed statistical analysis of 6418 participants who completed the Canadian initial programme (four lectures) and 2707 participants who returned the review information (at fifth lecture). At the review class, 64% indicated that their back pain had improved and 97% said the programme had been helpful. Occasional pain at the start of the programme correlated positively to good results, as did leg pain and the occurrence of pain-free intervals (as opposed to continuous pain). Previous use of multiple physiotherapy modalities and a high number of physicians consulted had negative prognostic value. The severity of pain and any previous back surgery, on the other hand, did not influence the outcome.

The data from this study are difficult to assess because there were no controls, it was based on subjective rating and only about 38% of patients did return for the six-month review. It must be concluded, however, that it is difficult (but not impossible) to perform good studies on the effect of a back-school programme. Apart from the difficulty of randomly assigning patients so that two (or more) groups are comparable, the outcome measures are

not easily assessed, and instructor influence is difficult to eliminate, as is additional treatment (such as rest, pain, medication etc.). In fact, the Volvo study involved some workplace adjustments, the importance of which is difficult to determine.

A superficial evaluation has also been made of the California Back School.[7] Reviewing the first 300 patients this author found that 89% sought no further medical treatment after their first month in the back school. Ninety-five per cent were able to resume normal activities after one month and retain that level of activity during the two-year study period.

Åberg[10] evaluated a more comprehensive back school where patients with chronic low back pain were rehabilitated as inpatients for a 6-week period. The study was prospective and patients were randomized, so that half of them were given the rehabilitation programme (with emphasis on schooling but with physical treatment also), while the other half were not admitted (but still cared for by the Health Care System). At 1 year, the return to work rate was the same in both groups. The school group was somewhat improved psychologically, however, with a more positive attitude.

The acceptance of the back school among patients is generally very high: 75% at the Volvo factory were satisfied with the programme, 97 and 96% at the California and Canadian back schools respectively.

A few studies have attempted to evaluate the usefulness of a back school in prophylaxis. The California Back School was used at the Southern Pacific Transportation Company, where 39 000 employees participated. The year after the 'school year' a 22% decrease in back injuries was noted, with a saving of US$1 million.[6] Nordin et al[11] reported on results from a back school programme modelled after the Swedish Back School, but adapted to the needs of the Boeing Company. Three half-hour lectures were given to 3424 employees, while 3500 constituted the control group. While the incidence of back pain and strain was similar in the two gorups, there was some difference in work loss time due to back pain: 4.2 days on average in the back school group compared to 5.3 days in the control group over the first five months. Another study was carried out at the PPG industries, where the Atlanta Back School was used as a preventive programme for 2000 workers. The injury rate in the ensuing two years was reduced by 70% and the cost by as much as 90%.[12] While these results are encouraging, longer follow-up periods would be needed for definitive analysis of results.

Although most of the back schools have some form of comprehension test, it is not known to what degree the 'students' actually do understand and use what is being taught. The purpose of the teaching programme is to make the student understand how the back functions, why it can be damaged, how to protect it and how to administer self-treatment. The students must not only learn a few facts, however, but should be guided to a proper understanding of the problem. Only then will they change their way of life according to the principles advocated. To determine how successful current back schools are in this last sense requires more profound evaluations than have been made hereto. Pedagogic evaluation is important if we are to derive the best from schools. At present, we do not know whether results are good or not because of the teaching system or the concept. Fundamental issues to consider in the design of such evaluation are:

1. The information should be structured from general concepts to details and not in the opposite direction,
2. The student should be able to identify with the visual material,
3. Questions and answers must be allowed.

Using these principles, the target group must be defined and the back school adapted to that group.

DISCUSSION

Back schools provide an important adjunct to other means of conservative treatment of low back pain. In addition, they may be useful in prophylaxis. While there is agreement on the concept and basic content, there are large differences among back schools with respect to specific content, format, teaching style and indications. This is important to remember when selecting from the ones available. Further, none of the schools is well-suited for primary prophylaxis. It is suggested that, when using an already existing back school, supplementary slides are used to help subjects identify with the situation presented.

Unfortunately, there is a lack of proper evaluation of the content and effect of back schools. We should not allow this to continue but make efforts to determine the true value of back schools. Only then will their proper place in helping back patients and providing prophylaxis be identified.

REFERENCES

1 Zachrisson Forssell M 1980 The Swedish Back School. Physiotherapy 66: 112–114
2 Zachrisson Forsell M 1981 The back school. Spine 6: 104–105
3 Hall H, Iceton J A 1983 Back school. Clin. Orthop. 179: 10–17
4 Hall H 1980 The Canadian Back Education Units. Physiotherapy 66: 115–117
5 Fahrni W H 1975 Conservative treatment of lumbar disc degenerations. Orthop. Clin. N. Am. 6: 93
6 White A 1979 Back school. AAOS instructional course lectures. Mosby, St Louis, p 184–189
7 Mattmiller A W 1980 The California Back School. Physiotherapy 66: 118–122

8 Fisk J R, DiMonte P, McKay Courington S 1983. Back schools. Past, present and future. Clin. Orthop. 179: 18–23
9 Bergquist-Ullman M, Larsson U 1977 Acute low back pain in industry. Acta Orthop. Scand. suppl 170
10 Åberg J 1980 How successful is back rehabilitation? Karolinska, Stockholm. Thesis (in Swedish)
11 Nordin M, Spengler D M, Frankel V H 1981 A preventive back care program for industry. Abstract. Int. Soc. for the Study of Lumbar Spine, Paris
12 Snook S H, White A H 1984 Education and training. In: Pope M H, Frymoyer J W, Andersson G B J (eds) Occupational low back pain. Praeger, New York, p 233–244

Indications for spinal surgery in low back pain

INTRODUCTION

Success in spinal surgery is a major challenge in the treatment of low back and leg pain arising from the spine. Surgery should be performed as part of a comprehensive programme of patient education and rehabilitation, and not as an isolated procedure. Success cannot be measured in months or years alone, but only if it achieves its aim, which is to return the patient to a normal lifestyle including occupation, hobbies and interests. This requires a detailed assessment of the clinical problem, including both the underlying spinal disorder and an understanding of the individual, with emphasis on a realistic expectation on the part of the patient and surgeon.

Historically spinal surgery began in the 19th century with the correction of deformity. In 1891 Hadra[1] operated to reduce a fracture dislocation of the cervical spine and used wires to retain the position. Surgery for spinal scoliosis was described by Hibbs[2] in 1911, and in the same year Albee[3] augmented the fusion with autogenous bone graft from the tibia. In 1931 Girdlestone[4] described a laminectomy for the evacuation of a tuberculous spinal abscess. In 1921 Dandy[5] first described the surgical treatment of a prolapsed intervertebral disc, but it was the classic paper by Mixter & Barr[6] in 1934 which stimulated 'the dynasty of the disc', a phrase coined by Macnab[7] in the 1960s.

Recent major advances in investigations, including the safe water-soluble contrast agents, computerized tomography and ultrasonic measurement techniques have enabled the surgeon to observe more precisely the pathological abnormalities and to evolve specific surgical procedures to deal with them.

FREQUENCY OF SURGICAL PROCEDURES

In an attempt to assess the application of surgery in the management of back pain disorders, Kane[8] reported the frequency of surgery of the spine in different countries, noting an incidence of 15 operations per 100 000 population in the United Kingdom, and up to 80 per 100 000 population in the Western States of the USA. If we assume that the incidence of pathology is similar, it is apparent that the indications for surgery vary widely. This may be explained on the basis of a different expectation on the part of the back pain sufferer or an unrealistic expectation on the part of the orthopaedic surgeon.

SELECTION FOR SURGERY

Surgery represents a potentially life-threatening procedure in the management of a symptom which for most patients never threatens life. The decision to operate, therefore, must be based on a sound anatomical and functional assessment in a patient who is realistic about the goals which can be achieved and who understands his or her role in after-care if a successful result is to be achieved.

CONSERVATIVE TREATMENT

While all clinicians would agree that conservative or non-operative methods of management should be used initially, there are certain situations in which the underlying disease warrants an early consideration of surgery. If surgery is delayed beyond a certain period, recovery will be impaired. For most patients, however, a period of conservative treatment consisting, at some stage, of two weeks bedrest, either at home or in hospital, with the avoidance of aggravating movements, is recommended.

DIAGNOSIS

Successful surgery demands that the surgeon has a full understanding of the cause of the pain and is sufficiently trained in spinal surgery to be able to tackle the different underlying abnormalities which he may meet. Experienced theatre and nursing staff, together with physiotherapists and occupational therapists, will ensure that the surgical procedure is augmented by skilled after care, thus leading to a successful outcome.

HISTORY

A careful history requires time and attention to detail, during which time the surgeon and the patient are gaining mutual confidence and trust. Studies on the reliability of the information obtained during history-taking have shown that much of it is imprecise and variable. Nevertheless, it remains the single most important tool available to the clinician in his or her assessment of the patient. The site, distribution, aggravating and relieving features of the pain should be carefully elucidated, and where possible the patient should be encouraged to outline the pain distribution on a pain drawing chart.

EXAMINATION

This is inevitably subjective and must be carried out without producing further pain. The whole spine should be examined, including the neck, thoracic and lumbar spine. A detailed neurological examination is essential to identify the slight changes in power or reflexes. A general examination should be included in order to exclude an extra-spinal origin for the pain.

INVESTIGATIONS

Plain X-rays

An AP lateral and two oblique films of the lumbar spine should be requested. These must be of good quality to show bone texture and details of the facet joints and pars interarticularis. Age-related changes may be demonstrated which have no relevance to the patient's symptoms, and great care must be taken in correlating the clinical diagnosis with the radiological findings.

Tomography

Conventional tomography in an anteroposterior and lateral plane may be requested to obtain further information about an existing abnormality. Midline tomography may be of help in obtaining measurements of the mid-sagittal spinal diameter, where ultrasonic scanning is not available.

Computerized axial tomography[9, 10]

This technique is now widely available and has made a major contribution to the evaluation of the spinal canal and its contents. It is essential to correlate the presumptive clinical diagnosis with the radiological findings. (See Chapter 13.)

Ultrasonic scanning[11]

This technique has now become firmly established as a safe, non-invasive and reliable method of obtaining information about the 15° oblique sagittal diameter of the spinal canal. (See Chapter 19.)

Contrast studies

Radiculography using the water-soluble medium (metrizamide) should be requested once the question of surgery has been considered. (See Chapter 12.)

Discography[12, 13]

Increasing experience with this technique in the hands of an experienced radiologist has shown that it can be of great help in the evaluation of painful disc syndromes which cannot be demonstrated by other techniques. The reproduction of the patient's symptoms preceding spinal fusion, and the assessment of a normal disc above a spondylolisthesis are two examples of its use. It may also help in evaluating the patient following failed spinal surgery. (See later.)

Radioactive bone scan[14]

When infection or tumour are suspected, this investigation may be of great value in identifying the abnormal lesion.

Disability

Until the clinician can measure pain accurately, he or she must lean heavily on the patient's description of the severity of the pain and the extent to which it interferes with the patient's life, occupation, hobbies and interests. Several disability questionnaires[15-17] have been developed to try and measure this modality more accurately. Unfortunately they tend to be directed at different groups of back pain sufferers, and therefore their value in any given individual may be limited. Ultimately if symptoms persist despite adequate conservative treatment in a patient whose condition is deemed to have a surgical solution by virtue of the history, examination and corroborative investigation, then surgery should be offered.

PHYSICAL FITNESS AND AGE

Concomitant disease of the cardiovascular and respiratory system may be a contra-indication for surgery, although patients with severe general illness are usually so limited in activities that back pain is rarely a problem. Individuals who are overweight should be encouraged to lose weight prior to surgery, in order to reduce the post-operative complications which are commonly associated with obesity, namely deep-vein thrombosis, urinary tract infections, etc.

Rarely is age itself a contra-indication,[18] as the elderly patient tolerates spinal surgery remarkably well provided early post-operative mobilization is emphasized. In the elderly, degenerative spondylosis and spondylolisthesis respond well to decompressive procedures. Care must be taken to exclude malignant disease as a cause of unexplained backache.

Occupation

Back and leg pain occur commonly throughout the population, but it is the heavy manual worker in whom back-pain disability can produce prolonged inability to work.[19] Every attempt should be made to adjust and modify the working environment, and even suggest a change of occupation, before embarking on extensive spinal surgery. It is in the heavy manual work field that spinal surgery is least likely to enable a patient to continue in his or her occupation. This is particularly so when spinal fusion has been undertaken. There is some evidence that in young patients spinal fusion at a single level for spondylolisthesis is compatible with a return to heavy work. However, nerve root decompression procedures, provided the remainder of the spine is normal, are compatible with a return to normal and heavy duties.

Personality and illness behaviour

Follow-up studies in problem back pain clinics in the United Kingdom and North America[19] have demonstrated that surgery is often undertaken because of pain and disability on the assumption that the symptoms and signs can be explained in terms of physical disease. Studies by Wadell et al[20] have attempted to evaluate the presence of inappropriate illness behaviour as part of the presenting clinical picture. In this way the clinician can treat the whole patient and not be tempted to operate too soon, too often or unnecessarily.

There have been many attempts to evaluate the precise role of psychological factors including depression, anxiety and hysteria in the evaluation of the back pain patient. There is much confusion in the literature and, while in North America the MMPI appears to be of value to the clinician,[21, 22] in the UK this test has had little success.[23]

INDICATIONS FOR SURGERY

The vast majority of back-pain sufferers do not require surgery. Their symptoms settle on simple measures; a moderate adjustment of their pattern of living is usually sufficient to prevent further problems. It has been estimated that in the United Kingdom about 10% of back-pain sufferers who see their doctors are referred to hospitals for specialist opinion,[24] and of these fewer than one in ten require surgery. In the United Kingdom a recent survey (Nelson, 1981)[25] revealed that about 8000 operations per year are performed for back pain and related disorders, and this represents about 15 per 100 000 population.

The purpose of spinal surgery is to relieve pain, relieve or prevent neurological damage and correct deformity where possible. This should permit the individual to return to a normal lifestyle without recourse to regular medication or regular treatment.

Pathological conditions

Pathological conditions for which surgery may be indicated are:

1. Lumbar nerve root compression
2. Lumbar instability
3. Infection
4. Tumour
5. Deformity

Surgery utilizes three principles which may be carried out individually or combined:

1. Decompression of nerve tissue (spinal cord and nerve roots)
2. Spinal fusion, that is the joining together of two or more mobile segments of the spine with bone to achieve bony continuity, and
3. Correction of deformity.

Lumbo-sacral nerve root compression syndrome

The nerve roots L1 to S1 emerge from the conus medullaris and pass down the lumbar spinal canal as the cauda equina. Each individual nerve passes along the intervertebral bony canal within a tube of dura and arachnoid which fuses to the intervertebral foramen, allowing the nerve to pass outside the canal and beyond.[26] It is during its passage through the spinal canal and nerve root canal that it may be irritated or compressed, and as a result the patient experiences a clinical syndrome comprising leg pain with or without back pain. There are a number of

important and significant conditions which can compromise the mobility of the spinal nerve and produce clinical syndromes[27] which, while being similar, can be indentified by detailed history and examination supplemented by investigations including plain X-rays, water-soluble myelography, nerve conduction tests, discography, computerized axial tomography and other investigations designed to localize the symptom arising from the nerves, such as nerve root block.[28]

The evaluation of leg pain. Pain in the leg due to nerve root irritation or compression may be difficult to evaluate. Clinical examination is unreliable, with a variable accuracy of 39%.[29] Straight-leg raising tests may be positive in only 80% of patients with a proven prolapsed intervertebral disc. Localization of the level by neurological examination is accurate in only 50% of patients.[30] In the presence of many previous operations, the diagnosis of leg pain may be notoriously difficult.[31] In this group Leyshon et al[32] have recommended that electrical studies may be of considerable help in recognizing individual nerve root compression and may guide the choice of surgery.

The syndromes which may cause nerve root compression include:

1. Lumbar disc prolapse
2. Nerve root canal stenosis (see spinal stenosis)
3. Central lumbar stenosis (see spinal stenosis)
4. Epineural fibrosis (arachnoiditis)
5. Spondylolisthesis.

The nerve roots are mobile structures of which the position and length alter with movements of the spine. They can compensate for chronic slow compression, but an acute compressive lesion such as a disc prolapse produces sudden-onset symptoms. The nerve root may be compressed from in front, from behind, from above or below, or circumferentially, resulting in a typical clinical presentation. Furthermore, there is a significant incidence of anomalous nerve roots, so that the typical clinical picture may be confused as a result of these variations.[33]

Lumbar disc prolapse

Acute lumbar disc prolapse was first described by Dandy[5] in 1929 when he removed loose cartilage from an intervertebral disc, noting that it simulated a tumour of the spinal cord. In 1934 Mixter & Barr[6] reported the results of surgery for rupture of the intervertebral disc within the spinal canal, and in so doing introduced the era of disc surgery which at one time postulated that all back pain was caused by a derangement of the disc. Recent studies have shown that disc prolapse is only one of a number of important causes of nerve root compression and that the surgeon aims to decompress the nerve root and remove all tissue, including the disc prolapse which might be compressing it.

Clinical features

Prolapsed intervertebral disc occurs maximally between the ages of 20 and 50. It is rare after the age of 60, but may occur in childhood and adolescence.[34] In a number of series an incidence of 3–11% of disc herniations have occurred in childhood and adolescence[35, 6] In the younger age group, trauma is a recognized precipitating factor, but this is less clearly seen in the adult. While disc disease occurs equally in the sexes, most series of surgical treatment show a preponderance in males.

History

Although the clinical picture may vary, the common presentation is of recurrent attacks of low back pain culminating in leg pain felt over the distribution of a lumbar nerve root, most commonly L5, then S1, and least commonly L3, L4. It is aggravated by activity and relieved by rest, and most patients at some stage record that coughing and sneezing increase the pain. Examination reveals impaired lumbar flexion and extension with normal rotation. Straight-leg raising is restricted, often severely, and there may be neurological deficit, including sensory and motor changes.[37]

Investigations

Plain X-rays may be normal or show narrowing of one or more disc spaces. Radiculography, which ideally should only be carried out once surgery has been decided upon, is a reliable technique for revealing the level and extent of the disc prolapse (Fig. 16.1). Other investigations which may be helpful include discography and the more recent 4th generation CAT scanners.[38]

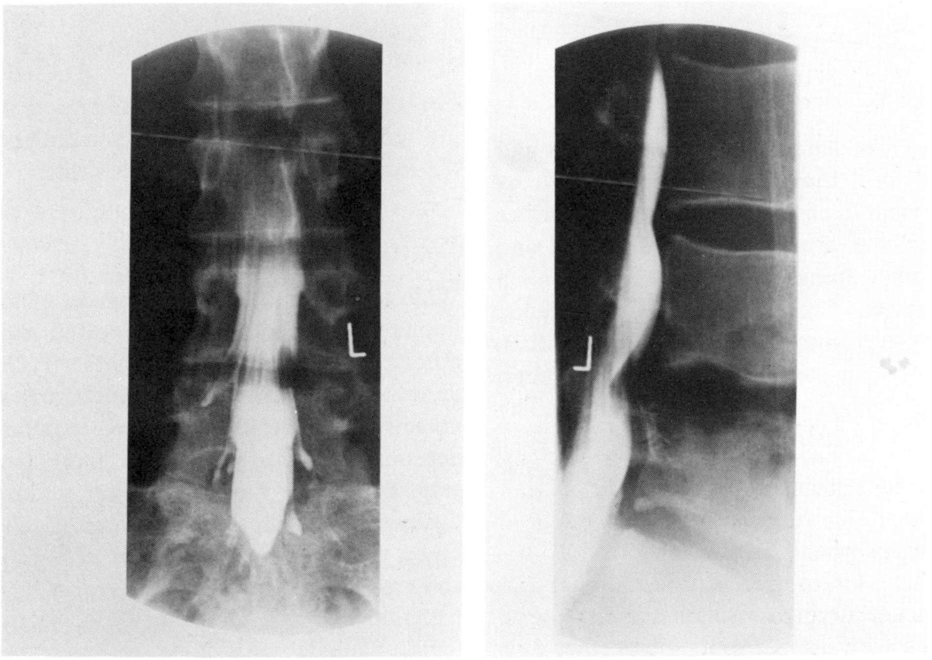

Fig. 16.1 AP and LAT radiculogram showing a posterolateral disc prolapse at L4–5 nerve root on the left

Indications for surgery

1. Sciatic pain felt along the distribution of a lumbar nerve root which fails to respond to conservative treatment, including a period of two weeks complete bed-rest, ideally in hospital
2. Recurrent attacks of sciatica which, while responding to bed-rest, result in a significant loss of work per year
3. Progressive neurological deficit despite bed-rest
4. Neurological involvement of the bladder or bowels.

Many patients may have temporary difficulty in passing urine when first put to bed, but any persistence of urinary or bowel difficulties associated with perineal numbness must not be ignored. Love & Emmett[39] described neurological disturbance of the bladder due to lumbar disc prolapse in the absence of back or leg pain. This occult disc lesion may, if untreated, lead to permanent bladder dysfunction. A large central disc prolapse presenting with bilateral leg pain and perineal numbness and weakness in the legs is an indication for urgent investigation and surgical decompression.[40, 41]

Nerve root canal stenosis

With the advent of water-soluble myelography and computerized axial tomography supplemented by ultrasonic measurement, there has been a greater understanding and awareness of the normal and abnormal lumbar spinal canal and lumbar spinal nerve root canal. Crock[26] presented a detailed description of the lumbar spinal nerve root canal, emphasizing that in contrast to the intervertebral foramen it is a tubular canal with a funnel shape. The nerve canal may be narrowed as a result of:

1. Developmental stenosis producing the characteristic trefoil spinal canal
2. Spondylolysis/spondylolisthesis
3. Degenerative osteoarthrosis of the lumbar facet joints occurring in isolation or in association with lumbar spondylosis (that is, narrowing of the disc spaces due to degenerative disease).

Crock suggests that the term lumbar spinal nerve root canal should be used to replace terms such as lateral recess, lateral canal and hidden zone.

Clinical presentation

The patient presents with a past history of recurrent low back pain which usually responds to rest or the wearing of a support. There is a recent history of atypical leg pain characteristically severe, often waking the patient at night, felt along the distribution of the nerve root and aggravated by walking. The patient often has difficulty in finding a comfortable position. Spinal flexion is often well retained, but extension is limited, with aggravation of the pain. Straight-leg raising may be normal in two-thirds of the patients, and neurological abnormality may be minimal.

X-rays of the lumbar spine show narrowing of the disc space with posterior facet arthritis, commonly at L5/S1. Radiculography may be normal and is often confusing. E.M.G. studies[32] may be of help in identifying the compressed nerve root. Computerized tomography may demonstrate the enlargement of the facet joints and the narrowing of the nerve root canals.

Treatment

Conservative treatment tends to be very disappointing because, whereas the back pain can be controlled, the leg pain continues to be disabling.

Surgery

Wide and adequate decompression of the affected lumbar nerve root canal is required and has been reported by a number of authors.[42-44] Getty et al[45] describe 78 patients who have undergone surgery for narrowing of the lumbar nerve root canal due to degenerative arthritis of the facet joints. They emphasized the importance of removal of the ligamentum flavum and osteotomy of the medial aspect of the facet joint in order to de-roof the canal and free the nerve root. They report 85% satisfied patients, with 59% achieving a good result. Interestingly, patients with good results experienced a reduction in the incidence of back pain from 89% to 33%. Twenty-eight (36%) of his patients had previous surgery, 25 of these for a prolapsed intervertebral disc without relief of symptoms.

Lumbar instability

This term has been widely used in the literature[46-48] in an attempt to describe intermittent mechanical failure of the spinal unit under load; the spinal unit comprising the vertebral body above, the disc and the vertebral body below, that is the motion segment. The clinical picture depends on the underlying cause and is characterized by low back pain related to activity and relieved by rest. The patients often describe a sudden catch of pain on walking or twisting, and characteristically cannot stand for any length of time without pain being produced. The syndrome may be associated with leg symptoms, but the latter are usually less severe than the former and do not produce a typical nerve root distribution. The syndrome may arise in association with a number of conditions,[49] such as:

1. Lumbar spondylosis, or chronic disc degeneration
2. Spondylolisthesis
3. Post-trauma
4. Post-infection
5. In association with spinal tumours
6. Following extensive decompression surgery.

SURGICAL APPROACH

The spinal canal may be approached from behind via a spondylotomy (literally, opening of the spinal canal). The extent of this procedure is dependent on the underlying pathology and may comprise:

Fenestration (interlaminar approach). The ligamentum flavum and the inferior margin of the lamina above are removed to expose the dura and the affected nerve root. Williams[50] described a microlumbar discectomy using the dissecting microscope and operating through a 2.5 cm skin incision using special instruments. He reported the results of 530 patients, emphasized the minimal disturbance of the epidural fat and nerve, and reported satisfactory results in 91% of patients.

The original fenestration procedure was described in 1939 by Love and Semmes independently.[51, 52]

Hemilaminectomy. Removal of the lamina on one side may be required to expose the nerve root more fully in order to ensure that it is completely freed and that disc excision is complete.

Laminectomy (bilateral laminectomy). This is a more extensive procedure which includes removal of the spinous process and both laminae, and may be extended proximally or distally as necessary. This procedure is used for decompressing the central part of the spinal canal in conditions such as spinal stenosis, or when infection is diagnosed. Mixter & Barr[6] originally described a wide bilateral laminectomy, but later limited their operation to hemilaminectomy. O'Connell[53] used both interlaminar (130 operations), hemilaminectomy (27 operations) and bilateral laminectomies (370 operations) and did not state any preference. Jackson[54] in 1971 routinely used a wide bilateral laminectomy and was unable to find any increased post-operative morbidity. However, Connolly & Newman[55] could not support Jackson's findings. It is the author's opinion that surgical exposure should be limited to that which is sufficient to see the pathology and to decompress the nerve root adequately.

Extent of disc removal

Nelson[25] reported the experience of UK orthopaedic surgeons and neurosurgeons who, when asked how much disc material they removed, recorded that 90% removed as much disc material as possible; one in ten only removed the loose disc fragment. Capanna et al[56] estimated the percentage of disc removal at operation on 12 cases and found that in their series it was no more than 6%. This may be of some significance when assessing re-operation incidence for repeated disc prolapse. Weir et al[57] found that recurrence took place within the first two years in 11% of cases, of whom 60% occurred at the same side and the same level, suggesting that a more complete disc evacuation could have avoided this complication.

Anaesthesia

Although the majority of patients are operated on under general anaesthesia, Silver[58] in 1976 reviewed 576 spinal operations performed under spinal anaesthesia and concluded that this was a safe and reliable technique.

Position

A patient may be operated in the prone, knee–elbow tuck or the lateral position. Eie[59] reported the complications of patients being operated on in the knee–elbow position and recorded in a series of 2690 patients an incidence of 5.5% of deep-vein thrombosis and pulmonary embolus (1.5%). Weir[57] in reporting the re-operation rate following lumbar discectomy favours the lateral position and attributes his low complication rate in a series of 560 patients to this position.

Post-operative epineural fibrosis — arachnoiditis

Animal experiments[60, 61] have demonstrated that free fat graft placed over the exposed dura and nerve roots is more effective in the prevention of nerve root adhesions than other materials, including gel foam, fascia and anti-inflammatory agents including steroids. Free fat grafts acquired a blood supply and effectively reduced haematoma formation and avoided epineural scarring.[61]

POST-OPERATIVE MANAGEMENT

Surgery is part of a programme of education and rehabilitation. Early mobilization of the patient following removal of the suction drain may be permitted. The patient is shown isometric abdominal exercises. Sitting is avoided until the 10th to 12th day, when the wound should be well healed and the sutures removed. During the follow-up period the patient should be carefully supervised and instructed on good back habits and encouraged to take gentle exercise, such as swimming and walking. The patients usually return to light work after about 6 weeks and heavier work within 3 months, provided spinal fusion has not been carried out.

COMPLICATIONS OF SURGERY

Although lumbar disc surgery is essentially a safe and reliable procedure for most patients, there is unfortunately a small but significant number of complications, some of which, such as vascular damage, may be fatal and others, such as infection, neural damage or dural damage, may prejudice an otherwise successful operation. Nelson[25] noted the following incidence of complications when reviewing the experience of orthopaedic and neurosurgeons in the UK and Northern Ireland in a questionnaire answered by 420 surgeons. Vascular damage was reported in two cases, an incidence of 0.5 per 1000. Infection was reported in 2.5% of cases. Dural damage was reported in 2.5–5% of cases, and damage to nerve tissue was reported in 0.8% of cases.

Vascular complications

Damage to the common iliac artery and the inferior vena cava may occur as the result of penetration of the anterior longitudinal ligament by the pituitary forceps or curette during the evacuation of the disc space. This injury should be suspected if:

1. There is an unexplained drop in blood pressure during the operation
2. There is excessive bleeding from the intervertebral disc space at the time of its removal
3. If following operation the patient complains of abdominal pains and an abdominal mass is palpable

There are many reports of vascular injuries associated with surgery in the literature.[62-67] Desaussure[68] in 1959 reported 106 vascular injuries from a questionnaire sent to neurosurgeons in the United Sates of America. In more than 50% of cases bleeding was noted through the interspace at the time of surgery. Early recognition was noted in 31 patients, in whom there was a 24% mortality. Delay in operation beyond 24 hours was associated with 50% mortality. All 25 patients in whom no operation was performed died. Awareness, early diagnosis and early expert surgical treatment of this complication are essential if the patient's life is to be saved.

Infection of disc space

Infection of a disc space following disc surgery is an important complication which may be noted early in the immediate post-operative period or may remain low-grade and present as increasing pain, weeks or months after the operation.[69-71] Lindholm[72] noted an incidence of 0.75% in a series of 3576 patients undergoing disc surgery.

Clinical features

Infection should be suspected if following operation the patient complains of increasing pain in the back and both legs, associated with a low-grade pyrexia and deterioration in previous progress. Movements of the spine are severely limited, with muscle spasm; straight-leg raising is restricted, the sedimentation rate is raised and may range from 45 to 130 mm/h.[73] Thibodeau[70] reviewed the clinical features in 100 cases, noting that blood culture was positive in very few.

Management

Bed rest, analgesics and antibiotics have been recommended by most authors. However, El-Gindi[73] explored all five cases of infection found in a series of 650 operations and noted pus and degenerative disc material, common organisms being *Staph. aureus* in four cases and *E. coli* in one.

Prognosis

Lindholm[72] followed 33 patients for an average of 7.5 years (range 1 to 16 years). Thirty-one out of 33 patients complained of spinal and pelvic pain, 24 out of 31 complained of sciatica, and 25 out of 31 had rigid backs. Only 6 had resumed previous work and 18 had retired from regular work.

X-rays

In 14 patients, spontaneous bony fusion had occurred but in others minor progressive degenerative changes were present at the disc space. It was stressed that this was a serious complication resulting in a significant degree of morbidity and that early diagnosis and treatment were essential to avoid a poor outcome.

Damage to meninges

Accidental damage to the dura and arachnoid may occur at the time of operation, allowing leakage of CSF. This complication may occur in as high as 5% of operations, particularly in the presence of epidural adhesion or during re-exploration.[25] This complication may present as:

1. Constant discharging wound
2. A subcutaneous cystic swelling or pseudocyst.

Muller[75] reported persistence of pseudocyst in 10 patients, most of whom had a dural tear rcorded at operation. All patients complained of backache. In 9 patients leg pain was also experienced.

Prevention

In the event of a breach of the dura and the arachnoid, which is recognized by the sudden release of CSF fluid, the surgeon should expose the dura more fully and attempt to close it with one or two sutures. If this is not possible, suturing of a patch of fat or fascia should be undertaken.

Treatment

CSF leak. The presence of a continuous CSF leak represents a risk of infection and meningitis. Once it has been established that the fluid is CSF by biochemical analysis, exploration excision of the tract and repair of the dura defect is indicated.

Persistent pseudocyst. If a pseudocyst persists and particularly if it gives symptoms, exploration and excision of the cyst with closure of the dural leak is indicated.

Neural damage. Eie[59] recorded an incidence of 6.8% of nerve root damage in a follow-up series of 943 patients in a total of 2690 patients operated. Nelson[25] noted an incidence of 0.8%.

Neural damage may occur at operation as a result of direct injury to the nerve root itself. This may occur as a result of traction, crushing or even severance. Furthermore, damage to the cauda equina may occur from excessive traction in the removal of a large midline disc prolapse or when the canal is very narrow.[74] In the latter situation a transdural approach with excision of the central disc followed by closure of the dura is the method of choice. An adequate exposure, both proximally and distally, to the proposed nerve root permits the surgeon to visualize the area and identify the structure before damage has occurred. Careful gentle retraction of the nerve root will minimize damage. The use of a microscope gives a better view of the nerve, and the added light which accompanies the microscope can be helpful in identifying the nerve and preventing damage. Morgan[74] described a patient who, following surgery for a L4/5 disc prolapse, recorded loss of perineal sensation, a hypotonic bladder and decreased and sphincter tone. This he attributed to excessive traction on the cauda equina.

Position

Careful positioning of the patient on the table is essential in order to reduce venous pressure in the abdominal veins and to minimize tension on the already compromised nerve root.[76,77].

In the UK, surgeons operate with the patient in one of three positions: the prone, the kneel position or the lateral tuck position. Nelson[25] noted that only 20% of UK surgeons preferred the side position, which was used equally by orthopaedic and neurosurgeons. The majority favoured the prone or crouch position. Eie[59] noted the complications in a series of patients operated upon in the knee–elbow position, and records that complications in this position are rare.

Results

Since 1934 there have been a number of large series reported of results of spondylotomy, ranging from fenestration to wide laminectomy for the treatment of prolapsed intervertebral discs (Table 16.1). Three out of four patients obtained complete relief of leg pain, and two out of three patients obtained relief of back pain.[6, 53, 54, 78–84]

Failed disc surgery

From the above figures it is apparent that roughly one in four patients continues to have or has a recurrence of sciatic pain following disc surgery, and one in three patients fails to obtain relief from back pain or has a recurrence of back pain following disc surgery. In an analysis of causes of failed back surgery it is important to stress that surgery for nerve root compression due to a disc prolapse aims to treat sciatic pain and not back pain, the cause of which is not due to the nerve compression but to other factors in relation to the degeneration of the underlying disc itself. The fact that many patients, as many as two-thirds, obtain relief from back pain is not clearly understood. Unfortunately, many patients undertake the operation on the understanding that all symptoms both back and leg pain will be relieved.

LUMBAR DISC HERNIATION IN CHILDREN AND ADOLESCENTS

The incidence of lumbar disc herniation in children and adolescents ranges from 0.8%[85] to 3.4%.[53] In Japan the incidence of surgically treated disc herniation varies from 7.8% to 22.3%.[86] Boys are affected more commonly than girls[87] and trauma is a significant factor in over 50% of patients.

Clinical Presentation

The initial presentation may be leg pain only in half the patients, but eventually back pain occurs in all. Clinical findings include an abnormal gait, loss of lumbar lordosis with a tilt, and gross limitation of straight-leg raising, both L4/5 and L5/S1 are

Table 16.1 Results of spondylotomy for prolapsed intervertebral disc

Author	No. of patients	Follow-up years	Relief of sciatica	Relief of back pain
Mixter & Barr[6]	94	1	77%	52% with fusion 73% without fusion
Spurling & Grantham[79]	259	N/S	79%	40%
O'Connel[53]	500	2–4	77.6%	60%
Jackson[54]	104	1–10	83%	53%
Naylor[83]	204	10–25	79%	
Weber[84]	60	4–10	75%	63%

commonly affected. Conservative treatment with bed-rest is less successful than in adults, and many patients come to surgery following diagnostic myelography.

Several reviews[85-89] record the results of surgery, giving an initial good to excellent result in 80–90%. Deorio et al[89] reported 50 patients and note that 12 had to have a second operation. Follow-up of all patients ranging from 5 to 30 years recorded excellent to good results in 73.5% and poor in 26.5%. The authors noted that lumbar disc excision in children and adolescents was recorded as 0.5% of all discectomies.

SPINAL STENOSIS SYNDROME

In 1945 Sarpyener[90, 91] first described congenital narrowing of the lumbar spinal canal in association with spina bifida occulta. Four years later Verbiest[92] linked the findings of a narrow lumbar vertebral canal with symptoms due to a disturbance of conduction of the cauda equina, including bilateral radicular pain, impairment of sensation and motor power in the legs. He noted the similarity and the possible confusion with intermittent claudication due to vascular insufficiency. Verbiest in 1954[93] and 1955[94] reported seven patients with symptoms in both legs, complaining of heaviness, numbness and tingling aggravated by walking and relieved by rest.

In 1961 Blau & Logue[95] coined the phrase 'intermittent claudication of the cauda equina' to describe this clinical syndrome, and subsequently many papers have confirmed this condition.[96-105]

Classification

In 1976 an agreed classification of spinal stenosis (Table 16.2) was published.[106] Eisenstein[107] made direct measurements of 2166 lumbar vertebrae in adult negro and caucasoid skeletons. He established the overall average lower limit of normal mid-sagittal diameter of the lumbar canal of 15 mm, and of the transverse diameter of 20 mm. He noted that, despite the fact that the negro spinal canal is narrower than the white spinal canal, spinal stenosis as a syndrome has never been reported in the literature and concluded that spinal stenosis as an exclusive cause of spinal stenosis syndrome may have been exaggerated. He emphasized that secondary narrowing by virtue of degenerative changes in the posterior facet joints further narrows an already narrowed canal and accounts for the onset of symptoms.

Clinical syndrome

The patient, usually a male in the fourth or fifth decade, presents with a history of many years' duration of low back pain and a more recent history

Table 16.2 Classification of spinal stenosis syndrome

1. *Congenital* (developmental)
   a.   Idiopathic
   b.   Achondroplastic

2. *Acquired*
   a.   Degenerative
        (i) Central portion of spinal canal
        (ii) Peripheral portion of canal, lateral recesses and
             nerve root canals (tunnel)
        (iii) Degenerative spondylolisthesis
   b.   Combined
        Any possible combination of congenital/developmental
        or degenerative stenosis
   c.   Spondylolisthetic/spondylytic
   d.   Iatrogenic
        (i) Post-laminectomy
        (ii) Post-fusion (anterior and posterior)
        (iii) Post-chemonucleolysis
   e.   Post-traumatic (late changes)
   f.   Miscellaneous
        (i) Paget's disease
        (ii) Fluorosis

of pain in one or both legs associated with heaviness, paraesthesiae and tingling. Three clinical presentations may be noted:

Bilateral symptoms

The symptoms are bilateral from the onset, with a feeling of heaviness, tingling, numbness and pain brought on by walking and relieved by rest. With the passage of time the walking distance has diminished, but the patients deny any leg symptoms when sitting. Often patients have sought treatment for back pain and have been prescribed various treatments, including lumbar supports.

Unilateral sciatica

In other patients the symptoms are unilateral, involving one leg only. Once again paraesthesiae, tingling, numbness and pain are related to activity and relieved by rest. Patients may describe that leaning forward or crouching gives them benefit, and extending the spine increases the pain.

Atypical[108]

In a small percentage of patients the presenting feature is a vague aching heaviness in the legs on walking and a feeling of coldness, also of the legs giving way and going dead, with no obvious pain and no backache.

Examination

Clinical examination may reveal a wide range of findings, from a stiff spine with limited extension, some limitation of straight-leg raising and depressed ankle jerks, to an essentially normal spine with good mobility, full straight-leg raising and no neurological abnormality. Palpation of the peripheral pulses reveals that they are full and bounding.

Diagnosis

The clinical presentation may be confused with intermittent claudication and occasionally may occur simultaneously with impaired circulation in the lower limbs.[109]

Plain X-rays

Routine AP and lateral radiographs of the lumbar spine may show some generalized disc narrowing and posterior joint changes. Careful inspection of the lateral films may reveal progressive shortening of the pedicles from L1 to L5, and this should suggest the possibility of spinal stenosis.

Ultrasonic scanning

Ultrasonic scanning of the lumbar spine is a simple non-invasive method of obtaining a reproducible 15° oblique measurement of the spinal canal and may indicate narrowing, prompting further investigation.

Tomography

In the absence of ultrasonic scanning, midline tomography in the AP and lateral planes may permit direct measurement of the spinal canal diameters.

Computerized axial tomography[110]

This investigation is the one of choice in assessing the spinal canal diameters. It provides accurate information concerning the capacity of the canal, together with the lumbar nerve root canal.

Contrast studies

Water-soluble radiculography may be used to identify the soft tissue components of the spinal canal stenosis, such as ligamentous thickening etc. Flexion and extension films, with the patient upright, may demonstrate intermittent blocking of the dural sac.

At operation the condition may be suspected on the finding of thickened closely approximated laminae, enlarged facet joints and a general lack of space when carrying out a spondylotomy.

Management

Conservative treatment

Physiotherapy with abdominal exercise, weight loss, the wearing of a lumbar support and alteration in job may help in the mild form in younger patients. When symptoms are severe, surgical treatment is usually necessary to achieve any significant improvement.[112]

Surgery (indications)

Severe and persistent back pain associated with limited walking distance and progressive neurological deficit are the main indications for surgical interference. In a fit patient age is not a contra-indication, and successful surgery can enable an elderly person to live a more active life.

Surgical technique

Surgical decompression. The operation must be designed to deal with the pathology found after investigation and should be confined to the levels involved and not carried out as a routine decompression from L1 to the sacrum unless this is clinically indicated. Most patients require a one- or two-level decompression with careful de-roofing of the lateral root canals and freeing of the constrained nerve roots. Most authors emphasize the importance of medial facetectomy, removal of the ligamentum flavum, but with preservation of the facet joints where possible. Increased subluxation may occur in patients who already demonstrate degenerative spondylolisthesis, and fusion may be required in the younger patient.[49]

Laminoplasty. Tsuji[111] in 1980 described a technique for enlargement of the spinal canal by laminoplasty in which the posterior elements, including spinous process and the laminae, are divided and levered backwards so as to increase the spinal canal size without laminectomy. He reports a preliminary series of 12 patients.

Spinal stenosis — results

Decompression laminectomy

Two out of three patients undergoing decompressive laminectomy for one- or two-level involvement have obtained good to excellent results with a follow-up of up to four years. Verbiest[113] reported 147 patients, of whom two-thirds were completely relieved of their symptoms. Leg pain was more successfully relieved than back pain and persisted most frequently in

reported cases. Russin & Sheldon[114] reported that 85% of 473 patients surveyed by questionnaire were satisfied with their results.

Paine[115] reviewed the results in 47 patients with a follow-up of 1–4 years. He noticed excellent to good results in 84% of patients undergoing a one-level decompression, and 58% of good results inpatients undergoing a two-level decompression. Tile[116] reported excellent to good results in 15 of 18 patients with developmental stenosis, 15 of 17 patients with central stenosis, and 9 of 9 patients with lateral recess stenosis. He obtained a total of 48 excellent results out of 70 patients, followed for a mean of 5 years (2–20).

Getty[117] in 1980 reviewed 30 patients, 28 of whom had degenerative spinal stenosis and 2 had idiopathic developmental spinal stenosis. Following surgical treatment he recorded 55% of the results as good, 84% of the patients being satisfied with their results.

Fusion in spinal stenosis

Extensive decompression of the spinal canal, particularly when resection of the posterior facet joints has been performed, is associated with a small but significant incidence of post-operative instability. White & Wiltse,[118] analysing a series of 182 patients in whom at least one part of the facet joint had been resected, showed that in 13 progressive spondylolisthesis developed post-operatively.

Hanraets[119] reviewed 6000 patients and found a 2% incidence of instability requiring fusion. White & Wiltse noted that, where only 2% of the spondylosis or disc patients had developed subluxation, 66% of the patients who already had degenerative spondylolisthesis slipped further. Wiltse[118] outlined the following guidelines for spinal fusion in spinal stenosis:

1. Patients under the age of 60 with degenerative spondylolisthesis and who lose stability due to removal of the articular processes
2. Patients under the age of 55 who have a midline decompression for degenerative spondylolisthesis with facet preservation
3. Patients under the age of 55 with isthmic spondylolisthesis if the posterior elements have been removed.

SPONDYLOLYSIS — SPONDYLOLISTHESIS

Although Kilian[120] first coined the term spondylolisthesis for a forward slip of one vertebra on another, the condition had been previously recognized many years earlier by an obstetrician, André, who in 1741 described subluxation of the vertebrae in what he called 'hollow back'.[121] Later Herbiniaux in 1782 noted a bony prominence in front of the sacrum as a cause of a narrow birth canal.[122] Meyerding[123] described a grade classification for the degrees of slip, from Grade 1 — less than 5% slip to Grade 4 — more than 75% of displacement.

Wiltse et al[124] produced a classification based on developmental and pathological aetiology as follows:

1. Dysplastic
2. Isthmic, of which there are:
   a. Lytic — a fatigue fracture of the pars
   b. an elongated but intact pars, and
   c. an acute fracture
3. Degenerative
4. Traumatic
5. Pathological.

Incidence and aetiology

Eisenstein[125] in 1978 found an incidence of spondylolysis in 3.5% of 485 macerated adult skeletons, of which 6 out of 18 were unilateral. Wiltse et al[126] found an incidence of approximately 5.8% in the general population (but only 1.9% in the Negro population and up to 60% in some isolated Eskimo communities). He described 12 children aged 5–19 with an isthmic spondylolisthesis. Wynne-Davies[127] undertook a radiographic study of 147 first-degree relatives of 47 patients with spondylolisthesis (12 dysplastic and 35 isthmic). She identified 19 relatives with spondylolysis. One-third of the relatives of patients with the dysplastic form were affected similarly, but only 15% of relatives of a patient with an isthmic form. Both these figures were significantly in excess of the estimated frequency of the general population of under 1% dysplastic and 5% isthmic.

Cyron[128] noted that the neural arch at the pars interarticularis is vulnerable to mechanical fatigue and this supported the fatigue fracture concept of aetiology of isthmic spondylolysis. Wertzberger et al[129] noted that there were many recorded descriptions of young children with a spondylolysis, but he was the first to describe an 18-month-old child who had normal X-rays at $7\frac{1}{2}$ months, 11 months and 15 months, and was then noted to have a spondylolysis at 18 months. Ravichandran[130] described six new cases of multiple spondylolysis i.e., two or more levels in the same patient.

Clinical Presentation

Low back pain

Although undoubtedly many patients have no greater incidence of backache than the normal population, low back pain is the most common symptom for which the patient seeks medical advice. It may be felt low in the back over one or both sacroiliac joints radiating into the buttocks and groin and into the front of the thighs. It is characteristically aggravated by standing and walking and when standing after sitting. It is relieved by rest and a reduction in activities. This pain is thought to arise from the annulus and posterior longitudinal ligament and is believed to be due to the abnormal movement occurring at the affected level.

Leg pain

Pain over the distribution of a lumbar nerve root may be experienced. When aggravated by coughing and sneezing and associated with limited straight-leg raising, it is probably due to an associated lumbar disc prolapse. Often the pain is less clearly defined, not affected by coughing and sneezing, and associated with relatively normal straight-leg raising. In the latter case it may be due to:

1. Impingement of the mobile bony element, or
2. Due to pressure of the fibrocartilagenous defect in the pars interarticularis.[131]

Referred symptoms

A vague heaviness in both legs, associated with numbness or tingling, related to standing and made worse by walking, may be experienced. These symptoms are similar to spinal claudication and may be due to the narrowing of the spinal canal, particularly in degenerative spondylolisthesis.

Deformity and waddling gait

When the degree of slip is severe, there is foreshortening of the trunk and an increased lumbar lordosis, often associated with a tilt to one side and accompanied by a waddling gait. These features are characteristic of the severe dysplastic form.

Dysplastic spondylolisthesis (Newman Group 1 congenital)[132]

The radiological features which are characteristic of this type are:

1. A moderate to severe lumbar sacral subluxation
2. Dysplasia of the sacral neural arch and superior articular facets
3. Attenuation and elongation of the pars interarticularis, with or without a defect.

Clinical presentation

The young patient aged between 9 and 19 presents with pain in the low back associated with a deformity and occasionally complains of leg symptoms. Girls usually present about $2\frac{1}{2}$ years before boys.

Indication for surgery

Severe low back pain, neurological involvement.

Treatment

Conservative treatment is of limited value in this age group once symptoms of a severe nature have occurred. Surgical stabilization with or without correction of the deformity is the treatment of choice.

There is considerable conflict as to whether stabilization alone without correction of the deformity is preferable to correction of deformity and stabilization, the latter procedure being associated with a higher incidence of complications. Dandy & Shannon[133] reviewed 25 patients out of an initial series of 46 patients who had undergone lumbosacral fusion using an intratransverse fusion with autogenous graft in the position of deformity. They noted that 24 of the 25 described their results as excellent. Many returned to active sport including football, etc. Verbiest[134] described surgical treatment of 11 patients with fourth-degree spondyloptosis. He noted that the ideal treatment was reduction, decompression and fusion, but considered reduction to be very dangerous and preferred an anterior strut graft using tibial cortex from the fifth lumbar vertebra to the sacrum. In 9 patients he obtained a solid fusion. Sijberandij[135] used a different method of reduction and stabilization of severe spondylolisthesis, and advocates reduction of Grades 3 and 4 using internal fixation and stabilization by an anterior and posterior approach.

Isthmic spondylolisthesis (Newman Group 2 spondylolytic spondylolisthesis)

Lytic spondylolisthesis

A defect in the pars interarticularis (Fig. 16.2) occurs in about 5% of the normal population and may be

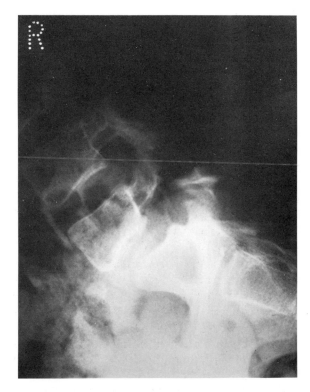

Fig. 16.2 LAT radiograph in flexion showing forward slip of a spondylolisthesis at L5–S1

asymptomatic. It is usually recognized following an injury and may cause difficulty when litigation is involved in determining its association to the injury.

Management depends on the age of presentation and the severity of symptoms.

Management in children. The natural history of spondylolysis and spondylolisthesis remains unclear. Fredrickson[136] carried out a prospective study of 500 unselected first-grade schoolchildren and reviewed them at 10 years, 15 years and 18 years. He noted an incidence of spondylolysis of 4.4% at the beginning of the study, which increased to 6% at the age of 18. Twenty-seven patients with spondylolisthesis were followed from childhood to adulthood. In 19 out of 22 children, a further slip occurred in about 16%, but only 4 out of 27 patients in 25 years of follow-up experienced low back pain (equivalent to 15% of the total). Thus, for the majority of children, the condition is painless and requires no treatment. If it is found incidentally, the question of limitation of activities arises. If the slip is of a minor degree, less than Grade 2, then normal activities should be permitted. If the slip is greater than Grade 2, then it has been suggested that patients should refrain from contact sports and high diving. Wiltse[138] advocates surgical treatment in asymptomatic children with a slip greater than 50%. Fredrickson[136] advises normal activities including all sports, provided the condition is asymptomatic.

Symptomatic spondylolisthesis in children. Initial conservative treatment with reduction in activities may be successful and no further active treatment required. If symptoms persist despite conservative treatment, Wiltse & Jackson[137] recommend inter-transverse or alar-transverse fusion. Some years earlier Buck[139] described a technique for a direct repair of the defect in spondylolysis using a screw supplemented by bone grafts. Turner & Bianco[140] noted that, of 114 patients reviewed with spondylolisthesis, 51 did not require surgical treatment, 50 underwent fusion and of these 80% obtained a sound fusion. There was a 26% pseudo-arthrosis incidence in posterior interlaminar fusion, whereas only 1 of the 19 patients treated by posterolateral inter-transverse fusion failed to fuse.

Management in adults. The vast majority of patients require simple conservative measures only, and no surgery is necessary.

Indications for surgery. Low back pain which persists, interfering with life and occupation; a persistent leg pain (see nerve root canal compression).

Surgical treatment. Decompression. Gill et al[141] describe the excision of a loose laminae with decompression of the nerve root as the treatment of choice in Grades 1 and 2 spondylolisthesis in the adult. Since then, several reviews have reported excellent results.[142, 143] Monticelli & Ascani[144] recommended the Gill procedure for patients over the age of 35, an age group in whom a further slip is not a likely possibility. However, in patients under the age of 35 they recommended a spinal fusion.

Elongated but intact pars articularis

This probably represents multiple stress fractures which have healed, and the treatment is similar to that for lytic spondylolisthesis.

Acute fracture of the pars

Fracture of the pars inter-articularis after trauma is rare and is often difficult to differentiate from a previous asymptomatic spondylolysis aggravated by the injury. If suspected, it is recommended that the patient should be rested until painfree, and then mobilised in a plaster jacket or similar external support until fracture healing has occurred.

Degenerative spondylolisthesis (Newman Group 4)

Junghanns[145] first described pseudo-spondylolisthesis or spondylolisthesis with an intact neural arch. This condition is three times more common in the female than the male and occurs predominantly at the L4/5 level, and rarely below the age of 40. It may be associated with peripheral features of osteoarthrosis including involving the knee and hands (Heberden's nodes).[146, 147]

Clinical presentation

1. A chronic low back pain related to activity and relieved by rest, commonly made worse by standing
2. Pain in the leg felt over the distribution of a peripheral nerve root associated with

reflex, motor and sensory changes, and consistent with a lumbar nerve root compression syndrome

3. Bilateral lower limb numbness, tingling and weakness suggesting spinal stenosis.

Treatment

Conservative treatment with rest, a moderation in activity and the wearing of a lumbar support may be helpful with the low back pain and diffuse lower limb symptoms.

Surgical treatment may be required if the symptoms are severe, particularly where nerve compression is present.

Investigations, including radiculography, may demonstrate evidence of a spinal block. Adequate decompression of the involved nerve roots and the nerve root canal are required.

Complications

White & Wiltse[138] reviewed the incidence of spondylolisthesis after extensive laminectomy and found an overall incidence of 2% among 182 patients. 76% of patients who underwent decompression laminectomy for degenerate spondylolisthesis underwent a further progressive slip. Lee[148] reported 27 patients following extensive posterior decompression. All four of his patients with pre-operative degenerative spondylolisthesis progressed further post-operatively. This occurred after the first 6 months of operation. Despite this the authors do not recommend routine spinal fusion at the time of decompression.

Traumatic spondylolisthesis (Newman Group 3)

A fracture of the base of the posterior element near to or passing through the pars interarticularis may occur after a fall, particularly on to the base of the sacrum. This may precipitate further slip with the passage of time.

Treatment

Following a period of bed-rest until the acute pain has subsided, the application of an external support, such as a plaster or polythene jacket, will allow the patient to mobilize. This is retained for 3–4 months until fusion can be determined radiologically.

Stabilization: if union fails to occur, the condition should be treated as an isthmic spondylolisthesis.

Pathological spondylolisthesis (Newman Group 5)

Generalized bone dysplasia or a localized bone disorder affecting the pars interarticularis may lead to a progressive elongation with an associated forward slip of one vertebral body upon another. This complication occurs most commonly in osteogenesis imperfecta, Albers-Schönberg disease, arthrogryposis congenita, Paget's disease and syphilitic disease.

ARACHNOIDITIS

Adhesive fibrosis of the lumbar nerve roots is reported under a number of different names. It was first described in the early 20th century. Phrases such as meningitis serosa spinalis[149], chronic spinal meningitis[150], adhesive spinal arachnoiditis[151], meningitis serosa circumscripta[152], spinal meningitis with radiculomyelopathy[153] and lumbosacral spinal fibrosis[154] are used to describe a progressive scarring found at operation and considered to be the cause of continued pain and disability.

Possible causes include:

1. Meningitis due to bacterial or viral infection
2. Trauma
3. Subarachnoid space injections of:
   a. contrast media
   b. steroids
   c. lumbar puncture
4. Previous spinal surgery:
   a. haemorrhage
   b. arachnoid tear
   c. infection
   d. haemostatic agents such as Gel-foam.

Burton[155] suggests a nomenclature to describe three stages in a progressive process:

1. Radiculitis in which there is inflammation of the pia-arachnoid with associated hyperaemia and swelling of the nerve root

2. Arachnoiditis recognized by progressive fibro-blastic formation and collagen deposition

3. Adhesive arachnoiditis, an end-stage with marked pia-arachnoid proliferation with dense collagen deposition encapsulating the nerve root which becomes ischaemic and undergoes progressive atrophy.

Clinical presentation

Persistent and disabling pack pain associated with unilateral or bilateral leg pain may come on slowly over a number of years following a precipitating cause such as outlined above. When previous surgery has been undertaken, the symptoms may appear after a short period of freedom from pain and may simulate the previous symptom, particularly with regard to lumbar nerve root compression. The patients have often had a considerable amount of conservative treatment, both physiotherapy and drug therapy, before presenting to the surgeon.

Clinical findings

These are variable and are often associated with an abnormal illness reaction, as described by Waddell.[156] Movements of the spine may be grossly limited in all directions, with widespread tenderness; straight-leg raising is severely restricted and there may be weakness, wasting and reflex changes.

Investigation

Plain X-rays may show previous surgery, radiculography may demonstrate loss of outline of the normal arachnoid space with impaired filling of nerve roots, but the appearances are by no means diagnostic, so that typical arachnoiditis is not usually diagnosed radiographically.

Management

Prevention

The water-soluble medium metrizamide appears to be associated with a very low incidence of arachnoiditis and should be used in preference to the oil-soluble media. Meticulous and careful surgery with minimal handling of the nerve roots, the avoidance of post-operative haematoma, the use of a free fat graft rather than artificial haemostatic agent, are all measures which experimentally can be shown to reduce the incidence of post-operative scarring.[157]

Treatment

Treatment is unsatisfactory. Both conservative and surgical treatment of this condition has been disappointing. Benoist[158] reported 38 patients upon whom excision of scar tissue and decompression of the nerve roots was attempted. He reports good results in 30 out of the 38 operations but gives no follow-up period. At the present time there appears to be no satisfactory long-term solution to lumbar arachnoiditis, and the author stresses the importance of prevention of this very disabling condition.

SPINAL FUSION

Whereas the indications for surgery for nerve root compression are relatively well defined and agreed by most surgeons, fusion of the spine as a treatment for intractable back pain is much more controversial. Nelson[25] noted that simultaneous spinal fusion at the time of disc surgery was never performed as a routine procedure by the orthopaedic and neurosurgeons reviewed. Half the orthopaedic surgeons used the procedure occasionally, whereas only 7% of the neurosurgeons ever used spinal fusion. 50% of the orthopaedic surgeons favoured an intertransverse approach, whereas 30% of the neurosurgeons preferred a posterior interbody or a posterior interspinous approach. It is apparent that the indications for and the techniques used in spinal fusion depend very much on the training of the surgeons and their experience, and there are wide differences in the surgical techniques favoured.

The principal of spinal fusion, that is the joining together by bone of two or more adjacent vertebrae, is based on the belief that the pain is arising from the abnormal movement of the vertebrae and that, by eliminating that movement by bony continuity, pain will be relieved.

Experimental studies on cadaveric spines have shown that rigid fixation of the anterior column still permits some movement of the posterior elements and vice versa, so that even after sound bony fusion has occurred by one of the normally used methods, some movement can be still demonstrated experimentally.[159, 160]

Indications

Persistent and disabling low back pain for which conservative treatment including bed-rest, physiotherapy, local immobilization by means of a corset or jacket, and various forms of injections and manipulations have failed to alleviate, is an indication.

Careful selection of patients is required to exclude illness behaviour and secondary gain. In the older patients it is essential to exclude malignant disease.

Conditions which may produce severe low back pain include:

1. Spondylolysis and spondylolisthesis
2. Acute and chronic disc degeneration
3. Trauma
4. Spinal infection
5. Post-laminectomy instability, particularly in children
6. Vertebral body destruction due to spinal tumours.

Technique

Albee & Hibbs[3, 2] first described posterior interlaminar fusion, and this remained the most commonly performed surgical fusion technique until Burns[161] described the anterior interbody fusion for spondylolisthesis. This technique was reported by other surgeons[162-165] who utilized both an anterior extraperitoneal and transperitoneal approach. A posterior interbody fusion technique was described by Cloward in 1945.[166, 167] The most popular and commonly used procedure today, namely the intertransverse and alartransverse fusion, was probably first described by Watkins in 1953.[169] Several series have reported the result of this technique since.[168, 170-172] The addition of internal fixation has been described by King,[179] Boucher,[180] Attenborough[181] and recently by Dove.[182]

Results

Posterior interlaminar fusion

A fusion rate of between 20 and 40% for single-level fusion and up to 50% for double-level fusion has been reported by various authors.[175-178] This technique is now confined to the cervical and thoracic region, and few surgeons use posterior interlaminar fusion routinely.

Posterior interbody fusion

In 1943 Cloward performed the first posterior lumbar interbody fusion, and in 1945 reported the results in 100 patients.[166] Lin[183] emphasizes the important biomechanical principle inherent in this technique as follows:

1. Preservation of the posterior portion of the motion segment
2. Integrity of the cortical end-plates
3. Maximal removal of disc material
4. A complete autogenous bone graft filling the disc space.

He reported a series of 465 cases with a follow-up period of one year and achieved a fusion rate of 88% and a satisfactory clinical result in 82%.

Hutter[184] reported a series of 500 patients treated by means of a posterior intervertebral body fusion with an average follow-up period of five years. 75% of his patients underwent primary excision of the disc with fusion, 11% had a spondylolisthesis and in 19% the operation was a secondary procedure after a failed disc operation. He reported a fusion rate of 90% with an 82% incidence of excellent or good clinical results. Despite these reports this operation is not widely used because of the technical difficulties encountered.

Anterior interbody fusion

Lane & Moore[185] described anterior interbody fusion in 36 patients. Harman[186] reported fusion rates between 80% and 90%. Freebody[187] and Sachs[188] had a similar success rate with this operation. Stauffer & Coventry[172] reserved the operation for a salvage procedure and noted a sound fusion in 56% of their 83 patients and a good or fair result in 56%. Fujimaki et al[189] report the results of anterior lumbar interbody fusion in 150 patients. They stress the importance of surgical technique and the low rate of complications. They record a fusion rate of 96%.

Inoue and colleagues[190] report the use of anterior

interbody fusion with disc excision as a primary procedure and record a fusion rate of 94.3%. In their first series of 200 cases ileus occurred in 5.5%, dry ejaculation in 5.9%, and phlebothrombosis in 6%; 5.5% had an abdominal hernia. In their second series of 179 cases, they reported a 2.2% incidence of phlebothrombosis and a 1.1% incidence of abdominal hernia. They recommend the operation for young adults, those doing physical labour with low back pain and sciatica, and patients with spinal instability.

Posterolateral fusion

Because of the unsatisfactory results of fusion of the posterior elements of the spine, Watkins in 1953[169] described a technique of intertransverse or alar-transverse fusion (Fig. 16.3). Excellent clinical and radiological results have been recorded by many authors. In 1972 Stauffer & Coventry[172] reviewed 177 patients who had undergone posterolateral fusion and noted 80% radiological and 81% good clinical results. The result in degenerative disc disease was 93% satisfactory results, and 95% fusion results compared with spondylolisthesis in which only 67% obtained radiological fusion, whereas 87% obtained a satisfactory clinical result.

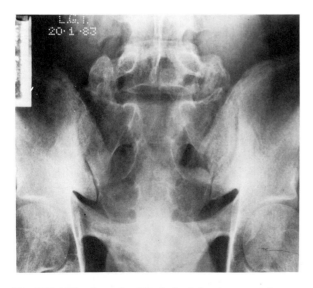

Fig. 16.3 AP lumbar spine (tilted view) showing a sound bilateral alar-transverse fusion

Conclusion

In the hands of experienced surgeons, anterior interbody and posterior interbody fusion can produce excellent radiological and clinical results. For the surgeon in normal clinical practice who will be carrying out no more than 5 to 10 spinal fusions a year, intertransverse or alar-transverse fusion is the operation of choice. This can be combined with decompression of the spinal canal by means of wide laminectomy without undue difficulty.

Post-operative management

The use of plaster beds and prolonged bed-rest following spinal fusion is no longer practised. Following the operation the patient is returned to bed, preferably a tipping bed; bedpans are avoided and the patient is turned gently from side to side over the next two to three days. Suction drainage reduces pain and the complication of haematoma formation.

At about 4–5 days the patient is tipped into the upright position, which is usually attained by the 7th to 10th day. At this time a plaster jacket or moulded polythene jacket is applied, which should include one hip and thigh to above the knee. The patient is allowed home, the polythene jacket being removed for showers. The external support is maintained until radiological fusion can be demonstrated, usually between the 10th and 12th weeks. Thereafter a lightweight lumbar support is worn and the patient can return to work, depending upon the nature of his or her job. The patient must be warned that the final clinical result may not be achieved until about a year following the operation, by which time bony consolidation has occurred and mobility has returned to the spine and the patient should be now undertaking normal activities.

FAILED SPINAL SURGERY SYNDROME (FSSS)

From the patient's point of view, and often from the referring doctor's point of view, a spinal operation is deemed to have failed if the patient has any residual pain in the back or leg, or has any recurrence of back or leg pain. Often the patient and the referring doctor have unrealistic expectations of surgery which may not have been clearly outlined by the surgeon.

Surgery for nerve root compression is carried out to relieve leg pain and not back pain. Thus residual back pain following a disc operation cannot be deemed to be a failure of that operation. Furthermore, occurrence of pain some years following a spinal operation is also in most cases not a result of failure of the operation but part of the underlying pathology present in the spine. It is unrealistic to expect a back operation to remove all pain in the back or the leg for the rest of the patient's life. Thus both patient and surgeon must have realistic expectations of the object of the surgery before it is undertaken.

Much of the literature of failed spinal surgery fails to take into account the original aims of the surgery and appears to assume that any residual back or leg pain represents a failure in the surgical procedure. In any consideration of the causes of failed spinal surgery, therefore, it is essential to recognize three possible situations:

1. Failure to relieve the presenting symptoms either in the back or in the leg
2. Failure to relieve back pain while relieving leg pain
3. Relief of back and leg pain for a period, but this is followed by:
    a. leg pain
    b. recurrence of back pain
    c. recurrence of back and leg pain.

Fager[191] reviewed the records of 105 patients who had undergone one or more operations and had persistent pain. He noted two groups of patients: Group 1, for whom the indications for operation were not clearly defined, and Group 2, in whom technical difficulties had led to an unsatisfactory operation.

Diagnosis

An accurate diagnosis of the cause of the persistent symptom is essential if a rational approach to the failed spinal surgery syndrome is to be effective. Unlike the initial presentation, the history is often less helpful, although a detailed history should always be taken. Patients who have had failure following spinal operations often demonstrate an abnormal illness behaviour which causes difficulty

in assessing the true characteristics of the pain. Where possible, precise details of the operation technique with previous X-rays should be obtained. Unfortunately these are often not available. Similarly, examination may be inconsistent, with considerable guarding and resistance to movements. Neurological examination may prove position, but the clinician cannot be certain whether the findings are recent or old.

Investigation

The clinician therefore has to lean very heavily on the results of investigations in order to make a diagnosis.

X-rays

Plain X-rays may be of limited value. They may, however, show the extent of the previous surgery, particularly if the surgeon has used radio-opaque markers at the time of surgery (Fig. 16.4).

Nerve conduction studies

These have been used by a number of workers who claim they can identify individual nerve roots still under compression.[32]

Radiculography

This may be helpful in identifying a recurrent disc, but the presence of post-operative scarring may cause difficulty in interpretation.

Computerized axial tomography

This investigation is of particular help in the failed back surgery syndrome. It enables the surgeon to identify the presence of spinal stenosis both centrally and laterally and, if the appropriate scanner is available, to identify soft tissues, including recurrent discs.

Discography

In experienced hands discography with the opportunity of reproducing the patient's symptoms and

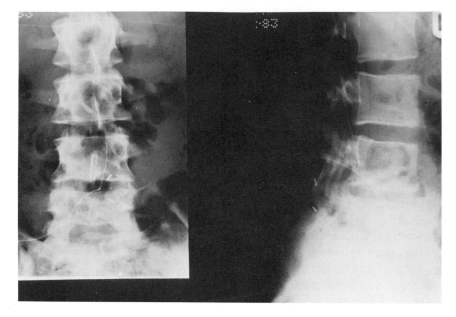

Fig. 16.4 AP and LAT radiographs of lumbar spine showing radio-opaque markers placed at the site of the laminotomy at the time of operation

obtaining a radiographic outline of the disc may be of help in determining the site of origin of pain.

Nerve root injection and facet joint injection

The use of local anaesthesia to anaesthetize the nerve roots individually and individual facet joints may be of help in localizing the site of origin of the pain.

Causes of failure of spinal surgery

1. Failure to relieve presenting symptoms either in the back or the leg:
    - a. Wrong diagnosis:
        - (i) ankylosing spondylitis
        - (ii) spondylolisthesis
        - (iii) tumour
        - (iv) abnormal illness behaviour
    - b. Technical error:
        - (i) operation at the wrong level
        - (ii) disc at another level missed
        - (iii) migration of disc fragment
        - (iv) associated spinal stenosis
        - (v) kinking of the nerve root around the pedicle
        - (vi) extra-foraminal lateral disc

2. Infection
3. Dural damage.

Failure to relieve back pain while relieving leg pain

1. Missed spondylolisthesis
2. Associated lumbar disc degeneration
3. Arachnoiditis.

Relief of back and leg pain for a period

1. Recurrence of disc prolapse
2. Development of nerve root canal stenosis
3. Development of central stenosis
4. Post-operative spondylolisthesis
5. Arachnoiditis
6. Infection

Management

This will depend on the probable cause of the pain and the results of the appropriate investigations. Weir & Jacobs[192] reviewed retrospectively 560 patients undergoing a first lumbar discectomy and noted that 63 underwent a second operation for recurrence, a re-operation rate of about 10%. The authors note that the major risk of recurrence occurs within the first three years. They stress the use of the lateral position, which in their opinion simplifies the operation, reduces blood loss and wound infection, and improves visibility. Moore[193] reported 107 cases of low back pain re-operated upon after disc excision only. Twenty-seven underwent spinal fusion, 6% had a recurrent disc. He concluded that 10% of all patients undergoing disc surgery will have a recurrence of symptoms sufficient to warrant re-operation. Frymoyer and colleagues[194] report the results in 45 patients who required a second operation after a previous lumbar disc operation. They reviewed these patients 10 years or more after the second operation. In the spinal fusion group (23 patients) 13 developed a pseudo-arthrosis, 1 an acquired spondylolysis, and 4 had a recurrent disc at the same level. Five had a recurrent disc at another level. In the disc excision group, 10 had a recurrent disc at the same level, 5 a recurrent disc at another level, and 7 demonstrated instability.

INFECTION OF THE SPINE

Tuberculosis

Despite major advances in management and chemotherapy, tuberculosis remains a widespread disease in many parts of the world. The thoracic and lumbar spine, and the sacroiliac joints, are commonly affected as part of a systemic spread of the disease. Over the last 10 years the Medical Research Council Working Party on Tuberculosis of the Spine have been supervising a number of collaborative controlled clinical trials in various parts of the world including Korea, Zimbabwe, South Africa and Hong Kong. The results of these trials have been reported in the literature.[195]

Diagnosis

When tuberculosis is endemic, the diagnosis of spinal infection is not difficult. But in the United Kingdom, where tuberculosis is becoming less common (although we still see it in the immigrant population and occasionally in the native population), diagnosis may present considerable difficulty due to its similarity to pyogenic non-tuberculosis infection. It is essential to identify the causative organism. This may require the use of

closed aspiration or open biopsy in order to obtain a sample for analysis.

Atypical presentation of spinal tuberculosis. Babhulak[196] noted that in 228 patients with tuberculosis of the spine, 22 presented with disease commencing in the neural arch and 10 with extra-dural extra-osseous disease. 206 presented with atypical disease of vertebral body destruction, deformity and occasional spinal cord involvement. He notes that the extra-dural extra-osseous TB was often not diagnosed until laminectomy, and was confused with an extra-dural tumour.

Management

With the introduction of chemotherapy, the initial hope that non-surgical treatment would be sufficient has not stood the test of time.[197, 198] Wilkinson[198, 199, 203] showed that, to eradicate bony involvement, direct drainage and removal of infected bone, together with chemotherapy, was required. The upper lumbar region is approached by an 11th rib incision, and the lumbo-sacral region by an extra-peritoneal renal approach. However, the lumbar spine may also be approached from behind by resection of a transverse process.[200, 201]

Results of surgical treatment

In 1970 Martin[204] recorded a 96.2% fusion rate in 80 patients undergoing radical surgery with chemotherapy. Bailey and colleagues[205] reported their experience of radical focal surgery in children and noted that radical resection of the tuberculous focus with anterior strut grafts gave results superior to those by other methods.

The eighth report of the Medical Research Council Working Party on Tuberculosis of the Spine[195] reviewed the 10-year follow-up of 119 patients distributed in two groups, 58 being subjected to a radical excision of the tubercular focus and repair with autogenous bone graft, compared with 61 patients subjected to open debridement but no bone graft. They noted that in the radical series a mean reduction in the angle of kyphosis of 1.4° in the thoracic region occurred compared to an increase of 9.8° in the debridement series. Both groups showed a high incidence of successful fusion amounting to

86% in the radical and 89% in the debridement group.

PYOGENIC INFECTION OF THE SPINE

Chronic back pain is the commonest presenting symptom of spinal non-tubercular infection in adults. In children, however, the presentation may be less characteristic, with the young child often refusing to walk and the older child complaining of hip or leg pain.

Pyogenic infection of the spine may present as:
1. Pyogenic osteomyelitis of the spine
   a. Pyogenic osteomyelitis of the vertebral body[206]
   b. Pyogenic infection of the intervertebral disc[207-212]
2. Epidural abscess.

Pyogenic osteomyelitis of the spine

Typical features

These are: an insidious onset of chronic low back pain of recent origin with minimal systemic signs and often associated with urinary tract infection, recent bowel surgery, diabetes or cutaneous sepsis. Digby et al[212] noted that 43% of their patients had had a urinary tract infection or recent urinary tract instrumentation. Griffiths & Jones[213] stressed the difficulty in diagnosis, stating that infection should always be considered in all patients with post-operative backache. They stressed the importance of muscle spasm, limited spinal movement, a raised sedimentation rate and typical radiological changes which may take weeks or months to appear.

Diagnosis

Identification of the causative organism is essential in order to select appropriate antibiotic therapy.

Blood culture. This was positive in 10 out of 20 children reported by Wenger et al,[226] but only 6 out of 18 patients reported by Digby.[212]

Erythrocyte sedimentation (ESR). This is consistently elevated and ranges from 30 to 130 mm/h. It is a most valuable investigation, both in diagnosis and in monitoring response to treatment.

Needle aspiration.[216] This is a simple and safe procedure and may avoid a more extensive operation to obtain a causative organism.

Open biopsy. If both blood culture and aspiration are inconclusive, an open operation is recommended to establish the true nature of the infection.

Radioactive bone-scanning. Technetium 99 polyphosphate or diphosphanate has provided an accurate, rapid and safe method for identifying early bone infection.

CT scan. Patients with suspected infection of the spine may show evidence of soft tissue involvement and it may be possible to identify early bone erosion. Bryant-Zawadzi.[217]

Infecting organisms

Staph. aureus is by far the commonest organism found. Infections by *E. coli, Proteus, Pseudomonas* and *Streptococcus haemolyticus* have been reported. The latter organisms are more likely to be responsible for spinal infection occurring with coincidental urinary instrumentation.[214,215,218,219]

Pyogenic infection of the intervertebral disc

Children

Many names have been used to describe an inflammatory condition of the intervertebral disc, including acute ostiitis of the spine,[220] discitis,[221] intervertebral disc infection and intervertebral disc space infection.[222]

In children under the age of 3, refusal to walk may be a presenting feature, whereas in the older child back and hip pain is noted. Clinical findings may be variable, but the sedimentation rate is universally raised. Spiegel et al[223] reported 48 children and noted the difficulty in diagnosis. In 43 children, X-rays showed disc narrowing but a definite pathological organism could be obtained in only a few. Treatment with immobilization and antibiotics gave excellent results. 25% developed an incomplete bony ankylosis at the infection site.

Adolescents and adults

In this age group the presentation is more insidious and diagnosis may be difficult. Kemp and colleagues[224] noted that a diagnosis may be delayed for many months and the routine pathological investigations may be unhelpful. However, radioisotope scanning can be very useful in diagnosis. In Kemp's series, 40% had some spinal cord involvement. He recommended anterior clearance of the disc space, together with antibiotics. Hooper et al[225] considered that infection in the adult and the child is all part of a broad spectrum of the same disease, and this view is echoed by Wenger and his co-workers.[226] They concluded that they were studying a widespread spectrum of one disease with variation in the resistance of the individual and the pathogenicity of the organisms. They suggest that the intact growth plate in the child may confine the infection to the immediate disc area, whereas in the adult the infection is free to spread into the intervertebral body.

Epidural abscess

In reviewing 100 patients operated on for suspected disc herniation Keon-Cohen[227] reported four cases of epidural abscess simulating a disc hernia. The condition should be suspected in a patient with an unexplained temperature, a recent history of skin sepsis, presenting with back and leg pain. The condition is more common in patients with diabetes. Early operation is indicated to avoid irreversible neural damage.

OTHER SPINE INFECTIONS

Brucellosis

Glasgow[228] reported three cases of brucellosis and stressed the difficulty in diagnosis. Samra[229] reported a further three cases, noted the delay in diagnosis and advocated treatment with tetracycline and streptomycin, and suggested surgical intervention only in the presence of spinal instability, progressive vertebral collapse or nerve root signs.

Vertebral echinococcosis

Carta et al[230] reported eight patients in whom spinal operations, including cord compressions, were required. Occasionally a repeated decompression was indicated.

Coccidiomycosis

Winter et al[231] reported their 26 years' experience, in which 12 patients with disseminated coccidiomycosis were treated. Surgical treatment ranged from the evacuation of abscesses and debridement to fusion.

Winston and colleagues[232] describe a patient presenting with a spastic paraparesis at T7/8 which was treated by thoracic laminectomy together with amphotericin and Ketoconazole®

Spinal hydatidosis

Duran and colleagues[233] reviewed 19 patients with osseous hydatidosis out of a total of 637 patients with hydatic disease treated during a 14-year period. Of these, 7 were in the thoracic region and 3 in the lumbar region. They advocate radical surgical removal of parasitic cysts with corticocancellous grafting of bony defects, augmented by internal fixation such as Harrington rods where necessary. The prognosis of hydatid disease is poor.

SPINAL TUMOURS

Tumours of the spine are rare. In the adult the vast majority are secondary from primary malignancies in the bronchus, breast, kidney, prostate and adrenal; less commonly Hodgkin's lymphoma may spread to the spine.[234–239] In the child, though equally rare, half the tumours are benign, for which the prognosis is excellent.

Primary benign tumours include neurinomata and meningiomata.[242] Cartilaginous tumours include osteochondromata, chondroblastomata, chondromyxofibromata,[241] haemangiomata,[242] osteoid osteomata,[243, 249] and aneurysmal bone cyst.[245]

Adults

Clinical presentation

In adults, there is severe unremitting backache of recent onset which does not respond to rest, as well as pain over the distribution of a lumbar nerve root, either unilateral or bilateral. There is motor, sensory and spincter involvement.

Investigations

Plain X-rays. These may show early erosion of the pedicle, collapse of a vertebral body or a soft-tissue shadow. However, in the early stages of the disease they may be normal.

Radio-active bone scan. This is the most important investigation and may show early bone involvement long before plain X-rays reveal any abnormality.

Contrast studies. A study of the subarachnoid space by means of a lumbar or cisternal puncture with injection of radio-opaque dye is essential to identify and define the site and extent of an extra-dural or intramedullary tumour.

Computerized axial tomography. This investigation, combined with contrast studies, can give very precise localization and extension of the lesion.

Treatment

Surgical intervention is indicated:

1. To relieve pain and identify the nature of the lesion
2. To decompress the cord and nerve root
3. To stabilize any unstable or potentially unstable segment.

Surgical procedures include decompressive laminectomy, anterior or anterolateral approach with excision of the lesion and bone grafting. This may be supplemented with radiotherapy, preferably after surgery. Stener[246] described total spondylectomy in a chondrosarcoma arising from the 7th thoracic vertebra. Kostuik[247] reported the results of anterior spinal cord decompression, bone grafting and anterior internal fixation for patients with tumours in association with kyphosis. Indications were progressive neurological deficit and deformity.

Children

Clinical features

These are: pain, stiffness and unwillingness to walk associated with deformity. Muscle spasm may precede the neurological deficit by some months.

Fraser and colleagues[248] review 40 cases of spinal tumour and note the long delay between the presentation and establishment of the correct diagnosis. The most common presenting feature was a limp, with pain localized in the back, and spincter disturbance.

Investigations

The authors noted pathological changes in 55% of the plain films.

Surgical treatment

Twenty-nine of the 40 children underwent laminectomy, with an average number of four laminae being removed. The authors stressed the importance of late onset of deformity following extensive laminectomy, with the more severe deformities occurring in the thoracic spine. They recommended the importance of appropriate bracing after laminectomy in order to prevent the deformity.

Benign tumours

Fraser and colleagues noted that 22 of the 40 cases of spinal tumours in children reviewed were benign, and these include osteoid osteoma, aneurysmal bone cyst, haemangioma, eosinophilic granuloma.

Osteoid osteoma

Kirwin et al[249] reviewed 18 cases of osteoid osteoma or osteoblastoma and noted an average delay of 19 months in diagnosis. Patients presented with marked spinal stiffness and scoliosis. Fifteen of the 18 tumours were in the pedicles. The average age of his series was 13.5 years, with a range of 8–19.5 years. Presenting features were pain, aggravated by activity and troublesome at night in all patients.

Investigations. In 6 patients the lesion was noted on plain X-rays, but in 12 patients a radioactive bone scan was necessary to identify it.[250]

Computerized tomography. Wedge et al[251] present two patients in whom CAT scanning was the investigation of choice.

Treatment. They describe a midline posterior approach with resection of the transverse process which was then removed, allowing the surgeon to approach the pedicle. In this way the pars interarticularis and the posterior facet joints were not interfered with and no fusion was required.

Eosinophilic granuloma

Green and colleagues[252] described three children who presented with pain and neural defect associated with the radiological appearance of a vertebra plana. They advocated needle biopsy and open biopsy if necessary and recommended immobilization and radiation. The prognosis is excellent.

REFERENCES

1 Hadra B 1891 Wiring of the vertebrae as a means of immobilisation in fracture and Pott's disease. Med. Times Register 22: 423–427
2 Hibbs R A 1911 An operation for progressive spinal deformities. New York Med. J. 93: 1013–1015
3 Albee R H 1911 Transplantation of a portion of the tibia into the spine for Pott's disease. JAMA 57: 885–886
4 Girdlestone G R 1931 The place of operation for spinal fixation in the treatment of Pott's disease. Brit. J. Surg. 19: 121–124
5 Dandy W E 1929 Loose cartilage from intervertebral disc simulating tumour of the spinal cord. Arch. Surg. 19: 660–663
6 Mixter W J, Barr J S 1934 Rupture of the intervertebral disc with involvement of the spinal canal. New Eng. J. Med. 211: 210–214
7 Macnab I 1977 Backache. Williams & Wilkins, Baltimore
8 Kane W J 1983 World-wide incidence of surgery for lumbar disc herniation. Presented to the International Society for the Study of the Lumbar Spine
9 Glenn W V, Rhodes M L, Altschuler E M, Wiltse L L, Kostanek C, Kuo Y M 1979 Multiplanar display computerised body tomography applications in the lumbar spine. Spine 4: 282–352
10 Teplick J G, Haskin M E 1983 CT and lumbar disc herniation. Radiol. Clin. N. Amer. 21: 259–288
11 Porter R W, Wicks M, Ottewell D 1978 Measurement of the spinal canal by diagnostic ultrasound. J. Bone Jt. Surg. 60B: 481–487
12 Holt E P 1968 The question of lumbar discography. J. Bone Jt. Surg. 50A: 720–726
13 Brodsky A E, Binder W F 1979 Lumbar discography. Spine 4: 110–120
14 Galasko C S B 1975 The pathological basis for skeletal scintigraphy. J. Bone Jt. Surg. 57B: 353–359
15 Roland M, Morris R 1983 A study of the natural history of back pain — Part I. Development of a reliable and sensitive measure of disability in low back pain. Spine 8: 141–143
16 Fairbank J C T, Cooper J, Davis J, O'Brien J 1980 The Oswestry low back pain disability questionnaire. J. Physiotherapy 66: 271–273
17 Lehmann T R, Brand R A, Gorman T W O 1983 A low back rating scale. Spine 8: 308–315
18 Epstein J A, Epstein B S, Lavine L S, Carras R 1967 Herniated discs and related disorders of the lumbar spine — surgical treatment in the geriatric patient. JAMA 202: 187–191
19 Waddell G, Kummel E G, Lotto W N, Graham J D, Hall H, McCulloch J A 1979 Failed lumbar disc surgery and repeat surgery following industrial injuries. J. Bone Jt. Surg. 61A: 201–207
20 Waddell G, Bircher M, Finlayson D, Main C J 1984 Symptoms and signs: physical disease or illness behaviour. Brit. Med. J. 289: 739–741
21 Southwick S M, White A A 1983 The use of psychological tests in the evaluation of low back pain. J. Bone Jt. Surg. 65A: 560–565
22 Taylor W P, Stern W R, Kubiszyn T W 1984 Predicting patients' perceptions of response to treatment for low back pain. Spine 9: 313–316
23 Lloyd G G, Wolkind S N, Greenwood R, Harris D J 1979 A psychiatric study of patients with persistent low back pain. Rheumatol. Rehabil. 18: 30–37
24 House D Personal communication
25 Nelson M A 1982 Survey of surgical management of lumbar disc prolapse in UK and N. Eire 1981. Presented to meeting of International Society for the Study of the Lumbar Spine, Toronto
26 Crock H V 1981 Normal and pathological anatomy of the lumbar nerve root canals. J. Bone Jt. Surg. 63B: 487–490
27 Macnab I 1971 Negative disc exploration: an analysis of the cause of nerve root involvement in 68 patients. J. Bone Jt. Surg. 53A: 891–903
28 Mooney V 1984 The role of spinal fusion. Spine 6: 304–305
29 Lansche W E, Ford L T 1960 Correlation of the myelogram with clinical and operative findings in lumbar disc lesions. J. Bone Jt. Surg. 42A: 193–206
30 Edgar M A, Park W M 1974 Induced pain patterns on passive straight leg raising. J. Bone Jt. Surg. 56B: 658–667
31 Coventry M B, Stauffer R N 1969 The multiply-operated back. In: American Academy of Orthopaedic Surgeons. Symposium on the Spine. Mosby, St Louis, p 132–142
32 Leyshon A, Kirwan E O G, Wynne-Parry C B 1981 Electrical studies in the diagnosis of compression of the lumbar root. J. Bone Jt. Surg. 63B: 71–75
33 Postacchini F, Urso S, Ferro L 1982 Lumbo-sacral nerve root anomalies. J. Bone Jt. Surg. 64A: 721–729
34 Epstein J A, Lavine L S 1964 Herniated lumbar intervertebral discs in teenage children. J. Neuro. Surg. 21: 1070–1075
35 Beks J W F, Terweeme C A 1975 Herniated lumbar discs in teenagers. Acta Neurochir. 31: 195–199
36 Grobler L J, Simmons E H, Barrington T W 1979 Intervertebral disc herniation in the adolescent. Spine 3: 267–278
37 Nelson M A 1975 Lumbar intervertebral disc lesions. Rheum. Rehab. 14: 163–166
38 Barmier E, Blinder G E, Sasson A A, Hirsch M 1983 Prone computed tomography metrizamide myelography — a technique for improved diagnosis of lumbar disc herniation. Clin. Radiol. 35: 479–481
39 Love J G, Emmet J L 1967 Asymptomatic protruded

lumbar disc as a cause of urinary retention. Preliminary report. Proc. Mayo Clin. 42: 249–251

40 Ross J C, Jamieson R M 1971 Vesical dysfunction due to prolapsed disc. Brit. Med. J. 2: 752–754

41 Scott P J 1965 Bladder paralysis in cauda equina lesion from disc prolapse. J. Bone Jt. Surg. 47B: 224–235

42 Briggs H, Krause J 1945 The intervertebral foraminotomy for relief of sciatic pain. J. Bone Jt. Surg. 27: 475–478

43 Schatzker J, Pennal G F 1968 Spinal stenosis — a cause of cauda equina compression. J. Bone Jt. Surg. 50B: 606–618

44 Shenkin H A, Hash C J 1976 A new approach to the surgical treatment of lumbar spondylosis. J. Neurosurg. 44: 148–155

45 Getty C J M, Johnson J R, Kirwan E O'G, Sullivan M F 1981 Partial undercutting facetectomy for bony entrapment of the lumbar nerve root. J. Bone Jt. Surg. 63B: 330–335

46 Hadley L A 1951 Intervertebral joint subluxation, bony encroachment and foramen encroachment with nerve root changes. Am. J. Roent. 65: 377–401

47 Lettin A W 1967 Diagnosis and treatment of lumbar instability. J. Bone Jt. Surg. 49B: 250–259

48 Kirkaldy-Willis W H, Farfan H F 1982 Instability of the lumbar spine. Clin. Orthop. 165: 110–123

49 Lee C K 1983 Lumbar spinal instability (olisthesis) after extensive posterior spinal decompression. Spine 8: 429–433

50 Williams R W 1978 Micro lumbar discectomy. Spine 3: 175–183

51 Semmes R E 1939 Diagnosis of ruptured disc without contrast myelography and comment upon recent experience with modified hemi-laminectomy for their removal. Yale J. Biol. Med. 11: 433–436

52 Love J G 1939 Removal of protruded intervertebral discs with laminectomy. Proc. Mayo Clin. 14: 800–805

53 O'Connell J E A 1951 Protrusion of the lumbar intervertebral discs. J. Bone Jt. Surg. 33B: 8–13

54 Jackson R K 1971 The long-term effects of wide laminectomy for lumbar disc excision. J. Bone Jt. Surg. 53B: 609–616

55 Connelly R, Campbell, Newman P H 1971 Lumbar spondylotomy. J. Bone Jt. Surg. 53B: 575–577

56 Capanna A H, Williams R W, Austin D C, Darmody W R, Murray-Thomas L 1981 Lumbar discectomy — percentage of disc removal and detection of anterior annulus perforation. Spine 6: 610–614

57 Weir B K, Jacobs G A 1980 Re-operation rate following lumbar discectomy. Spine 5: 366–370

58 Silver D J, Dunsmore R H, Dickson C M 1976 Spinal anaesthesia for lumbar disc surgery — a review of 576 operations. Anaesth. Analg. Curr. Res. 55: 550–554

59 Eie N, Solgaard T, Kleppe H 1983 The knee–elbow position in lumbar disc surgery — review of complications. Spine 8: 897–900

60 Jacobs R R, McClain O, Neff J 1980 Control of post-laminectomy scar formation. Spine 5: 223–229

61 Yong-Hing K, Reilly J, de Korompay V, Kirkaldy-Willis W H 1980 Prevention of nerve adhesions after laminectomy. Spine 5: 59–64

62 Linton R R, White P D 1945 Arteriovenous fistula between the right common iliac artery and the inferior vena cava. Arch. Surg. Chicago 50: 6–13

63 Holscher E C 1948 Vascular complications of disc surgery. J. Bone Jt. Surg. 30A: 968–974

64 Harbison S P 1954 Major vascular complications of intervertebral disc surgery. Ann. Surg. 140: 342–348

65 Seeley S F, Hughes C W, Jahneke E J Jnr 1954 Major vessel damage in lumbar disc operation. Surgery 35: 421–429

66 Mack J R 1956 Major vascular injuries incident to intervertebral disc surgery. Amer. Surg. 22: 752–763

67 Schumacker H B, King H, Campbell R 1961 Vascular complications of disc operations. J. Trauma 1: 177–185

68 De Saussure R L 1959 Vascular injury coincident to disc surgery. J. Neurosurg. 16: 222–229

69 Ford L T, Key J A 1955 Post-operative infection of intervertebral disc space. South. Med. J. 48: 1293–1303

70 Thibodeau A A 1968 Closed space infection following removal of lumbar intervertebral disc. J. Bone Jt. Surg. 50A: 400–412

71 Pilgaard S, Aarhus N 1969 Discitis (closed space infection) following removal of lumbar intervertebral disc. J. Bone Jt. Surg. 51A: 713–719

72 Lindholm T S, Pylkkanen P 1982 Disciitis following removal of intervertebral disc. Spine 7: 618–622

73 El-Gindi S, Aref S, Salama M, Andrew J 1976 Injection of intervertebral discs after operation. J. Bone Jt. Surg. 58B: 114–116

74 Morgan H C 1968 Neural complications of disc surgery. J. Bone Jt. Surg. 50: 411–417

75 Muller P R, Elder F W 1968 Meningeal pseudocysts (meningocele spurius) following laminectomy. J. Bone Jt. Surg. 50A: 268–275

76 Laurin C A 1969 Knee chest support for lumbo-sacral operations. Canad. J. Surg. 12: 245–250

77 Distepano V, Klein K S, Nixon J E, Andrews E T 1973 Intra-operative analysis of the effects of position and body habits on back surgery. J. Bone Jt. Surg. 55A: 1313–

78 Falconer M A, McGeorge M, Begg A C 1947/8 Surgery of lumbar intervertebral disc protrusion. Brit. J. Surg. 35: 225–249

79 Spurling R G, Grantham E G 1949 The end results of surgery for ruptured lumbar intervertebral discs. J. Neurosurg. 6: 57–64

80 Gurdjian E S, Ostrowski A Z, Hardy W G, Lindner D W, Thomas L M 1961 Results of operative treatment of protruded and ruptured lumbar discs. J. Nurosurg. 18: 783–791

81 Hirsch C, Nachemson A 1963 The reliability of lumbar disc surgery. Clin. Orthop. Rel. Res. 29: 189–194

82 Hakelius A 1969/70 Prognosis in sciatica. Acta Orthop. Scand. Suppl. 127

83 Naylor A 1974 The late results of laminectomy for lumbar disc prolapse. J. Bone Jt. Surg. 56B: 17–24

84 Weber H 1978 Lumbar disc herniation I and II. J. Oslo City Hosp. 23: 33–64, 89–120

85 Rugtveit A 1966 Juvenile disc herniations. Acta Orthop. Scand. 37: 348–356

86 Kurihara A, Kataoka O 1980 Lumbar disc herniation in children and adolescents. Spine 5: 443–451

87 Bradford D S, Garcia A 1970 Lumbar intervertebral disc herniations in children and adolescents. Orthop. Clin. N. Amer. 2: 583–592

88 Grobler L J, Simmons E H, Barrington T W 1979 Intervertebral disc herniation in the adolescent. Spine 3: 267–278

89   Deorio J K, Bianco A J 1982 Lumbar disc excision in children. J. Bone Jt. Surg. 64A: 991–995

90   Sarpyener M A 1945 Congenital stricture of the spinal canal. J. Bone Jt. Surg. 27: 70–79

91   Sarpyener M A 1947 Spina bifida aperta and congenital stricture of the spinal canal. J. Bone Jt. Surg. 29: 817–821

92   Verbiest H 1949 Sur certaines formes rares de compression de la queue de cheval. Hommage à cloris. Vincent, Paris, p 161–174

93   Verbiest H 1954 A radicular syndrome from developmental narrowing of the lumbar vertebral canal. J. Bone Jt. Surg. 36B: 230–237

94   Verbiest H 1955 Further experience on the pathological influence of a developmental narrowness of the body lumbar vertebral canal. J. Bone Jt. Surg. 37B: 576–583

95   Blau J N, Logue V 1961 Intermittent claudication of the cauda equina. An unusual syndrome resulting from central protrusion of an intervertebral disc. Lancet 1: 1081–1086

96   Epstein J A, Epstein B S, Lavine L 1962 Nerve root compression with narrowing of the lumbar spinal canal. J. Neurol. Neurosurg. Psych. 25: 165–176

97   Teng P, Paptheodorou C 1963 Myelographic findings in spondylosis of lumbar spine. Brit. J. Radiol. 36: 122–128

98   Graveleau J, Guiot G 1964 Congenital narrowness of the lumbar spinal canal and sensitive motor intermittent claudication syndrome of the cauda equina. Presse. Med. 72: 3344–3348

99   Joffe R, Appleby A, Arjona V 1966 Intermittent ischaemia of the cauda equina due to stenosis of the lumbar canal. J. Neurol. Neurosurg. Psych. 29: 315–318

100 Hancock D O 1967 Congenital narrowing of the spinal canal. Paraplegia 5: 89–96

101 Jones R A C, Thomson J L G 1968 The narrow lumbar canal. J. Bone Jt. Surg. 50B: 595–605

102 Schatzker J, Pennal G F 1968 Spinal stenosis, a cause of cauda equina compression. J. Bone Jt. Surg. 50B: 606–618

103 Ethni G 1969 Significance of the small lumbar spinal canal: cauda equina compression syndrome due to spondylosis. Part 4 — acute compression artificially induced during operation. J. Neurosurg. 31: 507–512

104 Ethni G 1969 Significance of the small lumbar spinal canal — cauda equina syndromes due to spondylosis. Part 1 — introduction. J. Nurosurg. 31: 490

105 Nelson M A 1973 Lumbar spinal stenosis. J. Bone Jt. Surg. 55B: 506–512

106 Arnoldi C C, Brodsky A E, Cauchoix J et al 1976 Lumbar spinal stenosis and nerve entrapment syndromes. Clin. Orthop. 115: 4–5

107 Eisenstein S 1977 The morphometry and pathological anatomy of the lumbar spine in South African negroes and caucasoids with special reference to spinal stenosis. J. Bone Jt. Surg. 59B: 173–180

108 Tile M et al 1976 Spinal stenosis — results of treatment. Clin. Orthop. 115: 104–108

109 Johansson J E, Barrington T W, Ameli M 1982 Combined vascular and neurogenic claudication. Spine 7: 150–158

110 Postacchini F, Pezzeri G, Montanaro A, Natali G 1980 Computerised tomography in lumbar stenosis. J. Bone Jt. Surg. 62B: 78–82

111 Tsuji H 1982 Laminoplasty for patients with compressive myelopathy due to so-called canal stenosis in cervical and thoracic regions. Spine 7: 28–34

112 Grabias S 1980 The treatment of spinal stenosis. J. Bone Jt. Surg. 62A: 308–313

113 Verbiest H 1977 Results of the surgical treatment of idiopathic developmental stenosis of the lumbar vertebral canal. J. Bone Jt. Surg. 59B: 181–188

114 Russin L A, Sheldon J 1976 Spinal stenosis — report of series and long-term follow-up. Clin. Orthop. 115: 101–103

115 Paine K W E 1976 Results of decompression for lumbar spinal stenosis. Clin. Orthop. 115: 96–103

116 Tile M 1976 Spinal stenosis. Clin. Orthop. 115: 104–108

117 Getty C J M 1980 Lumbar spinal stenosis. J. Bone Jt. Surg. 62B: 481–485

118 White A H, Wiltse L L 1977 Post-operative spondylolisthesis. In: Weinsein P, Ehni G, Wilson C B (eds) Lumbar spondylosis, diagnosis management and surgical treatment. Chicago Year Book Medical Publishers, p 184–194

119 Hanraets P R 1959 The degenerative back and its differential diagnosis. Trans M E Hollander. Elsevier, New York

120 Kilian H F 1854 Schilderungen neuer Beckenformen und ihres Verhaltens im Lehen. von Bassermann und Mathyl, Mannheim

121 Andre N 1741 cited by Keim H A. 1976 Grune & Stratton, New York. The adolescent spine

122 Herbiniaux G 1782 Traité sur divers accouchements laborieux et sur les polypes de la matrice. de Boubers, Bruxelles

123 Meyerding 1932 Spondylolisthesis. Surg. Gynae. Obst. 54: 371–377

124 Wiltse L L, Newman P H, Macnab I 1976 Classification of spondylolysis and spondylolisthesis. Clin. Orthop. 117: 23–29

125 Eisenstein S 1978 Spondylolysis. J. Bone Jt. Surg. 60B: 488–494

126 Wiltse L L, Widell E H, Jckson D W 1975 Fatigue fracture, the basic lesion in isthmic spondylolisthesis. J. Bone Jt. Surg. 57A: 17–22

127 Wynne-Davies R, Scott J H S 1979 Inheritance and spondylolisthesis. J. Bone Jt. Surg. 61B: 301–305

128 Cyron B M, Hutton W C 1978 The fatigue strength of the lumbar neural arch in spondylolysis. J. Bone Jt. Surg. 60B: 234–238

129 Wertzberger K, Peterson H A 1980 Acquired spondylolysis and sponylolisthesis. Spine 5: 437–442

130 Ravichandran G 1980 Multiple lumbar spondylolysis. Spine 6: 552–557

131 Tsuchihashihi A 1972 A clinical study of mechanism of pain in spondylolysis and spondylolisthesis. Nihon Seikei Geka Gakkai Zasshi 46: 387–403

132 Newman P H 1965 A clinical syndrome associated with severe lumbo-sacral subluxation. J. Bone Jt. Surg. 47B: 472–481

133 Dandy D J, Shannon M J 1971 Lumbo-sacral subluxation (Group I spondylolisthesis). J. Bone Jt. Surg. 53B: 578–595

134 Verbiest H 1979 The treatment of lumbar spondyloptosis or impending lumbar spondyloptosis accompanied by neurologic deficit and/or neurogenic intermittent claudication. Spine 4: 68–77

135 Sijbrandij S 1981 A new technique for the reduction and stabilisation of severe spondylolisthesis. J. Bone Jt. Surg. 63B: 266–271

136 Fredrickson B E, Baker D, McHolick W J, Yuan H A, Lubicky J A 1984 The natural history of spondylolysis and spondylolisthesis. J. Bone Jt. Surg. 66A: 699–707

137 Jackson A M, Kirwan E O'G, Sullivan M F 1978 Lytic spondylolisthesis above the lumbo-sacral level. Spine 3: 260–266

138 Wiltse L L, Jackson D W 1976 Treatment of spondylolisthesis and spondylolysis in children. Clin. Orthop. 117: 92–100

139 Buck J E 1970 Direct repair of the defect in spondylolisthesis. J. Bone Jt. Surg. 52B: 432–437

140 Turner R H, Bianco A J 1971 Spondylolysis and spondylolisthesis in children and teenagers. J. Bone Jt. Surg. 53A: 1298–1306

141 Gill G G, Manning J G, White H L 1955 Surgical treatment of spondylolisthesis without spine fusion. J. Bone Jt. Surg. 37A: 493–520

142 King A B, Baker D R, McHolick W J 1957 Another approach to the treatment of spondylolisthesis and spondyloschisis. Clin. Orthop. 10: 257–268

143 Cedell C A, Wiberg G 1969 The long-term results of laminectomy in spondylolisthesis. Acta Orthop. Scand. 40: 773–776

144 Monticelli G, Ascani E 1975 Spondylolysis and spondylolisthesis. Acta Orthop. Scand. 46: 498–506

145 Junghanns H 1930 Spondylolisesen ohne Spalt im zwischen Gelenstuck. Archiv für Orthopädische und Unfall-Chirurgie 29: 18–26

146 Macnab I 1950 Spondylolisthesis with an intact neural arch. The so-called pseudo-spondylolisthesis. J. Bone Jt. Surg. 32B: 325–333

147 Epstein J A, Epstein B S, Lavine L S 1976 Degenerative lymbar spondylolisthesis with an intact neural arch (pseudo-spondylolisthesis). J. Neurosurg. 44: 139–147

148 Lee C K 1983 Lumbar spinal instability (olisthesis-) after extensive posterior spinal decompression. Spine 8: 429–433

149 Mendal K, Adler S 1908 Zur Kenntnis der Meningitis serosa spinalis. Berl. Klin. Wochenschr. 45: 1596–1602

150 Horsley V 1909 Chronic spinal meningitis — its differential diagnosis and surgical treatment. Br. Med. J. 1: 513–517

151 Stookey B 1927 Adhesive spinal arachnoiditis simulating spinal cord tumor. Arch. Neurol. Psychiat. (Chicago) 17: 151–178

152 Elkington J 1936 Meningitis serosa circumscripta spinalis (spinal arachnoiditis). Brain 51: 181–203

153 Wadia N, Dastur D 1969 Spinal meningitis with radiculomyelography. J. Neurosurg. 8: 239–261

154 De La Porte C, Siegfried J 1983 Lumbo-sacral spinal fibrosis (spinal arachnoiditis). Spine 8: 593–603

155 Burton C H 1978 Lumbo-sacral arachnoiditis. Spine 3: 24–30

156 Waddell G, McCulloch J A, Kummelle 1980 Non-organic physical signs in low back pain. Spine 5: 117–125

157 Lee C K, Alexander H 1984 Prevention of post-laminectomy scar formation (dogs). Spine 9: 305–312

158 Benoist M, Ficat C, Baraf P, Cauchoix J 1980 Post-operative lumbar epiduro-arachnoiditis. Spine 5: 432–436

159 Rolander S D 1966 Motion of the spine with special reference to stabilising effect of posterior fusion. Acta Orthop. Scand. Suppl 90

160 Lee C K, Langrana N A 1984 Lumbo-sacral spinal fusion. Spine 9: 574–581

161 Burns B H 1933 An operation for spondylolisthesis. Lancet 1: 1233–1236

162 Mercer W 1936 Spondylolisthesis with a description of a new method of treatment and notes of 10 cases. Edin. Med. J. 43: 545–572

163 Lane J D Jr, Moore E S Jnr 1948 Transperitoneal approach to the intervertebral disc in the lumbar area. Ann. Surg. 127: 537–551

164 Harmon P H 1960 Anterior extraperitoneal lumbar disc excision and vertebral body fusion. A study of long term results. Clin. Orthop. 18: 169–198

165 Freebody D 1964 Treatment of spondylolisthesis by anterior fusion via the trans-peritoneal root. J. Bone Jt. Surg. 46B: 778

166 Cloward R B 1945 New treatment of ruptured intervertebral disc. Presented at the Annual Meeting of the Hawaii Territorial Medical Association

167 Cloward R B 1953 The treatment of ruptured lumbar intervertebral discs by vertebral body fusion. J. Neurosurg. 10: 154–157

168 James A J, Nesbit N W 1953 Posterior intervertebral fusion of the lumbar spine. J. Bone Jt. Surg. 35B: 181–186

169 Watkins M B 1953 Posterolateral fusion of the lumbar and lumbo-sacral spine. J. Bone Jt. Surg. 35A: 1014–1018

170 Kelly R P 1962 Intertransverse fusion of the low back. Trans. South. Surg. Assn. 74: 193–202

171 Wiltse L L, Bateman J G 1965 Experience with transverse process fusion of the lumbar spine. J. Bone Jt. Surg. 47A: 848–849

172 Stauffer R N, Coventry 1972 Postero-lateral lumbar spine fusion. J. Bone Jt. Surg. 54A: 1195–1204

173 Thompson W A L, Gristina A G, Healy W A 1974 Lumbo-sacral spine fusion. J. Bone Jt. Surg. 56A: 1643–1647

174 Harrold A J 1976 Limited intertransverse fusion using iliac grafts. Brit. J. Surg. 63: 920–923

175 Thompson W A L, Ralstone E L 1949 Pseudoarthrosis following spinal fusion. J. Bone Jt. Surg. 31A: 400–405

176 Shaw E G, Taylor J G 1956 The results of lumbo-sacral fusion for low back pain. J. Bone Jt. Surg. 38B: 485–497

177 Erikson B 1960 Lumbo-sacral fusion. J. Bone Jt. Surg. 42B: 660–661

178 Nelson M A 1968 A long term review of posterior spinal fusion. Proc. Roy. Soc. Med. 611: 558–559

179 King D 1948 Internal fixation for lumbo-sacral fusion. J. Bone Jt. Surg. 30A: 560–565

180 Boucher H H 1959 A method of spinal fusion. J. Bone Jt. Surg. 41B: 248–259

181 Attenborough C G, Reynolds M T 1975 Lumbo-sacral fusion with spring fixation. J. Bone Jt. Surg. 57B: 283–288

182 Dove J 1983 Stabilisation of the spine by the Luque method. Presented to the International Society for the Study of the Lumbar Spine. Cambridge, England

183 Lin P M, Cautilli R A, Joyce M F 1983 Posterior lumbar interbody fusion (PLIF). Clin. Orthop. 180: 154–168

184 Hutter C G 1983 Posterior intervertebral body fusion. Clin. Orthop. 179: 86–96

185 Lane J D Jnr, Moore E S Jnr 1948 Transperitoneal approach to the intervertebral disc in the lumbar area. Ann. Surg. 127: 537–551

186 Harmon P H 1960 Anterior extra-peritoneal lumbar disc excision and vertebral body fusion — a study of long term results. Clin. Orthop. 18: 169–198

187 Freebody D, Bedall R, Taylor R D 1971 Anterior transperitoneal lumbar fusion. J. Bone Jt. Surg. 53B: 617–627

188 Sachs S 1965 Anterior interbody fusion of the lumbar spine. J. Bone Jt. Surg. 47B: 211–223

189 Fujimaki A, Crock H V, Bedbrook Sir G M 1982 The results of 150 anterior lumbar interbody fusion operations performed by two surgeons in Australia. Clin. Orthop. 165: 164–167

190 Inoue S I, Watanabe T, Hirose A, Tanaka T, Matsui N, Saegusa O, Sho E 1984 Anterior discectomy and interbody fusion for lumbar disc herniation. Clin. Orthop. 183: 22–31

191 Fager C A, Friedberg S R 1980 Analysis of failure and poor results of lumbar spine surgery. Spine 5: 87–94

192 Weir B K A, Jacobs G A 1980 Re-operation rate following lumbar discectomy. Spine 5: 366–370

193 Moore J H 1970 Spinal cord decompression following unsuccessful disc surgery — surgical approach and technique. J. Bone Jt. Surg. 52A: 1259–1260

194 Frymoyer J W, Matteri R E, Hanley E N, Kuhlmann D, Howe J 1978 Failed lumbar disc surgery. Spine 3: 7–11

195 A 10-year assessment of a controlled trial comparing debridement and anterior spinal fusion in the management of tuberculosis of the spine in patients on standard chemotherapy in Hong Kong. 8th Report of M.R.C. Working Party 1982. J. Bone Jt. Surg. 64B: 393–398

196 Babhulkar S S, Tayade W B, Babhulkar S K 1984 Atypical spinal tuberculosis. J. Bone Jt. Surg. 66B: 239–242

197 Joiner D, Maclean K S, Pritchard E K, Anderson K, Collard P, King M B, Knox R 1952 Isoniazid in pulmonary tuberculosis; its use with and without streptomycin. Lancet 2: 843–846

198 Wilkinson M C 1952 The treatment of Pott's disease by curettage of the spinal lesion. J. Bone Jt. Surg. 34B: 153–154

199 Wilkinson M C 1955 The treatment of tuberculosis of the spine by evacuation of the paravertebral abscess and curettage of the vertebral bodies. J. Bone Jt. Surg. 37B: 382

200 Hodgson A R, Stock F E, Fang H S Y, Ong G B 1960/1 Anterior spinal fusion. The operative approach and pathological findings in 412 patients with Pott's disease of the spine. Brit. J. Surg. 48: 172–178

201 Hodgson A R 1964 Report on the findings and results in 300 cases of Pott's disease treated by anterior fusion of the spine. J. West. Pac. Orthop. Assoc. 1: 3–7

202 Arct M W 1968 Operative treatment of tuberculosis of the spine in old people. J. Bone Jt. Surg. 50A: 255–267

203 Wilkinson M C 1969 Tuberculosis of the spine treated by chemotherapy and operative debridement. J. Bont Jt. Surg. 51A: 1331–1342

204 Martin N S 1970 Tuberculosis of the spine. J. Bone Jt. Surg. 52B: 613–628

205 Bailey H L, Gabriel M, Hodgson A R, Shin J S 1972 Tuberculosis of the spine in children. J. Bone Jt. Surg. 54A: 1633–1657

206 Wilensky A O 1929 Osteomyelitis of the vertebrae. Ann. Surg. 89: 561–570

207 Kulowski J 1936 Pyogenic osteomyelitis of the spine. J. Bone Jt. Surg. 18: 343–364

208 Guri J D 1946 Pyogenic osteomyelitis of the spine. J. Bone Jt. Surg. 28: 29–39

209 Garcia A Jr, Grantham S A 1960 Hematogenous pyogenic vertebral osteomyelitis. J. Bone Jt. Surg. 42A: 929–436, 520

210 Robinson B H B, Lessoff M H 1961 Osteomyelitis of the spine. Guy's Hosp. Rep. 110: 303–318

211 Pritchard A E, Robinson M P 1961 Staphuylococcal infection of the spine. Lancet 2: 1165–1167

212 Digby J M, Kersley J B 1979 Pyogenic non-tuberculous spinal infection. J. Bone Jt. Surg. 61B: 47–55

213 Griffiths H E D, Jones D M 1971 Pyogenic infection of the spine. J. Bone Jt. Surg. 53B: 383–391

214 Bedow P H, Weisl H 1961 Skeletal infection as a complication of general surgery. Lancet 2: 743–745

215 Mitchell J P, Slade N, Linton K G 1962 Instrumental bacteraemia and its prevention. Brit. J. Urol. 34: 454–459

216 Ottolenghi C E 1969 Aspiration biopsy of the spine. J. Bone Jt. Surg. 51A: 1531–1544

217 Bryant-Zawadzi M, Burke V D, Jeffrey R B 1984 CT in the evaluation of spine infection. Spine 8: 358–364

218 Henson S W Jr, Coventry M B 1956 Osteomyelitis of the vertebrae as the result of infection of the urinary tract. Surg. Gynaec. Obst., 102: 207–211

219 Henriques C Q 1958/9 Osteomyelitis as a complication in urology. Brit. J. Surg. 46: 19–28

220 Bremner A E, Neligan G A 1953 Benign form of acute osteitis of the spine in young children. Brit. Med. J. 1: 856–860

221 Menelaus M B 1964 Disciitis — an inflammation affecting the intervertebral discs in children. J. Bone Jt. Surg. 46B: 16–25

222 Lascari A D, Graham M H, MacQueen J C 1967 Intervertebral disc infection in children. J. Pediat. 1967 70: 751–757

223 Spiegel P G, Kengla K W, Isaacson A S, Wilson J C 1972 Intervertebral disc space inflammation in children. J. Bone Jt. Surg. 54A: 284–295

224 Kemp H B S, Jackson J W, Jeremiah J D, Hall A J 1973 Pyogenic infections occurring primarily in intervertebral discs. J. Bone Jt. Surg. 55B: 698–714

225 Hooper J, Griffin P 1976 Pyogenic osteomyelitis of the spine. Aust. N.Z. J. Surg. 46: 367–371

226 Wenger D R, Bobechko W P, Gilday D L 1978 The spectrum of intervertebral disc space infection in children. J. Bone Jt. Surg. 60A: 100–108

227 Keon-Cohen B T 1968 Epidural abscess simulating disc hernia. J. Bone Jt. Surg. 50B: 128–130

228 Glasgow M M S 1976 Brucellosis of the spine. Brit. J. Surg. 63: 283–288

229 Samra Y, Hertz M, Saked Y, Zwas S, Altman G 1982 Brucellosis of the spine. J. Bone Jt. Surg. 64B: 429–431

230 Carta F, Perria C, Davini V 1974 Vertebral echinococcosis. J. Neurosurg. Sci. 18: 228–232

231 Winter W G, Larson R K, Zettas J P, Libke R 1978 Coccidiodal spondylitis. J. Bone Jt. Surg. 60A: 240–244

232 Winston D J, Kurtz T O, Fleischmann J, Morgad D, Batzdorf U, Stern W F 1983 Successful treatment of spinal arachnoiditis due to coccidiodomycosis. J. Neurosurg. 59: 328–331

233 Duran H, Ferrandez L, Gomez-Castresana F, Lopez-Duran L, Mata P, Brandau D, Sanchez-Barba A 1978 Osseous hydatidosis. J. Bone Jt. Surg. 60A: 685–690

234 Martin N S, Williamson J 1970 The role of surgery in the treatment of malignant tumours of the spine. J. Bone Jt. Surg. 52B: 227–237

235 White W A, Patterson R H Jnr, Bergland R M 1971 Role of surgery in the treatment of spinal cord compression by metastatic neoplasm. Cancer 27: 558–561

236 Hall A J, Mackay N N S 1973 The results of laminectomy for compression of the cord or cauda equina by extradural malignant tumour. J. Bone Jt. Surg. 55B: 497–505

237 Jameson R M 1974 Prolonged survival in paraplegia due to metastatic spinal tumours. Lancet 1: 1209–1211

238 Boland P J, Lane J M, Sundaresan N 1982 Metastatic disease of the spine. Clin. Orthop. 169: 95–102

239 Constans J P, De Divitiis E, Donzelli R, Spaziante R, Meder J F, Hayes C 1983 Spinal metastases with neurological manifestations. J. Neurosurg. 59: 111–118

240 Iraci G 1972 Intraspinal neurinomas and meningiomas. Int. Surg. 56: 289–303

241 Bell M S 1971 Benign cartilaginous tumours of the spine. Brit. J. Surg. 58: 707–711

243 Witwicki T, Siedlik J, Daniluk A 1974 Haemangiomas of the spine. Chir. Narzed. Ruchu 39: 223–229

243 MacLellan D I 1967 Osteoid osteoma of the spine. J. Bone Jt. Surg. 49A: 111–121

244 Lassman L P, Michael James C C 1967 Lumbo-sacral lipoma. J. Neurol. Neurosurg. Psychiat. 30: 174–181

245 Hay M C, Paterson D C, Taylor T K F 1978 Aneurysmal bone cysts of the spine. J. Bone Jt. Surg. 60B: 406–411

246 Stener B 1971 Total spondylectomy for chondrosarcoma arising from the 7th thoracic vertebra. J. Bone Jt. Surg. 53B: 288–295

247 Kostuik J P 1983 Anterior spinal cord decompression for lesions of the thoracic and lumbar spine. Spine 8: 512–531

248 Fraser R D, Paterson D C, Simpson D A 1977 Orthopaedic aspects of spinal tumours in children. J. Bone Jt. Surg. 59B: 143–151

249 Kirwan E O'G, Hutton P A N, Pozo J L, Ransford A O 1984 Osteoid osteoma and benign osteoblastoma of the spine. J. Bone Jt. Surg. 66B: 21–26

250 Rinsky L A, Goris M, Bleck E E, Halpern A, Hirshman P 1980 Intra-operative skeletal scintigraphy for localisation of osteoid osteoma in the spine. J. Bone Jt. Surg. 62A: 143–144

251 Wedge J H, Tchang S, MacFadyen D J 1981 Computerised tomography in localisation of spinal osteoid osteoma. Spine 6: 423–427

252 Green N E, Robertson W W, Kilroy A W 1980 Eosinophilic granuloma of the spine with associated neural defect. J. Bone Jt. Surg. 62A: 1198–1202

Chemonucleolysis

INTRODUCTION

Since it was first isolated by Jansen & Balls[1] in 1941, chymopapain has followed a chequered course to widespread clinical acceptance. After 1963, when Smith[2] first reported its clinical use in the treatment of lumbar disc herniations, chymopapain was widely used in Canada, Great Britain, France, Germany and the United States. However, an American double-blind study in 1975[3] led to the withdrawal of chymopapain from clinical use in the United States. Subsequent double-blind studies by Fraser,[4] Smith Laboratories[5] and Travenol Laboratories[6] led the FDA to reconsider its position, and chymopapain was again released for general use in 1982. Surgeons, accustomed to surgically excising space-occupying pathology, were reluctant to embrace the concept of injecting discs with chymopapain, a constituent of meat tenderizer. Further, six deaths and 37 serious neurological complications[7] have occurred in the United States in approximately 80 000 injections done over a timespan of 18 months (ending time, 1984). Unfortunately, these events have served to undermine chymopapain as a clinical tool.

One manufacturer's claim that chymopapain is as good as surgery (92% success rate)[8] and unsupported claims of product superiority by competing firms fostered more credibility problems for this drug.

Despite the on-going controversy which surrounds chymopapain, the author continues to be convinced of its clinical efficacy.

PHARMACOLOGY

Chymopapain is an extract of latex of the tropical fruit, papaya. Of the proteolytic enzymes in papaya, chymopapain is the most specific in its activity on nucleus pulposus and the least antigenic. Despite its being less antigenic than papain, it is still a foreign protein to the human body and can precipitate allergic reactions. It is a sulphur-containing enzyme and, therefore, reducing agents such as cystine hydrochloride are required to stabilize the product. Chelating agents (EDTA) are also contained in one product (Discase®) to stabilize the enzyme. The enzyme is very heat-sensitive and must be kept refrigerated before reconstitution. It must be reconstituted immediately prior to use and is good for only one hour. After that, the enzyme digests itself and is no longer pharmacologically active.

MECHANISM OF ACTION

Tissue can be classified into two basic components — cells and non-cellular matrix. The cartilage connective tissue of nucleus pulposus contains, obviously, cartilage cells; the matrix is made up of collagen and proteoglycan water complexes. This non-cellular matrix of nucleus pulposus can be thought of as collagen-reinforcing bars laid in a visco-elastic base of proteoglycan and water. It is a very pliable structure, and through the various effects of trauma and ageing can be displaced, in whole or in part, from the disc space cavity, to lie in the spinal canal.

Chymopapain effects the proteoglycan–water aggregates of nuclear tissue. A proteoglycan aggregate is made up of many proteoglycan monomers (Fig. 17.1). A proteoglycan monomer is a protein core with glycosaminoglycan (mucopolysaccharide) side chains. Chondroitin sulphate and kerato-sulphate make up almost all of the glycosamino-

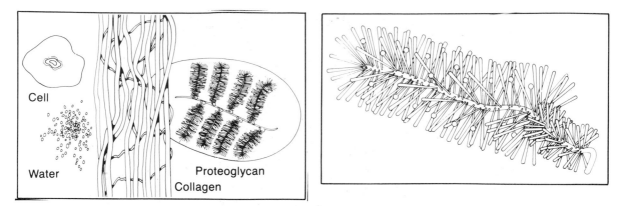

Fig. 17.1 (Left) The four components of connective tissue. (Right) The proteoglycan *monomer* appearing as a bottle brush. Numerous proteoglycan monomers are linked to a hyaluronic acid central core to form the proteoglycan *aggregate*.

glycan side chains. A number of monomers then link to a central chain (hyalaronate) to form a proteoglycan aggregate. This proteoglycan aggregate imbibes water and cements itself amongst the collagen fibers to give the nucleus pulposus its visco-elastic structure. Proteoglycans are negatively charged. Because of the chemical make-up of proteoglycan and its fluid nature, it has the ability to absorb and dissipate water, thereby absorbing and dissipating forces across the disc space.

On displacement of nuclear material of a disc into the spinal canal, three local components can then contribute to the symptom of sciatica (Fig. 17.2). Chymopapain, positively charged, has a direct effect on the negatively charged proteoglycan aggregate by splitting off the glycosaminoglycan side chains, interfering with the ability of proteoglycan to hold water. This hydrolysis deflates the nuclear bulge and thus reduces pressure on the nerve root. Since collagen is not directly affected, there is still some mass of disc tissue present for weeks or months after chemonucleolysis (Fig. 17.3).

To understand further the action of chymopapain, one must appreciate that there are three types of nuclear displacement (Fig. 17.4). In addition to the free fragment location of a disc *sequestration*, the histological make-up of this mass of material lying free in the spinal canal is almost uniformly collagenous. At the other end of the spectrum is a disc *protrusion*, which probably contains a considerable amount of proteoglycan. In between is the *extruded* disc with various degrees of proteoglycan and collagen in its mass. Since chymopapain affects only the proteoglycan component of nuclear material, it will not affect a sequestered disc. Thus, the combination of a free fragment and the collagenous nature of that fragment makes chymopapain injection for a sequestered disc a 'fruitless endeavour'.

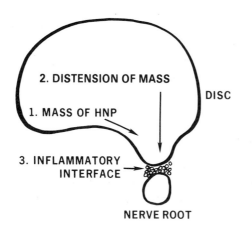

Fig. 17.2 There are three *local* components that contribute to the symptoms and signs of sciatica: (1) Mass of nuclear material. (2) Proteoglycan-water distension within mass of HNP. (3) Inflammatory interface between HNP and nerve root.

TOXICOLOGY

Except for subarachnoid injection, chymopapain enjoys a wide margin of safety between the effective therapeutic dose and the toxic dose.[9] In animal experiments there is a 100-fold margin of safety between the effective therapeutic dose and the toxic

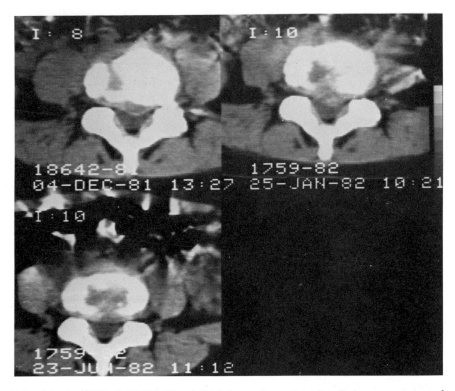

Fig. 17.3 (Top left) Pre-injection HNP, L4-5 left. (Top right) One month post-injection. Patient was symptom-free yet mass of HNP was still present, theoretically minus its distension. (Bottom left) Six months post-injection; with no further treatment and continued work, the mass has disappeared.

dose. Because chymopapain has no effect on collagenase structures such as bone, ligaments, muscle, nerve and epidural tissue, it is very safe and has virtually no local complications when properly injected. Rydevik[10] reported adverse effects on nerve tissue in rabbit tibial nerves, but this has not been borne out with clinical work.[11]

Chymopapain is very dangerous when injected into the subarachnoid space. It dissolves the basement membrane of the pia arachnoid vessels, resulting in subarachnoid haemorrhage. This haemorrhage can cause a local phenomenon such as arachnoiditis and cauda equina syndrome, or it can spread to the entire CSF space and cause the serious intracranial neurological complications of subarachnoid haemorrhage.

In addition, there seems to be some sinister, albeit iatrogenic, delayed, possibly hypersensitive effect of chymopapain in the subarachnoid space which has caused transverse myelitis in humans. These topics will be covered in the Complications section.

INDICATIONS AND CONTRA-INDICATIONS

As with any surgical procedure, it is difficult to obtain a good result to a treatment modality if one cannot recognize the patients that will respond to that treatment. There are very clear indications and contra-indications to the use of chymopapain and they are summarized below.

Indications

There is only one indication for chemonucleolysis with chymopapain — the herniated nucleus pulposus. The diagnosis is based on the following five criteria:

1. The leg pain (including buttock discomfort) is of greater severity than the back pain: it follows a typical radicular distribution and affects one leg.

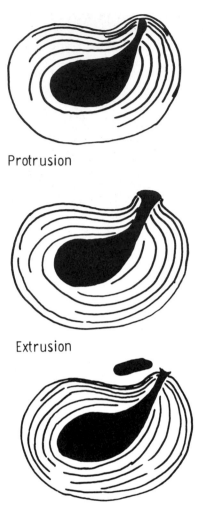

Protrusion

Extrusion

Sequestration

Fig. 17.4 Types of HNP.

2. Paraesthetic sensations, incriminating a single nerve root, are present in the leg and/or foot (e.g. pins and needles or tingling in the lateral calf and/or dorsum of the foot for 5th lumbar root involvement).
3. Root tension signs: any one or combination of the following:
   a. SLR is less than 50% of normal (due to reproduction of pain in the leg)
   b. Pain crosses into the symptomatic leg when the well leg is lifted (crossed straight-leg raising)
   c. Proximal (or distal) radiating leg discomfort is present when pressure is

applied to the tibial nerve in the popliteal fossa (bowstring test)
4. Two of four neurological signs (wasting, weakness, sensory loss or reflex alteration) are present.
5. An investigative study in the form of a myelogram and/or a CT scan is positive and the defect corresponds to the clinical level of root involvement.

There is considerable controversy as to whether one can do a chemonucleolysis on the basis of a CT scan alone. If the patient has the classic syndrome as described above, with the first sacral nerve root incriminated, and a quality CT scan clearly shows an L5–S1 disc herniation, then I see no reason to proceed to myelography. However, if there is some difficulty in diagnosis (e.g. a midline component to the disc herniation causing bilateral leg pain, double root involvement on clinical examination, congenital lumbosacral anomalies with some confusion as to the level of the disc herniation, or a poor-quality scan), then it is important that a myelogram be done before the discolysis procedure. Indeed, the ultimate investigation is a combined CT/myelogram (Fig. 17.5).

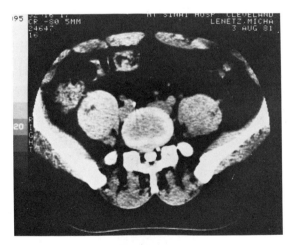

Fig. 17.5 Contrast CT (CT/myelogram) showing HNP, L5-S1 right.

Four or five of the above criteria must be met before one makes the diagnosis of an HNP and considers chemonucleolysis.

Sequestered disc

Within these five criteria there is the contra-indication of a *sequestered* disc. This is a very difficult clinical diagnosis. We have reviewed 50 consecutive sequestered discs (documented at surgery), looking at all aspects of the patient's history and physical examination.[12] Age, sex, type of work, level of disc herniation, side of disc herniation, smoking, onset of symptoms, location of pain, nature of pain, aggravating factors, relieving factors, associated symptoms, progression of symptoms, nerve root tension findings and neurological signs offered no clue as to whether or not the disc was sequestered. With a few clinical exceptions, the diagnosis of a sequestered disc is best made on the basis of investigative studies. The following findings point to a sequestered disc, and discolysis is contra-indicated.

1. Cauda equina syndrome with bladder and bowel involvement
2. A large myelographic or CT defect that is in association with a significant neurological deficit
3. The defect on CT or myelogram lies largely behind the vertebral body (Fig. 17.6)

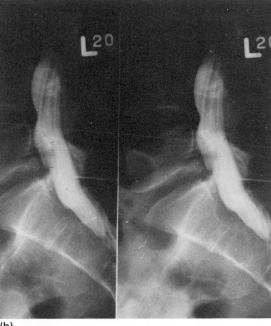

(b)

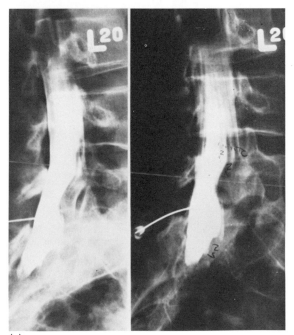

(c)

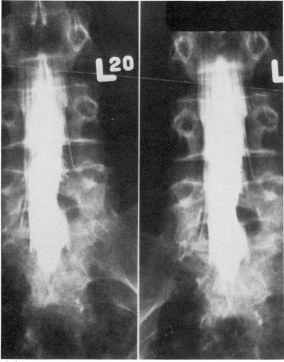

(a)

Fig. 17.6 (a) AP myelogram. (b) Lateral myelogram. (c) Oblique myelogram. The HNP was largely behind the vertebral body. The patient had both lumbar 5 and sacral 1 root involvement, which is often a clinical clue to a disc sequestration.

4. A foraminal disc herniation (Fig. 17.7)
5. A pedicular disc herniation (Fig. 17.8)
6. A pedunculated disc herniation (Fig. 17.9)
7. A complete block on myelography or total obliteration of the spinal canal by disc material on any single CT scan cut
8. A fragment of disc material lying free in the spinal canal (Fig. 17.10)

The following investigative findings suggest that a protrusion or extrusion is present and chymopapain injection may be of benefit.

1. A defect exactly opposite the disc space (Fig. 17.11).

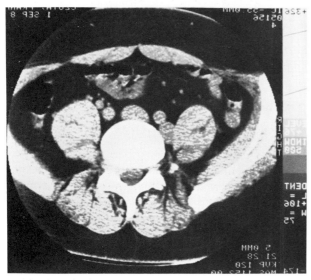

Fig. 17.7(a) A foraminal HNP, L5-S1 left, with predominantly 5th lumbar root findings.

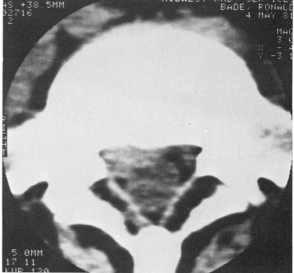

Fig. 17.8 A pedicular disc herniation. The disc fragment has migrated down from the L5-S1 space (the most common direction for fragments to travel) and lies adjacent to the 'pedicle' of S1.

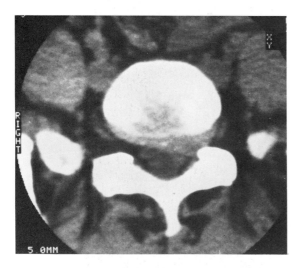

Fig. 17.7(b) Far lateral foraminal disc herniation, L5-S1 left. Note this HNP is opposite the disc space with a portion of the disc herniation directly behind the disc space. This patient did not have a sequestered disc and, in fact, did well with chemonucleolysis.

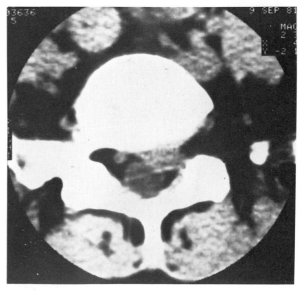

Fig. 17.9 A pedunculated disc herniation. The depth of the disc protrusion into the canal was at least as much as the width of the base of the HNP.

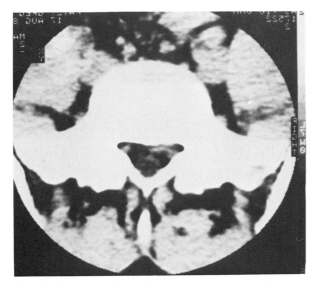

Fig. 17.10 A free fragment, L5-S1 right.

2. A shallow defect with more breadth than depth (Fig. 17.12).

Relative contra-indications

Spinal stenosis

Spinal stenosis affecting the canal or lateral recess will never respond to chemonucleolysis. Occas-

ionally, these bony defects will be complicated by a disc herniation; it is highly unlikely that these combined conditions will be favourably altered by chemonucleolysis.

Previous surgery

Patients who have had previous surgery and who suffer from recurrent disc herniations at the same level/same side should not have chemonucleolysis. Patients who have had previous surgery who suffer from a disc herniation at a different level or opposite side may benefit from chemonucleolysis.

Strong contra-indications

Degenerative disc disease and facet joint disease

Patients with back pain predominantly due to mechanical instability either within the disc space or within the facet joint will not respond to chymopapain injection.

Spinal instability

Patients with spondylolisthesis will not benefit from the injection of chymopapain at the slip level. In fact, the temporary instability that occurs at a disc space level after the injection of chymopapain[13] could

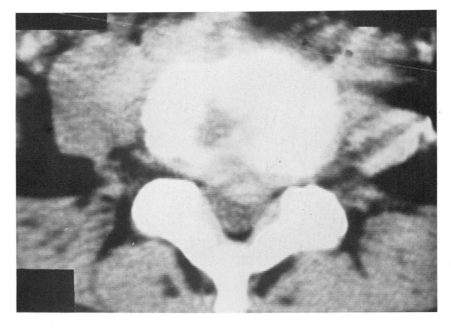

Fig. 17.11 The defect was exactly opposite the disc space, L4-5 left.

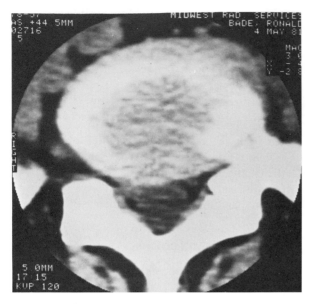

Fig. 17.12 A shallow defect that has more breadth of attachment to disc space than depth of penetration into canal.

result in an increase in the listhesis. This contra-indication applies to both lytic and degenerative spondylolisthesis. There is always a possibility that a patient with spondylolisthesis has a symptomatic disc herniation at a level away from the slip, and that patient would qualify for chymopapain injection, provided he or she fulfils the criteria for the diagnosis of a soft disc herniation causing sciatica.

Absolute contra-indications

Sensitivity to chymopapain

A patient may give a history of an allergy to the ingestion of meat tenderizer or foods containing chymopapain (beer, cheese and some toothpastes). These patients are at risk for an allergic reaction and should not be considered for chymopapain injection. Obviously, a patient with a positive skin test[14] for chymopapain sensitivity is a contra-indication to chymopapain injection. A patient who has had a previous chemonucleolysis may, after a long latent interval, develop another disc herniation at another level. Manufacturers are recommending against a second chymopapain injection. However, if that patient has a negative skin test, a repeat chemo-nucleolysis (different level) could be considered.[14]

Disc herniations at cord levels

To date, there is no recommendation for chymo-papain to be injected into disc herniations at cord levels. The cord level that one might consider could be a thoracic disc. Unfortunately, most of these are calcified, and a chymopapain injection would be of no benefit. In the cervical spine, most radicular problems are due to osteophyte encroachment on the nerve root canal rather than an actual soft disc herniation. When research on these infrequent soft disc herniations is completed, a recommendation for or against injection into soft cervical or thoracic discs can be made.

Neurological lesion of unknown aetiology

It is unreasonable to risk plant enzyme aggravation of a neurological problem of obscure aetiology (e.g. multiple sclerosis).

Pregnant women

Non-organic spinal pain[15]

Provided that the patient fulfils the criteria for the diagnosis of an HNP causing sciatica, age and duration of symptoms do not play a role in the response to chemonucleolysis. There is a tendency for the older patient or the patient with many years of symptoms to have diagnosis such as spinal stenosis, but these patients, in general, do not fulfil the clinical criteria for the diagnosis of an HNP.

PREPARATION OF PATIENT

Conservative treatment

All patients who are considered for chemonu-cleolysis must have failed to respond to excellent conservative therapy (including at least two weeks of complete bed-rest). It is reasonable for a patient to spend three months attempting conservative care before opting for chymopapain injection. There are some patients with persistant sciatica that interferes significantly with their pattern of living or who have a pattern of living that does not allow for two weeks of bed-rest. Early chemonucleolysis may be considered in this patient population. However, this represents a short-cutting of conservative care therapy and is really not consistent with our treatment philosophy.

Aim of therapy

Since most disc ruptures occur at single levels, chemonucleolysis should be done only at single levels. Almost all of the failures to chymopapain injection should go on to surgical intervention, because most of those patients will be found to have a sequestered or extruded disc. Thus, in selecting patients for chymopapain injection, it is obvious that only those patients in whom you would expect a good surgical result are candidates for chymopapain injection. Chymopapain is not to be used as a catch-all for those patients that you reject for surgery.

Pre-operative investigation

The author prefers the CT scan alone as the pre-operative investigation. However, in the following circumstances, a myelogram, alone or in combination with a CT scan, is essential.

1. Any doubt about the diagnosis, clinically or radiologically
2. Older patients (over age 50–55 years)
3. Bilateral symptoms suggesting a midline defect
4. Previous surgery at another level (with or without metal)
5. Obese patient who will not fit properly in the scanner gantry, thereby contributing a poor scan.

Thus, CT scanning alone, as a pre-operative test, is limited to the patient with a classic HNP:

1. Young patient
2. No previous surgery
3. The classic story of unilateral, dominant leg pain with marked reduction in SLR and with neurological symptoms and signs and a scan that shows an HNP at the clinical level.

A final contra-indication to any investigative procedure is poor technique. In this age of outstanding CT scan technology, the author still sees poorly performed scans and scans done on machines that are technically outdated.

Pre-operative chymopapain sensitivity testing

The best strategy for coping with chymopapain sensitivity and anaphylaxis is to identify the patients who are at risk and exclude them from the injection of chymopapain. We have experimented with a sensitive and sufficiently specific skin test, the prick test.[14] We are now over 1000 consecutive patients who have had a negative skin test who have not had an anaphylactic or other immediate hypersensitivity reactions. We feel confident enough to recommend the chymopapain skin test to detect chymopapain sensitivity (see Appendix).

Tests for chymopapain antibody level (IgE), such as chymoFAST® and RAST®, are also available but are not considered as reliable as skin testing.

TECHNIQUE OF CHEMONUCLEOLYSIS

Considerable confusion arose when one manufacturer[16] originally recommended the use of general anaesthesia, pre-medication, a needle insertion site 8 cm from the midline, a 45° angle to approach the disc space, single-needle technique to get into the L5-S1 disc space, and the use of contrast material for discographic assessment for disc integrity. With the occurrence of the complications following the release of chymopapain in the USA, a critical review suggested that a safer protocol was in order. For this reason, there have been some changes recommended in the technique of chemonucleolysis.[17] They are essentially the recommendations published by numerous authors[18,19] in the past and include the use of local neuroleptic anaesthesia, the selection of a needle insertion site at adequate distance from the midline (12 cm average), the use of a double-needle technique at the L5-S1 disc space, and the avoidance of discography using contrast material.

This last recommendation has caused considerable confusion among users of chymopapain. To assist in clarifying this issue, consider discography in light of its four parameters:

1. The volume of test material that can be injected into a disc
2. The resistance to the injection of test material
3. The patient's response to injection
4. The pattern of contrast material.

It is possible to omit contrast material and key on the other three parameters. This is known as water or saline acceptance test, or discometry. With an awake patient under local neuroleptic anaesthesia, it is possible to measure the volume of test material, the resistance, and the patient's response to injection of test material, thereby obtaining information about the integrity of the disc space without using contrast material. However, once this information is obtained, then its role in the selection of the disc space for injection needs critical review. It is likely that this discometric approach to the assessment of disc space integrity offers little more than verification of needle-tip position. The information does not appear to play a prognostic role.

The basic technical rule is: you must know exactly where the needle tip lies before injecting chymopapain. If that requires the use of contrast material, then you must use contrast material. The author feels that, with proper needle insertion technique and good radiography at 90° to each other, routine use of contrast material is not necessary to localize needle tip position.

Local vs general anaesthesia

Local (augmented with neuroleptic agents) is the anaesthetic of choice.

1. It is safer
2. It is efficient: it shortens OR time and the patient's length of stay in hospital
3. The patient avoids the complications of general anaesthesia and intubation
4. It allows for earlier intervention in the event of a complication, e.g. anaphylaxis
5. It preserves discometry or discography as a test.

In the face of a negative skin test, it is slightly unlikely that a patient will experience a hypersensitivity reaction, and thus the main reason for suggesting general anaesthesia is eliminated.

Pre-medication — test dose regimen[8]

The author does not pre-medicate, or test dose. Rather than assume all patients are at risk and pre-medicate, the better approach is to try to identify reactors with an allergic history, and skin test. Other tests, such as RAST® or chymoFAST®, are available.

The reasons for *not* pre-medicating are:

1. The incidence of anaphylaxis is low (0.35%),[20] and lower still with skin testing.
2. There is no scientific evidence that pre-medication lowers the incidence below the figure in our experience.[7]
3. Any treatment regime in medicine considered to be prophylactic in nature should contain the most effective agent — in anaphylaxis this is epinephrine. Obviously, it cannot be included in a prophylactic program.
4. Patients who have been pre-medicated according to recommendations have experienced severe anaphylactic reactions.[7]
5. Patients who have received an intradiscal test dose (not skin test) of chymopapain have experienced severe anaphylactic reactions.[7]
6. Anaphylaxis requires aggressive treatment as follows:
    a. The doses of cortisone and antihistamines required to treat anaphylaxis are much greater than the recommended doses in the pre-medication regime.
    b. The addition of epinephrine.
7. The best defence against anaphylaxis is:
    a. Identification and exclusion of the hypersensitive patient (skin test).
    b. An alert, well-prepared team of assistants.

Operating room or radiology department

The OR has the greatest concentration of skilled personnel for managing the complications of discolysis. Generally speaking, life-threatening emergencies such as anaphylaxis severely stress a radiology department. On the other hand, if your operating room image intensifier capabilities are not good, you will have to consider the radiology department.

Prone or lateral position?

The lateral position is the choice of most users. The prone position is acceptable, provided you do not get too far laterally with your puncture site. Theoretically, the bowel has not fallen away from the lateral abdominal gutter in the prone position. In the lateral position, the bowel falls away from the lateral gutter, and a 10–12 cm insertion site is very safe.

Principles of the lateral approach

1. Maintain proper position of the patient. If you are doing the procedure in the lateral position, there is a tendency for the awake patient to roll out of the perfect lateral position. This is the most common mistake made by the beginner trying to get a needle into a disc space.

2. Select the correct disc. It is very important to see the front of the sacrum before selecting the disc space for injection. One can inadvertently put a needle into the L3-4 disc space, believing it to be at the L4-5 level. View the front of the sacrum before counting levels. Four or six lumbar vertebrae, or other congenital lumbosacral anomalies, may confuse the selection of the disc space to be punctured.[21]

3. Select the correct insertion site. This has been covered earlier in this chapter. It is important to get far enough from the midline. For the average patient, 12 cm from the midline, adjacent to the iliac crest, is the correct insertion site. For a larger patient, you sometimes have to go further than 12 cm from the midline, and for a smaller patient you would select a needle insertion site closer to the midline.

4. Approach the disc at the proper angle. The angle of approach to the disc space is closer to 60° than 45°. However, at all times it is important to remember that the needle must not penetrate the foramen and enter the spinal canal to puncture the subarachnoid space. (It is advisable to leave the stylet out of the needle as an additional precaution. Inadvertent puncture of the subarachnoid space is then heralded by the immediate flow of CSF, signalling abortion of the procedure and rescheduling in two to three weeks.)

5. Position the needle tip in the centre of the disc. The centre of the disc space is defined as the middle third of the disc space on lateral X-ray and superimposed on the spinous process on AP X-ray (Fig. 17.13).

6. Appreciate all the intricacies of discometry (discography). See discussion above.

7. Inject the proper amount of active chymopapain into a clean disc space. The dose of

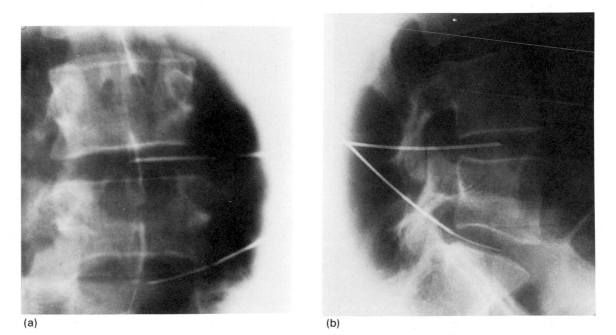

(a)   (b)

Fig. 17.13(a) AP showing perfect needle position at L4-5, L5-S1. (b) Lateral showing perfect needle position at L4-5, L5-S1. Needles were placed in two disc spaces for demonstration purposes. Chemonucleolysis is a single disc space injection procedure.

chymopapain ranges from 1.5 to 2 cc (depending on the brand). This is equivalent to 3000–4000 units.

It is important that chymopapain be reconstitued just prior to injection. After 30–60 minutes, the enzyme, at room temperature, will start to digest itself and lose its activity.

If more than five passes of the needle have occurred, without entry to the disc space being achieved, abort the procedure. Similarly, if you penetrate the nerve root (i.e. cause severe leg pain), abort the procedure. Never abandon the lateral approach for the midline transdural approach.

POST-OPERATIVE CARE

The most important thing to recognize about post-operative management of the patient is the tremendous variation in patient response to the procedure and recovery from the chemical disc excision. Approximately 20% of the patients will have significant back pain (back spasms) immediately after the procedure. This is best managed with an intravenous or intramuscular dose of steroids. This back spasm usually settles within a few hours to a few days after the procedure. The pain is very severe and is usually more severe than pain patients experience following surgical intervention. However, 80% of the patients do not have excessive back pain and their symptoms can be controlled by moderate doses of oral analgesics. Most patients benefit from a light canvas corset support to help them ambulate in the first few weeks following chymopapain injection.

Patients follow one of three courses in regard to post-injection leg pain. Often, there is very dramatic relief of leg pain, but most patients destined for a good result will notice a gradual reduction in their leg pain. Leg cramping and paraesthetic discomfort in the leg are the last to disappear. The latter paraesthetic discomfort often takes many weeks to go away. Occasionally, a patient will notice a dramatic increase in leg pain immediately after injection. In this case, a large extruded disc has been made worse by injection. This patient requires swift surgical intervention (within a day or two of the procedure) to remove the extruded or sequestered fragment of disc material. This will occur in approximately 1 in 100 patients.

Following chymopapain injection, patients are usually discharged from hospital the same day or within one or two days. Analgesic and/or muscle-relaxant medication are usually required for one to two weeks after discharge. The patient who is self-employed may feel compelled to return to work within the first week after injection. However, it is prudent for the patient with light occupational demands to wait two to four weeks before considering a return to work. Patients who have heavier work demands should convalesce for the same period as a patient who undergoes the standard laminectomy/discectomy. The return to leisure activity varies according to its form. The first leisure activity usually available to patients is swimming, which can be started two to four weeks after injection.

It is advisable to see the patients at one month for assessment, including an X-ray. Those patients who have lost most of their leg pain, who have improved in SLR ability and who show disc space narrowing on a plain lateral X-ray, are destined for an excellent result. Patients with some improvement in leg discomfort and some improvement in SLR may be observed for a further one to two months before a decision about future treatment intervention is made. However, those patients who persist with unaltered leg pain one month after the procedure usually have persisting SLR reduction and can be considered a failure. These patients need immediate surgical intervention. As mentioned earlier, most of these patients have an extruded or sequestered disc and will benefit from microsurgical[22] intervention. If you have been careful in selecting your patients and have had the assistance of a CT scan, most cases of lateral recess stenosis will have been promptly and correctly diagnosed. However, if myelography has been your only available method of evaluating patients, a significant number of your failures will be found to have lateral recess stenosis. These patients will require appropriate decompression.

RESULTS

Results vary all the way from 'no good' to 90–95% good. The author has experienced approximately a 70% good result rate,[23] slightly higher for younger patients, and at the L5-S1 level.

Failure is obvious within six weeks of injection,

and almost every failure to the injection of chymopapain should go on to surgical intervention. The most common cause of failure is a sequestered or extruded fragment of disc material that has not been dissolved by chymopapain. Since the nuclear contents of the disc space have been dissolved by the chymopapain, very little work needs to be done within the disc space itself during surgery. In fact, microsurgery dealing solely with the spinal canal pathology is the treatment of choice in these patients. Chemonucleolysis has not compromised surgical intervention in over 200 personal cases.

It is obvious that the 70% good result rate is going to be improved upon only by promptly identifying the patient with a sequestered disc. Following failed conservative treatment, the intervention of choice in this patient is microsurgery, not chemonucleolysis.

COMPLICATIONS

Anaphylaxis

Anaphylaxis occurs in 0.35% of patients who have not been pre-screened. It is manifested by a profound drop in blood pressure and requires very vigorous immediate resuscitation to save the patient's life.[20] The cornerstone of treatment for anaphylaxis is appropriate doses of epinephrine, large volumes of intravenous fluids, steroids and antihistamines.

With the use of skin testing, anaphylaxis is becoming a less frequent problem. The author has experience with 1000 cases of chymopapain injection preceded by skin testing for chymopapain sensitivity. To date, there has not been an anaphylactic reaction in a patient who has had a negative skin test. This represents unpublished data and is a combined study in Berlin, Germany, and Akron, Ohio.[24] Thus, the management of anaphylaxis has moved into the best medical realm, that of prophylaxis. Any patient with a positive skin test is eliminated from treatment with chymopapain.

Neurological complications

Chymopapain, with or without contrast material, injected into the subarachnoid space is almost certain to cause a disaster. Thus, it is extremely important that the needle tip does not cross the subarachnoid space on insertion into the nuclear

cavity. If there is any question about the needle tip crossing the subarachnoid space at the time of needle insertion, the procedure should be aborted.

The possibility of a connection between the disc space and the subarachnoid space is the one drawback to not using contrast material at the time of needle placement. It is obvious, on injecting contrast material into the disc, that when it appears in the subarachnoid space (Fig. 17.14), there is a connection between the disc cavity and the subarachnoid space. The most common cause of this connection is crossing the subarachnoid space on needle insertion. It is the author's opinion that whenever there is any degree of resistance to injection of test material into the nuclear cavity, it is highly unlikely that there is a connection between the disc space and the subarachnoid space. For this reason, it is possible to use a water acceptance test rather than contrast material at the time of chymopapain injection.

Injection of chymopapain (with or without contrast material) into the subarachnoid space may cause subarachnoid haemorrhage with cerebral complications, a cauda equina syndrome, or a delayed traverse myelitis. Recent preliminary experimental[8] work suggests that it is not chymopapain alone but rather the combination of chymopapain and contrast material in the subarachnoid space that is causing the serious neurological complications. Other research[9] would suggest that chymopapain alone is capable of causing subarachnoid haemorrhage and serious neurological complications.

Causes of subarachnoid injection

1. Direct injection. The needle tip is in the subarachnoid space at the time of injection. Appropriate X-rays should be taken to ensure that the needle tip is in the disc space and not in the subarachnoid space (Fig. 17.14).

2. Indirect injection. Indirect injection into the subarachnoid space can occur when there is a connection between the nuclear space and the subarachnoid space. This occurs in three situations:

a. The needle you are using to inject chymopapain has violated the subarachnoid space. Injected chymopapain can then leak along the outside of the needle or drip off the end of the needle on withdrawal. Therefore do not use the midline to do discolysis with chymopapain. Always be sure you are

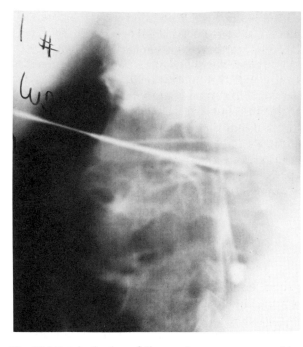

Fig. 17.14(a) At the time of discography, contrast appeared in the subarachnoid space. Abort the chemonucleolysis procedure at this stage.

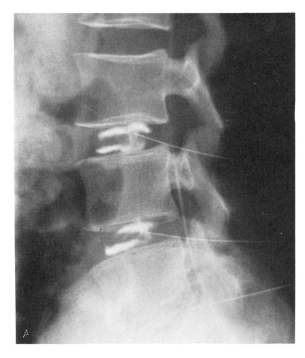

Fig. 17.14(b) At the time of discography, contrast material appeared in the epidural space. This is not a contra-indication to chemonucleolysis.

far enough away from the midline when selecting your site for needle insertion. Avoid using the stylet in your needle (except possibly to penetrate the skin).

b. A prior investigation (myelogram or midline discogram) has penetrated the dura, leaving a dural puncture that is slow to seal (multiple punctures or punctures with a large needle). Thus, chymopapain injected into a disc space that is host to an extruded or sequestered disc may leak into the epidural space and gain entry to the subarachnoid space through the unsealed dural puncture. It is advisable to wait at least 24 hours between myelography and chemonucleolysis.

c. Prior surgery has left dura scarred to the annulus, and a recurrent disc herniation, same level, same side, actually penetrates the dura. Although this is rare, it presents a slightly increased risk to a patient with previous surgery and a recurrent herniated nucleus pulposus.

Acute tranverse myelitis (ATM)

A sinister, delayed complication known as acute transverse myelitis (ATM) has occured in six North American patients following chemonucleolysis.[7] The syndrome is manifested by ascending paralysis, usually striking the mid-to-upper thoracic cord regions, occurring approximately 10–24 days after chymopapain injection. Most patients have ended up totally paralysed in a transected cord fashion. The levels have been in the watershed area of blood supply of the spinal cord (mid-to-lower thoracic).

It is too early to have complete and accurate data on these patients, but the following information has been gathered.

These patients probably have had some transgression of the subarachnoid space during the procedure as evidenced by the subarachnoid haemorrhage that has preceded ATM in some patients or the xanthochromic CSF seen at the time of presentation of ATM in other patients.

Most ATM has occurred 10–24 days after chymopapain injection, which is the time when chymopapain antibody production has reached its peak. The syndrome occurs suddenly (over a period of hours) after a period of continuing post-chemonucleolysis improvement. Initial symptoms are either a girdle-like radicular pain at the level of the cord lesion and/or radiating leg pains. Paralysis quickly follows.

One case of ATM has undergone spinal angiography which failed to reveal an artery of Adamkiewicz. That patient had a partial recovery of paralysis after administration of massive doses of steroids.[25]

Theory for ATM

The following theory is reconstructed from preliminary information. At the time of chemonucleolysis, chymopapain inadvertently enters the subarachnoid space. If the dose is large enough, immediate side-effects such as subarachnoid haemorrhage will occur. If the dose of chymopapain entering the subarachnoid space is small, it will cause no immediate damage.

The chymopapain protein is not broken down by anything in the subarachnoid space. Outside of the CSF space the serum contains alpha-2-macroglobulins which inhibit chymopapain in the general circulation. However, the level of alpha-2-macroglobulins is thought to be very low in CSF and, as a result, the chymopapain protein is not neutralized. It becomes deposited in the perivascular tissues of the spinal cord.

Chymopapain antibodies, produced at approximately 10–24 days, cross the blood–brain barrier and seek out the dormant chymopapain antigen. The resulting antigen–antibody reaction produces a vasculitis that leads to a rapidly progressive cord infarct and the syndrome of ATM.

The basic assumption of this theory is that ATM results from the technical error of placing chymopapain in the subarachnoid space and is not a complication inherent to the drug.

Treatment of ATM

The only drug available today that might alter the reaction of ATM is steroid in massive doses, administered immediately on receiving a patient early in the syndrome.

Miscellaneous complications

Two miscellaneous complications require consideration. The first is root damage from penetration of the nerve root at the time of needle insertion. This usually occurs under general anaesthesia when one is attempting to get the needle into the L5–S1 disc space.[26] Under local neuroleptic anaesthesia, this is a very rare complication. Root penetration has led to some permanent causalgic syndromes.[26]

A second complication is discitis. This is either a low-grade infective discitis or a chemical discitis that results in a prolongation of the patient's back pain and a typical X-ray picture (Fig. 17.15). It is infrequent that one has to deal with a fulminating septic discitis with systemic manifestations. When this does occur, the basic principles of management of any infective discitis apply.

FAILURES

It is possible with any surgical therapy to select a patient with non-physical disability, to make the wrong diagnosis or to do the wrong operation and end up with a poor result. This has happened, and continues to happen, with selection of patients for chymopapain injection. Assuming a very infrequent complication rate which causes failure, it becomes obvious that true failures to chymopapain injection

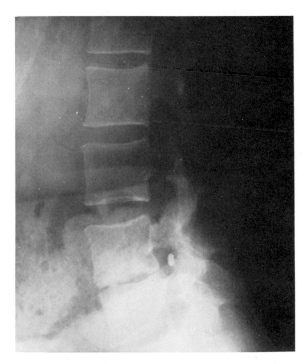

Fig. 17.15 Low-grade post-discolysis infection. Prolonged antibiotic therapy and time produced resolution.

are almost always due to pathology within the spinal canal, and almost always this pathology is an extruded or sequestered disc.

It should be possible to determine that a patient has failed to respond to chemonucleolysis at 4 to 6 weeks post-injection. Subsequent surgery is not compromised by chemonucleolysis. In fact, there is a discolysis advantage because within a number of weeks of injection of chymopapain into the disc space, the disc space narrowing offers some degree of stability. Further, there is no nuclear material left within the disc space and thus no extensive disc space dissection is needed. Finally, the absence of nuclear material within the disc space and the surgical removal of nuclear material within the spinal canal should result in an extremely low recurrence rate.[22]

CONCLUSIONS

Chemonucleolysis with chymopapain represents the least-invasive, lowest-risk, lowest cost surgical intervention for a patient with a herniated nucleus pulposus causing sciatica. In spite of the recent serious complications and deaths, there is still a wide margin of safety between chemonucleolysis and surgical intervention for disc disease (Table 17.1). In the properly selected patient, there is at least a 70% chance of a successful result.

In the author's hands, chemonucleolysis with chymopapain has been a safe, simple and effective treatment modality. The patient does not end up with an incision in his or her back. The patient is in hospital for a shorter length of time and, in some cases, a faster return to work is possible. Two long-term studies[27,28] by the author suggest that the long-term results are excellent and the recurrence rate is

extremely low. Finally, a failure to respond to chymopapain injection does not compromise any future surgical considerations.

APPENDIX

Ingredients and instructions for mixing skin test solution

Ingredients

Buffer:	Albay buffered saline and phenol diluent for allergenic extract — 4.5 ml vials
Glycerol:	99.5% — any local pharmacy should have this.
Discase®:	Manufactured by Omnis Surgical Inc. Obtain through your hospital pharmacy.
Dropper bottles:	Two (2) small (1 oz) sterile dropper bottles.

Skin test

Do not mix Discase® with sterile water as indicated by the package insert. This is only for disc injection purposes. For the skin test, use 1 cc of buffer to mix Discase® and withdraw from the vial and put into one dropper bottle. Add 1 cc of glycerol and shake. This skin test solution should set at room temperature for the first 24 hours so that the active enzymatic component is spent.

Control solution

In the second dropper bottle, combine 1 cc of glycerol and 1 cc of buffer. You now have your control solution. Both of these solutions should be refrigerated when not in use.

Test

Standard prick test — one drop of each solution on skin and prick. Positive is a wheal of 5 mm or more with a surrounding flare of 10 mm or more at the Discase® test site much greater than that of the control site. Read in 15 minutes.

Table 17.1

Complication	Surgery %	Chemonucleolysis USA %	Europe %
Mortality	0.3[29]	0.02[32]	0.0[33]
Morbidity			
Serious	0.02[29-31]	0.05[33]	0.04[33]
Anaphylaxis	0.00	0.5[32]	0.06[33]
Less serious	2.0[29, 30, 33]	0.03[32]	0.8[33]
General	2–3	Extremely low	

REFERENCES

1   Jansen E F, Balls A K 1941 Chymopapain: new crystalline proteinase from papaya latex. J. Biol. Chem. 137: 459

2   Smith L 1964 Enzyme dissolution of nucleus pulposus in humans. J.A.M.A. 187: 137

3   Schwetschenau P R, Ramirez A, Johnston J et al 1976 Double-blind evaluations of intradiscal chymopapain for herniated lumbar discs: Early results. J. Neurosurg. 45: 622

4   Fraser R D 1982 Chymopapain for the treatment of intervertebral disc herniation. Spine 7: 608

5   Javid J J, et al 1983 Safety and efficacy of chymopapain (chymodiactin) in herniated nucleus pulposus with sciatica. J.A.M.A. 249: 2489

6   Travenol Laboratories Inc: New Drug Application 18-625. (Submitted to United States Food and Drug Administration on 24 April 1981)

7   Data from post-marketing surveillance: Smith Laboratories Inc, 2211 Sanders Road, PO Box 3044, Northbrook, Illinois 60062, USA

8   Smith Laboratories Inc, 2211 Sanders Road, PO Box 3044, Northbrook, Illinois 60062, USA

9   Macnab I, et al 1971 Chemonucleolysis. Can. J. Surg. 14: 280

10 Rydevik B, et al 1976 Effects of chymopapain on nerve tissue. Spine 2: 237

11 Wiltse L L, Widell E H, Hansen A Y 1975 Chymopapain chemonucleolysis in lumbar disc disease. J.A.M.A. 231: 474

12 McCulloch J A Unpublished data

13 Wakano K, Kasman R, Chao E Y, Bradford D S, Oegema T R Jr 1983 Biochemical analysis of canine intervertebral disc after chymopapain injection: a preliminary report. Spine 8: 59

14 McCulloch J A, Dolovich G, Canham W Skin testing for chymopapain allergy: a preliminary report. Annals of Allergy. October 1985

15 Waddell G, McCulloch J A, Kummel E, et al 1980 Non-organic physical signs in low-back pain. Spine 5: 117

16 Smith Laboratories Inc, 2211 Sanders Road, PO Box 3044, Northbrook, Illinois 60062, USA

17 Product information letter (July 1984) Smith Laboratories Inc, 2211 Sanders Road, PO Box 3044, Northbrook, Illinois 60062, USA

18 Parkinson D, Shields C 1973 Treatment of protruded lumbar intervertebral discs with chymopapain. J. Neurosurg. 39: 203

19 Weiner D S, Macnab I 1970 The use of chymopapain in degenerative disc disease: a preliminary report. Can. Med. Assoc. J. 102: 1252

20 Hall B B, McCulloch J A 1983 Anaphylactic reactions following the intradiscal injection of chymopapain under local anesthesia. J. Bone Joint Surg. 65A: 1215

21 McCulloch J A 1984 Congenital anomalies of the lumbosacral spine. In: H Genant (ed) Spine Update. Radiology Research and Education Foundation, San Francisco, p 43-49

22 Kitaoka H, McCulloch J A Microdiscectomy for failed chemonucleolysis. Presented to Canadian Orthopaedic Association 40th Annual Meeting, 14 June 1984

23 McCulloch J A 1983 Outpatient discolysis with chymopapain. Orthopedics vol 6 12: 1624

24 McCulloch J A, Brock M Unpublished data

25 Whisler W Personal communication

26 Wiltse L L 1975 Chymopapain chemonucleolysis in lumbar disc disease. J.A.M.A. 233-1164

27 McCulloch J A 1981 Chemonucleolysis for relief of sciatica due to a herniated intervertebral disc. Can. Med. Assoc. J. 124: 880

28 Lorenz M, McCulloch J A 1985 Chemonucleolysis for herniated nucleus pulposus in adolescents. Presented to American Academy of Orthopaedic Surgeons, Las Vegas Submitted for publication

29 Spangfort E 1972 The lumbar disc herniation. Acta Orth. Scand. Suppl 142

30 Mayfield F H Complications of laminectomy. In: Clinical neurosurgery, ch 32

31 McLaren A C, Bailey S I 1983 Cauda equina syndrome: a complication of lumbar discectomy. Presented at the American Academy of Orthopaedic Surgeons Meeting, Atlanta

32 Morris J 1984 Complications of chemonucleolysis. Presented at Spine Update, San Francisco

33 Bouillet R 1983 Complications of discal hernia therapy, comparative study regarding surgical therapy and nucleolysis by chymopapain. Acta Orth. Belg. vol 49, suppl 1, p 48

Facet joint syndrome

INTRODUCTION

The facet joint syndrome is one of the most vague yet tantalizing aspects of low back disease. I hope to clarify the current status, but unhappily our gaps in knowledge will still leave dissatisfaction. This presentation will be divided into five sections. Background information will be provided by a survey of the historical development of facet syndrome, current understanding of the facet joint, and its neuro-anatomy will be reviewed. Clinical studies of the facet syndrome will be summarized. Finally, the author's current concept of the facet joint role in the diagnosis and treatment of low back problems will be summarized.

HISTORICAL BACKGROUND

It was Ghormley[1] in 1933 who coined the expression 'facet syndrome'. In fact, his paper pointed to the role of the facet joints in creating nerve root pressure and thus providing a source of sciatica. He did not consider referred pain. This indeed is somewhat different from our current use of the term 'facet syndrome'. Probably the first investigator to suggest facet joints as a major source of back pain and sciatica was Goldthwait.[2] Here again, current concepts are different from the hypothesis he proposed in that he observed that asymmetry of the facet articulations is a common event and he assumed that the supposed abnormal stress is the source of pain. (This has never been confirmed in that studies comparing X-rays with disability show no greater incidence of back pain and leg pain in those with than those without asymmetry of the facet joints[3].)

Other clinicians of this time also recognized the

abnormal articulations of the facet joint and suggested this non-symmetrical anatomy must be related to back pain.[4,5] Perhaps Putti[6] deserves the first credit for recognition that the degenerative process about the articular facets has an important role in back ache and sciatica. Putti's main interest was the explanation of sciatica. For years he maintained that sciatica is a neuralgia caused by a pathological condition of the intervertebral foramina and especially of the intervertebral articulations — the articular facets. Writing before the definition of the herniated intervertebral disc, he felt that idiopathic sciatica was essentially the result of vertebral arthritis involving chiefly the articular facets. He could not define the exact pathophysiology of the sciatic pain, however. Nor could he specifically pinpoint the source of disease of the apophyseal joints. He too preferred to think that the problem was related to asymmetry of articulations and the abnormal forces achieved by these congenital variations.

The first major paper to discuss the role of the articular facets in relation to low back pain and sciatica after the identification of the ruptured disc by Mixter & Barr[7] was by Carl Badgley[8] in 1941. He pointed out that in his series of low back problems 'less than 20 per cent show any neurological evidence of direct nerve irritation'. He presented two illustrative cases of individuals with sudden onset of back pain and sciatica who improved with conservative care. He too was impressed that the asymmetry of the facets was the most significant anatomical aspect contributing to their complaints, and he also pointed out that there was a correlation of arthritic changes noted pathologically and radiographically with advancing age, but he could not draw a direct correlation between these pathologic changes and back pain with sciatica. The underlying inciting cause of the pain remained mysterious.

Sources of pain implied specific innervation. Pain pathways of the lumbar spine were poorly understood. Up to the 1940s it was thought that a portion of the facet joint innervation came from a recurrent branch of the anterior-primary division. Dissections of this area by McCotter and Strong were reported by Badgley, who identified a medial branch of the posterior-primary ramus that consistently innervated the capsule and the periosteum of the joints. Based on this information, Badgley[9] suggested the hypothesis that irritation of the capsule of the lumbar facets could well produce stimuli which, through primary posterior division, could return to the central nervous system and produce referred pain through the dermatomes of the involved nerve which correspond exactly to the pathway of sciatic radiation, i.e., the 4th and 5th nerves. The failure of Badgley to pursue his ideas is reflected in a lack in the literature from the early 1940s into the 1970s of any significant paper referring to the lumbar facet joints as a cause of back pain or sciatica. However, the subject of referred pain as related to other specific anatomic sources began to be noted. The dermatome distribution of innervation was defined by Foerster.[10] Kelgren[11] noted that stimulation of connective structures such as muscle caused referral distally, not as precisely as the dermatomes. He identified these referral areas as sclerotomes.[11,12] Referred pain from skeletal structures was identified by Inman & Saunders.[13]

What seemed to be a very precise theory was thrown into some question when specific anatomical localization was attempted. Various authors found insufficient consistency between normal subjects to support the concept of a specific pattern with considerable overlap in referral location.[14,15] Not only was there confusion as to the specificity of the areas of referred pain, but also there was some doubt as to the specificity of origin of the symptoms. Steindler & Luck[16] suggested that referred pain could come from the facet joint. They injected local anaesthetic percutaneously into the joint and were able to relieve back pain. However, they did not specifically identify the anatomical structure injected other than by inference of needle location. Whether the material was inject intracapsularly or extra-capsularly could not be defined without radiographic control which was not available at that time. It was clear from these various studies, however, that pain could be perceived to be present at various locations which were remote from the anatomical source. The nerve root itself need not be stimulated to produce perception of distant pain, and various anatomical locations give similar and sometimes overlapping distributions of pain.

There seems to be a void in the literature concerning the symptomatic facet joint in the 1940s, 1950s and 1960s. All discussions related to back pain and leg pain were focused on the disc. The surgical literature discussed various approaches to the ruptured disc and perhaps consequences for the narrowed spinal canal.

Eventually interest in the facet joint as a clinically significant source of pain was rekindled by Rees of Australia.[17] He proposed the concept of surgical denervation of the facet joint by a percutaneous method which cut the intertransverse ligament with the supposed result of severing the posterior primary ramus — the nerve supply to the facet. He reported fantastic results with over 900 cures out of 1000 cases. Nonetheless, he did develop the concept that pain was arising from the facet joint and this was the cause of the lumbago and sciatica of which the patients were complaining. In spite of the potential validity of that concept, his idea of antomy was totally in error, at least by our current understanding of formal anatomical dissections. He probably achieved his successful results by the wide infiltration of the posterior structures with local anaesthetic.

Struck by the reported success of this denervation approach, Shealy, a neurosurgeon who previously had been interested in pain control by central nervous system counter-stimulation, observed the Rees technique. Failing to achieve anatomical denervation without considerable morbidity using the Rees method, he used a more discreet instrument to achieve the supposed methods of facet joint denervation. Using a standard neurosurgical tool known as a lesion maker, he created soft-tissue destruction by radio frequency thermal effect.[18] The author observed Dr Shealy's spectacular and nearly instant relief of pain in several patients using the radio frequency lesion maker. Shealy indicated that at that time, 1972, this was his method of choice for treatment of back pain and sciatica.

From the standpoint of an orthopaedic surgeon, it seemed irrational to attempt to denervate a painful joint. Historically, attempts at denervation of various other joints with painful arthropathy such as the hip and the elbow had always resulted in only short-term relief. Eventual return of pain — frequently with a greater degree of complaints — always occurred. On the other hand, minor arthropathy of various other joints of the body had been successfully relieved of pain by the injections of steroids, and therefore it seemed rational to care for the painful facet joint by a similar steroid injection directly into the assumed painful site of joint arthropathy. Based on Shealy's radiographic localization techniques, we decided to proceed with various studies focused at identifying the relationship of the lumbar facet joints to back pain and sciatica. Specifically, we decided to approach the painful facet joint as in other locations and inject local anaesthetic into the joint.[19] In normal subjects, after initial localization with arthrography, irritative solutions were injected into the joint. Both manoeuvres confirmed the lumbar facet joint as a potential source of pain of lumbago and sciatica.

ANATOMY AND BIOMECHANICS

The anatomy of the facet-joint is well described in many standard anatomical texts. Its characteristics are the same as any diarthroidal joint. The first detailed analysis of this joint was in 1969.[20] The first question to be answered regarding the clinical significance of facet joint arthropathy is the degree to which this joint can participate in the deterioration of the lumbar spine motion segment. It was very tempting for the various earlier authors to suggest that anatomical asymmetries were the 'horse' which pulled the 'cart' of degenerating motion segments. However, as suggested earlier, no radiographic study has confirmed that asymmetry leads to a greater incidence of back disease.[21] It is clear from their anatomic orientation, however, that a major function of the lumbar facet joints is the control and stabilization against torsional forces. Farfan,[22] with a series of elegant anatomical studies, has shown that the torsional forces are probably the major source of disc degeneration. However, no one has been able to identify a particular role of the facet joints in

influencing the gradual progression of this degencration first as circumferential and later radial tears.

The interrelationship between the discs and the facet joints, of course, is anatomically apparent. Excluding trauma which is of such severity that actual fracture and malalignment of the facet joints occur, it seems more likely to assume that the degeneration first occurs at the disc. To what degree the degenerating disc creates abnormal stress transfer and secondarily excessive loading on the facet joints has not been defined. One can only suspect that, because of the interrelationship, excessive loads do occur at the facet joint on the occasion of minor disruptions within the discs.

The relationships of load-bearing characteristics with alignment of the facet joints has been identified.[23] According to this study, under normal loading circumstances the facet joints apparently take about 20% of the axial load. With facetectomy on one side, the facet is free to move away and thus it takes far smaller loads, demonstrating the important role facets must take in supplying stability to the spine. As would be predicted from an anatomical analysis, with extension, the loads on the facet joints greatly increase.[24] No study is available which has analysed the stresses on the facet joint in the living individual. The role of compliance and stiffness of associated ligamentous and capsular structures is likewise unknown. Thus, at this time we truly have no scientific understanding as to the loads that the facet joints must tolerate in the living environment and the degree to which these joints are submitted to stresses with subluxation and capsular tear. When we observe the trained athlete with a fantastic range of movement in the lumbar spine, it is difficult to conceive that there might be major physiological limits to the mobility of the facet joint. On the othr hand, with the progressive stiffness of inactivity, overload certainly must be possible.

When we look to the specific anatomical aspects of the facet joint, there are several interesting concepts which should be understood. There is a relatively capacious capsule. A radiographic study using arthrography found that the facet joint without degenerative disease can take 2–3 cc of fluid before bursting.[25] The most complex issue is the relationship between facet disease and disc degeneration. In a study of 86 cadavers, Lewin[26] found that intersegmental arthritis of the facet joints occurred occasionally, independently of disc degeneration. Another study has shown that facet degeneration can precede any evidence of disc rupture. In this study the patients had a complaint of pain with no neurological deficit, and in only 20% of the subjects was a suggestion of disc herniation noted, whereas 40% showed facet joint changes.[27]

So, from a mechanical aspect we are left with the dilemma of trying to identify the role that the unstable or traumatized facet joint might have as the source of pain. In multiple dissections of the lumbar facet joints, Paris[28] noted that the facet joint capsule is a significant structure which can be lax, and indeed on manipulation can infold into the joint. The synovial lining of the joint covers the non-articular parts of the synovial joints and projects into the crevice between joints, sometimes as fat pads and sometimes as a miniscule type of structure. Adhesions can develop between the capsule and the joint itself. These adhesions have been observed directly and may be the source of limited movement range of the facet joint.

One of the difficulties in understanding the relationship of noxious stimuli coming from the stressed anatomical structures of the facet joint versus its relationship to nerve root irritation resides in the very 'tight' anatomy of this region. In the illustration from Rauschning (Fig. 18.1), we can see all the structures well outlined. We note in addition the very close approximation of the neural structures to the superior articular facet of the motion segment. No one has yet identified the degree to which mechanical irritation of this neurological structure is a source of pain rather than noxious stimuli arising from overstressed connective tissue structures related to the joint such as its synovium and capsule. All these points await further definition.

NEURO-ANATOMY — FACET-JOINT PAIN

Gross anatomical innervation

The neuro-anatomy of facet joints can be considered at two levels. First is the gross anatomical innervation which has been described by various dissectors and most recently in the most comprehensive description by Paris.[28] Results of his dissections are displayed (Figs 18.2(a), 18.2(b)) and described below.

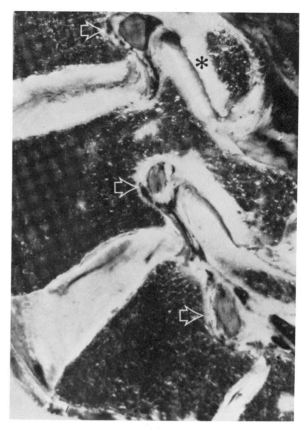

Fig. 18.1 The relationship between neural structures and the facet joint capsule is clearly illustrated in these anatomical specimens from Rauschning.[29] The arrows point to the neural structures; the asterisk identifies the facet joint. The capsule is in very close relationship to the nerve.

The features of innervation which are pertinent to a discussion of the facet syndrome are, first of all, the profuse innervation of the posterior articular structures, and, second, the anatomical juxtaposition of the nerve root and spinal ganglion to the facet joint and its capsule, and especially the highly innervated ligamentum flavum.

The profuse and in particular overlapping nature of the innervation is especially important when the question of potential for denervation is considered. A particular feature of the dissections of Stanley Paris is the definition of an ascending branch of the posterior primary ramus. It is found at all lumbar levels of L1 through L5, where it leaves the medial branch of the posterior primary just prior to passing through the foramen bounded laterally by the intertransverse ligament. This ascending branch is

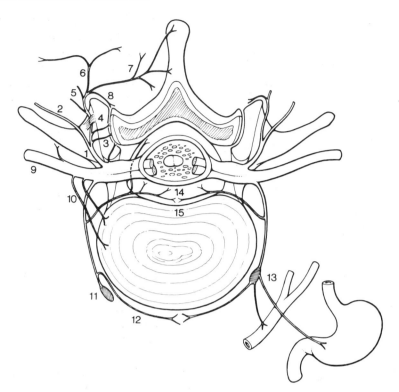

Fig.18.2(a) Neuro-anatomical definition of the lumbar motion segment (redrawn from Paris[28])

1. Posterior primary rami
2. Lateral branch of the posterior primary rami to skin and muscles
3. Muscular branches to multifidus and to facet capsule
4. Medial branch posterior primary rami
5. Branch to the posterior sacroiliac joint
6. Muscular and cutaneous branches
7. Muscular and ligamentous branches — large to multifidus
8. Local branch to facet
9. Anterior primary rami
10. Branches to the disc from the anterior primary rami
11. Sympathetic chain
12. Recurrent grey rami communicans
13. Branches to blood vessels and viscera
14. Branches to dura
15. Branches to posterior longitudinal ligament

well clear of the transverse process as it ascends to the facet above. Thus, in standard manoeuvres to denervate the joint, related to sites associated with the transverse process, it would be quite possible for this nerve not to be damaged. Even the S1 branch gives an ascending branch leaving the neuroforamen of the first sacral segment. Thus, for the denervation of one segment, three levels of destruction would be necessary. This overlapping denervation has been confirmed by other authors.[30]

A constant branch of the posterior primary ramus is the medial branch, which comes to lie on the posterior superior and medial aspect of the transverse process, fitting snugly against the root of the superior articular process. It passes dorsally and

caudally into the deep groove formed between the mammalary process of the superior articular process and adjacent accessory process to the transverse process. There is a fibrous ligament which may be cartilaginous and on occasions even ossified to form a bony foramen for the passage of the nerve at the superior portion of the transverse process as it joins the body. Once the nerve emerges from beneath the ligament, it sends off muscular branches to the multifidus ligamentous branches to the inter- and superspinous ligaments, a small articular branch to the adjacent facet and a somewhat larger articular branch to the superior aspect of the facet capsule below. On occasions there may be several articular descending branches from the medial branch of the

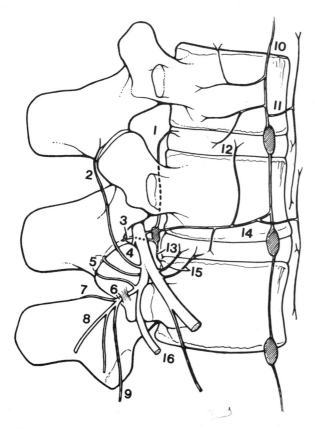

Fig. 18.2(b) Neuro-anatomical definition of the lumbar motion segment (redrawn from Paris[28])

1. Ascending branch of sinuvertebral nerve
2. Ascending facet branch
3. Sinuvertebral to facet
4. Direct branch to facet
5. Branches to multifidus
6. Medial branch of posterior primary ramus
7. Local facet branch
8. Descending facet branch
9. Branch to sacroiliac
10. Sympathetic chain
11. Branch under anterior longitudinal ligament
12. Branches from grey ramus to disc
13. Sinuvertebral to disc
14. Grey ramus communicans
15. Branches from anterior primary ramus to disc
16. Lateral branch of posterior primary ramus

posterior primary ramus. This is diagrammatically displayed in Figure 18.2(a).

Figure 18.2(b) demonstrates the somewhat selective nature of facet joint innervation, contrasted to spinal canal innervation. Clearly, a branch emerges from the anterior primary ramus to innervate the spinal canal and dura. This is a recurrent branch which returns to the spinal canal from the neuro-

foramen and thus could be embarrassed by stenotic events. On the other hand, only the posterior primary branch innervates the facet joint, in the overlapping manner described above. It is clearly understandable why, with at least three different neurological segments innervating the structure, a very blurred pain pattern arises from noxious stimuli emerging from this joint.

Microscopic anatomy

The second aspect of the examination of the source of pain is the microscopic anatomy. Referred pain must be based on irritation of innervated structures. One major investigation into this area was by Hirsch et al in 1963.[31] In this study, using methylene blue, nerve endings in the joint capsular structures of the lumbar facet were identified as similar to those of the annulus of the lumbar disc. In this study also, 11% hypertonic saline injection was used to evaluate the pain sources in normal volunteers comparing the lumbar discs with the intervertebral facet joints. These authors' studies seemed to indicate that the disc is the more sensitive of the two areas, but indeed the vertebral facet joints could be a source of pain which was referred to the buttock and thigh. The posterior ligamentous structures which were also injected with hypertonic irritant solution did not produce evidence of lumbago.

A similar study, focused specifically on the facet joints, was undertaken more recently.[19] Under 3 cc of hypertonic saline were injected into the facet joint, once the needle location had been defined by an arthrogram. After several seconds, the pain was located in the low back region, lateral thigh area and in some patients even down the lateral calf. Another aspect of the study was that those patients and volunteers who had slightly larger amounts of injections seemed to have greater pain distribution. In none of these studies was the pain resulting from the injection of irritant solution into the facet joint associated with a neurological deficit such as sensory loss or motor weakness. Neither was there a clear definition of the pattern of pain referral. L3 facet joint injections usually caused pain referral slightly more lateral on the leg.

More recent studies from Oswestry,[32] have shown that provocation studies at the L1-2 level and at the L4-5 level demonstrate a significant overlap of pain referral, but the more caudal location generally creates more caudal pain. Probably the most significant aspect of this study on normal volunteers was the demonstration that injection intracapsularly versus pericapsularly caused very similar areas of pain referral. In an effort by the same institution[33] to clarify the issue from another angle, a group of patients who had back pain for no more than three months were injected at the site of greatest tenderness under radiographic control. Those who responded seemed to have a wider spinal canal, which suggested that disc irritation of the nerve root was not a factor. No other characteristic could separate these two groups. Thus, once again, it was difficult to differentiate those patients whose pain arose from the facet joints and those who had it from some other anatomical location. In none of these studies did the pain referral caused by injection of irritant solution cross the midline, nor did pain relief from one anatomical site injected with one local anaesthetic cross the midline.

None of these studies is truly definitive; they are only suggestive. It seems likely that pain may arise from the facet joint in that there is clearly profuse innervation of this site. The site can be irritated by appropriate agents such as chemical irritants. Pain can be relieved in some patients who have pain which seems to be arising from this location. Unhappily, in all of these settings, there is a significant number of non-responders, which suggests that there are likely to be other sources of painful stimuli to explain the syndrome of lumbago and sciatica.

CLINICAL STUDIES

This will be a survey of current clinical studies which demonstrate various results from treatment of the lumbar facet joint. None of the studies is satisfactory in that disease entity itself is so poorly defined. Subjective pain complaints are basically the only criteria for diagnosis, and pain relief is the only criterion for success. Until more objective measurements of function and disability become available, unhappily this will remain the index of success or failure. In addition, problems of analysis exist because each author has varying criteria for success or failure based on pain complaints. Thus, one can only get a most general view of efficacy.

Denervation

There are two basic techniques for treating the facet joints — denervation and desensitization by local anaesthetic/steroids. The method with the longest history is denervation, as initiated by Shealy. In 1973 Shealy[34] made his initial presentation of a large series of cases. He reported good and excellent results in 80% of patients with no previous surgery. However, in those who had previous surgery, only a 40% success rate was obtained. Since that time other investigative authors have reported their results, with roughly similar findings. A large series by Oudenhoven[35] of 801 facet rhizotomies showed that, at 6 months follow-up, 80% of virgin backs had a good result, but again only about 57% of surgical backs were doing well. However, when the patients were followed for a longer period, the success rate gradually deteriorated, so that eventually only about 68% of the virgin backs and 35% of the post-surgical backs seemed to be doing well.[35] It is interesting to note also that in Oudenhoven's reports he specifically tested for denervation of the paraspinal musculature by e.m.g. to demonstrate that the procedure had been technically well done. This, of course, is appropriate on an anatomical basis in that the posterior primary ramus not only innervates the facet capsules but supplies motor innervation to the extensor musculature. On the other hand, it leaves one with some concern about a procedure which is destructive not only of the sensory aspects of the motion segment but the motor aspect as well.

Some authors have tried to be more specific in their estimate of success and failure. One report[36] indicated that 41% were successfully treated when the criterion for success was a 50% reduction in pain and an activity level twice the pre-operative level (a fairly harsh standard for painful back syndromes). In this series the authors admitted that pain gradually returned, but were pleased to report that high activity level and lower narcotic use persisted.

It is interesting to note that very few reports of this type of care are now presented at meetings and in the literature. Dr Shealy himself has, in general, given up the procedure.[37]

There are alternative ways to denervate the articular nerve, and these have been explored as well. Injection of phenol into the nerve has been advocated in an effort to create less destruction to surrounding tissue than was the case with radio frequency. A report of this procedure on patients who had already been successfully treated by facet joint injection with steroids demonstrated a 70% success rate in virgin backs at 6 months follow-up.[38] Due to the deterioration of success, however, as the patients were followed for longer periods, the procedure has been given up by the authors.

Another way to achieve denervation is the use of a cryoprobe method of tissue destruction. It was anticipated that this method would cause less destruction than the radio frequency probe and thus return of pain secondary to scarring would be less likely to occur. As in all the earlier reports, the short-term results were good and the long-term results have not been presented.[39] In none of these studies has the patient apparently been made worse. There have been no reports of neurological deficits created by any of these methods. The burden rests on the question of whether this minor destructive treatment can affect the course of disease.

Desensitization

An alternative therapeutic approach is, of course, to expect that the source of the pain is arthropathy of the facet joint itself, and therefore anti-inflammatory medication should have a positive effect. In the initial series using this approach,[19] 62 patients out of 100 patients with non-specific back and leg pain had relief of pain. At 6 months follow-up, 20 of the initial 62 felt that they still maintained complete relief of pain; however, half of the patients who had initial success still required pain medication to control their disability. Again, the method of selection of the ideal candidate remained vague. The patient was considered appropriate if he had low back or leg pain for over 3 months and no neurologic deficits. In this series, all three lower segments were injected on the painful side because our studies suggested that it was impossible to differentiate the painful segment at one level alone based on patient complaints.

More precise studies have been reported. A French study[40] took the view that interarticular injection of steroids should be accomplished without local anaesthetic so that the anti-inflammatory effect could be the only therapeutic event. They pointed out that flow of local anaesthetic through the surrounding soft tissues may confound the perception of results if this is injected at the time of steroids. Using this method in one group, about 80% of those with sciatica but no neurological deficit improved for at least three days, while about 70% improved if there was back pain only. The authors were using this approach chiefly to evaluate further methods of care. It was thus considered a specific diagnostic study.

Two recent studies have looked at the therapeutic potential of facet joint injections. A very precise study of 223 consecutive patients was reported by Jackson & Craven.[41] Their study group included 80 private and 118 Workman's Compensation cases who had low back pain and sciatica averaging 24 weeks. Choice of the site to be injected was defined as those with tenderness overlying the facet joint. For ideal patients, i.e., more normal psychological status as identified by pain drawings and private pay financial arrangements, the pain relief was as high as 67%. Pain relief deteriorated, however, if other factors such as Workman's Compensation and excessive psychological overlay were demonstrated. The study was important in that it showed that prior success with manipulation and pain on hyperextension were not good predictors for success of facet injection.

Another study was presented by Shroeder.[39] In this study, overall 56% of the patients had improvement when their facet joints were injected with local anaesthetic and steroids. Only 26%, however, had continued improvement. The results were better in those who had had no previous surgery and with shorter pain histories. A good prognostic sign was the production of the patient's pain by stimulation of the anatomical site to be injected. As had been demonstrated by previous studies, radicular patterns did not result from the stimulation but rather the vague sensation of pain in the buttock and thigh. It was diffuse and somewhat delayed in its definition. It seldom went below the knee.

Thus, to summarize these clinical studies, a high success rate could not be anticipated and perhaps only 20% of the patients had persistent relief of pain complaints. The results of this treatment programme are certainly no better than a multitude of other methodologies used to relieve back and leg pain. Thus, what is its current role?

CURRENT STATUS OF FACET SYNDROME

After this review of the historical developments, current understanding of neuro-anantomy and various clinical reports, it is apparent that we still do not know exactly what is meant by the facet syndrome. In the Jackson series,[41] two parameters which intuitively we would have felt to be significant proved not to be so. Tende— ss overlying the facet joints in hyperextension did not provide a good prognostic indicator of facet disease. Even though from a neuro-anatomical standpoint there is no question that noxious stimuli can arise from derangement of this joint, to what degree is this clinically significant as a source of back pain? The clinical studies suggest that the more definite the degenerative changes noted in facet joints radiographically, the more likely a response from injection can be obtained. The French study[40] clearly indicated that it is not just the local anaesthetic which can relieve the pain, but apparently the true anti-inflammatory effect of the steroids is of benefit. Again, unfortunately we do not know specifically what is accomplished when we inject steroids into a synovial space. The studies from Oswestry[32] do support the view that noxious stimuli arising from the capsule are as significant as intra-articular stimuli in that the authors found no difference in efficacy, whether the injection was intra-articular or merely at the capsule.

The whole concept of denervation as achieved by rhizotomy seems to reinforce the view that back pain and sciatica can arise from these articular structures. If the sciatica were due to irritation of the anterior primary ramus in the neuroforamen, denervation of the facet joint should not be effective in reducing this mechanical irritation, if the irritation is on a structural basis, as would be suggested by the anatomy so vividly displayed in the figures from Rauschning.[29] The failure for the pain relief to be persistent following facet-joint rhizotomy again reinforces the concept that it is a source of back pain which once again will return with re-innervation and the assumption that no basic change has occurred in the deranged mechanics of this joint which was the source of pain to start with.

Probably the most tantalizing problem regarding facet-joint pain is its relationship to pain arising from the disc. We must assume that this pain is derived from noxious stimuli due to the innervation of the annulus and the posterior longitudinal ligament which arrives at the dorsal root ganglion by the recurrent nerve. Theoretically, the cells innervating the facet joints are in juxtaposition to the cells innervating the spinal canal and destabilization of the membrane potentials of either one could affect the other. Therefore, stimuli arising from the facet joint in general should be perceived as only one of several sources of pain. Alternative sources are impacting at the dorsal root ganglion. Perhaps it is the reduction of noxious stimuli below a critical level which is the source of pain relief observed following facet joint injection. At present, this concept remains totally theoretical.

At a clinical level, however, it seems clear that stimuli from the deranged facet joint can affect the neurological status of the individual. We have demonstrated in several patients that, following radiographically controlled facet injection, a depressed ankle jerk returns to normal. We have also observed improvement in muscle strength and change in subjective statement of dysaesthesia in the leg and foot following radiographically controlled facet injections at either L4-5 or L5, S1. We have never observed an absent ankle jerk return; significant motor weakness or atrophy has never resolved. Nerve root tension signs have never recovered, and objective dermatome sensory changes have never resolved. Thus, from the clinician's view, it seems that noxious stimuli arising from the facet joint can have an inhibitory effect on the neurological function at a segmental level. There has never been an effect on definite neurological signs, however.

Thus, what is the role of facet-joint injections in current clinical practice? From my standpoint they serve two significant functions: a diagnostic tool, and a mechanism to buy time. The more significant role is that of a diagnostic tool.

Technique for facet injection

The technique for facet injection is quite simple, but does require a fluoroscopy unit for needle localization. It is possible, of course, to make an assumption as to the location of the needle purely on 'feel' of the needle to the bony relationships of the spine — but one is never certain exactly where the medication might be injected without radiographic localization. Thus, my own technique is as follows:

The patient is brought to the radiology suite without pre-medication. The patient is requested to lie prone on the fluoroscopy table and prepared in the usual manner. Local anaesthetic is injected in the subcutaneous area, approximately 2-3 cm lateral to the midline over the presumed length of the injections, depending upon the number anticipated. In our experience, the pain does not cross the midline and therefore, if unilateral pain is to be treated, only that side will be injected. We hope that for diagnostic purposes the least number of segments can be injected. Sometimes this is not possible due to a lack of definable clues as to the abnormal segment. At a site 2–3 cm lateral to the spinous process of the appropriate vertebra, a disposable 20 gauge spinal needle is inserted perpendicularly. The patient is then rotated into the oblique position, with the involved side superior. This oblique position brings the obliquely-oriented facet joints into profile. Frequently some adjustment in the degree of obliqueness is required to account for the natural variation. This is easily accomplished by rolling the patient's pelvis more or less to the side-lying position. Forty-five degrees is usually an appropriate starting point.

The needle is passed down till the bone is struck. Once the skin has been anaesthetized, this is generally not uncomfortable. In my experience the patient pain response when the facet joint is struck has not been a good predictor as to the efficacy of the injection. At this point, the position of the needle is viewed on the fluoroscopy screen and adjusted. Figure 18.3 demonstrates the usefulness of the vertical approach contrasted to an oblique approach of the needles. The needle at the L3-4 level was inserted more lateral and at about 45° obliqueness. This does approach the parallel joint surfaces from a more physiological angle, but the potential for obliteration of radiographic features is evident. The needles at the L4-5 and L5, S-1 levels show appropriate localization at the facet joint without the potential for obliteration of skeletal detail due to the overlying needle. Also, for obese patients, one can use a shorter needle if the joint is approached perpendicular to the posterior facet capsule. Usually, one can 'feel' perforation of the capsule and entry into the joint. This is especially the case in the

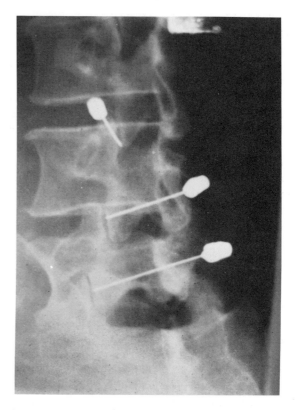

Fig. 18.3 A three-level facet-joint injection was accomplished in this subject. No clinical criterion was available to identify which of the potential levels was the source of pain. Needles were passed oblique to the joint, but perpendicular to the spine, L4-5 and L-5, S-1, or directly into the joint as at L3-4. The potential for overlying metallic obliteration of detail is noted at the L3-4 level.

younger individual without significant degenerative changes. In fact, in the aged individual with significant degenerative changes, it may be impossible to localize the needle within the joint itself.

Figure 18.3 represents the 'shotgun' approach to facet joint injection. From previous work we recognize that there is a significant overlap in pain complaint from each of the segmental levels. Therefore, when a patient is complaining of back, buttock and leg pain, any one of the three lower lumbar levels statistically could be a source of pain. If one is only trying to identify whether segmental dysfunction is the source of the pain — and there are no physical findings to point to any specific level — then all three levels must be injected as is seen in this figure. This is not ideal. Unhappily, currently there are no specific findings which point to the painful

source in the largest group of back pain patients —
those with no neurological deficits and without
significant radiographic findings.

One can be more specific in the injection, as is
indicated in Figure 18.4. Here, the L4-5 level was
injected in a 45-year-old female with chronic back
pain for 5 years unresolved by various medications
and physical therapy. There were no specific
radiographic findings, but at a statistical level L4-5
was thought to be the most likely painful segment.
This was indeed confirmed in this individual, who
achieved 10 month's relief with this injection. She
returned on a later occasion to be injected once more
at that level and remains pain-free to the present
time.

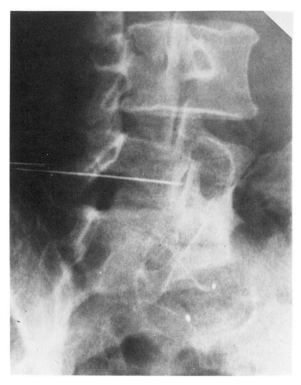

Fig. 18.5 The L4-5 level alone was injected in this individual
at the potentially symptomatic segment which is also
represented by degenerative changes radiographically. L-5, S-1
injection achieved significant long-term relief in this
individual.

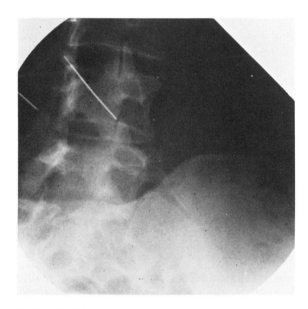

Fig. 18.4 L4-5 level has been injected bilaterally in this case.
Pain relief over a prolonged period suggests this is the
symptomatic mobile segment.

When there are degenerative changes, fewer
injections can be accomplished. Figure 18.5 demonstrates early reactive changes at the L-5, S-1 level.
These are extremely minor. Whether they are
symptomatic remains uncertain until the occasion of
the injection. Certainly, degenerative changes of the
lumbar spine are frequent and often not associated
with back pain, or perhaps the painful segment is at
L4-5 not L5-1, due to progressive stiffening at the
L4-5 level. These questions can be answered by the
injection. In this particular individual, who was a 45-

year-old truck driver, following the injection pain
relief did occur which had remained persistent until
then.

The ideal application of radiographically-
controlled facet-joint injections is in a setting where
there are significant radiographic changes and
consideration about further therapeutic procedures
is necessary. Figure 18.6 demonstrates significant
changes at the L2-3 level in a 30-year-old female who
had a past history of significant trauma in her youth.
She had become progressively more disabled and
could not carry out housework activities. Was her
back pain related to this injury? Facet-joint injection
was accomplished bilaterally, which gave her significant relief for 2 months. Following this, the pain
returned in spite of bracing and appropriate physical
therapy, and the pain could not be relieved.
Eventually she proceeded to have an interbody
fusion at that level with good long-term relief of
pain. Thus, these are examples of the potential of the

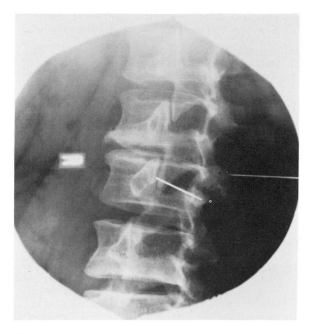

Fig. 18.6 The L2-3 level is injected bilaterally in a 30-year-old female with persistent back pain following trauma. Successful relief of pain after these injections led eventually to a successful lumbar fusion.

technique to provide specific localization of the problem and to give relief.

Unhappily, the pain is seldom relieved indefinitely. This is not surprising, in that we are treating a chronic degenerative disease for which there is no greater potential for cure than is for greying hair and wrinkles. The problems described reflect our experience in which significant relief of pain can be achieved immediately in those with persistent pain for many months. This allows them to proceed with more natural activities.

Once pain relief has been achieved, progress to physical therapy exercise programmes is organized. At this time we are uncertain as to the best type of exercise programme. Nonetheless, it seems reasonable to expect that a joint able to pass through a greater range of movement and associated with smoother motion would be a less likely source of noxious stimuli than a stiff joint surrounded by weakened stiff soft tissues. Thus, if a specific manoeuvre can improve the function of the lumbar area to allow progress into more physiological activities, there seems potential that this might benefit the patient.

SUMMARY

This discussion I have developed the concept that the lumbar facet joints can be a source of pain. This pain can be relieved specifically by radiographically controlled injection of local anaesthetic, and the persistence of pain relief is coincidental with the use of steroids. We do not have a clear predictor to identify patients whose pain complaints arise mostly from the facet joints contrasted to other potential sources. Clinical medicine awaits differentiation of the lumbar syndrome into the category in which dysfunction of the facet joints can be identified as the principal problem versus dysfunction of the disc itself. Injection of the facet joint itself, however, is a valuable tool for a diagnosis and short-term symptomatic relief. I personally continue to use it and find it a very helpful adjunct to clinical care. Once better definition of the lumbar syndrome is available, its predictive use in rational therapeutics can be more clearly outlined.

REFERENCES

1   Ghormley R K 1983 Low back pain with special reference to the articular facets, with presentation of an operative procedure. J. A. Med. A. C.I., 1773
2   Goldthwait J E 1911 The lumbosacral articulation. An explanation of many cases of 'lumbago, sciatica and paraplegic'. Boston Med. Surg. J. 164: 356–372
3   LaRocca H, MacNab I 1969 Value of pre-employment radiographic assessment of the lumbar spine. Canad. Med. Assoc. J. 101: 383
4   von Lackum H L 1924 The lumbosacral region, an anatomic study and some clinical observations. J. Am. Med. Assoc. LXXXII: 1109

5   Danforth M S, Wilson P D 1925 The anatomy of the lumbosacral region in relation to sciatic pain. J.B.J.S., E11: 109
6   Putti V New conceptions in the pathogenesis of sciatic pain. Lancet 2: 53–60
7   Mixter W J, Barr J S 1934 Rupture of the intervertebral disc with involvement of the spinal canal. New Eng. J. Med. 211: 210
8   Badgley C E 1941 The articular facets in relationship to low back pain and sciatic radiation. J. Bone Joint Surg. 23A: 481–496
9   Badgley C E 1936 A new theory to explain radiation of

pain. Read before the annual meeting of the American Academy of Orthopedic Surgeons, St Louis, 14 January 1936, but never published

10 Foerster 1933 The dermatomes in man. Brain 56: 1–39

11 Kelgren J J 1938 Observation on referred pain arising from muscle. Clin. Sci. Mol. Med. 3: 175–190

12 Kelgren J H 1939 On the distribution of pain arising from deep sematic structures with charts of segmental pain areas. Clin. Sci. Mol. Med. 4: 35–46

13 Inman V T, Saunders J B 1944 Referred pain from skeletal structures. J. Nerv. Ment. Dis. 99: 660–667

14 Sinclaire D C, Feindel W H, Weddell G, Falconer M A 1948 The intervertebral ligaments as a source of segmental pain. J.B.J.S. 30B: 515–521

15 Hockaday J M, Whitty C W N 1967 Patterns of referred pain in the normal subject. Brain 90: 481–496

16 Steindler A, Luck J V 1938 Differential diagnosis of pain in the low back: allocation of the source of pain by procaine hydrochloride method. JAMA 110: 106–113

17 Rees W E S 1971 Multiple bilateral subcutaneous rhizolysis of segmental nerves in the treatment of the intervertebral disc syndrome. Ann. Gen. Practice 26: 126–127

18 Shealy C N 1975 Percutaneous radiofrequency denervation of spinal facets and treatment for chronic back pain and sciatica. J. Neurosurg. 43: 448–451

19 Mooney V, Robertson J 1976 The facet syndrome. Clin. Orth. 115: 149–156

20 Lewin T, Moffett B, Viidik A 1969 The morphology of the lumbar synovial intervertebral joints. Acta Morph. Neur. Scand. 4: 299–319

21 Horal J 1969 The clinical appearance of low back disorders in the city of Gothenburg, Sweden. Acta Orth. Scand. Suppl. 118

22 Farfan H F 1973 Mechanical disorders of the low back. Lea & Febiger, Philadelphia

23 Lorenz M, Patawardhan A, VanDerby R 1983 Load bearing characteristics of lumbar facets in normal and surgically altered spinal segments. Spine 8: 122–130

24 Tencer A F, Ahmed A M, Burke D L 1982 Some static mechanic properties of the lumbar intervertebral joint, intact and injured. J. Biomech. Eng. 184: 193–201

25 Dory M A 1981 Arthrography of the lumbar facet joints. Radiology 140: 23–27

26 Lewin T 1964 Osteoarthritis of the lumbar synovial joints: a morphologic study. Acta Orth. Scand. Suppl 73: 6–112

27 Carrera G F, Williams A L, Waughton V M 1980 Computed tomography in sciatica. Radiology 137: 433–437

28 Paris S B 1983 Functional anatomy of the lumbar spine. PhD thesis, University of Atlanta

29 Rauschning W 1983 Computed tomography and cryomicrometry of lumbar spine specimens (a new technique of multi-planer anatomic correlation). Spine 8: 170–180

30 Stillwell D L 1956 Nerve supply of vertebral column. Anat. Rec. 125: 139–142

31 Hirsch C, Ingelmark V E, Miller N 1963 The anatomic basis for low back pain: studies on the presence of sensory endings in ligamentous capsular and intervertebral disc structures in the human lumbar spine. Acta Orth. Scand. 33: 1–17

32 McCall E W, Park W M, O'Brien J P 1979 Induced pain referral from posterior lumbar elements in normal subjects. Spine 4: 441–446

33 Fairbank J C T, Park W M, McCall I W, O'Brien J P 1981 Apophyseal injection of local anesthetic as a diagnostic aid in primary low back syndromes. Spine 6: 598–605

34 Shealy C N, Prieto A, Burton C V, Long D N 1973 Articular nerve of Luschka rhizotomy for the relief of back and leg pain. Presented at the Annual Meeting of the American Association of Neurologic Surgeons, Los Angeles

35 Oudenhoven R C 1981 Results of facet denervation. Presented at the International Society of the Study of the Lumbar Spine, Paris

36 Igneizi R J, Cummings T W 1980 A statistical analysis of percutaneous radiofrequency lesions in the treatment of chronic low back pain and sciatica. Pain 8: 181–187

37 Shealy C N Personal communication

38 Mooney V, Selby D 1981 Phenyl injection into the facet articular nerve. Abs. Intern. Soc. Study Lumbar Spine, Gothenburg

39 Shroeder W F 1984 The facet syndrome: diagnosis and treatment. Exhibit presented at the American Academy of Orthopedic Surgeons, Atlanta

40 Theron J, Blais M, Casaco A, Courteoux P, Adam Y, Derlon JN, Houteville J P 1983 Lumbar spine: therapeutic radiology. J. Neurorad. 10: 223–230

41 Jackson R P, Craven S D 1984 Facet joint injections in mechanical low back pain: a prospective statistical study. Abst. Intern. Soc. Study Lumbar Spine

Spinal stenosis in the central and root canal

We use the term spinal stenosis to define any symptomatic condition where the limitation of space within the vertebral canal is a significant factor. There are many clinical syndromes encompassed by the term 'spinal stenosis', the variable presentation depending on the site of compromise within the vertebral canal, the age of the patient and factors other than the canal's size and configuration. We shall consider first the normal variations in the vertebral canal, and then two clearly defined clinical syndromes where space is significant.

THE VERTEBRAL CANAL

The anatomy of the vertebral canal

The term 'vertebral canal' refers to a highly complex anatomical space posterior to the vertebral bodies and discs, within the neural arch, which widens and narrows at each vertebral level in both coronal and sagittal planes. There is not only regional variation at each vertebral level, but also considerable individual variation within a population.

The vertebral canal is arbitrarily divided into the central canal and the root canal (Fig. 19.1). At the pedicular level the central canal is bounded laterally by the two pedicles, anteriorly by the posterior surface of the vertebral body, and posteriorly by the cranial aspect of the laminae and the medial aspect of the superior apophyseal joints. Between each pedicular level the central canal has an artificial boundary. It extends from one pedicular level to the next, and contains the cauda equina within the dural envelope.

The root canal is that space lateral to the central canal, in the intervertebral region between pedicular levels. Anteriorly it is bounded by the posterior surface of the vertebral body above, the posterolateral aspect of the disc, and the posterior surface of the vertebral body below. Superiorly it is bounded by the pedicle of the vertebra below. Its posterior relations are the lateral aspect of the lamina, and the superior articulation of the apophyseal joint of the vertebra below. Medially it

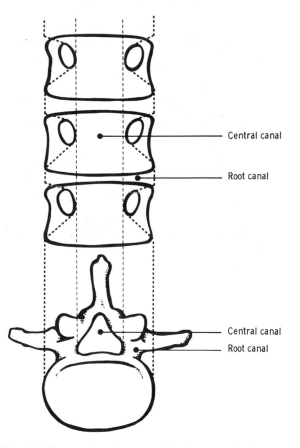

Fig. 19.1 The central and root canals in the coronal and transverse planes

opens into the central canal, and laterally it ends at the intervertebral foramen.

The lateral recess is that lateral part of the central vertebral canal at the pedicular level, anterior to the medial aspect of the superior apophyseal facet.[1] It is only trefoil-shaped canals that have a lateral recess, because dome-shaped canals have a continuous concave posterior surface to the canal with no lateral recess at all. The root canal has been loosely but inaccurately called the lateral recess.

In the sagittal plane the central canal pursues a serpentine course (Fig. 19.2). It is indented posteriorly by the cranial aspect of each lamina, and anteriorly by each intervertebral disc. In the coronal plane the vertebral canal is narrowest at each pedicular level, widening into each root canal and narrowing again at the next pedicular level.

The general dimensions of the vertebral canal tend to follow a constant pattern from the first to the fifth lumbar levels.[2] In the mid-sagittal plane at the pedicular level, it is generally widest at L1, reducing to L4 and widening again at L5. In the coronal plane, the interpedicular diameter measurements are fairly constant from L1 to L3, widening a little at L4 and then considerably at L5. The total cross-sectional area at the pedicular levels reduces from L1 to L4 and then increases again at L5 to an area equal or even greater than at L1. Measurements from 241 spines are shown in Figure 19.3. Eisenstein,[3] measuring the mid-sagittal diameter of Caucasoid and Negro spines, found similar absolute measurements with a slight racial difference. The racial variation may have some significance when we are considering the incidence of back pain syndromes.

The range of measurements in any population is greater at L5 than at other levels, with more variability in both size and shape of the canal. Eisenstein[4] described that 14% of canals trefoil at L5. The trefoil configuration is a relative term caused by posterolateral indentation of the neural arch. The canal of many spines changes to a trefoil shape from L2 to L5.

One would expect the cross-sectional area of the canal to decrease caudally, as there is a gradual reduction in the volume of the neural contents. As first sight, the increased cross-sectional area at L5 (Fig. 19.3(c)) may seem surprising, until we consider the trefoil shape of the canal. A larger cross-sectional area will be advantageous when the surface area of the canal increases and, in addition, the lordotic curve, most marked at L5/S1, places some vulnerability on the neural elements unless the cross-sectional area is increased.

Unfortunately the trefoil-shaped canal is unhealthy if that spine is affected by pathological change. Not only are the L5 nerve roots at risk from encroachment of disc or osteophytes into the lateral recess, but the cross-sectional area of trefoil canals is generally less than for non-trefoil canals, and the mid-sagittal diameter is often reduced.[3]

We know little about the cause of the trefoil-shaped canal. It is not influenced by the angle of the apophyseal facets. nor by the degree of degenerative change. Baddeley[5] noted a relationship between the trefoil shape and a vertebra in which the pedicle height was small and the apophyseal joints close together. We found a correlation of 0.35 ($p < 0.05$)[2] but though of interest, this is not sufficient to predict

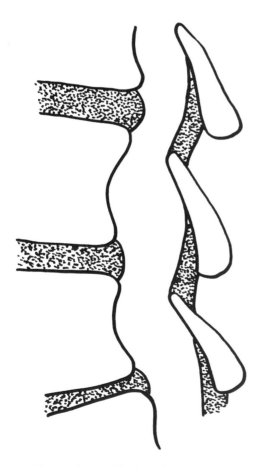

Fig. 19.2 The vertebra canal in the sagittal plane

MID-SAGITTAL (mm)

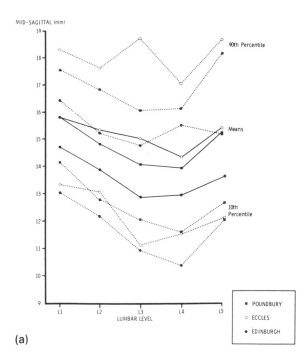

(a)

INTER-PEDICULAR (mm)

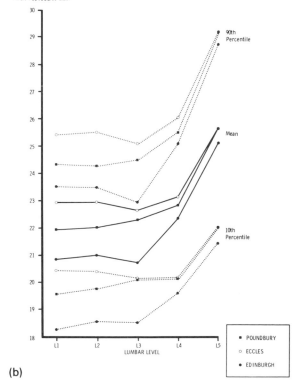

(b)

AREA (cm²)

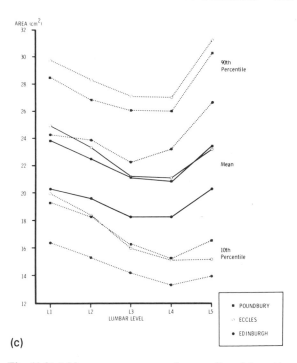

(c)

Fig. 19.3(a) Mean measurements and percentiles of the mid-sagittal diameter of the vertebral canal from 119 Romano-British skeletons from Poundbury, 61 Anglo-Saxon skeletons from Eccles, and an Edinburgh collection of 61 contemporary skeletons from the Indian sub-continent. (b) Measurements of the inter-pedicular diameters of the three populations. (c) Measurements of the cross sectional area of the vertebral canal in the three populations.

the trefoil shape from a radiograph. There is a better correlation of 0.5 ($p < 0.05$) between the trefoil shape and the degree of wedging of the vertebral body at L5. It cannot be assumed from a radiograph that a spine with an acute lumbosacral angle has a trefoil canal, but it does suggest that lumbar lordosis is a factor in the development of the trefoil shape.

The trefoil shape is uncommon in children under 10 years of age, and when it does develop it becomes apparent in the mid-teens. If a pliable triangular tube is gradually bent, it will develop a trefoil configuration, which may in fact be the mechanism of some spines becoming trefoil with the development of the secondary curve of lumbar lordosis (Fig. 19.4).

We are surprisingly ignorant about the normal size of the vertebral canal during growth,[6,7] but the sagittal diameter does not appear to vary significantly.[8] Ultrasound measurements of children's spines suggest that the sagittal diameter is relatively

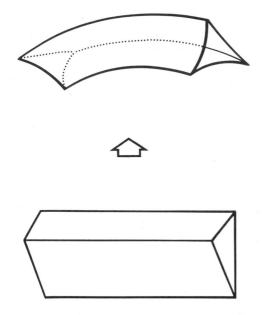

Fig. 19.4 Bending a triangular tube will produce a trefoil configuration

large even in the very young.[9] The vertebral canal of children appears to be relatively large when compared with the size of the vertebral body. The size of a child's skull is also relatively large, however, and presumably the spinal contents require adequate space. The mid-sagittal and the interpedicular diameters of the vertebral canal have approached adult size by the age of 10 years, but if the shape is to change, it does so in the years around puberty.

Significance of canal size

An obvious argument against the vertebral canal being a significant factor in the pathogenesis of back pain is that, although the canal does vary in size and shape from one individual to another, this variation is probably adequate for each subject. In other words, the neural contents may be greater with a large canal, and smaller with a small canal. The lordotic curve, and the range of movement for one individual, may also be reflected in the canal's dimension and be satisfactory for that person. The neural contents undoubtedly influence the dimensions of the vertebral canal to some degree,[10] much as the brain determines epigenetically the size of the skull in hydrocephalus and microcephalus.[11] In the spine, however, this is not the only factor. There

must be other influences at work, both genetic and environmental, because clinical observations show great variation in the proportion of intradural to extradural space. We know from CT scans and surgical experience that many patients with back pain have a canal with a small mid-sagittal diameter, a trefoil shape and a tightly-packed cauda equina. In fact, the canal will often determine the pattern of symptoms from any particular pathology.

Sarpyener,[12] Schlesinger & Taveras,[13] Verbiest,[14] van Gelderen,[15] the Epsteins,[16] Ehni,[17] and many others have described how spinal pathology in the presence of a shallow vertebral canal can produce a variety of back pain syndromes. These include neurogenic claudication, root entrapment from lateral stenosis, and symptoms associated with herniation of the nucleus pulposus. Nearly half of the patients with symptomatic disc protrusion have canal measurements in the bottom 10% of the population. It is reasonable to assume that subjects with wider canals are equally vulnerable to develop disc pathology, but many do not experience root symptoms because there is sufficient space within the vertebral canal for the roots to avoid involvement. It is the sagittal diameter rather than the interpedicular diameter that is critical, the exception being in achondroplasia, when a narrow interpedicular diameter can cause stenotic symptoms.[19,20] The argument that the canal size is insignificant because it reflects the contents and is adequate for that individual runs contrary to anatomical and clinical observations.

Factors which influence the canal's development

Anthropometric measurements may have given a clue to the canal's variable shape, but studies to date have not really shown any useful correlations. We may expect a tall person to have a large spinal canal, but this is not in fact the case. There is a relationship between the length of the long bones and the size of the vertebral bodies, and also a relationship between the size of the bodies and the interpedicular diameter of the vertebral canal. A tall individual does have a wide interpedicular diameter. However, there is no correlation between the mid-sagittal diameter and any vertebral or other skeletal measurement.

There is a weak correlation between the AP and

lateral diameters of the skull and the mid-sagittal diameter of the canal, but this is not sufficient to predict accurately the canal size from skull measurement. Perhaps it reflects a weak epigenetic influence of the neural contents on canal's size.

The clinically important mid-sagittal diameter of the vertebral canal is independent of other anthropometric measurements — it cannot be predicted, and must be measured directly.

The vertebral canal almost reaches adult capacity by late infancy, and therefore factors which disrupt growth in the first few years of life may have a profound and irreversible effect on the adult canal size.[21]

Malcomb[22] has suggested that, because body tissues are crystalline in structure, it is to be expected that their growth would resemble that of crystals and liquid crystals. Crystal spinals are logarithmic, as in the spiral growth commonly found in sea shells, and the shape of the human ribs fits well into a hexagonal logarithmic spiral. Spirals may occur of opposite sense and when conjoined produce a variety of forms, and re-entrant angles can be a source of self-perpetuating growth steps. He suggests that the complicated shape of the vertebrae may be explained in terms of crystal growth. It may yet account for variations in form.

Pathological change

There is no evidence that the mid-sagittal or the interpedicular diameters of the vertebral canal reduce with age after puberty. However, degenerative change at the margins of the apophyseal joints can encroach into the vertebral canal, especially the root canal, and osteophytes develop from the cranial edge of the laminae into the ligamentum flavum. A posterior vertebral bar can develop at the cranial or caudal aspect of the posterior surface of the vertebral bodies, generally in association with disc degeneration, but the central bony canal is probably not reduced in diameter by age-related processes. Skeletal studies have not shown any reduction in canal diameters in older spines, nor have in vivo studies of different occupational groups.

Soft-tissue changes can certainly reduce the capacity of the vertebral canal. CT imaging has shown that the ligamentum flavum may become thickened and buckle into the posterior margin of the central canal and root canal. The anterior margin of the canal may be indented by the posterior longitudinal ligamentum overlying bulging degenerate discs or by previously sequestrated disc material, and iatrogenic scarring can also reduce the canal's capacity.

The canal is also deformed by segmental movement, or vertebral displacement in any of the three planes of rotation. Thus, although the bony canal does not become narrower with age, age-related processes, degeneration and injury can significantly compromise an already narrow canal.

The vertebral canal is one factor that cannot be ignored when attempting to understand the mechanism of a patient's back pain. What is its size and shape? Could there be clinically significant disproportion between the contents and the capacity of the central or the root canal? How important are the soft tissues, vertebral displacement or unnatural segmental movement? It is only as these questions are answered that the diagnosis of a patient's back pain, and eventually its management, becomes possible.

CLINICAL SYNDROMES

There are several clinical syndromes where a shallow vertebral canal has significance. A disc herniation is more likely to produce symptoms if a root is compromised in a shallow, trefoil central canal (Fig. 19.5) or laterally in the root canal. Segmental instability in the presence of a tight dural sac may result in dural pain especially in extension, and root pain on rotation. But the two syndromes where spinal stenosis is accepted as a major contributing factor are neurogenic claudication from central canal stenosis and root entrapment syndrome from lateral stenosis.

Neurogenic claudication

The term 'claudication of the spinal cord' was first used by DeJerine[23] to describe three patients with claudication symptoms but normal peripheral pulses. Van Gelderen[15] reported a patient with symptoms of lumbar root compression which appeared on walking and were relieved by rest, which he thought was due to thickening of the

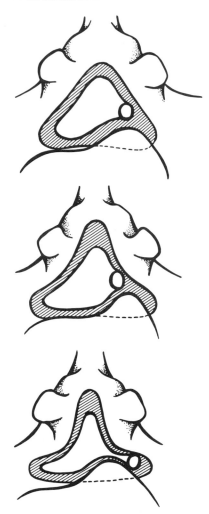

Fig. 19.5 A nerve root can be spared by a disc protrusion into a triangular central canal but is soon compromised if the canal is of trefoil shape

ligamentum flavum. Bergmark[24] described 'intermittent spinal claudication', attributing a neurospinal origin to the walking pains of two patients. It was Verbiest[14] in 1954 who recognized that structural narrowing of the vertebral canal could compress the cauda equina and produce claudication symptoms, and since that time there have been numerous publications on the subject.[7,25-27]

Clinical presentation

This intriguing syndrome usually affects men over 50 years of age who have been heavy manual workers. They complain of discomfort in the legs when walking, affecting both legs equally, usually in the thighs, calves and feet. Describing the discomfort is difficult, but they describe the legs as feeling 'heavy' or 'tired', as though it is difficult to drag one leg after another. One man said his legs felt like those of a deep-sea diver, another as though he had cricket pads on his legs. There is usually a threshold distance when the discomfort develops and a tolerance when they have to stop, and the tolerance is about twice the threshold. The distance can vary during the day, from one day to the next, and even during one stretch of walking. The second period of walking can be longer than the first after a short rest. Often the sufferers find they gradually reduce the walking speed and stoop forward until they finally stop — the stoop test.[28] They will lean forward on a wall, or stoop forward to tie up a shoelace to save embarrassment, and after a few minutes the legs recover sufficiently to start walking again. The flexed position seems to relieve the discomfort and for that reason the sufferers may be able to walk better up a hill leaning forward than down a hill leaning back.

Extending the spine in the standing position can precipitate symptoms in severely disabled patients. They say they can cycle for miles and climb a ladder and stairs, but not come down stairs easily. As the condition progresses, the walking distance reduces, sometimes to only 20 metres. It is probably not neurogenic claudication if a man can walk more than a mile at a reasonable pace.

Nights are usually troublesome, with sleep being disturbed by restless legs and night cramps. The sufferers disturb their wives, and will often get up and walk about at night.

Back pain is a common but not an invariable accompaniment. There is usually a long history of back pain, sometimes with previous surgery, and claudication symptoms for a number of years before help is sought. Apart from the spinal posture, the examination is remarkable for its lack of gross abnormality. The subjects may be able to flex well forward with extended knees, though lumbar extension is usually absent. In fact, it may be difficult for them even to stand erect, and these patients adopt a 'simian stance'[29] with hips and knees slightly flexed (Fig. 19.6). This can be corrected with an effort, but it quickly returns as they relax. If this posture is not present at rest, it tends to develop with walking, the will co-exist. A treadmill enables us to establish an objective record of walking pain, noting the distance at which symptoms develop, the distribution of discomfort, the speed of walking, the changing posture and the tolerance. The impression gained from the patient's history can be completely different from an objective assessment of walking. For measuring a response to treatment, a treadmill is invaluable.

A plain radiograph may raise the suspicion of a shallow vertebral canal, and perhaps show a degenerative spondylolisthesis, present in half the men with neurogenic claudication. A myelogram is essential to confirm the diagnosis. It will show one or several segmental filling defects, or even a complete block (Fig. 19.7). The lack of space in the central canal can make injection of the contrast medium very difficult, and the myelogram may have to be abandoned at the lower lumbar level.[17,30] When myelography is difficult, epidural venography will show the extent of the stenosis.[31]

Ultrasound measurements confirm a reduced mid-sagittal diameter of the vertebral canal. 57% of our patients with neurogenic claudication had measurements below the tenth percentile. A narrow canal supports the diagnosis, but obviously narrow canals exist without neurogenic claudication symptoms. A wide canal is incompatible with the diagnosis.

Differential diagnosis

Intermittent claudication, a phrase coined by Charcot[32] in 1858 to describe ischaemic pain from peripheral vascular disease, is difficult to distinguish from neurogenic claudication by the history alone. It is not affected by posture, and the patient does not find himself stooping forward the further he walks. He finds climbing hills worse than descending them, and he can neither cycle nor walk. The bicycle test of van Gelderen[33] modified by Dyck & Doyle[34] is helpful in differentiating between these two types of claudication. The patient is asked to cycle with the spine first extended and then flexed. The distance is the same in intermittent claudication, whilst in neurogenic claudication the flexed position allows greater exercise tolerance (Figs 19.8 and 19.9). His walking threshold and tolerance are generally much the same from one day to the next. One leg may be

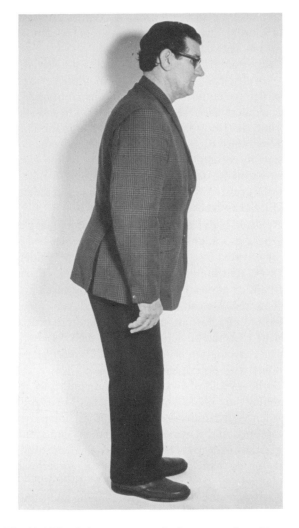

Fig. 19.6 The simian stance — a classic posture adopted by patients with neurogenic claudication, with flexed hips and knees.

patient gradually stooping further forward until he has to stop. The 'stoop test' makes use of this phenomenon in diagnosing claudication of neurogenic origin, the leg symptoms being relieved by the patient stooping forward at the point of walking tolerance, and returning by his standing upright again.

The lumbar spine is often tender over several segments. SLR is generally full, the reflexes normal, the power and sensation also normal. It has been suggested that re-examination after exercise alters the neurological examination. The peripheral circulation is normal, but not infrequenlty arterial disease

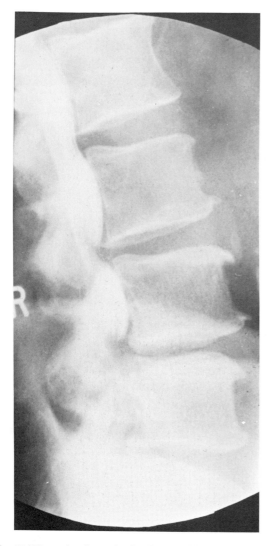

Fig. 19.7 Lateral radiograph of a 63-year-old man with neurogenic claudication. There is a degenerative spondylolisthesis at L4/5, with the metrizamide column completely blocked at the level of displacement, and partially occluded at L3/4

intermittent claudication.[35] To confuse the issue, intermittent claudication and neurogenic claudication may coexist.[36]

Lamerton et al[37] described sciatic claudication as an insufficiency of the inferior gluteal artery, producing claudication in a sciatic distribution from ischaemia of the sciatic nerve. The claudication is in a root distribution, but spinal examination and myelography are normal. It is an important condition to recognize. Endarterectomy of the aorto-iliac segments can relieve the symptoms, whilst an arterial graft, by disturbing the inferior gluteal artery and its anastomoses, will be ineffective.

Referred pain from the lower lumbar region in the buttocks and thighs, even up to the upper calves, can be aggravated by walking. 18% of Crock's[38] patients with isolated lumbar disc resorption had increasing leg pain or paraesthesia on walking distances up to 500 metres. We can recognize referred pain from its proximal distribution, not beyong the upper calves, and its presence in activities other than walking. A normal myelogram is compatible with referred pain but not with neurogenic claudication.

Some types of root pain and multiple root pathology are made worse by walking,[39] probably if segmental instability is a factor in producing the root symptoms, and if venous engorgement contributes to restriction of space in the root canal. There may be little or no pain at rest, but walking precipitates unilateral leg pain with a variable threshold and tolerance, which is relieved by stopping and leaning forwards. Root claudication may be the remaining symptom after a classical disc protrusion has settle down, or it may occur in the older patient with root entrapment from lateral bony stenosis.

Claudication pain is sometimes a symptom of distress. Abnormal behaviour patterns are common in patients who have a long history of back pain, and not infrequently a symptom inappropriate to the underlying organic problem in the spine is pain in the legs when walking. There are usually inappropriate signs also.

It is difficult to assess accurately the claudicating patient who also has a ligation problem. One can exclude a peripheral vascular lesion and, if the myelogram is normal, exclude neurogenic claudication. An equivocal myelogram is a problem. Although the diagnosis would be suspect with more than one inappropriate sign, these signs may mask a

more affected than the other, and perhaps only the calves. These, however, are generalizations, and in practice the difference between the two is not always straightforward. Impalpable peripheral pulses and femoral bruits will suggest peripheral vascular disease. If clinical examination is difficult, a Doppler scan may be more objective, but it can take an arteriogram to be certain of the relative importance of the peripheral arterial circulation. Cerebral somatosensory evoked potential after walking may help to differentiate neurogenic from vascular

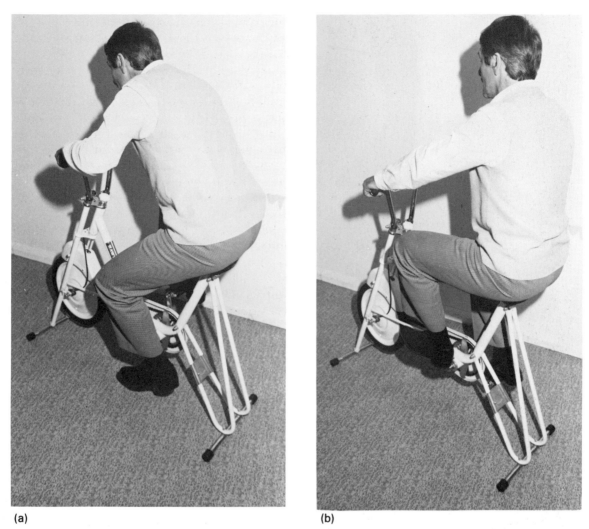

(a)   (b)

Fig. 19.8 The cycle test. The cycling distance is the same in intermittent claudication whether the spine is flexed (left) or upright (right). The extended spine limits the cycling distance in neurogenic claudication

genuine underlying problem. Ligation can so confuse the issue that it may not be possible to decide how many of the symptoms are organic, and whether the organic element of the leg pain is neurogenic claudication, multiple root pathology, or referred pain.

Pathology

Verbiest[14] recognized that neurogenic claudication was associated with a shallow vertebral canal. In fact the term 'spinal stenosis' has unfortunately become synonymous with neurogenic claudication, when in fact a shallow canal is only one factor in the

pathology. Symptoms develop after middle life, but there is no evidence that the vertebral canal becomes narrower with age. There can be a little encroachment into the canal from hypertrophy of the apophyseal joints and marginal osteophyte formation, but this is more into the root canal than the central canal. Also posterior vertebral bar formation on the lower and upper posterior margins of the vertebral bodies can reduce the sagittal diameter to some degree. In general, however, the central canal retains the same cross-sectional diameter throughout life. An individual with spinal stenosis and neurogenic claudication has therefore had a narrow canal for many years before the development of leg

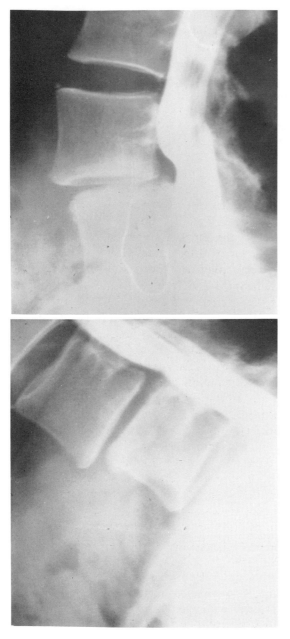

Fig. 19.9 (Left) Lateral radiograph of a 56-year-old man with a degenerative spondylolisthesis at L4/5. The myelogram shows partial soft tissue encroachment into the vertebral canal in extension. (Above) Flexion of the spine reduces the encroachment.

symptoms,[18,40,41] and many patients with stenotic canals never have claudication pain. The canal is therefore but one factor in the pathology.

A second factor is degenerative disease of the lumbar spine associated with heavy manual work. The majority of patients with neurogenic claudication have been involved in heavy work. Few have been sedentary workers. It would seem that the cumulative effects of the mechanical stress of labouring work plays a part in pathology rather than the degenerative process from one disc insult in the earlier life of a sedentary worker.

The high male incidence of 9 to 1 may be due to heavier manual work, or indicate that hormonal factors are significant. Degenerative spondylolisthesis effectively reduces the canal size at the level of displacement.[42,43] Although degenerative spondylolisthesis is more common in women, half of the men with neurogenic claudication in our series had a degenerative spondylolisthesis.[44] Women with degenerative displacement rarely develop claudication symptoms.

Neurogenic claudication must be very unusual in children, but Birkensfield & Kasdon[45] described it in two adolescent boys with congenital lumbar ridges producing ventral defects on myelography.

Symptoms are probably the result of inadequate oxygenation of the cauda equina, but the mechanism is at present purely speculative. There may be arterial ischaemia or venous engorgement which just permits adequate nerve function at rest, but inadequate function during exercise. The fact that patients are generally over 50 years of age, when arteriosclerosis is becoming more common, is compatible with an ischaemic component to the pathology. Many claudicating patients have a stenosis at L3/4 level.[46] This may have a neuro-ischaemic explanation. The proximal third of the cauda equina is an area at risk, being supplied by an astomosis of both proximal and distal radicular arteries.[46] If the supply is just adequate for its needs,[47] then deprivation could precipitate claudication symptoms at this level.

Fifty years ago, Reichert et al[48] described ischaemia of the spinal cord due to arteriosclerotic involvement of the lumbar arteries, giving weakness of the lower limbs on exertion. They noted similar temporary weakness in dogs by ligating the lumbar artery. Cauda equina ischaemia may have a similar mechanism.

There is probably localized vasodilatation of the radicular arteries in response to exercise. Exercising the single limb of a mouse will produce vasodilatation of the ipsilateral region of the spinal cord.[49] In addition, the selective paralysis in poliomyelitis is probably related to the vasodilatation of the anterior horn in response to muscular activity in the pre-paralytic stage of the disease.[50] Should the vessels of the cauda equina likewise dilate with exercise, they will be vulnerable to ischaemia if space is at a premium.

A vascular steal syndrome could explain the claudication symptoms of some patients with claudication and Paget's disease when the vertebral canal may not appear significantly narrow.[51-53]

Iatrogenic neurogenic claudication can follow spinal surgery, more so after a spinal fusion than discectomy. The patient is at risk whose developmentally narrow canal is fused. It was previously thought that bony ingrowth from the posterior fusion mass compromised the canal causing symptoms, but it is more likely that symptoms arise at the segment proximal to the fusion. It can become unstable, and the narrow canal, segmental instability and ischaemia from iatrogenic scarring combine to produce symptoms.

Claudication must be related to the dynamic activity of walking. There are probably three processes caused by walking which precipitate symptoms in a cauda equina already deprived and vulnerable. Segmental rotation, which accompanies walking, especially with segmental instability, will reduce the available space in an already narrow canal. Secondly, the increased venous return from the exercising lower limbs will be accompanied by engorgement of the pelvic veins and of Batson's venous plexus, reducing the available space for the cauda equina. Thirdly, the arterial system of the cauda equina, responding to the increasing demands of exercise, may do so inadequately when space is limited. Nutriments fail to reach the nerve roots, metabolites are not removed, and function is affected.

The first process is probably the most critical, because it is not the exercise of the lower limbs that produces the symptoms, but rather the torque and posture of the spine at the time of that exercise. A fourth mechanism may be responsible if there exists an intra-osseous arterial shunt.[54,55] In health, the intra-osseous arterial branches of the lumbar arteries may vasoconstrict and shunt blood to the radicular branch, during the activity of walking or running. If there is already incipient ischaemia of the nerve roots from restricted space in the vertebral canal, and if in addition the vertebral shunt should fail as a result of bony degenerative pathology, neurogenic claudication symptoms would develop in times of physiological stress.

As yet, we do not know how important is the cerebrospinal fluid in the normal function of the cauda equina. It is possible that this is the key to the mechanism of the symptoms of neurogenic claudication.[56] The cauda equina probably needs to be bathed in a free circulation of cerebrospinal fluid for its nutrition, for removal of metabolites and for insulation. When the fluid is deficient from reduced space in the canal, and especially when there is a closed sac of fluid distally, the circulation will be deficient. Magnaes[57] was able to record a high cerebrospinal fluid pressure in claudicating patients distal to a stenosis segment and related to posture. One can imagine a claudicating patient stopping after a few hundred metres, leaning forward on a wall for a minute and, as the fluid above the stenosis is permitted to exchange with the closed sac below, the discomfort rapidly clears from the legs.

It is interesting that neurogenic claudication does not usually occur from stenosis at L5/S1 alone. It is usually from segmental narrowing at the two or three more proximal segments, which permits a closed sac of dura distally. If the sac is too large from stenosis at the thoracolumbar level, claudication symptoms are rare. Although L3/4 interspace is the most common level of stenosis in neurogenic claudication,[1,58] it is still possible for a central disc protrusion at L5/S1 to produce the same symptoms, if there is a large distal dural sac.

Management

Patients with neurogenic claudication are either offered surgical decompression or are advised to live with their symptoms. If symptoms are not too severe, or if surgery is contra-indicated, simple reduction of activities, alteration of job, together with instruction on the correct postures for lifting and carrying, may enable the patients to live within their limitations.[39] Once the syndrome is well established, however, conservative management rarely improves the quality of life.[40]

The beneficial effects of calcitonin on the paraparesis of patients with spinal Paget's disease was noted by Walpin & Singer,[59] Herzberg & Bayliss,[53] Ravichandran[51] and Douglas et al.[52] Many of their patients, besides losing the Paget's pain, also found that their walking improved dramatically and suddenly. Calcitonin can also significantly increase the walking distance for patients with neurogenic claudication but without evidence of Paget's disease.[44]

It is uncertain whether the mechanism is vascular or a placebo response, but a course of Calsynar® (100 units four times a week for eight weeks) is recommended for those patients who are a poor operative risk, for post-operative recurrence of claudication or as a pre-operative trial.

When claudication symptoms are sufficiently severe, they are generally relieved by surgical decompression[46,60,61] (Fig. 19.10). Most patients are immediately impressed with the improved sensation in their legs and are soon walking long distances. Not a few relapse as a laminectomy membrane of fibrous tissue develops over the posterior dura. Their walking distance again becomes reduced. Verbiest[60] recorded that 70 out of 74 of his patients with neurogenic claudication were relieved by decompression. Russin & Sheldon[62] and Lassale et al[63] likewise recorded excellent long-term follow-up results of stenotic symptoms by decompression

This probably depends on careful patient selection and adequate decompression. Advanced age is no contra-indication to decompression; it will often improve the quality of life for the elderly.[40] Some results are less satisfactory, and in these it is claimed that decompression was less than adequate, that arachnoiditis spoilt the results, or that long-standing ischaemia of the nerve roots became irreversible. Most operative series have a hard core of failures.

The spinal decompression must be adequate.[1,64] It must extend sufficiently proximally to permit a free flow of cerebrospinal fluid to the distal cauda equina, and it must be sufficiently lateral to ensure there is no occlusion of the nerve roots. It usually involves removing three laminae, with the spinous processes, sometimes two and occasionally four. The results of one- or two-level decompression for localized segmental stenosis seem to give better long-term results than a more extensive three-, four- or five-level decompression for multi-level disease.[65] The canal will have been narrow for years prior to the development of symptoms and, although there may be stenosis at multiple levels, the symptomatic pathology is probably localized. The operative dilemma is to ensure that this critical segment is effectively decompressed. One tends to rely upon a clinical impression that the tight dura and roots are given adequate space, and on the grounds of safety

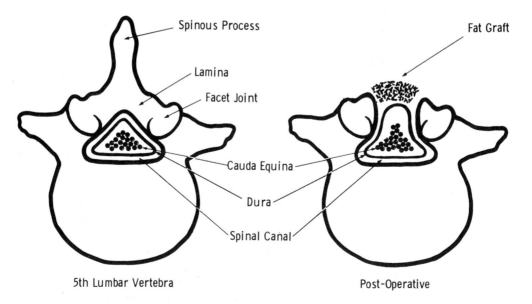

Fig. 19.10 Decompression of the cauda equina by removal of the neural arch, undercutting of the facets and application of a fat graft. The extent of undercutting required is indicated from a pre-operative CT scan.

one may at times be more radical than is necessary. Somatosensory evoked potentials may have a place as an intra-operative diagnostic aid to the extent of decompression.[66]

If there is a degenerative spondylolisthesis, it is essential not to increase the instability of that segment unnecessarily,[67] but forward post-operative displacement is unusual, even with wide decompression, and even with a pre-existing degenerative spondylolithesis.[65,68] The integrity of the apophyseal joints is not disturbed, though the medial third of the joint must often be removed and the facet undercut. It is necessary to perform a decompression wide enough to ensure a completely free dura,[64] but not too wide to produce either instability or such a shallow spinal gutter that a laminectomy membrane will soon compress the dura to a ribbon. Provided there is no degenerative spondylolisthesis, it is legitimate to sacrifice the major part of the apophyseal joint on one side in order to obtain satisfactory decompression, and not jeopardize stability.

A fat graft applied over the decompressed dura reduces the risk of post-operative fibrous compression. To ensure that the fat survives, and is revascularized, it is applied as thin postage-stamp-size grafts, rather than one large cube of fat. This is obtained from the subcutaneous layer at the operation site, but in thin men it may have to be dissected from a separate buttock incision. One should obliterate 'dead space' and secure haemostasis.

Patients are pleased to be mobilized early. In fact, it is difficult to restrain them. They find their own limitations and many remain highly satisfied.

Root entrapment syndrome — lateral canal stenosis

Entrapment of the lumbar nerve root in the root canal produces a clinical syndrome distinct from that of the acute disc lesion. In this condition, the root is usually affected by bony and soft tissue encroachment into a narrow root canal or in the lateral recess of the central canal. By contrast, the disc protrusion affects the root in the central canal and uncommonly in the root canal. Though both cause pain in the leg, their presentation and management are distinctly different.

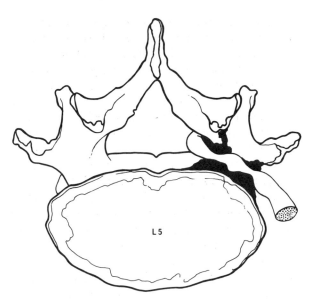

Fig. 19.11 The L5 root in the root canal below the broad pedicle, showing its vulnerability to bony degenerative change.

Pathology

The site of the lesion can be very variable, but the root most commonly involved is the 5th lumbar, probably because of the frequency of degenerative change at L5/S1, and the length of the root canal at L5, below the broad pedicle (Fig. 19.11). The L4 and L3 roots are occasionally affected in their root canals. In the central canal the L5 root can be involved from degenerative changes at the L4/5 disc space, and the S1 root anterior to the cranial lip of the upper sacral lamina.[61]

The original size of the root canal is variable and must be highly significant. The root canal will be further reduced by a posterior vertebral bar on the inferolateral border of the body, or by osteophytes from the margins of the apophyseal joints (Fig. 19.12). The overhanging medial lip of the superior facet is a common site for subarticular entrapment, with the root tightly stretched against the pedicle in the lateral recess. Bony encroachment may follow ossification of spinal ligaments. In spite of the gross degenerative change sometimes encountered in the lower lumbar spine, it is surprising how the nerve root tunnel is always preserved. It may be reduced, but never occluded. If a CT scan should give the impression that the canal is non-existent, this is but an artefact of the mathematical display.

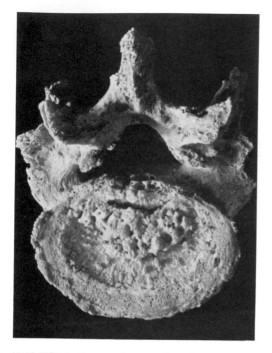

Fig. 19.12 Fifth lumbar vertebra seen from below, showing advanced degenerative changes of the vertebral body margins and apophyseal joints, with a large osteophyte encroaching into the left root canal.

Soft-tissue involvement of the root canal adds to the bony encroachment. Organization of an annulus after a disc protrusion, or fibrosis of extruded or sequestrated nucleus, reduces the available space for the root. The posterior longitudinal ligament can thicken, the ligamentum flavum infold,[69] the apophyseal joint capsule hypertrophy and soft tissue of a lytic pars proliferate until space for the nerve root is at a premium. Venous engorgement in the root canal may critically affect the function of the nerve root.

Segmental movement of the spine adds a dynamic factor.[70] Extension and rotation further reduce available space and are both limited and painful in this syndrome. It becomes particularly significant when there is posterior or rotational displacement of the vertebra.[71] Several dynamic factors can be responsible for symptoms. Postural movement, especially extension, can compromise the root and precipitate symptoms. The activity of walking can produce root symptoms by both intervertebral segmental rotatory movement and by the epidural venous engorgement associated with exercise. The dynamic factors involved in normal root excursion in activities such as walking and bending can assume significance in a pathological root.

Just as the tunnel is never occluded, the root is never trapped. There is some excursion, even if at operation the root gives the impression of being tight. The lumbar roots have an excursion of a few millimetres, limited by proximal and distal attachments.[72] These attachments probably make the root vulnerable to traction symptoms in the presence of pathological change. A mobile root in a restricted space will produce root irritation and ischaemia. Friction on a tethered root or anomalous root with limited excursion will have similar results.[73] The root then becomes considerably thicker, harder and inelastic from fibrosis.

There are many pathological changes that can cause lumbar root pain in the middle-aged and older patient. The most common site of these changes is in the root canal, related to disc pathology of a previous decade.

Clinical presentation

Though the pain from root entrapment is in the same distribution as the sciatica from a disc lesion, from the buttock, thigh, calf to the foot, its character is different. It is described as a severe pain, often unremitting day and night. Whilst the pain from a disc is frequently relieved by lying down, this pain is so troublesome at night that the patient will walk about. Sitting is uncomfortable, driving far impossible, as though the whole length of the sciatic nerve is over-sensitive. Unlike root pain of disc origin, it is unaffected by coughing and sneezing.

The periodicity of the pain is variable. One patient may experience constant severe pain, and present at the consulting room after many sleepless nights. Another may have mild pain with episodes of severe pain in relation to posture, especially to sitting or standing for long. Another may say that walking is the main cause of pain. If walking only produces pain, one should suspect a vascular component, either venous engorgement around the root or arterial insufficiency.

The past history is also variable. There has usually been previous disc pathology, but the previous disc symptoms may have been either classical, with root pain, or have produced only back pain. They may even have been entirely occult. The degree of original disc symptoms years before depends much on the size of the central vertebral canal. There may have been no symptoms at all from a disc protrusion into a wide dome-shaped central canal, but, with disc space narrowing over the years, bony and soft tissue degeneration and perhaps slight vertebral displacement, the root becomes compromised in the root canal. The very first symptom of the silent lesion years before is now severe root pain from root canal entrapment.

The progress of the root pain, once it has developed, is unpredictable. It can develop and subside in weeks, months or years, and patients may therefore present with long or short histories. It has no typical pattern, sometimes being severe and gradually resolving, and at other times getting steadily worse, requiring surgery.

The abnormal signs are generally few. Many patients are able to reach down to the floor and have good straight-leg raising, normal reflexes and no abnormal motor or sensory signs. Only one-third of Getty's patients with root entrapment[74] had significant restriction of straight-leg raising, and this was similarly recorded by Macnab.[75] Spinal extension is often restricted, but for many patients with little to find clinically, the diagnosis therefore begs a good history. Most patients have some radiological evidence of degenerative change, reduction of L5/S1 disc space being the most consistent finding. There is a greater incidence of abnormal neurological signs in those patients who have had previous surgery, and in those referred for surgery from other units because of the intensity and duration of root symptoms.

In expert hands, electromyography can provide objective evidence of impaired root function, and it will sometimes identify the root affected.[76] Other studies with electromyography have not confirmed the ability of this investigation to predict which nerve roots are responsible for symptoms,[77] probably because of the variable anatomy of root innervation. Electrodiagnostic methods can complement other investigations and help in the overall evaluation but probably have limited value, especially after previous laminectomy.[78] Radiculography has a poor sensitivity for root entrapment syndrome,[79] but it will exclude other pathology in the severely disabled patient.

CT scan is advisable if surgery is being seriously considered. Bony encroachment may of course not be the cause of the symptoms, but a CT scan is an essential adjunct to surgery (Fig. 19.13).

Management

Most patients presenting to an orthopaedic surgeon with root entrapment syndrome can be managed by a careful explanation of the cause of pain, and advice.[80] They certainly need to be given time to discuss the probable cause of the pain, and to understand that, if aggravating factors can be avoided, it will probably settle. If sitting for long and standing increase the symptoms, the position should be quickly changed. The mechanical stress on the spine should be kept to a minimum, and if this is not understood, it is reinforced with a back school programme. Patients are told that symptoms will probably remain for a long time, but will reduce in intensity and eventually settle.

187 of our patients with root entrapment described their symptoms after two years.[80] Three-quarters of them still had some root pain, but it was less troublesome, and only 12% had either returned in those two years or sought help elsewhere.

For some patients the pain is so intense that it is not reasonable to offer advice only. It is difficult to obtain statistical evidence that an epidural injection is better than placebo, but there is strong circum-

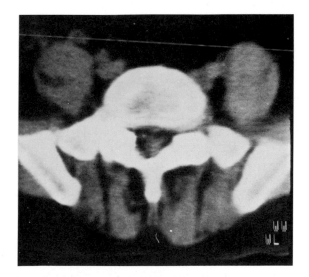

Fig. 19.13 A CT scan of a 52-year-old woman with severe root pain, showing bony encroachment at L5. (Published with kind permission of Dr P. Butt, Leeds).

stantial evidence that this is perhaps the best indication for an epidural.

For a few patients, surgical decompression of the root canal or lateral recess is essential. There should, however, be an adequate period of observation over several weeks lest the condition will resolve either naturally or with the help of one or two epidural injections. When the diagnosis is clear, the pain severe and of long duration, when it is not settling and there is no evidence of exaggeration, surgical decompression of the root can be rewarding. Getty recorded early relief of leg pain in 68 per cent of his operated patients.[81]

Decompression of the root requires adequate exposure of the root over the length at risk.[82] The site of compression may be suspected pre-operatively by conventional radiography, by CT scan, or occasionally by myelography. Electrical studies may identify the root. The area is exposed surgically, and the root followed proximally and distally until there is no question at all that it is free and mobile. However, there is sometimes uncertainty about the area of pathology and about the root which is involved, and it may be necessary to explore the lower lumbar central canal and two root canals fairly extensively.

The confidence with which one views the investigations will determine the extent of surgical exploration. Many feel that a wide decompression is generally necessary, removing the spinous process and laminae at L5, occasionally at L4 if the 4th lumbar root is suspect, and following the L5 root well into the root canal, undercutting the lamina to ensure complete freedom for the root. The L5 root may be obviously thickened and tough, with perineural fibrosis, and there is then no doubt about the root involved. Bony hypertrophy in the 5th lumbar root canal should not cause us to suspect the root automatically. The S1 root may be the cause of symptoms, and removal of the upper sacral lamina may, in fact, reveal compression under the cranial lip.

Others more confident of the site of the lesion may be happy to perform a limited decompression, removing the window of the lamina and part of the apophyseal joint, undercutting the lamina and removing ligamentum flavum.[81] There are obvious advantages in a more limited exposure, provided the decompression is adequate. Most patients experience early post-operative relief of their leg pain, but not a few have persisting symptoms of varying degree, perhaps the result of irreversible root pathology.

REFERENCES

1 Schatzker J, Pennal G F 1968 Spinal stenosis. A cause of cauda equina compression. J. Bone Joint Surg. 50B: 606–618
2 Porter R W, Hibbert C, Wellman P, Langton C 1980 The shape and the size of the lumbar spinal canal. Proc. Inst. Mech. Eng. 51–58
3 Eisenstein S 1977 Morphometry and pathological anatomy of the lumbar spine in South African negroes and Caucasoids with specific reference to spinal stenosis. J. Bone Joint Surg. 59B: 173–180
4 Eisenstein S 1980 The trefoil configuration of the lumbar vertebral canal. J. Bone Joint Surg. 62B: 73–77
5 Baddeley H 1976 Radiology of lumbar spinal stenosis. The Lumbar Spine and Back Pain, 2nd edn. Pitman Medical, Tunbridge Wells, p 151–171
6 Haworth J B, Keillor G W 1962 Use of transparencies in evaluating the width of the spinal canal in infants, children and adults. Radiology 79: 109–114
7 Bowen V, Shannan R, Kirkcaldy Willis W H 1978 Lumbar spinal stenosis. Child's Brain 4: 257–277
8 Larsen J L, Smith D 1981 The lumbar spinal canal in children. Eur. J. Radiol. 1: 163–170
9 Porter R W, Hibbert C, Wellman P 1980 Backache and the lumbar spinal canal. Spine 5: 99–105
10 Roth M 1973 The relative osteo-neural growth. A concept of normal and pathological (tetrogenic) skeletal morphogenesis. Gegenbaurs Morph. Jahrb., Leipzig 119: 250–274
11 Lindborgh J V 1972 The role of genetic and local environmental factors in the control of post natal craniofacial morphogenesis. Acta Morphol. Neth Scand. 10: 37–47
12 Sarpyener M A 1945 Congenital stricture of the spinal canal. J. Bone Joint Surg. 27: 70–79
13 Schlesinger E B, Taveras J M 1953 Factors in the production of cauda equina syndromes in lumbar discs. Trans. Am. Neurol. Assoc. 78: 263
14 Verbiest H 1954 A radicular syndrome from developmental narrowing of the lumbar vertebral canal. J. Bone Joint Surg. 36B: 230
15 van Gelderen V 1958 Ein orthotisches (lordotisches) Kaudasyndrom. Acta Psychiatr. Neurol. Scand. 23: 57
16 Epstein J A, Epstein B S, Levine I 1962 Nerve root compression associated with narrowing of the lumbar spinal canal. J. Neurol. Neurosurg. Psych. 25: 165–176
17 Ehni G 1969 Significance of the small lumbar spinal canal: cauda equina compression syndrome due to spondylolysis. J. Neurol. 31: 490–494
18 Salibi B S 1976 Neurogenic claudication and stenosis of the lumbar spinal canal. Surg. Neurol. 5: 269–272
19 Epstein J A, Malis L I 1955 Compression of spinal cord and cauda equina in achondroplastic dwarfs. Neurology 5: 875–881
20 Nelson M A 1970 Orthopaedic aspects of the

chondrodystrophies. Ann. Roy. Coll. Surg. Engl. 47: 185–210

21 Clark G A, Panjabi M M, Wetzel F T 1984 Infant malnutrition and adult spinal stenosis. Presented to the International Society for Study of the Lumbar Spine, Montral

22 Malcomb J E 1981 Crystalline structure of the vertebral column: thoracic region. J. Anat. 133: 148–150

23 DeJerine J 1911 La claudication intermittente de la moelle épinière. Presse Méd. 19: 981

24 Bergmark 1950 Intermittent spinal claudication. Acta Med. Scand. 246 (suppl): 30

25 Gathier J C 1959 A case of absolute stenosis of the lumbar vertebral canal in adults. Acta Neurochir (Wien) 7: 344–349

26 Brish A, Lerner M B, Braham J 1964 Intermittent claudication from compression of the cauda equina by a narrowed spinal canal. J. Neursurg. 21: 207–211

27 Dyck P, Pheasant H D, Doyle J B et al 1977 Intermittent cauda equina compression syndrome: its recognition and treatment. Spine 2: 75–81

28 Dyck P 1979 The stoop test in lumbar entrapment radiculography. Spine 4: 89–92

29 Simkin P A 1982 Simian stance: a sign of spinal stenosis. Lancet: 652–653

30 Williams R W 1975 The narrow lumbar spinal canal. Australas. Radiol. 19: 356–360 Bestawros O A, Vreeland O H, Golman M L 1979 Epidural venography in the diagnosis of lumbar spinal stenosis. Radiology 131: 423–426

32 Charcot J M C 1858 Sur la claudication intermittente observée dans un cas d'oblitéteration complète de l'une des artères iliaques primitives. Comptes Rendus Soc. Biol. 10: 225–238

33 van Gelderen C 1948 Ein orthotisches (lordotisches) Kaudsyndrom. Acta Psychiatr. Neurol. 23: 57–68

34 Dyck P, Doyle J B 1977 Bicycle test of van Gelderen in diagnosis of intermittent cauda equina compression syndrome: case report. J. Neursurg. 46: 667–670

35 Larson S J, Milwaukee W I 1983 Somato-sensory evoked potentials in lumbar stenosis. Surg. Gynaecol. Obst. 157: 191–196

36 Johansson J E, Bazrrington T W, Ameli M 1982 Combined vascular and neurogenic claudication. Spine 7: 150–158

37 Lamerton A J, Bannister R, Withrington R, Seifert M H, Eastcott H H G 1983 Claudication of the sciatic nerve. Br. Med. J. 286: 1785–1786

38 Venner R M, Crock H V 1981 Clinical studies of isolated disc resorption in the lumbar spine. J. Bone Joint Surg. 63B: 491–494

39 Jayson M I V, Nelson M A 1979 Spinal stenosis and low back pain. Rheum. Dis. 70: Arthritis and Rheumatism Council

40 Ami Hood S, Weigl K 1983 Lumbar spinal stenosis: surgical intervention for the older person. Israel J. Med. Sci. 19: 169–171

41 Critchley E M R 1982 Lumbar spinal stenosis. Br. Med. J. 284: 1588–1589

42 Rosenberg N J 1976 Degenerative spondylolisthesis. Clin. Orth. Rel. Res. 117: 112–120

43 Wilson C B, Brill F R 1977 Spinal stenosis. The narrow lumbar spinal canal syndrome. Clin. Orth. 122: 244–248

44 Porter R W, Hibbert C 1983 Calcitonin treatment for neurogenic claudication. Spine 8: 585–592

45 Birkensfield R, Kasdon D L 1978 Congenital lumbar ridge causing spinal claudication in adolescents. J. Neurosurg. 49: 441–444

46 Parke W W, Gammell K, Rothman R H 1981 Arterial vascularisation of the cauda equina. J. Bone Joint Surg. 63A: 53–61

47 Domminisse G F 1976 Arteries and veins of the lumbar nerve roots and cauda equina. Clin. Orth. 115: 22–29

48 Reichert F L, Rytand D A, Bruck E L 1934 Arteriosclerosis of the lumbar segmental arteries producing ischaemia of the spinal cord and consequent claudication of the thighs. Am. J. Med. Sci. 187: 794–806

49 Blau J N, Rushworth G 1958 Observations of blood vessels of the spinal cord and their responses to motor activity. Brain 81: 354–363

50 Buchthal F 1949 Problems of the pathologic physiology of poliomyelitis. Am. J. Med. 6: 587–591

51 Ravichandran G 1981 Spinal cord function in Paget's disease of spine. Paraplegia 19: 7–11

52 Douglas D L, Duckworth T, Kanis J A, Jefferson A A, Martin T J, Russell R G G 1981 Spinal cord dysfunction in Paget's disease of bone: has medical treatment a vascular basis? J. Bone Joint Surg. 63B: 495–503

53 Herzberg L, Bayliss E 1980 Spinal cord syndrome due to non-compressible Paget's disease of bone: a spinal artery steal phenomenon reversible with calcitonin. Lancet 2: 13–15

54 Pooley J, Pooley J E, Stevens J 1984 Evidence for an intraosseous arteriovenous shunt operating in long bones during exercise conditions. Presented to the British Orthopaedic Research Society, Stanmore

55 McCarthy I D, Davies R, Hughes S P F 1984 The response of the microcirculation in bone to the administration of noradrenaline and ATP. Presented to the British Orthopaedic Research Society, Stanmore

56 Porter R W 1982 Relief work, spinal decompression. Nurs. Mir. 42–44

57 Magnaes B 1982 Clinical recording of pressure on the spinal cord and cauda equina. J. Neurosurg. 57: 57–63

58 Weisz G M 1983 Lumbar spinal canal stenosis in Paget's disease. Spine 8: 192–198

59 Walpin L A, Singer F R 1979 Paget's disease: reversal of severe paraparesis with calcitonin. Spine 4: 213–219

60 Verbiest H 1977 Treatment of idiopathic developmental stenosis of the lumbar vertebral canal. J. Bone Joint Surg. 50B: 181–188

61 Crock H V 1981 Normal and pathological anatomy of the lumbar spinal nerve root canals. J. Bone Joint Surg. 63B: 487–490

62 Russin L A, Sheldon J 1976 Spinal stenosis. Report of series and long term follow up. Clin. Orth. 115: 101–103

63 Lassale B, De Burge A, Benoist M 1984 Long term results of surgical treatment of lumbar stenosis. Presented to the International Society for the Study of the Lumbar Spine, Montreal

64 Wiltse L L, Kirkaldy-Willis W H, McIvor G W D 1976 The treatment of spinal stenosis. Clin. Orth. 115: 83–91

65 Grabias S 1980 Current concepts review the treatment of spinal stenosis. J. Bone Joint Surg. 62A: 308–313

66 Kiem H A, Hajdu M, Gonzales E, Brand L, Balasubramaniam 1984 Somato-sensory evoked potentials as a diagnostic aid in the diagnosis and intra-operative management of spinal stenosis. Presented to the International Society for the Study of the Lumbar Spine, Montreal

67   Lin P M 1982 Internal decompression for multiple levels of lumbar spinal stenosis: a technical note. Neurosurgery 11: 546–549

68   Shenkin H A, Hash C J 1976 A new approach to the surgical treatment of lumbar spondylosis. J. Neurosurg. 44: 148–155

69   Towme E B, Reichert F L 1931 Compression of the lumbosacral roots of the spinal cord by thickened ligamenta flava. Ann. Surg. 94: 327–336

70   Panjabi M M, Takata K, Goel U K 1983 Kinematics of lumbar intervertebral foramen. Spine 8: 348–357

71   Krayenbuhl H, Benini A 1979 Die Enge des Recessus lateralis im Lumbalen bereich der Wirbelsaule a la Ursache der Nerven Wurzelkompression bei Bandscheiber Verschamlerung. Z. Orthop. 117: 167–171

72   Spencer D L, Irwin G S, Miller J A A 1983 Anatomy and significance of fixation of the lumbosacral nerve roots in sciatica. Spine 8: 672–679

73   Kadish L J, Simmons E H 1984 Anomalies of the lumbosacral nerve roots: an anatomical investigation and myelographic study. J. Bone Joint Surg. 66B: 411–416

74   Getty C J M 1980 Lumbar spinal stenosis: the clinical spectrum and the results of operation. J. Bone Joint Surg. 62B: 481–485

75   Macnab I 1977 Backache. Williams & Wilkins, Baltimore

76   Leyshon A, Kirwan E O'G, Wynn Parry C B 1980 Is it nerve root pain? J. Bone Joint Surg. 62B: 119

77   Merriam W F, Smith N J, Mulholland R C 1982 Lumbar spinal stenosis. Br. Med. J. 285: 515

78   Eisen A, Hoirch M 1983 The electrodiagnostic evaluation of spinal root lesions. Spine 8: 98–106

79   Euinton H A, Locke T J, Barrington N A, Getty C J M, Davies G K 1984 Radiological diagnosis of bony entrapment of lumbar nerve roots using water soluble radiculography. Presented tothe International Society for Study of the Lumbar Spine, Montral

80   Porter R W, Hibbert C, Evans C 1984 The natural history of root entrapment syndrome. Spine 9: 418–422

81   Getty C J M, Johnson J R, Kirwan E O'G, Sullivan M F 1981 Partial undercutting facetectomy for bony entrapment of the lumbar nerve root. J. Bone Joint Surg. 63B: 330–335

82   Scoville W B, Corkhill G 1973 Lumbar disc surgery: technique of radical removal and early mobilisation. J. Neurosurg. 39: 265–269

'Fibrositis' and soft tissue pain syndromes

PERSPECTIVE

In this book the enormous personal and economic burden of low back pain is well documented. Most of the attention is centred around the acute episode and the importance of recognizing nerve root pressure associated with acute protrusion of disc material. Root pressure is dramatic and important, but fortunately involves less than 10% of those patients disabled with back pain. The rest have recovered to the extent that signs of nerve pressure have disappeared, or have never had such signs. The great majority of back pain sufferers need another system of diagnosis, and another system of therapy.

What of the other 90–95% Are they to continue to remain essentially undiagnosed, and shunted off to back classes for a routine, prepackaged programme of education and behaviour modification? This dismissive approach is often ineffective, and the patients turn to non-surgical consultants for help.

When they come to me, I may find medical problems such as unrecognized spondylitis, osteoporosis, or DISH. But far more commonly there will be one or both of two syndromes. The most common is abdominal muscle weakness, easily detected by the graded sit-up. This is important, but not the subject of this chapter. The other is the presence of a pain amplification syndrome (Table 20.1). Understanding of these syndromes follows easily from the discovery of tender points, and effective therapeutic opportunities often arise from the application of simple but unfamiliar clinical assessment techniques.

PAIN AMPLIFICATION SYNDROMES

The term 'amplification' implies that the increase in pain or tenderness has resulted from altered neuro-

Table 20.1 Pain amplification syndromes

Group 1: Tenderness at "Fibrositic" sites
1. Referred pain syndromes
2. "Fibrositis" syndrome
3. Experimental sleep deprivation
4. Narcotic withdrawal
5. Others
Group 2: Tenderness of different distribution
1. Reflex dystrophies
2. Tender shins of steroid therapy

physiological mechanisms, independent of psychological influences. The effect is selective, not diffuse. Certain sites become tender, but background pain threshold is unaltered.[1] The tenderness is quite pronounced: typically 50% greater than the tenderness of an inflamed rheumatoid joint, best demonstrated when both conditions coexist in the same patient. It still remains difficult for patients and their physicians to accept that there is not a local inflammatory lesion, particularly in the absence of full definition of the pain mechanism. It is frustrating also that technology in the form of biochemistry, histology and radiology has so far been of so little help. The best evidence comes from a careful examination of the clinical findings.

The point count

The clinician must have a systematic and effective approach to the examination of the peripheral joints, the spine and the non-articular regions. There must be a practised familiarity with the sites in which tenderness is likely to occur, and a technique which measures the quantity of tenderness, allowing for differences among individuals in general responses to pain stimulus. One approach is to do a 'point count', analogous to the 'joint count' used in assessing changes in the severity of peripheral joint inflammation. The basic idea is simple enough, and to the novice examiner there are only two methodological problems: where to press, and how hard to press.

A list of 14 sites at which tenderness may be found has been published,[2] and is reviewed below and in Figure 20.1.

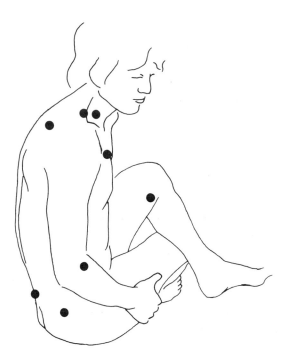

Fig. 20.1 Fourteen tender points. The tenderness can be quite localized. Skill and care in this assessment is rewarded.

The point count: 14 tender sites

— Low cervical: anterior aspects of intertransverse spaces C5-7
— Trapezius: midpoint of upper fold
— Costochondral: just lateral to 2nd junction, on upper surface
— Supraspinatus: above scapular spine, near medial border
— Lateral elbow: 'tennis elbow' site, 4 cm distal to epicondyle, in lateral intermuscular septum, moves with radius, deep to extensor to long finger
— Low lumbar: interspinous ligaments L4-S1
— Gluteus medius: deep in upper outer buttocks
— Medial fat pad: over ligament, proximal to joint line

This list is not all-inclusive and certainly not immutable. The firmness of pressure is determined by using as reference sites clinically 'silent' areas — the lower ribs, the forearm or thigh muscles, the fat pad medial to the knee. In order to be humane as well as precise, one works at the threshold of tenderness, reducing the stimulus for generally tender individuals. Pressure over the target site should be somewhat less firm, about 80% of the pressure over adjacent non-tender areas, and the site scored positive only if very distant tenderness is reported. This comparison of two sites, target and reference, may have to be done with some care, as the patient often assumes that the exquisite tenderness is due to deliberate roughness, and must be assured that the pressure on the 'target' site is in fact less than on the 'reference' area.

Numerical methods help. The use of a simple dolorimeter to record the pressure used is of value clinically as well as in investigation (Fig. 20.2). The quantity of tenderness may also be scored in terms of the number of tender points, and the distribution of these points examined for clues as the underlying mechanisms. A small number of points, clustered in a single region, unassociated with diffuse aching stiffness and fatigue, suggests a referred pain syndrome. A large number of tender sites, spread widely and symmetrically, with systemic symptoms, suggests the 'fibrositis' syndrome. The absence, presence, number and distribution of these points is of such help in clarifying otherwise ill-defined pain syndromes that I urge that some variation of this count be taught and used as part of the standard routine clinical examination.

Referred pain and associated phenomena

When a finger is injured, the patient can accurately localize the site of the pain and identify the nature of the stimulus. He or she can summon up an image of the finger, and draw a picture of the part and the site of injury. This kind of detailed knowledge of the position and environment of the hand is essential to function, and a large area of the cerebral cortex is assigned to this task.

However, we have no comparable need for information about deeply lying structures, and no similar cortical mechanism exists. We have no 'body image' of these deeply lying structures, and pain

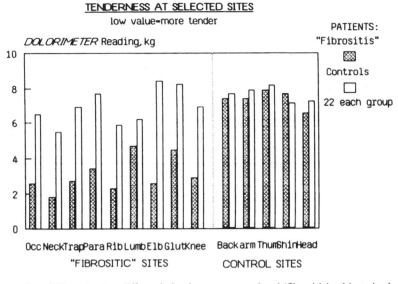

Fig. 20.2 Dolorimeter readings.[1] There is clear differentiation between normal and 'fibrositic' subjects in the readings at 'fibrositic' sites, and clear separation between 'fibrositic' and control sites, but *no* excess tenderness of 'fibrositic' subjects at control sites.

arising in them cannot therefore be accurately located. The pain must be referred, misinterpreted as arising in other structures, usually muscular areas and bony prominences sharing the same nerve supply and familiar enough to be included in the 'body image'. This misinterpretation is very persistent: the brain continues to insist that the problem is in the leg even after the intellect has understood that the real trouble is in the low back. The spread of pain is not dependent on nerve root compression, and the electric numbness in the fourth and fifth fingers produced by trauma to the ulnar nerve is not a good general illustration of the nature of referred pain. The areas to which pain is referred often develop secondary reflex changes, misguided but protective in intent. These include deep tenderness and hyperaesthesia, circulatory changes, and muscular splinting with inhibition of voluntary movement. These changes are enhanced by chilling, sleep deprivation, tension and fatigue.

Quality of referred pain

The quality of referred pain is determined more by the site to which it is referred than by the nature of the original pain stimulus. Anginal pain is of course not localized to the myocardium, as we have no body image of the heart muscle. It may be felt in the precordial region, where it is appreciated as a heaviness or a crushing pressure. It may be referred to the shoulder region, where it is felt as a deep ache, perhaps exacerbated by a draught. It may be referred to the forearm or hand, which may be described as dead, numb, woody or swollen. The same pain, arising in the same area of heart muscle, and travelling by the same pathways to association areas in the cerebral cortex, may simultaneously give three very different kinds of sensory impression to the patient struggling to find words to describe accurately the nature of his or her distress.

Pain equivalents

The qualities of deadness, numbness or swelling associated with distal referral should be particularly noted, as they are common to many pains referred distally in the limbs, and commonly are misinterpreted as evidence of neural involvement. Similarly, the patient may be absolutely convinced that the part is swollen, pointing to a perfectly normal fatty fullness, so that it is mistakenly accepted that an inflammatory process has been present.

Clustered distribution of referred tenderness

Tenderness ('hyperalgesia') in areas to which pain is referred is part of all the classic descriptions of referred pain.[3-6] These accounts placed emphasis on the development of skin tenderness, 'cutaneous hyperalgesia'. Deep referred tenderness is much more common than skin tenderness. The sites that become tender are the sites described above, i.e. exactly the same sites that become tender in the 'fibrositis' syndrome. The distribution is asymmetric and clustered in the often broad region of reference of the deep primary site. Pathology in any deep structure, visceral or musculoskeletal, can give rise to referred pain, but the neck and low back are the origin in the great majority of cases.

The cervical syndrome as a source of referred pain

The neck is vulnerable for a variety of reasons, of which the most important are compressive and shearing stresses arising in the unsupported arch of the cervical spine during sleep. Its importance as a source of referred pain and reflex dystrophic disorders has been much underestimated, because few observers know where to find the tenderness, including myself until a few years ago. The interspinous ligaments, posterior joints and muscles are relatively non-tender, and indeed massage of these structures often feels good to the patient with a stiff neck. The real tenderness is in the front of the lower neck, quite precisely located in the anterior aspects of the interspinous ligaments between C5 and C7. The dolorimeter can sample this by pressing through the lower sternomastoid muscle, but the tip of the examiner's thumb is more subtle, as it can be insinuated behind the muscle, well centrally, to localize accurately the sites of maximum tenderness. The patient is usually unaware of this tenderness, and has to be convinced that the examiner is not deliberately trying to hurt. The dolorimeter can help convince the patient and third parties that the tenderness is very real, and greater than at any other site tested.

Neck pain, referred pain or pain equivalents, neck tenderness, and referred tenderness at characteristic sites make up the cervical syndrome; loss of range of movement occurs only in late, severe cases. But sometimes the patient minimizes or even denies neck pain, and presents with headache, or pain about the shoulder region, lateral elbow, anterior chest or interscapular region. They may complain of pain and numbness of the hands, especially at night. The strong temptation is to make a local diagnosis, such as tennis elbow or costochondritis. Systematic point counts reveal the multiple, clustered distribution of tender points (Fig. 20.3), with unsuspected but marked asymmetrical tenderness deep in the neck, indicating the presence of a *silent cervical syndrome*. Perhaps microtrauma may have produced an undocumented inflammatory process at the tennis-elbow site; but once marked tenderness has also been shown in the lower neck, and in the mid-trapezius and costochondral junctions, and the lateral elbow tenderness is found to be maximum at precisely the site affected in referred pain syndromes, then why add an additional diagnosis? At least concede that measures to help the neck are appropriate if local measures fail. Knowledge of additional sites is helpful in the analysis of these cases. Two common ones are the tip of the coracoid (giving rise to frequently erroneous diagnoses of bicipital tendinitis), and the medial elbow.

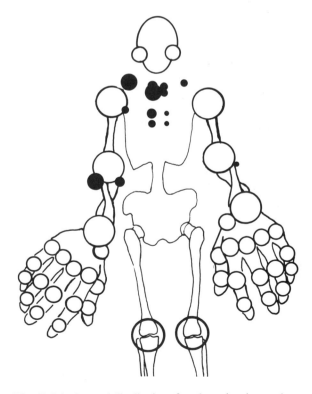

Fig. 20.3 A clustered distribution of tender points in a patient with a cervical strain syndrome, asymmetrical and concentrated in one region.

The low back syndrome

The low back syndrome may be similarly defined, consisting of low back pain, referred pain or pain equivalents, low back tenderness and referred tenderness. Again, this diagnosis is easy when back pain is prominent, or when there is a band of referred pain extending continuously from buttock to posterolateral thigh, calf and foot. But the referred symptoms may differ so markedly in quality from the back pain, or be separated from it in time or distribution, so that the diagnosis is not obvious, again a *silent low back syndrome*. Furthermore, in the low back we do not have access to the deep spinal structures, and there is no lumbar equivalent to the low anterior neck tenderness. We must make do with the interspinous ligament tenderness, and with the characteristic pattern of multiple, asymmetrical distant referred tenderness. Gluteus medius tenderness is nearly always present, and often more marked than the interspinous tenderness. The medial fat pad tenderness is even better, because it is not central to an area of pain and is totally unsuspected by the patient. Tenderness here does not result from knee-joint pathology, and it may be important to demonstrate to the patient the absence of stress pain or tenderness in the knee, in contrast to the asymmetrical and marked tenderness of the fat pad. The patient often has a conviction that there is arthritis in the knee, reaffirmed by the brain's stubborn refusal to relate the knee region pain to the back, so that the evidence and its interpretation must be demonstrated with care to the patient. Again, knowledge of additional characteristic sites may be very helpful in establishing the multiplicity and asymmetry of unsuspected points. The insertion of soleus into Achilles' tendon, and in the medial instep the origin of the short flexor muscle to the great toe, are two additional sites commonly affected.

THE 'FIBROSITIS' SYNDROME

17% of adults complain of musculoskeletal pain, and many do not have degenerative or inflammatory joint disease. Their pain is distressing, but examination reveals no swollen joints, no injured or damaged tissues. In the study of such patients, localized points of acute tenderness are both the

mystery and the solution. In the referred pain syndromes, pain arising from a deep central source is felt in another, more peripheral site. A special kind of enhanced pain sensitivity has developed in the involved segments as part of the neurological response to chronic regional pain.

The enhancement of pain transmission may be central rather than segmental, with effects that are general rather than regional. When multiple regions are chronically involved, with diffuse aching and stiffness, and a wide distribution of tender points, the clinical descriptive term 'fibrositis syndrome' is used.

The cardinal features of 'fibrositis' are:
1. A rheumatic pain syndrome
2. A wide distribution of tender points
3. The sleep disturbance
4. The irritable everything syndrome
5. The personality.

The rheumatic pain syndrome

The pain or aching is widespread, poorly circumscribed and deep, referred to muscles or bony prominences. When central, it has an aching character; when peripheral, pain may be replaced by pain equivalents, with swelling, stiffness or numbness. The stiffness is an increase of a sense of tissue tension or of muscular effort required towards the extremes of range. These symptoms are concentrated in the broad areas of reference of the cervical and lumbar segments and tend to shift with time, so that the patients recurrently present with 'new' sites of complaints. The stiffness is worse in the morning and is increased by weather changes, cold, tension, fatigue or excess use. Simple analgesics are disappointing, but heat, massage or a holiday may give relief.

The wide distribution of tender points

The individual tender points are precisely the same in 'fibrositis' as in referred pain syndromes, and the difference lies in the number of points, the widespread distribution and the association with other general manifestations. Many of the points are unknown to the patient and are situated in areas with little cortical representation or emotional significance. The pattern is impossible to feign. Dolorimetry can be helpful; in psychogenic pain syndromes the tenderness is diffuse or variable, while in 'fibrositis' it is predictable, focal and constant. Old[7,8] and new[9] studies may describe subtle pathologies, but they have failed to show any local inflammation. The tenderness should appreciated as an alteration in neurological function, not the result of immunological or other damage.

The sleep disturbance

The exhaustion may be most disabling and not clearly related to lack of rest. It is often marked in the morning, and paralyses as well as punishes initiative. The patients emphasize their exhaustion, but may minimize their sleep disturbance. They may have been light sleepers for years and relate their frequent and prolonged wakefulness to pain. Virtually all arise feeling unrefreshed (this is the key question to ask), more exhausted than at bedtime the night before. After stress, they may spend whole nights without sleep. (See Table 20.2).

Key studies have provided evidence of a specific disturbance in sleep physiology. In the first,[10] 'fibrositic' subjects showed a decrease in stages 3 and 4 slow-wave sleep, with intrusion of a rapid alpha rhythm, as determined by computer analysis of the energy-frequency spectra (see Fig. 20.3), and all showed an overnight increase in tenderness measured by dolorimeter. These observations have since been confirmed and extended in a large number of other patients. High-energy bursts of alpha intruding into slow-wave sleep were described by Hauri[11] as alpha-delta sleep, and its association with aching, fatigue and stiffness was also described.[12] This more florid pattern can be read by eye, and was recognized in 8 or 26 'chronic pain' patients.[13]

Table 20.2 Symptoms of sleep disturbance (after Campbell et al[2])

Symptom	"Fibrositis" group (n = 22) %	Control group (n = 22) %
Waking with aching, stiffness	100	23
Tired during the day	100	41
Waking tired	95	32
Waking frequently	68	59
Difficulty falling asleep	36	23
Waking early	36	36

In another study,[14] experimental reproduction of aspects of the 'fibrositis' syndrome was achieved in healthy university students. After control nights, for three nights they were deprived either of rapid-eye movement (REM), or stage 4 non-REM sleep by a buzzer, supplemented when necessary by hand arousal. The buzzer caused a rapid alpha rhythm to appear in the e.e.g. superimposed on the slow wave pattern, mimicking the pattern seen in the 'fibrositis' patients. No increase in tenderness was associated with REM deprivation, but disturbance of slow-wave non-REM sleep was associated with a marked overnight increase in tenderness scores and symptoms of anorexia, overwhelming physical tiredness and heaviness. (See Fig. 20.4.)

The irritable everything syndrome

'Fibrositis' patients do not simply report pain, they express it in urgent verbal and body language. Pressure on a tender point may result in a dramatic twisting total body response, the 'leap' sign. The perception of sensations other than pain is also much enhanced in 'fibrositis' patients. They may be hypersensitive to cold, noise and environmental irritants of all kinds, and to internal stimuli such as drug effects, cough, bladder fullness. The irritable bowel syndrome may be the GI manifestation of 'fibrositis'.[15] They have often had inappropriate investigation and therapy because of headaches, chest pain, urinary frequency. As with the tenderness, the hypersensitivity is widespread but not general. Patients with rheumatoid arthritis and 'fibrositis' have much more tenderness at their points than their joints.

The 'fibrositis' personality

These patients set high standards, as demanding of themselves as of others. They are caring, honest, tidy, committed, moral, industrious. Their vices are their virtues carried to excess. They hate to complain, they respectfully doubt, they forgivably fail to comply, they loyally reject. Their perfectionism can by trying, but they are often very effective in their chosen field of activity and have unusual loyalty from employers and family. Queen Victoria's husband, Prince Albert, was a classic case: 'excessively conscientious on quite minor matters'.[16]

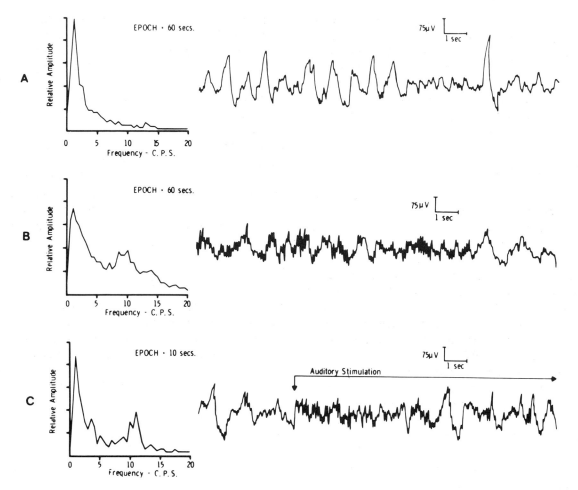

Fig. 20.4 E.e.g.s with computer analysis of frequency spectra during deep non-REM sleep in A, a normal subject; B, a 'fibrositic' subject; C, a normal subject disturbed by a buzzer. Note the alpha intrusion in B and C, indicated by energy at about 10 cycles per second.[10]

'Fibrositics' are not abnormal, just characteristic. They deeply resent any suggestion that they are using their illness as a crutch, as they drive themselves harder than most, and dislike other crutches, such as alcohol and prescribed medication. They are not depressed,[17,18] and the concept of 'masked depression' may have arisen because of the response of 'fibrositic' symptoms to tricyclic medication.

The association of 'fibrositis' and other diseases

Therapy is often determined by the urgency of the patient's complaints, and not by the severity of the underlying disease. Patients with rheumatoid arth-ritis, cervical or lumbar disc disease, or a whole host of other conditions may have amplification of their symptoms by 'fibrositic' mechanisms. The 'point count' allows rapid recognition of this complication and avoidance of the excess of therapy which might otherwise follow. Moldofsky & Chester[19] identified a subgroup of 'paradoxical responders' among hospitalized rheumatoid patients, identified by worsening mood with improving disease. When first admitted, these patients seemed cheerful and cooperative, but they became depressed, complaining and agitated as treatment progressed. They were more likely to receive prolonged hospitalization, extensive investigation and hazardous medical and surgical therapies, with increased morbidity and even mortality. 'The squeaky wheel gets the grease.'

Almost half the hospitalized rheumatoid patients showed this pattern, and on examination the 'fibrositic' sites were characteristically more tender than their swollen joints.

Prevalence, classification and nomenclature

Figure 20.5 shows the number of tender points recorded in an unselected group of rheumatic disease patients.[20] Clearly the prevalence of 'fibrositis' will be dependent on the point count criterion chosen. In published studies, the criteria have varied from 4 of 53 points[15] to 12 of 14.[10] The 20% with 4 or more points will include a majority with simple referred pain syndromes, without the exhaustion, stiffness and personality associated with large numbers of points, and it seems inappropriate to apply the same name, be it 'fibromyalgia' or 'fibrositis', to these very different groups. These archaic names are probably beyond rehabilitation, and Moldofsky[21] has suggested the 'rheumatic pain modulation syndrome' for the generalized syndrome associated with non-restorative sleep. The referred pain syndromes associated with tender points can simply be named according to the source pathology. 'Localized fibrositis' disappears into 'tender point'.

One may wish to reserve judgment, but there seems to be little need for the concept of 'secondary fibrositis'. The data collected by Wolfe[21] and Moldofsky[22] suggest that the 'fibrositic' symptoms seen in patients with rheumatoid arthritis or osteoarthritis are identical in their pathogenesis and manifestation to 'primary fibrositis', and rarely a polymyalgic extension of the underlying disease.

Treatment

In 'fibrositis', multiple factors combine to produce the symptom complex, and explanations may involve:
1. Referred pain and reflex responses
2. Mechanical stresses in neck and low back
3. The sleep disturbance
4. The irritable everything syndrome, and
5. Attitudes and expectations.

The pain is neurological but not neurotic in origin. The distress arises from an interaction between segmental and central factors, with referred pain and reflex tenderness, aggravated and prolonged by tension and sleep deprivation.

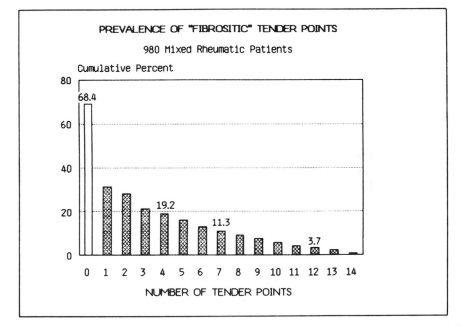

Fig. 20.5 Number of tender points found in unselected rheumatic disease patients.[20] The estimated prevalence of 'fibrositis' or 'fibromyalgia' is very sensitive to this criterion. In general, patients with fatigue and stiffness will tend to have more, diffusely distributed points; and those with referred pain will have fewer, clustered points.

Recommendations

Simple analgesic methods can do much to break the vicious cycles described above. These may include enteric coated aspirin, 600–900 mg four times daily for continuous, background pain relief, with added propoxyphene 65 mg, or codeine 15 mg, sparingly as needed for peaks. Since no inflammation is involved, anti-inflammatory drugs are not indicated. Prednisone has been found to be ineffective in the 'fibrositis' syndrome.[23] Heat, liniments, massage or other counterirritant therapy give real if short-lived relief.

Mechanical stresses in neck and low back

The vast majority of mechanical problems affecting the spine arise in the lower neck, or two lower lumbar levels. The key to success in treating the neck is support for the arch of the cervical spine during sleep. A pair of cervical ruffs, made by enclosing 20 by 60 cm (8″ by 24″) gauze pads within tubes of 7.5 cm (3″) stockinette, tied loosely in front, are quite effective for acute therapy. However, many patients stop wearing their ruffs when they begin to feel better, and so fail to prevent the next attack. Neck-support pillows are cooler and more comfortable for prolonged use.

The low back is at the extreme range of hyperextension in the standing position in virtually all patients with low back problems, and many have such weak abdominal muscles that they can neither improve their posture nor use a positive intra-abdominal pressure to spare their back. Weak abdominals should be recognized and corrected by specific progressive sit-up exercises, with hips and knees bent to eliminate the lumbar lordosis, and feet held. Avoid straight-leg raising or push-ups, which strongly compress the hyperextended lower spine. The safe posture for the low back is that of an athlete with knees bent and back flat, not the erect ideal of parents or teachers.

The sleep disturbance

Oxazepam 15 mg or flurazepam 15–30 mg, may be used as night sedatives but do not restore the normal sleep pattern. Tricyclic agents such as imipramine or amitryptiline, 10 or 75 mg early in the evening, are more effective, at the cost of more side-effects. All the tricyclics currently available are too long-lasting, with 30-hour half-lives. 'Fibrositic' patients tend to be very sensitive to the hangover somnolence associated with these drugs, and the drugs are best reserved for crises.

Attitudes and expectations

These patients are often perfectionists, with high standards of performance for themselves, their families and their therapist. They are particularly resentful of any suggestion that they are 'quitters' or 'fakers'. They have often been unusually effective, but at too high a cost.

Tension normally and necessarily accompanies major effort. Consider an athlete preparing for a 4-minute mile, or an actress for a first night, or a student facing a final examination. The mother who must guide three explosive children while protecting a civilized moment for herself and her husband, and the loyal but unappreciated office worker, have less dramatic but more chronic and equally demanding roles. The defect in patients with fibrositis is not the build-up of tension, but the failure to 'get out from under'.

Tension and aching are built-in reaction patterns for such patients, and complete long-term freedom from symptoms is unlikely. The anatomical prognosis is excellent, and the prospect of partial relief is also good. The patients should continue to be involved; they are not helped by restricting activities, and it is extremely important that work patterns not be interrupted. We set realistic goals, and keep investigation and treatment patterns simple. Do not interrupt employment for medical care. Advise tension-dissipating routines, such as exercise, saunas, massage, cocktails or a holiday. The activities should be social, and represent pleasure rather than duty. A night out, a weekend away, or other part-time escape from four walls or imprisoning interpersonal situations may often have to be specifically prescribed.

Fitness

There is accumulating evidence that a most effective way of controlling the pain is to achieve a high degree of general fitness, especially cardiopulmonary fitness. With other joint diseases, joint protection must be stressed, and caution used in exercise. With 'fibrositis', exercise is strongly urged, even at the cost of early increase in pain.

Responsibility

Despite (or because) of their perfectionism, 'fibrositic' patients often comply poorly. They don't use their neck supports, don't do their sit-ups, don't take their prescribed medicines (all for the best of reasons), don't get involved in fitness activities, don't adjust their schedules and attitudes, and return for the second appointment feeling no better. This makes it easy for the doctor. All that need be done is to go over the ground again, assure them that they will not improve until they follow the appropriate programme, and assure them also that the responsibility for improvement is theirs. This is not the time to prescribe tricyclic drugs, a strategy which makes the doctor primarily responsible for all outcomes, good and bad. The therapist points the way, and is a forgiving friend and counsellor, wary of the temptation to become a healer, accepting the crucial transfer of responsibility. It is the patient's job to improve.

REFERENCES

1   Campbell S M, Clark S, Tindall E A, Forehand M E, Bennett R M O 1983 Clinical characteristics of fibrositis. Arth. Rheum. 26: 817–824
2   Smythe H A, Moldofsky H 1977 Two contributions to understanding of the 'fibrositis' syndrome. Bull. Rheum. Dis. 28: 928–932
3   Kellgren J H 1949 Deep pain sensibility. Lancet 1: 943–949
4   Kellgren J H 1938 Observations on referred pain arising from muscle. Clin. Sci. 3: 174–190
5   Kellgren J H 1939 On distribution of pain arising from deep somatic structures with charts of segmental pain areas. Clin. Sci. 4: 35–46
6   Lewis T, Kellgren J H 1939 Observations relating to referred pain, visceromotor reflexes and other associated phenomena. Clin. Sci. 4: 47–71
7   Simons D G 1975 Muscle pain syndromes — Part 1. Am. J. Phys. Med. 54: 289–311
8   Simons D G 1976 Muscle pain syndromes — Part 2. Am. J. Phys. Med. 55: 15–42
9   Kalyan-Raman U P, Kalyan-Raman K, Yunus M B, Masi A T 1984 Muscle pathology in primary fibromyalgia syndrome: a light microscopic, histochemical and ultrastructural study. J. Rheumatol. 11: 808–813
10 Moldofsky H, Scarisbrick P, England R, Smythe H 1975 Musculoskeletal symptoms and non-REM sleep disturbance in patients with 'fibrositis syndrome' and healthy subjects. Psychosomat. Med. 37: 341–351
11 Hauri P, Hawkins D R 1973 Alpha–delta sleep. Electroencephalogr. Clin. Neurophysiol. 34: 233
12 Hauri P 1977 The sleep disorders. Upjohn, Kalamazoo, p 51
13 Wittig R M, Zorick F J, Blumer D, Heilbronn M, Roth T 1982 Distributed sleep in patients complaining of chronic pain. J. Nerv. Ment. Dis. 170: 429
14 Moldofsky H, Scarisbrick P 1976 Induction of neurasthenic musculoskeletal pain syndrome by selective sleep stage deprivation. Psychosomat. Med. 38: 35–44
15 Yunus M, Masi A T, Calabro J J, Miller K A, Feigenbaum S L 1981 Primary fibromyalgia (fibrositis): clinical study of 50 patients with matched normal controls. Semin Arth Rheum 11: 151–171
16 James R R 1984 Prince Albert. Knopf,
17 Clark S, Campbell S M, Forehand M E, Tindal E A, Bennett R M 1985 Clinical characteristics of fibrositis. II. A 'blinded' controlled study using standard psychological tests. Arth Rheum 28: 132–137
18 Smythe H A 1984 Problems with the MMPI. J Rhematol 11: 417–418
19 Moldofsky H, Chester W J 1970 Pain and mood patterns in patients with rheumatoid arthritis. Psychosomat Med 32: 309–318
20 Wolfe F, Cathey M A 1983 Prevalence of primary and secondary fibrositis. J Rheumatol 10: 965–968
21 Moldofsky H 1982 Rheumatic pain modulation syndrome: the interrelationships between sleep, central nervous system serotonin and pain. In: Critchley M, Friedman A P, Sicuteri F (eds) Advances in neurology, vol 33. Raven Press, New York, p 51–57
22 Moldofksy H, Lue F A, Smythe H A 1883 Alpha EEG sleep and morning symptoms in rhematoid arthritis. J Rheumatol 10: 373–379
23 Clark S, Tindall E, Bennett R B 1984 A double blind crossover study of prednisone in the treatment of fibrositis. (Abstract). Arth Rheum 27 (supp), S76

Chronic inflammation and fibrosis in back pain syndromes

INTRODUCTION

Although back pain is most commonly of mechanical cause, it can arise due to inflammatory, neoplastic or metabolic disorders. Mechanical or structural problems are by far the most common. These include prolapsed intervertebral disc, lumbar spondylosis, spondylolisthesis etc. The majority of patients suffer recurrent attacks of back pain, but each individual attack usually gets better within a comparatively short period. However, some patients suffer chronic back pain with resulting severe disability. In patients with chronic back pain for whom infective metabolic and neoplastic causes have been excluded, it is commonly difficult or impossible to make a precise diagnosis. Radiographs may show evidence of lumbar spondylosis, but the correlation between radiological evidence of lumbar spondylosis and back pain is poor. Lawrence[1] conducted surveys on whole populations, comparing the frequency of back pain with radiological evidence of lumbar spondylosis. He found some increase in prevalence of back pain in patients with the grossest radiological changes compared with those with normal or virtually normal radiographs, but the difference in prevalence rate was quite small, and indeed only accounted for some 12% of the problem. We frequently see patients with gross evidence of lumbar spondylosis but no back symptoms, and vice versa. In ankylosing hyperostosis there is very marked evidence of osteophyte formation, but this syndrome is not associated with back pain.

It therefore appears that the presence of degenerative changes alone is not enough to account for the severity of chronic back problems, and other factors, presently poorly identified, must play an important role in the development of back pain.

ARACHNOIDITIS AND NERVE ROOT SHEATH FIBROSIS

Thickening and scarring of the membranes surrounding the spinal cord and nerve roots may in turn lead to nerve root damage. It is a recognized cause of severe back and nerve root problems, and particularly occurs in patients who have undergone invasive procedures in the spine. The first description is attributed to Quincke in 1893. Early reports suggested it might follow meningitis due to infections from viruses,[2] *Neisseria meningitis*,[3,4] *Haemophilus influenzae*,[5] syphilis, gonorrhoea, tuberculosis and middle ear-infections.[3,6,7] The use of spinal anaesthetics has also been implicated.[8] However, it is most commonly recognized in patients who have undergone myelography, particularly using an oil-based medium[9] and/or have undergone one or more laminectomies.[10]

The recognition of arachnoiditis and nerve root sheath fibrosis is difficult and commonly requires specialist imaging techniques such as further radiculography or CAT scanning. Without such studies it can be impossible to recognize the presence of this problem. However, the recognized spectrum of arachnoiditis probably represents only the 'tip of the iceberg'.[11] The patients with non-specific back pain without definite nerve root abnormalities are unlikely to undergo radiculography or CAT scanning, and in many such cases it is not known whether arachnoiditis or nerve root sheath fibrosis of clinical significance is present. The secondary development of scar tissue formation could account for the development of chronic back and nerve root pain and its variable presence for the relatively poor association with radiological evidence of degenerative disease of the spine.

Pathology

In disc prolapse, pain arising in the nerve root distribution is thought to be a consequence of mechanical pressure on the nerve root. There is however evidence of secondary inflammatory changes occurring in the perineurium. Lindhal and Rexed[12] examined ten specimens of nerve root and found several cases of hyperplasia and chronic inflammatory changes in the perineurium. It is possible that the development of scar tissue in such cases is responsible for the persistence of pain in those patients that fail to improve. The stages in the development of arachnoiditis have been classified by Burton[13] as follows:

Radiculitis. Inflammation of the pia-arachnoid with associated hyperaemia and swelling of the nerve roots of the cauda equina. This stage is characterized by a minimal fibroblast proliferation and the beginning of deposition of strands of collagen between nerve roots and pia-arachnoid.

Arachnoiditis. Progression of fibroblast proliferation and collagen deposition. Nerve root swelling has decreased. Nerve roots are now adherent to each other and to the pia-arachnoid.

Adhesive arachnoiditis. The end stage of the inflammatory process. Marked pia-arachnoid proliferation with dense collagen deposition has produced complete encapsulation of the nerve roots with are now hypoaemic and have undergone extensive atrophy. This process can involve the nerve root sleeves alone, or extend to involve the sub-arachnoid space.

There may also be loculated cysts containing spinal fluid and/or residual oily medium from previous myelography. When large, these cysts can also produce compression of local nervous tissue.

It is of particular relevance that, in the early stages, arachnoiditis is characterized by a fibrinous exudate with a negligible cellular component and without notable injection of the blood vessels within the arachnoid.[14] The development of adhesive arachnoiditis is suggested as similar to adhesions elsewhere in which fibrin-covered roots and redundant arachnoidal membranes stick together during the stage of resolution of the inflammation. Bands of fibrinous adhesions become the bridges for proliferating fibrocytes which lay down collagen, converting them into collagenized adhesions. This eventually leads to adhesive arachnoiditis.

Our own observations in a number of biopsy specimens have shown the presence of extensive collagenous tissue with relatively little or no inflammatory infiltration but with masses of fibrin intimately blending with the excessive collagen (Fig. 21.1).

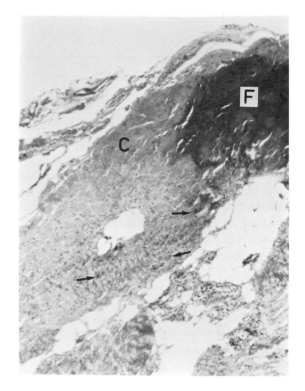

Fig 21.1 Meninges and peri-menigeal fat showing the interface between fibrin (F) and collagenous fibrous tissue (C). Fibrin is also seen distributed within the collagen (arrows). MSB×64. (By courtesy of Dr A. J. Freemont).

The role of fibrin in chronic inflammation

Deposition of fibrin is a common process in association with chronic inflammation. A possible pathogenic role in the chronicity of such problems has been suggested. In particular, the first experimental models of arthritis in animals[15] were produced by the intra-articular injection of both autologous and heterologous fibrin in sensitized rabbits. There is evidence that the persistence of fibrin deposited in vessel walls leads to failure of nutrients or oxygen to diffuse into the tissues, or, alternatively, if it is deposited around capillaries, it may block the diffusion of oxygen with consequent ischaemia of the nerve roots.[16] Elevated fibrinogen levels in the blood can be associated with elevated blood viscosity and poor perfusion of tissues. All these mechanisms may be responsible for the development of chronic tissue damage.

The fibrinolytic system

The fibrinolytic system is a complex cascade of reactions responsible for cleaving fibrin to fibrin degradation products. The system is summarized in Figure 21.2. Briefly, plasminogen activator is released from vessel walls and damaged tissues to activate plasminogen to form plasmin, and plasmin is responsible for cleaving fibrin to fibrin degradation products which can be eliminated. The whole system is controlled by a series of inhibitors, the most important of which are α-2-macroglobulin and α-2-antiplasmin. Defective fibrinolytic activity can arise due to reduction of circulating plasminogen, release of plasminogen activator or increase of the inhibitors α-2-antiplasmin and α-2-macroglobulin.

There are important analogies with other disorders in which chronic inflammation and fibrosis develops and in which there is excess of fibrin deposition in tissues. In particular, in venous lipdermatosclerosis (post-phlebitic leg syndrome),[16] chronic fibrosis and inflammation in the calf is associated with fibrin deposition in the tissues and with defective fibrinolytic activity. Similarly, in cutaneous vasculitis[17] and in systemic sclerosis similar pathological changes are associated with defective fibrinolytic activity.

These observations have led us to undertake studies of fibrinolytic activity in patients with severe chronic back pain syndromes, including patients with post-myelography and post-laminectomy back pain, and also including patients with lumbar spondylosis and spinal stenosis. Measurements are performed under standard basal conditions at the same time each morning with the subjects resting, not having smoked or eaten for at least ten hours. Measurements are made of the euglobulin clot lysis time[18] and fibrin plate lysis area,[19] which are direct measures of fibrinolytic activity. We also measure the fibrinogen levels[20] and the plasminogen, α-2-antiplasmin and α-2-macroglobulin by using chromogenic substrate assays and immunodiffusion techniques.

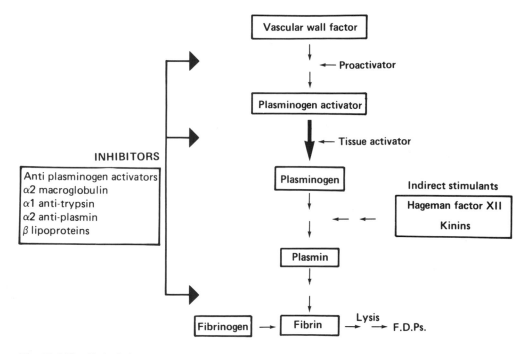

Fig. 21.2 The fibrinolytic system.

Fibrinolytic studies in chronic back pain patients

In our initial studies[21] we have demonstrated significant defective fibrin activity with prolongation of the euglobulin clot lysis time (ELT), reduction of fibrin plate lysis area (FPLA) and plasminogen (Pg) levels and increases of the inhibitors α-2-macroglobulin (α-2M) and α-2-antiplasmin with normal fibrinogen (Fg) levels (Table 21.1).

We have now extended these observations to a much larger series of patients and obtained similar results from separate groups of post-laminectomy, post-myelography, lumbar spondylosis and spinal stenosis groups of patients. It therefore appears that defective fibrinolytic activity is a common problem in patients with severe chronic back pain syndromes. This could be responsible for the persistence of fibrin deposits in tissues and the chronicity of chronic fibrosis in involved areas.

The cause of this fibrinolytic defect is unknown. It is possible that it preceded the particular back problem but its presence led to the persistence of fibrin and the chronicity of the pain. Alternatively, some patients may develop a persistent fibrinolytic defect following injury, and this serves to perpetuate the back problem.

Sequential measurements

In order to elucidate the sequence of events, we have undertaken sequential measurements in patients presenting with acute back pain and sciatica and compared them with matched control subjects. Following the sequence of events in eight subjects (Table 21.2), we have found that at presentation the sciatica patients had a prolongation of the euglobulin clot lysis time but a normal fibrin plate lysis area. Two weeks later there was a non-significant fall in the fibrin plate lysis area. At three months the fall in fibrin plate lysis area had become statistically significant. By six months, although the mean increase in euglobulin clot lysis time and decreased in fibrin plate lysis area were unchanged, the differences from controls had become non-significant.

The difficulty with these data is that they include some patients in whom back pain cleared completely but others who had persistent problems. By examining data from individual subjects, the sequence of

Table 21.1 Fibrinolytic activity in chronic back pain patients and matched controls

	ELT min	FPLA (mm²)	Fg (mg/dl)	Pg (%)	α-2-antiplasmin %	α-2M (%)
Controls (18)	125.2 ±57.0	103.4 ±25.7	278.1 ±100.5	108.8 ±18.4	110.8 ±12.7	101.0 ±15.2
Patients (18)	265.5 ±135.4	78.2 ±36.8	263.3 ±123.0	99.0 ±16.5	124.1 ±23.5	125.3 ±32.8
P(2-tail) Mann-Witney U	<0.01	<0.05	NS	<0.05	<0.05	<0.05

Table 21.2 Sequential measurements in patients presenting with acute sciatica compared with matched controls

		Sciatica patients	Controls	Significance P
Entry	ELT	244.0 ± 121.5	93.9 ± 27.9	<0.05
	FPLA	113.4 ± 43.8	104.5 ± 30.4	NS
2 weeks	ELT	270.5 ± 69.3	90.8 ± 34.1	<0.01
	FPLA	65.0 ± 35.2	105.5 ± 32.9	NS
3 months	ELT	261.9 ± 77.7	93.9 ± 27.9	<0.025
	FPLA	76.6 ± 11.9	104.5 ± 30.4	<0.05
6 months	ELT	255.4 ± 85.9	90.9 ± 34.1	NS
	FPLA	70.2 ± 16.0	105.5 ± 32.9	NS

events has become clearer. Figure 21.3 illustrates the sequence of changes in a patient presenting with acute sciatica which rapidly improved after a couple of weeks. The patient developed significant abnormalities of the euglobulin clot lysis time and fibrin plate lysis area, which rapidly improved back to normal. In contrast, Figure 21.4 shows the sequence of events in a patient who developed acute sciatica which failed to resolve. The abnormalities in fibrinolytic activity have persisted and indeed have become somewhat worse.

These data may explain certain associations of chronic back pain that have been identified in epidemiological surveys. Frymoyer et al[22] found a significant increase in smoking in sufferers from severe back pain compared with asymptomatic controls. Suggestions regarding the cause of this association have included excess coughing, emotional, recreational and environmental factors, but Frymoyer et al[22] also speculated that cigarette smoke or one of its constituents might have a direct adverse physiological effect on the spine. It is known that smoking is associated with a defect in fibrinolytic activity.[23] It is therefore possible that smoking is associated with chronic back pain by this mechanism.

Similarly, Westrin[24,25] and Gyntelberg[26] found a higher prevalence of ischaemic heart disease in back pain sufferers. Ischaemic heart disease is associated with defective fibrinolytic activity, so that a common mechanism may explain the association with chronic back pain.

Fibrinolytic enhancement therapy

The management of the patient with arachnoiditis is unsatisfactory. In particular, symptoms are poorly controlled by analgesics and anti-inflammatory agents, and physical therapy only offers marginal relief. It is possible to remove scar tissue surgically, and this procedure may be enhanced by the use of the dissecting microscope.[27] The operation may produce some short-term improvement but commonly the scar tissue recurs, with recurrence of symptoms. If the hypothesis of a defective fibrinolytic mechanism underlying the chronicity of back pain problems is correct, stimulation of fibrinolytic activity may offer a new approach to treating such problems.

In the condition venous lipodermatosclerosis, there is chronic inflammation and fibrosis in the

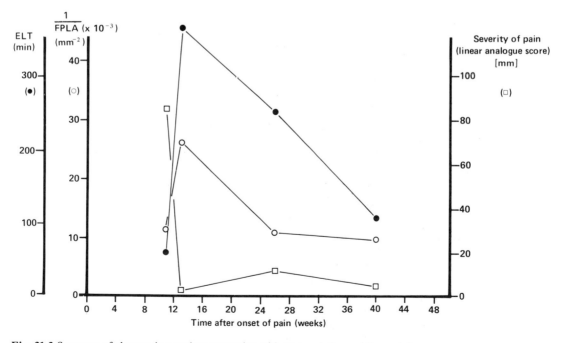

Fig. 21.3 Sequence of changes in a patient presenting with acute sciatica rapidly resolving

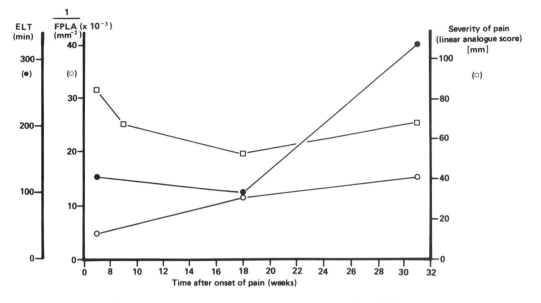

Fig. 21.4 Sequence of changes in a patient who developed acute sciatica which failed to resolve

tissues of the calf associated with fibrin deposition and similar evidence of defective fibrinolytic activity. A controlled trial of fibrinolytic enhancement therapy using stanozolol not only corrected the biochemical defect in the blood but also reduced the area of liposclerosis, with a significant improvement in symptoms.[16] Similarly, in systemic sclerosis, we have found that fibrinolytic enhancement will produce a significant improvement in microcirculatory blood flow,[28] and fibrinolytic enhancement has been found effective in cutaneous vasculitis.[17]

These results have led us to undertake preliminary studies with patients with severe chronic back pain syndromes. The drug used, stanozolol, is a non-virilizing anabolic steroid. It has the property of stimulating fibrinolytic activity. In some female patients it may produce mild androgenic side-effects and may occasionally disturb liver function. At the present time I do not believe that it should be used for back pain patients except where a fibrinolytic defect has been demonstrated and the course of the patient has been followed under strictly controlled conditions.

We now have a number of anecdotal cases treated in this way, with apparently marked improvement in the clinical parameters associated with correction of the fibrinolytic defect.

Representative case

A 36-year-old female schoolteacher had suffered from chronic back pain for ten years and was severely disabled. Examination showed all spinal movements to be limited. On investigation the ESR was 2mm/h with a normal blood count and biochemical profile. Tissue type was negative for HLA B27. X-ray of the lumbar spine showed minor spondylotic changes only. Fibrinolytic assessments showed gross evidence of defective activity with a prolonged ELT, reduced FPLA, elevated fibrinogen, low plasminogen, normal α-2-antiplasmin but elevated α-2-macroglobulin. She was treated for three months with stanozolol 5 mg bd, with gradual improvement of her symptoms and normalization of the fibrinolytic parameters. At that stage she had developed some mild androgenic problems, with disturbance of menstruation. She therefore discontinued the drug. Over the subsequent six months the symptoms gradually recurred and the fibrinolytic abnormality redeveloped. She then decided to go back onto stanozolol and again there was improvement in symptoms and normalization of fibrinolytic activity (Table 21.3).

Cases such as this suggest that this form of treatment may be effective for some such patients.

Table 21.3 Treatment with stanozolol in a representative case

	Initial	\multicolumn{5}{c}{Months}				
	Initial	1	2	3	9	11
ELT	177	74	67	62	128	72
FPLA	86	144	147	143	140	147
Fg	225	200	92	125	115	130
Pg	72	98	100	119	75	142
α-2-antiplasmin	95	95	116	115	108	100
α-2M	158	95	105	81	98	86
Stanozolol						

However, a double blind controlled trial is required to validate this approach and is currently in progress.

HYPOTHESIS OF A MECHANISM FOR CHRONICITY OF LOW BACK PAIN

The various tissue within the spine may be damaged by a wide variety of events. These include trauma, surgery, myelography, spondylosis etc. The actual damage produces localised inflammation with fibrin deposition. Normally this resolves so that the pain is only a transient event. For some patients, however, there is a defect in fibrinolytic activity. This defect may be a consequence of the injury, the chronic inflammation or even its treatment, or may be due to other unrecognized problems. The defect leads to failure to clear fibrin and persistence of chronic inflammation and scar tissue, and in turn this leads to chronicity of the back pain (Fig. 21.5). This

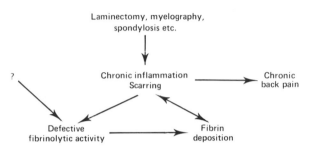

Fig. 21.5 Hypothesis of a mechanism for the chronicity of low back pain.

hypothesis may explain why scar tissue recurs after surgical treatment of arachnoiditis and also the association of chronic back pain with smoking and ischaemic heart disease. If correct it suggests that fibrinolytic enhancement may offer a new approach in the management of such problems.

REFERENCES

1 Lawrence J S 1977 Rheumatism in populations. Heinemann, London, p 68–97
2 Barker L F, Ford F R 1937 Chronic arachnoiditis obliterating the spinal arachnoid space. JAMA 109: 785
3 Elkington J St C 1936 Meningitis serosa circumscripta. Brain 59: 181
4 Gotshall R A 1972 Conus medullaris syndrome after meningococcal meningitis. New Eng. J. Med. 286: 882
5 Glista G G, Sullivan T D, Brumlik J 1980 Spinal cord involvement in acute bacterial meningitis. JAMA 243: 1362
6 Horrax G 1924 Generalised cisternal arachnoiditis simulating cerebellar tumour: its surgical treatment and end results. Arch. Surg. 9: 95
7 Stookey B 1927 Adhesive spinal arachnoiditis simulating spinal cord tumour. Arch. Neurol. Psychiat. 17: 151
8 Arner O 1952 Complications following spinal anaesthaesia. Acta Chir. Scand. suppl 167
9 Hansen E B, Fahrenburg A, Praestholm J 1978 Late

meningeal effects of myelographic contrast medium with special reference to metrizamide. Br. J. Radiol. 51: 321–327
10 de la Porte C, Siegfried J 1983 Lumbosacral spinal fibrosis (spinal arachnoiditis). Spine 8: 593–603
11 Hoffman G S, Ellsworth C A, Wells E E, Frank W A, Mackie R W 1983 Spinal arachnoiditis. What is the clinical spectrum? II. Arachnoiditis induced by Pantopaque/autologous blood in dogs, a possible model for human disease. Spine 8: 541–551
12 Lindhal O, Rexed B 1951 Histologic changes in spinal nerve roots of operated cases of sciatica. Acta Orth. Scand. 20: 215–225
13 Burton C V 1978 Lumbosacral arachnoiditis. Spine 3: 24–30
14 Quiles M, Marchisello P J, Tsairis P 1978 Lumbar adhesive arachnoiditis. Etiologic and pathologic aspects. Spine 3: 45–50
15 Dumonde D C, Glynn L E 1962 The production of

arthritis in rabbits by an immulogical reaction to fibrin. Br. J. Exp. Path. 43: 373–383

16   Browse N L 1983 Venous ulceration. Br. Med. J. 286: 1920–1922

17   Cunliffe W J, Dodman B, Roberts B E, Tebbs E M 1975 Clinical and laboratory double-blind investigation of fibrinolytic therapy of cutaneous vasculitis. In: Davidson J F, Samara M M, Desnoyers P C (eds) Progress in chemical fibrinolysis and thrombolysis. Raven Press, New York, p 325–332

18   Cash J D, Leaske E 1965 Automatic determination of euglobulin lysis time. J. Chem. Path. 18: 821–823

19   Haverkate F, Brakman P 1975 Fibrin plate assay. In: Davidson J F, Samama M M, Desnoyers P C (eds) Progress in chemical fibrinolysis and thrombolysis. Raven Press, New York

20   Clauss A 1975 Rapid physiological coagulation method in determination of fibrinogen. Acta Haematol. 17: 237–246

21   Jayson M l V, Keegan A, Million R, Tomlinson I 1984 A fibrinolytic defect in chronic back pain syndromes. Lancet 2: 1186–1187

22   Frymoyer J W, Pope M H, Clements J H, Wilder D G, MacPherson B, Ashikaga T 1983 Risk factors in low back pain. J. Bone Joint Surg. 65A: 213–218

23   Meade T W, Chakrabarti R, Haines A P, North W R S, Stirling Y 1979 Characteristics affecting fibrinolytic activity and plasma fibrinogen concentrations. Br. Med. J. i: 153–156

24   Westrin C G 1970 Low back sick-listing. Acta Soc. Med. Scand. 2–3: 127–134

25   Westrin C G 1973 Low back sick-listing. Scand. J. Soc. Med. suppl 7

26   Gyntelberg F 1974 One year incidence of low back pain among male residents of Copenhagen aged 40–59. Den. Med. Bull. 21: 30–36

27   Johnston J D H, Matheny J B 1978 Microscopic lysis of lumbar adhesive arachnoditis. Spine 3: 36–39

28   Jayson M I V, Keegan A L, Holland C D, Longstaff J, Gush R 1985 A study of stanozolol therapy for systemic sclerosis and Raynaud's phenomenon. In: Davidson J F, Donati M B, Coccheri S (eds) Progress in fibrinolysis VII. Churchill Livingstone, Edinburgh, p 111–112

Understanding the patient with back pain

INTRODUCTION

Backache is the common presenting symptom of a variety of low back conditions. In a few patients we can identify a spinal fracture, compression of the spinal nerve roots or more serious disease such as infection or tumour,[1] but in most patients with non-specific backache we have neither the biomechanical nor pathological knowledge to reach a meaningful diagnosis.[2]

Consider for a moment the contrast between one patient with chronic backache and another with hip replacement for osteoarthritis.[3] In backache the doctor frequently cannot identify the cause or source of the pain. The patient does not understand what is wrong. Worst of all, if backache becomes chronic, the patient soon realizes that the doctor does not know what is wrong. In contrast, with arthritis, the problem is clearly evident to doctor and patient, and moreover can be seen objectively by both on X-ray.

Treatment of backache is not only empirical but has a high failure rate. Treatment of arthritis is based on a clear rationale and, although failures and complications can occur, they are uncommon, and the reason for failure is usually self-evident. When treatment for backache fails, the doctor is tempted to look for psychological or other excuses and the patient becomes defensive; both patient and doctor may become mutually hostile. If the doctor is reluctant to admit or the patient to accept the limitations of treatment for backache, then it is easy to understand why some patients may develop psychological problems.

HISTORICAL PERSPECTIVE

Disc surgery has survived the test of time for more than half a century[4] because at least 70% of patients obtain good results (Table 22.4). When the number of disc operations escalated after World War 2, however, it was soon realized that the failures were equally dramatic,[5,6] and one of the pioneers was forced to conclude that 'no operation in any field of surgery leaves in its wake more human wreckage than surgery on the lumbar spine'.[7] As many as 15% of patients undergoing low back surgery will sooner or later come to repeat surgery, and the success rate of repeated operations progressively deteriorates.[8] Problem Back Clinics are full of such multiply-operated back cripples, and every study for the last thirty years has stressed the association of surgical failure with psychological disturbances and their importance when considering further salvage surgery.[8]

Psychological studies have confirmed and identified psychological disturbances in patients with chronic pain compared with acute pain,[9] in chronic disability as well as pain[10] and associated with repeated failed treatment.[3,11] Less clear-cut psychological differences have been suggested[12] between patients with no physical findings to account for their persisting pain and those with a confirmed disc prolapse and proportionate pain and disability.

In 1975 Wiltse & Rocchio[11] demonstrated that pre-operative psychological tests could predict how patients would respond to treatment (Table 22.1). Indeed, this study suggested that psychological factors are *more* important than physical factors in predicting symptomatic relief. Following this, a number of prospective studies have shown that psychological factors influence how patients respond to physical treatment, whether by physiotherapy,[13,14] rehabilitation,[15,16] chemonucleolysis,[11,17] surgical decompression,[18,19] fusion,[20] repeat spinal surgery[21]

Table 22.1 Pre-operative psychological test predicting symptomatic relief from chemonucleolysis for lumbar disc prolapse. (Reproduced with permission from Wiltse & Rocchio[11] and the Journal of Bone and Joint Surgery)

Pre-operative Hs and Hy scores on the MMPI*	% good or excellent symptomatic relief
85 and above	10
75–84	16
65–74	39
55–64	72
54 and below	90

* The mean score for 'normal' people is 50. See Appendix.

or pain tract surgery,[22] although none of these studies have found psychological factors to be as powerful influences on outcome as the original Wiltse & Rocchio study on chemonucleolysis.[11]

There is no doubt that psychological factors are important in backache but, before we go any further, it is important to clear away some common misconceptions.

Firstly, patients with backache are not personality-deficient or psychopathic; they are no different from the rest of us, and personality tests have not identified any pre-morbid personality type.[10,23]

Secondly, patients with backache are not mad or psychotic; they rarely have any psychiatric illness, and referral to a traditional psychiatrist is rarely of any help.[9] Terms such as hysteria and hypochondriasis have been so variously used, misused and abused, particularly by clinicians, that they should be completely discarded in the context of chronic pain.[24,25]

Thirdly, we cannot divide pain artificially into physical or psychogenic, organic or non-organic, real or imaginery.[9] Physical disorders and emotional reactions co-exist. They are not alternatives, and failure to identify a physical disorder does not mean that the problem is psychological any more than the presence of a psychological disturbance excludes a treatable physical problem. All our clinical analyses[23,25] suggest that, contrary to psychoanalytical theories or psychosomatic hypotheses, the vast majority of backache starts with a physical source for pain in the back. From a pragmatic clinical viewpoint, accepting a physical cause for backache is not only more realistic and safer but also promotes a better doctor–patient relationship. Our frequent

inability to identify or localize the source of the pain is not the patient's fault, but rather reflects our limited biomechanical and pathological understanding. Diagnosis of psychological disturbance must be based on positive emotional and behavioural assessment.

Finally, we must recognize that patients cannot help how they react to illness. They do not want to have pain, they do not choose to be psychologically disturbed, and malingering is uncommon. The doctor's role is not to sit in judgement, but rather with compassion to understand the problem, both physical and psychological, in order to provide the best possible management for both the backache and the patient.

DISTRESS

From an extensive review of previous work[26–28] and his own detailed clinical studies[9,29–32] Sternbach concluded that the most important psychological disturbances associated with pain were anxiety in acute pain and depression in chronic pain.

In our own analysis of chronic backache and disability[23,25] we found that the most important psychological factors were increased bodily awareness,[33] which is related to anxiety, and symptoms of depression.[34] These completely overshadowed other psychological measures of personality traits or fears and beliefs about illness. In particular, increased awareness and reporting of bodily functioning appeared to be a much more powerful clinical concept than theories of hypochondriasis based on fears or beliefs about illness, while depressive symptoms appeared to be part of an emotional reaction to pain and disability rather than a primary psychiatric illness.

These psychological disturbances of anxiety, increased bodily awareness and depression are best regarded clinically as forms of distress, a simple emotional reaction to pain and disability.

If we now reconsider the MMPI[35,36] (see Appendix), the psychological questionnaire most widely used in backache and for most of the studies on treatment quoted earlier, we find that the common MMPI disturbance seen in backache and related to the outcome of treatment is the 'neurotic triad'.[9,11,29,30] Although loosely labelled 'neurotic' and originally derived from psychiatric ideas of 'hypochondriasis', 'depression' and 'hysteria', these labels have never been clinically valid, and the MMPI disturbance seen in backache again makes more clinical sense if it is interpreted as distress.

There is thus no need for esoteric psychological theories in backache. Patients with backache are generally not personality-deficient, neurotic, hypochondriacal, hysterical nor mad, but simply distressed by their physical problem. The next step is to consider how that distress presents to the doctor.

ILLNESS BEHAVIOUR

All good clinicians use the clinical interview and examination not only to diagnose physical disease but also to learn about the patient and his or her response to illness. Firstly, we must recognize that

the patient is ill, not only by what is said but also by certain changes in the whole pattern of behaviour which we recognize as 'sick' or 'illness behaviour'. Unfortunately, most medical training concentrates on disease, while assessment of the patient is learned by experience and is largely based on subconscious impressions which are unreliable, difficult to evaluate and impossible to teach. What is necessary is to distinguish these clinical symptoms and signs which do portray physical disease from those which reflect illness behaviour.

Pain

Clinical observation of illness behaviour is most simply illustrated by the pain drawing (Fig. 22.1). Patients willingly record their pain on an outline of the body, but the *way* in which they draw the pain is strongly influenced by their distress.[37] Thus the

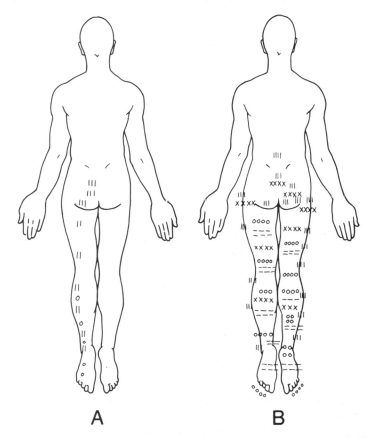

Fig. 22.1 Pain drawing. Patient A describes the physical pattern of S1 sciatica from a disc prolapse. Patient B with simple backache is communicating distress. Many patients do both to varying degrees. (|| = pain; 0 = pins and needles; X = ache and == = numbness.) Reproduced with permission from the British Medical Journal.[46]

patient's apparently straightforward description of the anatomical pattern of pain provides both physical information about the pain and psychological information about their response to it.

Similarly, the adjectives which patients use to describe pain[38] fall into two distinct categories — words which describe the sensory qualities of the pain and other words which describe the affective or emotional qualities of the pain experience.[39,40]

Inappropriate descriptions of symptoms

Interpretation of a medical history is based on the occurrence of common and hence recognizable patterns of symptoms. The way in which patients describe their symptoms usually approximates to anatomical and pathological patterns of disease. Occasionally, however, patients offer descriptions which clearly do not fit clinical experience. Certain symptoms appear to be physically inappropriate but are more related to the patient's emotional response.

A large number of such inappropriate symptoms can be identified in the clinical and medico-legal literature or in a Problem Back Clinic, but we have shown[25] that a small group of inappropriate symptoms common in and specific to backache can provide useful clinical information:

Specific questions

1. Do you get pain at the tip of your tailbone?
2. Does your *whole* leg ever become painful?
3. Does your *whole* leg ever go numb?
4. Does your *whole* leg ever give way?
5. In the past year have you had *any* spells with very little pain? (NO is scored as 1.)

Information gathered in routine history

6. Intolerance of or reactions to treatments.
7. Emergency admission(s) to hospital with backache.

These are each scored as present (1) or absent (0) and added together. Although such 1/0 scoring is very simple, it is easy to use in routine practice, it fits clinical thinking, and the final score out of seven is statistically highly satisfactory.[25] Isolated symptoms are of no significance and behavioural assessment,

just like physical diagnosis, must be based on the whole clinical picture.

These inappropriate symptoms are clearly separable from the common symptoms of physical disease and closely related to other psychological features. In rare cases they can occur in relation to serious spinal pathology such as tumour, infection or paraparesis. This particular group of symptoms are therefore only inappropriate to non-specific or mechanical backache and may not be inappropriate in other situations. They should not be regarded as inappropriate until spinal pathology has been excluded.

Non-organic signs or inappropriate responses to examination

In the same way we have identified and standardised a group of non-organic or inappropriate signs.[41] Physical findings on examination are frequently regarded as objective, but when one human being examines another human being in pain, and in the process may deliberately elicit pain, then the examination should not only detect objective physical abnormality but also provide information about the patient's response. Inappropriate responses to examination include:

1. Tenderness — superficial, non-anatomical
2. Simulation — axial loading, simulated rotation
3. Distraction — straight-leg raising
4. Regional — weakness, sensory disturbance
5. Over-reaction to examination

Tenderness

Tenderness related to physical disease is usually localized to a particular skeletal or neuromuscular structure. Non-organic tenderness (Fig. 22.2) may be either superficial or non-anatomical.

Superficial tenderness. The skin is tender to light pinch over a wide area of lumbar skin. A localized band in a posterior primary ramus distribution may be caused by nerve irritation and should be discounted.

Non-anatomical tenderness. Deep tenderness over a wide area is not localized to one structure and often extends to the thoracic spine, sacrum or pelvis.

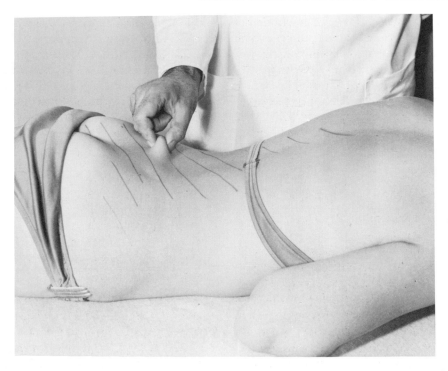

Fig. 22.2 Non-organic tenderness showing technique of testing superficial skin tenderness and the area (shaded) frequently involved in widespread non-anatomical tenderness. Reproduced with permission from Spine.[41]

Simulation tests

These give the impression that a particular manoeuvre is being carried out when in fact it is not. Usually this is based on movement producing pain. On formal examination a particular movement causes the patient to report pain. That movement is then simulated without actually being performed. If pain is reported it is likely to be inappropriate. It is essential to minimize suggestion.

Axial loading. Low back pain may be reported on vertical loading over the standing patient's skull by the examiner's hands (Fig. 22.3). Neck pain is common and should be discounted, but organic lumbar pain is surprisingly rare, even in the presence of serious spinal pathology.

Simulated rotation. Back pain is reported when the shoulders and pelvis are passively rotated together in the same plane as the patient stands relaxed with the feet together (Fig. 22.4). In the presence of nerve irritation, leg pain may be produced and should be discounted.

Distraction tests

A positive physical finding is demonstrated in the routine manner, and this finding is then checked while the patient's attention is distracted. Distraction must be non-painful, non-emotional and non-surprising. In its simplest and most effective form, this consists of indirect observation — simply observing the patient throughout the period that he or she is in the examiner's presence, while he or she is unaware of being examined. During examination, parts of the body other than the particular part being formally tested should also be observed. Any finding that is consistently present is likely to be physically based. Findings that are present only on formal examination and disappear at other times may have a non-organic component.

Straight-leg raising. Straight-leg raising is the most useful distraction test. A patient with distress or limited pain tolerance may show marked improvement in straight-leg raising on distraction, compared with formal testing. There are several variations

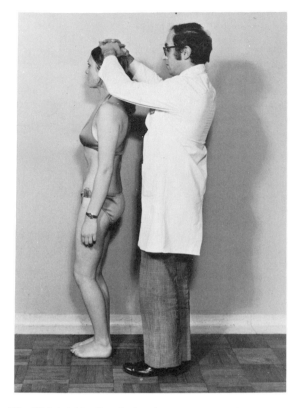

Fig. 22.3 Axial loading: back pain on vertical loading on the standing patient's head. Reproduced with permission from Spine.[41]

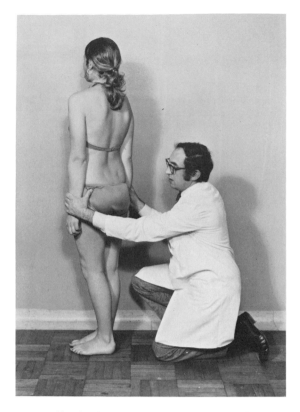

Fig. 22.4 Simulated rotation: back pain when shoulders and pelvis are passively rotated in the same plane. Reproduced with permission from Spine.[41]

based on sitting (Fig. 22.5). This is commonly known in North America as the 'flip test'.

Regional disturbances

Regional disturbances involve a widespread region of neighbouring parts such as the whole leg. The essential feature is divergence from accepted neuroanatomy.

Weakness. Weakness is demonstrated on formal testing by jerky 'giving way' of many muscle groups which cannot be explained on a localized neurological basis.

Sensory. Sensory disturbances (Fig. 22.6) include diminished sensation to light touch, pinprick and sometimes other modalities fitting a 'stocking' rather than dermatomal pattern. 'Giving way' and sensory changes commonly affect the same area and there may be associated non-anatomical regional tenderness. Care must be taken, particularly in patients with spinal stenosis or who have had repeated spinal

surgery, not to mistake multiple nerve root involvement for a regional disturbance.

Over-reaction

Over-reaction during examination may take the form of disproportionate verbalization, facial expression, muscle tension and tremor, collapsing or sweating (Fig. 22.7). The response to procedures such as venepuncture or myelography provides additional information. Judgements should, however, be made with caution and minimizing the examiner's own emotional reactions: there are considerable cultural variations and it is very easy to introduce observer bias or to provoke this type of response.

These inappropriate signs are again clearly separable from the standard signs of physical disease and are closely related to distress. Although they can occur in medico-legal situations, they are also commonly present in the Problem Back Clinic in

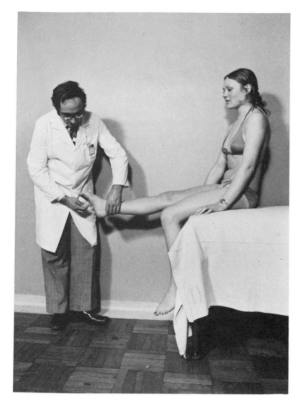

Fig. 22.5 Straight-leg raising improving with distraction, as when testing the plantar reflex in the sitting position. Reproduced with permission from Spine.[41]

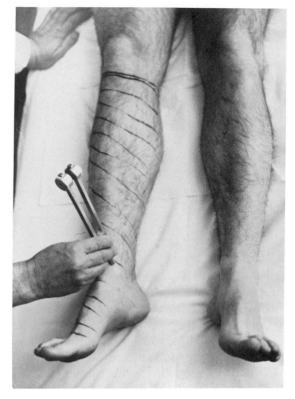

Fig. 22.6 Non-anatomical sensory alteration in a 'stocking' distribution affecting light touch, pinprick and sometimes other modalities. Reproduced with permission from Spine.[41]

patients with no medico-legal or compensation factors. They form part of complex emotional and behavioral patterns and should not be interpreted simplistically as faking.

Both the inappropriate symptoms and inappropriate signs provide clinical methods of assessing illness behaviour or, more specifically, illness presentation in the context of a medical interview and examination. Many of the inappropriate symptoms and signs are vague and ill-localized and fit what Walters[42] has described as regional or body image patterns rather than neuroanatomical patterns (Table 22.2).

There is a considerable overlap between the inappropriate symptoms and signs and distress[25] and also between the pain drawing and MMPI measures of distress.[37] Analysis of the inappropriate symptoms and signs themselves (Table 22.3) suggests that they are the result of the severity and chronicity of the physical problem, the amount of distress and some

social and medical influences. The inappropriate symptoms are more common in women and associated more with increased bodily awareness, while the inappropriate signs are more common in men and associated more with depressive symptoms. They may best be regarded as a magnified presentation or communication of the patient's problem and of the need to do something about it or, more simply, as the clinical equivalent of psychological distress.

Having looked at several of its clinical manifestations, we may now define illness behaviour more precisely as 'observable and potentially measurable activities and conduct which express and communicate the individual's own perception of disturbed health'[43-45] This is obviously a broad concept of one important aspect of illness, but it can be assessed clinically by the description of pain and the symptoms and signs elicited by the perceptive doctor. Abnormal, inappropriate or magnified illness behaviour may then be recognized clinically as

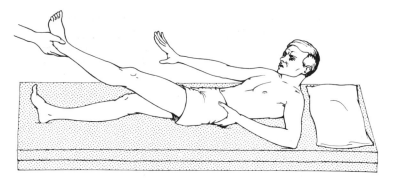

Fig. 22.7 Over-reaction to examination; disproportionate verbalisation, facial expression, muscle tension and tremor, collapsing or sweating. Reproduced with permission from Spine.[41]

'illness behaviour which is out of proportion to the underlying physical disease and related more to associated psychological disturbances than to the actual physical disease'.[46] Some illness behaviour is normal. Abnormal illness behaviour may originally develop as a socially productive 'cry for help' but, unfortunately, in the absence of due help, it may itself add to disability and become counter-productive.

A CONCEPT OF ILLNESS

'A pain, an ache, a discomfort — these are the common complaints of those who seek the doctor's help. Pain issues a warning with kindly intent. She calls to action and, pointing the way, brooks no delay. And thus the ancient cycle is served, from pain to cause, to treatment to cure.'[47] It is easy to forget that it is only in historically recent times, since

Table 22.2 A comparison of the symptoms and signs of physical disease and magnified illness behaviour in chronic backache

	Physical disease Normal illness behaviour	Magnified or inappropriate illness behaviour
Pain drawing[37]	Localized Neuroanatomical Proportionate	Poor anatomical localization Expansion or magnification Additional emphasis
Pain adjectives[38]	Sensory	Affective Evaluative
Symptoms:[25]		
Pain	Localized	Whole-leg pain Tailbone pain
Numbness	Dermatomal	Whole-leg numbness
Weakness	Myotomal	Whole-leg giving way
Time pattern	Varies with time	Never free of pain
Response to treatment	Variable benefit	Intolerance of treatment Emergency admissions to hospital
Signs:[41]		
Tenderness	Localized	Superficial, widespread, non-anatomical
Axial loading	No lumbar pain	Lumbar pain
Simulated rotation	No lumbar pain	Lumbar pain
Straight-leg raising	Limited on distraction	Improves with distraction
Sensory	Dermatomal	Regional
Motor	Myotomal	Regional, jerky giving way
General response	Appropriate pain	Over-reaction

Table 22.3 Analysis of the causes of magnified illness behaviour. (Reproduced with permission from the British Medical Journal[25])

Identifiable influences	Extent to which these influence	
	Inappropriate symptoms (%)	Inappropriate signs (%)
Physical severity	20	27
Distress	10	8
Duration	6	5
Amount of and failure of treatment	17	<1
Medico-legal proceedings	<1	9
Total identified*	57	50

* Due to the inaccuracies of clinical observation it is unusual to be able to identify such a high percentage of any biological phenomenon.

Pasteur suggested that infectious disease was caused by microbes and Virchow proposed the concept of cellular pathology, that medicine has been about disease:

1. Recognise patterns of illness behaviour — symptoms and signs
2. Infer underlying pathology — diagnosis
3. Physical therapy to underlying pathology — treatment
4. Expect illness to improve — cure

The success of such an approach, for example in the surgical treatment of disc prolapse[48] depends on a clear-cut physical problem, an effective physical treatment and accurate diagnosis (Table 22.4). Conversely, we have seen that the success of treatment is influenced by psychological factors (Historical perspective), while several independent studies[17,21,49,50] have shown that the success of treatment for sciatica is inversely proportional to abnormal illness behaviour (Table 22.5), and eleven comparative studies have shown that the result of any form of treatment in compensation patients is one-third poorer than in non-compensation patients.[8]

Concentration on the understanding, investigation and treatment of disease has led to the tremendous advances of the past century but also underlies the major humanitarian criticisms of modern medicine. This has led to increasing recognition that medicine must return to dealing with all the physical, psychological and social aspects of illness. Tragically, though we may all agree in theory with the principle of treating the whole person, we too often get on in practice with treating the perceived disease.

Disability

The present analysis has identified the most important clinical elements of illness as the physical disorder, distress, illness behaviour and invalidism, each of which can be clinically defined, assessed and measured. The analysis shows that they are all interrelated and combine to provide a broad description of illness.[25] If we now analyse disability in chronic backache,[25,51] we find that the physical

Table 22.4 Relief of sciatica and back pain related to the degree of herniation found at operation. (Recalculated from the data of Sprangfort[48])

Operative findings	Relief of sciatica		Relief of back pain (%)
	Complete (%)	Partial (%)	
Complete herniation	90	9	75
Incomplete hernation	82	16	74
Bulging disc	63	26	54
No herniation	37	38	43

Table 22.5 Outcome of physical treatment for sciatica related to pre-existing illness behaviour. (Reproduced with permission from the British Medical Journal[46])

Treatment	Success rate of treatment (%) in patients with:	
	No inappropriate signs	Multiple inappropriate signs
Chemonucleolysis for disc prolapse[17]	57	11
Compensation Board patients:[21]		
First lumbar surgery	78	48
Repeat lumbar surgery	65	38
Rehabilitation (unsuitable for surgery)	54	4
Laminectomy for disc prolapse (based on the pain drawing[49])	94	28
Calcitonin for neurogenic claudication[50]	65	0

disorder accounts for almost half the total disability, while distress and illness behaviour together account for an additional one-third (Table 22.6).

The Glasgow illness model (Fig. 22.8) provides a visual representation of this analysis. It is an over-simplification to regard disability as the sum of physical disorder plus distress plus abnormal illness behaviour, and the model attempts to show the overlap and interaction between these elements.[25] The model also illustrates that, while illness may start with the physical disorder, its presentation to the doctor is largely in the form of illness behaviour.

Analysis of treatment[46] suggests that, in a poorly understood condition such as backache, even after every allowance is made for physical factors, distress and illness behaviour are the most powerful influences on the amount of conservative treatment received (Table 22.7). This may be one example of a more general hypothesis that social interactions may be related more to illness behaviour than to disease. Certainly, time off work is very poorly explained by physical severity, distress and abnormal illness behaviour (Table 22.6) but may depend more on social factors.

Finally, although the analysis is based on a large group of patients, clinical assessment of the individual patient may be represented by variation of the same basic model (Fig. 22.9). Most patients with backache can be understood and treated as a predominantly physical disorder with normal and proportionate illness behaviour (Fig. 22.9a). Occasional patients, however, may develop distress and illness behaviour out of all proportion to the original physical disorder and this may even become the major management problem (Fig. 22.9b).

Conclusions

This concept of illness does not lead to a new test or a new treatment for backache: instead it demands and offers a fundamental reconsideration of medical practice. Medicine is about human illness, not

Table 22.6 Analysis of the causes of disability and time off work[25]

Main elements of illness	Extent to which these influence:	
	Disability (%)	Time off work (%)
Physical severity	40	22
Distress / Abnormal illness behaviour	31	7
Social interactions	—	?
Total identified*	71	29

* See footnote to Table 22.3

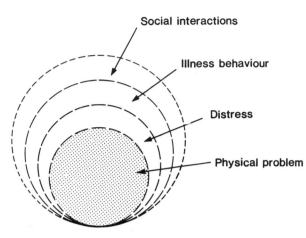

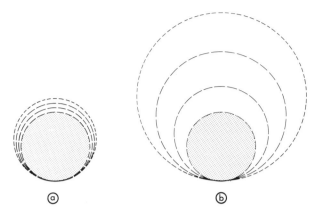

Social interactions

Illness behaviour

Distress

Physical problem

Fig. 22.8 The Glasgow illness model. A diagrammatic representation emphasizing that the outward expression of physical disease is illness behaviour and that the symptoms and signs of illness behaviour must be distinguished from those of physical disease. Adapted with permission from Spine.[25]

Fig. 22.9 Variation of the relative importance of the different elements of illness in individual patients.

disease, and it may be necessary to redefine health and illness. The World Health Organization definition[52] quite rightly points out that health is 'not only the absence of disease' but then goes on to the idealistic social goal of 'a state of complete physical, mental and social well-being'. This reflects the unrealistic expectation that there should be a medical answer for all the ills of life, even unhappiness or social problems, and some of the current abuses of medicine appear to be based on this misconception. A more pragmatic definition of illness would be 'a variable combination of disease, distress about health, illness behaviour and invalidism', while health would be not the absence of disease but 'freedom from illness'.

Medicine cannot confine itself to disease nor abandon the patient in distress, and the doctor's role as healer cannot be separated from his or her more ancient role as personal adviser and comforter in illness.[53] If, however, physical disease and illness behaviour are distinguished, then physical treatment can be directed more appropriately to physical disease, while improved understanding of illness will provide an equally scientific basis for the practice as well as the technology of medicine. The aims are to alleviate disease, relieve distress, reduce illness behaviour and restore social function.

Physical therapy should be administered efficiently and without delay and prolonged only if it is beneficial. Potentially harmful physical treatment should be reserved for clear-cut physical disease where there is a reasonable prospect of it being successful. Treatment is directed to physical disease, but also affects the patient, and every decision about treatment should consider not only its physical effect but also its effect on the patient's distress, illness behaviour and social function. There is no benefit in treatment which improves the disease but worsens the illness, and failed treatment may be worse than no treatment at all. Conversely, it may be possible to help the patient by reducing distress and illness behaviour and improving function, even when physical cure of the disease is not possible.

At all times we must remember that the aim of medicine is to make the patient better: treatment of disease is only a means to this end and not an end itself. Quite simply, we must treat patients rather than diseases, and this means treating patients as human beings. Time to listen and talk to patients

Table 22.7 Analysis of those elements of illness influencing how much conservative treatment patients received for backache. (Adapted with permission from the British Medical Journal[46])

Identifiable influences	Extent to which these account for the amount of treatment received (%)
Duration of symptoms	14
Physical severity	11
Distress	9
Abnormal illness behaviour	15
Total identified*	50

* See footnote to Table 22.3

provides simple psychotherapy by allowing them to talk out their problems and fears, develop a satisfactory doctor–patient relationship, and providing reassurance, advice and encouragement. It also permits the clinical application of the more basic virtues of faith, hope and caring. For many patients physical treatment alone is enough, some need physical treatment and better management of the whole illness, but for some the role of adviser and comforter may meet the most important need of all. The challenge facing medicine now is to improve our treatment of patients to match our ever-increasing ability to treat disease.

ACKNOWLEDGEMENTS

The critical research reported here was generously supported by the Medical Research Council and the Back Pain Association, and much of the material has already been published in Spine and the British Medical Journal. I am deeply grateful to Dr C J Main, to my Spinal Research Fellows Messrs M Bircher, M Di Paola, D Finlayson and E W Morris and to my Consultant colleagues who referred patients to the Problem Back Clinic.

APPENDIX: PSYCHOLOGICAL TESTS

Psychological tests usually take the form of questionnaires which the patient fills in himself or herself. The answers are then scored, and groups of related questions are added together to provide measures or scales of different psychological characteristics. Such questionnaires have the advantage over clinical or psychiatric interviews in that they can be carefully designed and tested, they eliminate observer variation and bias, give a numerical measure of each psychological characteristic and give a reproducible assessment to compare different patients or changes with time. Their weakness is that their content is limited to specific questions or characteristics which have been built in, and they may completely miss other important features which would be detected and explored further in interview. Psychological tests are, therefore, complementary rather than alternatives to clinical assessment.

Three main types of psychological questionnaires

have been used in backache — personality tests which attempt to assess underlying personality traits, measures of current psychological distress and measures of attitudes, fears and beliefs about illness. These have been reviewed in detail elsewhere.[23,54]

MMPI

The most widely used psychological questionnaire in backache, particularly in North America, where most psychological studies have been done, is the Minnesota Multiphasic Personality Inventory, or MMPI.[35,36] This suffers from a number of major disadvantages. It is long, cumbersome and time-consuming. It is American both in language and culture, many of the questions are obviously completely unrelated to backache or illness, and some are offensively intrusive. Because of these problems, 30% of backache patients in a British pilot study either could not or would not complete it or provided invalid answers. More fundamentally, the MMPI was originally derived from selected groups of psychiatric patients and aimed to study basic personality characteristics not particularly relevant to physical illness. Attempts to pick out a new group of questions from the MMPI which would provide a 'Low Back Scale'[12] have not overcome this fundamental limitation.

Despite its hallowed position and vested interests, the role of the MMPI in chronic pain is increasingly under question, and there is little doubt that questionnaires specifically designed and directed to the psychological features of illness provide much more useful clinical information.

MSPQ and Zung

We would suggest two simple psychological questionnaires assessing distress[55] — the Modified Somatic Perception Questionnaire or MSPQ (Table 22.8)[33] and a slightly modified version of the Zung Depression Inventory (Table 22.9).[34] Both questionnaires are filled in by the patient using an unstarred version reproduced in normal type size without the scores. Care should be taken to make sure that the patient understands that he or she has to make a grading of 'none', 'little', 'moderate' or 'major', though the headings on the columns provide additional guidelines. After instruction, the patient

Table 22.8 MSPQ. Reproduced with permission from C J Main[33,55,56] and the Journal of Psychosomatic Research.

Please describe how you have felt during the PAST WEEK by making a check mark ($\sqrt{}$) in the appropriate box. Please answer all questions. Do not think too long before answering.

	Not at all	A little/ slightly	A great deal/ quite a bit	Extremely/ could not have been worse
Heart rate increase				
Feeling hot all over	* 0	1	2	3
Sweating all over	* 0	1	2	3
Sweating in a particular part of the body				
Pulse in neck				
Pounding in head				
Dizziness	* 0	1	2	3
Blurring of vision	* 0	1	2	3
Feeling faint	* 0	1	2	3
Everything appearing unreal				
Nausea	* 0	1	2	3
Butterflies in stomach				
Pain or ache in stomach	* 0	1	2	3
Stomach churning	* 0	1	2	3
Desire to pass water				
Mouth becoming dry.	* 0	1	2	3
Difficulty swallowing				
Muscles in neck aching	* 0	1	2	3
Legs feeling weak	* 0	1	2	3
Muscles twitching or jumping	* 0	1	2	3
Tense feeling across forehead	* 0	1	2	3
Tense feeling in jaw muscles				

* Only these 13 items are scored

Table 22.9 Modified Zung. Reproduced with permission from C J Main[33,55,56] and Current Concepts of Pain, from Zung[34] © W Zung 1965, 1974. All rights reserved. Adapted and reproduced with permission of the author.

Please indicate for each of these questions which answer best describes how you have been feeling recently.

	Rarely or none of the time (less than 1 day per week)	Some or little of the time (1–2 days per week)	A moderate amount of time (3–4 per week)	Most of the time (5–7 days per week)	
1. I feel downhearted and sad	0	1	2	3	
2. Morning is when I feel best	3	2	1	0	*
3. I have crying spells or feel like it	0	1	2	3	
4. I have trouble getting to sleep at night	0	1	2	3	
5. I feel that nobody cares	0	1	2	3	
6. I eat as much as I used to	3	2	1	0	*
7. I still enjoy sex	3	2	1	0	*
8. I noticed I am losing weight	0	1	2	3	
9. I have trouble with constipation	0	1	2	3	
10. My heart beats faster than usual	0	1	2	3	
11. I get tired for no reason	0	1	2	3	
12. My mind is as clear as it used to be	3	2	1	0	*
13. I tend to wake up too early	0	1	2	3	
14. I find it easy to do the things I used to	3	2	1	0	*
15. I am restless and can't keep still	0	1	2	3	
16. I feel hopeful about the future	3	2	1	0	*
17. I am more irritable than usual	0	1	2	3	
18. I find it easy to make a decision	3	2	1	0	*
19. I feel quite guilty	0	1	2	3	
20. I feel that I am useful and needed	3	2	1	0	*
21. My life is pretty full	3	2	1	0	*

Table 22.9 (Cont.)

	Rarely or none of the time (less than 1 day per week)	Some or little of the time (1–2 days per week)	A moderate amount of time (3–4 per week)	Most of the time (5–7 days per week)	
22. I feel that others would be better off if I were dead	0	1	2	3	
23. I am still able to enjoy the things I used to	3	2	1	0	*

* Note that the scoring is reversed in these questions.

should be left undisturbed to fill in the questionnaires alone without 'help' from friends, relatives or staff. The answers are then scored by the examiner from 0 to 3 using the 13 starred questions only from the MSPQ and reversing the scores on the starred items of the Modified Zung. The 'marks' are then added to give total scores for bodily awareness (MSPQ) and depressive symptoms (Modified Zung).

Normal values and suggested cut-offs are given in Table 22.30. It should, however, be emphasised that such tests must not be over-interpreted and will not in themselves turn a clinician into an amateur psychologist. Advice on their use should be sought from a Clinical Psychologist and background reading is essential.[33,34,56] A manual giving further normative data is available from C J Main.[56]

Table 22.10 The identification of psychological distress in patients with chronic backache[55,56]

	Score out of	Normal asymptomatic people*	Routine referrals to an orthopaedic clinic with backache*		Suggested 'normal' range† in backache	
			Male	Female	Male	Female
MSPQ	39	1.8 ± 2.1	3.3 ± 3.5	4.8 ± 4.7	Up to 7	Up to 10
Modified Zung	69	12.2 ± 7.8	18.8 ± 7.3	19.8 ± 6.7	Up to 27	Up to 29
Inappropriate symptoms	7	0.6 ± 1.0	0.8 ± 1.0	1.7 ± 1.5	0–2	0–3
Inappropriate signs	8	0.1 ± 0.4	0.6 ± 1.5	1.1 ± 1.6	0–1	0–2
					Higher in elderly patients	

* Mean ± SD
† Note that there is not a sharp boundary between 'normal' and 'abnormal' and the clinical significance of minor degrees of psychological disturbance is a matter of clinical judgement.

REFERENCES

1 Waddell G 1982 An approach to backache. Hos. Med. 28: 187–219
2 Editorial 1979 Back pain — what can we offer? Brit. Med. J. i: 706
3 Gray I C M, Main C J, Waddell G 1985 Psychological assessment in general orthopaedic practice. Clin. Orth. 194: 258–263
4 Mixter W J, Barr J S 1934 Rupture of the intervertebral disc with involvement of the spinal canal. New Eng. J. Med 211: 210–215
5 Greenwood J, McGuire T H, Kimbell F 1952 A study of the causes of failure in the herniated vertebral disc operation. J. Neurosurg. 9: 15–20
6 Kelly J H, Voris D C, Svien H J, Ghormley R K 1954 Multiple operations for protruded lumbar vertebral discs. Proc. Staff Meetings Mayo Clinic 29: 546–550
7 De Palma A F, Rothman R H 1970 The intervertebral disc. Saunders, Philadelphia
8 Waddell G, Kummel E G, Lotto W N, Graham J D, Hall H, McCulloch J A 1979 Failed lumbar disc surgery and repeat surgery following industrial injuries. J. Bone Joint Surg. 61A: 201–207
9 Sternbach R A 1974 Pain patients: traits and treatment. Academic Press, New York
10 Naliboff B D, Cohen M J, Yellen A N 1982 Does the

MMPI differentiate chronic illness from chronic pain? Pain 13: 333–341

11 Wiltse L L, Rocchio P D 1975 Preoperative psychological tests as predictors of success in chemonucleolysis in the treatment of low back syndrome. J. Bone Joint Surg. 57A: 478–483

12 Hanvik L J 1951 MMPI profiles in patients with low back pain. J. Consulting Psychol. 15: 350–353

13 Brown T, Barr J S, Nemiah J C, Barry H 1954 Psychological factors in low back pain. New Eng. J. Med. 251: 123–128

14 Bergquist-Ullman M, Larsson U 1977 Acute low back pain in industry. Acta Orth. Scand. (suppl) 170

15 Beals R K, Hickman N W 1972 Industrial injuries of the back and extremities. J. Bone Joint Surg. 54A: 1593–1611

16 Flynn R J, Salomone P R 1977 Performance of the MMPI in predicting rehabilitation outcome: a discriminant analysis, double-cross validation analysis. Rehab. Lit. 38: 12–15

17 McCulloch J A 1977 Chemonucleolysis. J. Bone Joint Surg. 59B: 45–52

18 Pheasant H, Gilbert D, Goldfar J, Herron L 1979 The MMPI as a predictor of outcome of low-back surgery. Spine 4: 78–84

19 Oostdam E M, Duidenvoorden H J, Pondaag N 1981 Predictive value of some psychological tests on the outcome of surgical intervention in low back pain patients. J. Psychosom. Res. 25: 227–235

20 Wing P C, Wilfling F J, Kokan P J 1973 Psychological, demographic and orthopaedic factors associated with prediction of outcome of spinal fusion. Clin. Orth. 90: 153–160

21 Doxey N 1983 Unpublished data. Workmen's Compensation Board, Ontario

22 Blumetti A E, Modesti L M 1976 Psychological predictors of success or failure of surgical intervention for intractable back pain. In: Bonica J, Albe-Fessard D (eds) Advances in pain research and therapy, vol 1. Raven Press, New York

23 Main C J, Waddell G 1982 Chronic pain, distress and illness behaviour. In: Main C J (ed) Clinical psychology and medicine: a behavioural perspective. Plenum Press, New York

24 Slater E 1965 Diagnosis of 'hysteria'. Brit. Med. J. i: 1395–1399

25 Waddell G, Main C J, Morris E W, Di Paola M, Gray I C M 1984 Chronic low back pain, distress and illness behaviour. Spine 9: 209–213

26 Engel G L 1959 'Psychogenic' pain and the pain-prone patient. Am. J. Med. 26: 899–918

27 Szasz T S 1968 The painful person. Lancet 88: 18–22

28 Merskey H, Spear F G 1967 The concept of pain. J. Psychosom. Res. 11: 59–67

29 Sternbach R A, Wolf S R, Murphy R W, Akeson W H 1973 Aspects of chronic low back pain. Psychosomatics 14: 52–56

30 Sternbach R A, Wolf S R, Murphy R W, Akeson W H 1973 Traits of pain patients: the low back 'loser'. Psychosomatics 14: 226–229

31 Sternbach R A, Timmermans G 1975 Personality changes associated with reduction of pain. Pain 1: 171–179

32 Sternbach R A 1977 Psychological aspects of chronic pain. Clin. Orth. 129: 150–155

33 Main C J 1983 The modified somatic perception questionnaire (MSPQ). J. Psychosomat. Res. 27: 503–514

34 Zung W W K 1965 A self-rating depression scale. Arch. Gen Psychiat. 12: 63–70

35 Dahlstrom W G, Welsh G S 1960 An MMPI handbook: a guide to clinical practice and research. University of Minnesota Press, Minneapolis

36 Graham J R 1977 The MMPI: a practical guide. Oxford University Press, New York

37 Ransford A O, Cairns D, Mooney V 1976 The pain drawing as an aid to the psychologic evaluation of patients with low back pain. Spine 1: 127–134

38 Melzack R 1975 The McGill pain questionnaire: major properties and scoring methods. Pain 1: 277–279

39 Melzack R, Wall P D 1982 The challenge of pain. Penguin, Harmondsworth

40 Main C J 1984 Unpublished data

41 Waddell G, McCulloch J A, Kummel E, Venner R M 1980 Non-organic physical signs in low back pain. Spine 5: 117–125

42 Walters A 1961 Regional pain alias hysterical pain. Brain 84: 1–18

43 Fordyce W E 1966 Behavioural methods for chronic pain and illness. Mosby, St Louis

44 Mechanic D 1968 Medical sociology. Free Press, New York

45 Pilowsky I 1978 A general classification of abnormal illness behaviour. Brit. J. Med. Psychol. 51: 131–137

46 Waddell G, Bircher M, Finlayson D, Main C J 1984 Symptoms and signs: physical disease or illness behaviour? Brit. Med. J. 289: 739–741

47 Penfield W 1959 Foreward. In: White J C, Sweet W H. Pain and the neurosurgeon. Thomas, Springfield

48 Spangfort E V 1972 The lumbar disc herniation. A computer-aided analysis of 2504 operations. Acta Orthop. Scand. (suppl) 142: 1–95

49 McCoy C E, Selby D K, Lawlis G F, Mooney V, Mayer T 1983 Pain drawing grid. Presented to the International Society for the Study of the Lumbar Spine, Cambridge

50 Porter R W, Hibbert C 1983 Neurogenic claudication treated with calcitonin. Presented to the International Society for the Study of the Lumbar Spine, Cambridge

51 Waddell G, Main C J 1984 Assessment of severity in low back disorders. Spine 9: 204–208

52 World Health Organization Constitution. 1946

53 Merskey H 1979 The analysis of hysteria. Baillière Tindall, London

54 Southwick S M, White A A 1983 The use of psychological tests in the evaluation of low back pain. J. Bone Joint Surg. 64A: 560–565

55 Main C J, Waddell G 1984 The detection of psychological abnormality in chronic low back pain using four simple scales. Current Concepts in Pain 2: 10–15

56 Main C J, Waddell G 1984 Manual. The identification of psychological abnormality in patients with chronic low back pain. Available from Dr C J Main, Top-grade Clinical Psychologist, Hope Hospital, Salford M6 8HD

Psychological approaches to management and treatment of back pain

INTRODUCTION

As early as 1911 it was suggested that some cases of low back pain (LBP) have an 'emotional' cause,[1] and discussion about causes or influences other than tissue pathology on the presentation of pain symptomatology has been evident in the compensation and medico-legal literature for many decades. Indeed, selected physical signs which appeared to have predominantly non-physical interpretation were described early in this century.[2-4] But although attempts have been made to explain the discrepancy between the level of disability and the degree of physical pathology on the basis of 'functional overlay', a wide variety of approaches has been taken to the definition and quantification of such psychological features, and much of this confusion has resulted in turn from the adoption of quite different psychological models. It seems possible, however, to identify three major perspectives which can be described as the 'mental illness' model, the 'personality' or 'attitudinal' model and the 'environmental' model, although the advent of complex statistical methodology has allowed the development not only of more sophisticated variants of these, but also of models incorporating features of more than one of them. Both the 'mental illness' and the 'personality' or 'attitudinal' models can be seen as examples of psychosomatic theory; the 'environmental' model is closer to a sociopsychosomatic or even sociosomatic theory.

Perhaps fortunately, investigation into the psychology of back pain is relatively recent, in comparison for example with peptic ulcer, and therefore has been encumbered less with the extravagant psychodynamic theorizing so prevalent in the early psychosomatic literature. The attractiveness of identifying underlying mental illness as the 'missing link' is obvious, since it not only offers a diagnosis but also possibilities for treatment. In a large general population study, an association was found between low back pain and history of psychological illness, and patients with and without LBP could be differentiated according to history of diagnosis of 'anxiety', although no differences were found in the incidence of depression.[5] In another study[6] an association was found between a history of psychiatric illness, low social class and insidious onset of back pain. Non-specific physical diagnoses are correlated with a history of psychological or psychiatric treatment.[7] A recent study,[8] however, showed no differences in psychiatric diagnosis between patients with and without physical abnormalities, and psychiatric and chronic pain patients do not endorse the same pattern of items on psychological symptom scales.[9,10]

Major psychiatric illness such as schizophrenic psychosis and manic depressive psychosis are extremely rare in patients presenting with chronic backache, although organic psychoses can be produced by acute systemic diseases such as infection or disseminated malignancy, and so physical pathology must be excluded prior to psychiatric assessment. The association between depressive symptomatology and chronic pain, however, has long been recognized.[11] In a study of 200 consecutive admissions to a psychiatric clinic, 53% of the patients included pain as one of their complaints, and of those with a diagnosis of depression 56% had pain as one of their symptoms.[12] In a study of pain clinic patients, 10% of the patients were classified as having a depressive syndrome.[13] There are undoubted similarities between the chronic pain syndrome and the depressive syndrome,[14-16] and it has been suggested that pain and depression may share a common pathogenesis.[17]

Antidepressants have been used in the management of chronic pain for many years, but the relationships between their antidepressant action and their effect on pain remains the subject of debate.[18] Many studies on chronic pain contain patients with diagnoses other than that of chronic back pain, and the results of the few on back pain specifically are inconclusive. In a double-blind comparison between Tofranil® and placebo, no significant advantage of antidepressant over placebo was found.[19] (Indeed, the most interesting feature of the study was that, for various reasons, 30 of the original 59 patients were rejected from the study.) In another study[20] no significant difference in initial or change in depression scores were found between imipramine and placebo, and neither could any linear relationship be found between serum drug levels and symptomatology. In a recent study[21] of volunteers with major affective or dysthymic disorder and chronic back pain, both drugs produced significant decreases in depression, with an overall response rate of 70%, but while baseline pain, depression and anxiety were correlated, treatment changes in these measures did not correlate. CSF beta-endorphin levels did not change with treatment.

The 'mental illness' model

Differences in methodology, and particularly in types of assessment, make it difficult to assess the worth of the 'mental illness' model in chronic low back pain. It has been claimed[22] that there is a substantial proportion of mental illness in new pain clinic attenders, and that both the presence and severity are significantly underestimated by anaesthetists. There would seem to be general agreement that symptoms of anxiety and depression are a common feature of back pain, with relative preponderance of anxiety symptoms in the more acute stages, and depressive symptoms in the more chronic stage.[15] A distinction must be made, however, between the presence of symptoms of psychological distress and psychiatric illness of a severity meriting psychiatric treatment.

Antidepressant medication is not the treatment of choice for the chronic back pain patient, although in the small minority of patients with severe depressive symptomatology, or in whom there is evidence of a clear endogenous illness (assuming one accepts the validity of that diagnosis), then it would appear sensible to treat depression in the first instance, prior to reassessment. A dimensional rather than a categorical model of distress in back pain would seem appropriate in general orthopaedic or rheumatological clinics where it has been suggested[23] that chronic pain patients' depressive problems may be best construed as a form of learned helplessness[24] rather than as a fully blow depressive syndrome.[25] In a comment on sadness and depression in terminal illness[26] attention was drawn to the distinction between sad or depressed mood in the context of an extremely difficult life situation and a depressive illness. With slight modification, the same perspective can be brought to bear on chronic low back pain.

Although the 'mental illness' model has considerable problems in the diagnostic sense of providing an alternative or a supplement to a physical diagnosis, psychodynamic concepts have produced a treatment impetus in leading to the development of a variety of counselling techniques and psychotherapies sometimes offered to chronic back patients. These will be discussed later in the chapter.

A fundamental tenet of much such therapy is the concept of 'conversion hysteria'. In the context of low back pain, the pain is considered an emanation of psychological distress of which the patient is unaware or is unwilling to confront. Attempts to evaluate such theoretical models are bedevilled by problems of definition and difficulties in the adequate description or quantification of such psychological constructs, and it is easy to sympathize with the view that such psychological edifices may have more to do with the psychologist or psychiatrist's perception of the patient's world than that of the patient. The construction of a causal pathway from the individual's unconscious conflicts (established in the very early years of childhood) to the persistence of chronic low back pain seems difficult indeed, and it will be argued that such an exercise is not only theoretically hazardous, but in general unnecessary, since for the vast majority of chronic low back pain and for even those with fairly high levels of emotional distress, less speculative or extravagant theoretical models are available. As far as psychological methods of treatment are concerned, therefore, the 'mental illness' model has made little impact.

The 'personality' model

Of more importance is the 'personality' model, here used in a very general sense to encompass the measurement of attitudes and emotion. The development of statistical methodology, particularly in the field of mental testing, offers much more refined assessment instruments than were previously available, and sophisticated psychological tests permit the investigation of a wide range of attitudes and beliefs. As far as the identification of a 'functional' component in back pain is concerned, the most widely used test is the Minnesota Multiphasic Personality Inventory or MMPI,[27] a 566 item test yielding scores on ten clinical scales and three validity scales. Since then a large number of additional scales have been derived, including a 'low back' scale[28] and a DOR[29] also intended to differentiate 'functional' from 'organic' back pain. It has also been suggested that the low back and DOR scales used in conjunction are superior to either alone.[30] Findings using these scales have been seriously criticized on methodological grounds[30,31] and, in general, the failure to find consistent relationships between various personality dimensions and the presence or absence of organic impairment in chronic pain patients has led to a shift in emphasis in the use of the MMPI.

The test has been also used descriptively, and elevations on the hysteria, hypochondriasis and depression scales are frequently found in chronic pain patients. A particular profile, the so-called 'Conversion-V', is often used to identify 'somatization of psychic distress'.[32] It can be argued that the distress identified by the first three clinical scales (consistently but not powerfully) may be a function of a normal reaction to chronic ill-health rather than an inappropriate or neurotic reaction. Quite simply, patients with chronic health problems are almost invariably found to have elevated neurotic triad (hysteria, hypochondriasis and depression) scores. Such elevations may result from the scales containing items about ability to work, physical health, past and present symptomatology and pain. In a recent review, it was concluded, 'The data do not support attempts at defining a low back pain or chronic pain personality profile apart from the emotional disturbance associated with chronic limitation and disruption of activity.'[33]

The importance of psychological factors in chronic low back pain can be taken as established, therefore, although their precise significance is remains unclear. A natural sequela of this recognition has been an extension to the investigation of psychological methods of treatment directed not simply at pain itself, but also at response to physical methods of treatment and to the reduction of disability and invalidism.

For the purpose of this chapter, psychological treatment has been divided into four main areas: stress reduction techniques with primary physiological focus; stress reduction techniques with a primary cognitive or emotional focus; behavioural approaches; and the incorporation of psychological techniques within multidisciplinary pain programmes (with the exception of back schools which are reviewed earlier in the book), although it must be recognized that in clinical practice there is frequently overlap among these techniques. The chapter concludes with a brief discussion of implications for assessment, treatment and research with a consideration of the design of health care delivery for back pain sufferers and suggestion of a modification to the traditional disease model in back pain.

STRESS REDUCTION I — PHYSIOLOGICALLY FOCUSED TECHNIQUES

Physiological changes resulting from sympathetic activity in the autonomic nervous system are well recognized in individuals placed in situations of alarm and danger. Pain has an alarming effect in human (and animal) physiology. In the treatment of chronic stress problems, the treatment approach frequently is designed to reduce physiological over-arousal (whether by pharmacological or psychotherapeutic means) and improve emotional well-being. It is easy to construe chronic pain as a stressor, not only because of the unpleasant nociceptive input, but also, particularly with chronic low back pain, because of the associated disability and disruption to personal life.

Although stress-reduction techniques are employed by all sorts of professionals, the theoretical basis and much of the experimental work has derived from psychology, and it is easy to understand how such approaches have become an important feature of clinical psychology. Psychophysiological studies have shown that subjects who report high autonomic reactivity in general have higher levels of sympathetic activity,[34] but that individuals not only vary in the extent to which they react physiologically to stress, but also can be classified according to the relative response of different physiological variables.[35] Some individuals tend to show increased cardiovascular activity (e.g. heart rate increase), some increased galvanic skin response, while others show heightened muscle activity. Stress reduction techniques are designed to redress the posited autonomic imbalance. In chronic back pain, there may be not only an increased level of sympathetic activity in general (with or without a specific muscle focus), but also there may have become an established pain-tension cycle. It has been observed[36] that in chronic back pain patients, even though the original injury may have healed, a response to organic insult increases tension in muscles surrounding the area, and the pain–tension cycle is quite capable of perpetuating the pain itself. Very often, with an increase in pain, neighbouring muscle groups will also be tensed, which will increase pain and so on. Anxiety will further exacerbate the problem.

General procedures

The most widely known 'physiological' stress reduction technique is Jacobsonian systematic muscle relaxation training[37] which consists in training the patient to systematically tense and relax specific muscle groups in turn. Such techniques have been particularly important in the treatment of anxiety,[38] although whether the major mechanism is the induction of mental rather than physical relaxation[39] is a matter of debate[40] since one can be muscularly relaxed, yet autonomically aroused.[41,42] Many variants of muscle relaxation training are practised, but most involve progressively tensing

and relaxing various muscle groups throughout the body.[43]

Most studies evaluating relaxation training with chronic pain syndromes have consisted of studies of tension headache,[44] and there have been several reports of significant reduction in tension headache frequency.[45–47] In a controlled comparison of progressive muscle relaxation with frontalis electromyographic (e.m.g.) biofeedback and a placebo medication, both active treatments were shown to be superior to placebo.[48] Similar results were found in another study.[49] Relaxation training has also been effective for migraine.[50,51] In a study of facial pain, relaxation training in combination with haloperidol was found to be effective.[52] In a study of acute ischaemic pain, relaxation training was effective in reducing stress, but the magnitude of the effect was determined by cognitive factors.[53]

Few studies have examined the specific effectiveness of relaxation training for chronic back pain, since it is usually offered as simply one part of a therapeutic package. Thus in one study, systematic relaxation training was given in combination not only with educational advice, but also with general and paraspinal biofeedback, making it impossible to disentangle the specific value of the relaxation training component in a successful behavioral treatment programme for chronic low back patients.[54] In combination with an operant activity programme, it has been found to be superior to both traditional rehabilitation and a waiting list control.[55] In an interesting study examining different behavioural treatment components in an additive, order-balanced fashion, relaxation training was found to be more important than social reinforcement for increased activity, assertion training or a functional pain-behaviour analysis.[56] Finally, in a controlled comparison of group progressive-relaxation training and cognitive behavioural therapy for chronic low back pain, both relaxation training and cognitive behavioural therapy patients improved significantly on self-report measures of pain, depression and disability (waiting list controls did not); and a marked reduction in health care use was found at $1\frac{1}{2}$–2 year postal follow-up.[57]

Other techniques such as autogenic training (relaxation-inducing self-statements) are found in multidisciplinary pain programmes and have been reported to enhance the value of biofeedback training[58] but to the author's knowledge have not been systematically evaluated for back pain. Transcendental meditation has been found to decrease the distress associated with the experience of acute experimental pain (cold pressor test),[59] and it has been recently claimed to produce significant, reproducible and long-term improvements in pain and psychological status for chronic pain patients,[60] but specific studies of its value for low back pain have not as yet appeared in the literature.

Electromyograpic feedback

A more specific type of stress reduction is biofeedback, in which physiological events (frequently electromyographic) are electronically monitored, usually by means of surface electrodes, and the information is displayed visually or aurally in order that the patient can learn to bring under control processes normally under involuntary control. Its application to pain is based on assumptions that a physiological disorder (usually an aspect of sympathetic overactivity) at least contributes to the severity of the pain problem and that, using various analogue or digital representations of physiological activity, patients can learn to change such activity and thereby ameliorate pain. Four types of biofeedback have been identified[44] in the treatment of chronic pain syndromes:

1. Electroencephalogram (e.c.g.) feedback to help the subject produce alpha (8–13 Hz) brain activity, a relaxed state hypothesised to be incompatible with pain
2. Skin temperature feedback to increase finger temperature in patients with migraine headaches
3. Cephalic blood volume pulse feedback (BVP) to reduce the blood volume pulse of the cephalic temporal artery in migraine headache patients, and
4. Electromyographic (EMG) feedback to reduce muscle tension.

As far as pain patients are concerned, biofeedback has been seriously evaluated only for headache, where it would appear to be of comparable efficacy to relaxation training.[48,49] As far as back pain is concerned, the type of feedback is almost always EMG. EMG is used diagnostically to identify sites of specific muscle tension and suitable sites for electrode placement, or therapeutically either as a form of general stress reduction (usually from the frontalis muscle) or to decrease lateral imbalance in the correction of gait or decrease muscle spasm in cervical or lumbar paraspinal muscles.[61,62]

An EMG scanning procedure designed to identify bilateral EMG sites suitable for various chronic pain problems is described.[62] Perhaps unsurprisingly they identify frontalis and masseter muscle groups as being of prime importance for headache, and right–left discrepancy in lumbar and cervical paraspinal muscle groups as being important for low back pain. They comment further on the importance of site of electrode placement and the relationship with posture. Their EMG Diagnostic Scan Protocol would seem to merit further investigation.[62]

Another study evaluated EMG biofeedback for a group of patients having either tension headache, jaw pain or back pain, but although evidence of reduction in frontalis EMG was found in all groups, only one of the eight low back pain patients derived benefit. In a fairly large study of biofeedback relaxation training[63] a number of predictors of positive response to biofeedback were identified, but since only 7 of the 54 patients had low back pain, and it was commented that patients with head pain had better outcomes than those with back pain, the result can hardly be taken as conclusive. A study of EMG assisted relaxation training, however, showed that in a study of 18 patients with low back pain, after six sessions (supplemented by home practice) 15 patients reported a regular decrease in pain, and at one year follow-up, 9 of the 13 contacted had maintained initial therapeutic gains.[54]

In the last few years, more attention has been paid to EMG biofeedback from the paraspinal lumbar muscles. In a study of eight male patients with low back pain attributed to muscle spasm, four of the patients following treatment showed at least a 50% reduction in muscle tension levels with concomitant increase in activity levels.[64] In a controlled trial of EMG biofeedback, a creditable pseudotherapy, and conventional medical treatment in patients with chronic rheumatic back pain, biofeedback proved superior in reducing EMG levels, pain levels and health care use, although since patients also received a cognitive model emphasizing the relationship between appraisals of stress, increased muscle tension and pain, and physical therapy, it may have been that the EMG feedback was superior only in combination with the aforementioned additional therapeutic ingredients, since no group received EMG alone.[65] In an interesting single-case study[66] a patient was given 15 sessions of paraspinal lumbar EMG over 5 weeks. Training was provided while the patient was standing, during trunk movements and for movement patterns known to exacerbate the pain problem. Specific joint ranges of motion and pain ratings were recorded at each session. Joint ranges increased over time while subjective pain drug intake and EMG variability was reduced. Fifteen weeks after the first session, the patient was still able to minimize variability in EMG activity in specific positions.

The theoretical basis for lumbar biofeedback for back pain, however, has been questioned. Attention has been drawn to a number of studies[67-70] showing that paraspinal EMG levels can be either elevated or reduced in patients with chronic back pain, and levels of paraspinal EMG activity can be at the extreme ends of the spectrum even among patients who have allegedly identical diagnoses stemming from similar pathophysiological process. A series of Japanese studies seemed to demonstrate higher back muscle tension in low back pain subjects in comparison with normals during various movements and in various static postures.[71] It has also been found that, with prolonged standing, low back pain subjects show increases in paraspinal EMG readings in contrast to normal subjects who show decreases.[72] In a study of psychophysiological response patterns during static posture and stress tasks, low back pain patients were found in general to be autonomically more reactive than normal controls but showed no tendency to develop asymmetrical or differential EMG increases in physically stressful tasks in comparison with the normals.[73] In a study employing EMG paraspinal feedback to reduce standing levels of pain, the experimental group, in comparison with a waiting list control group showed a significant decrease in EMG but no significant pain reduction[74] An investigation of EMG differences between low back pain patients and normals in various positions and during various tasks[75] showed that each person with low back pain had a distinctive muscle contraction pattern. In a recent interesting study,[76] chronic back patients, unlike non-chronic

back patients or healthy controls, displayed paravertebral muscle elevation to personally stressful situations but not to other tasks, raising the possibility of a particular muscular response stereotype in specific situations.

Conclusions

It is difficult to draw conclusions about such disparate findings. It has been suggested that chronic low back patients may respond specifically to certain types of EMG feedback (binary rather than analogue), although it is difficult to see why this might be so.[77] Following a discussion of some of the specific problems encountered in producing a satisfactory theoretical integration of EMG findings, it has been suggested[78] that 'expectation of personal mastery' (essentially a belief in the therapeutic value of biofeedback) may be a vital component. It may be that, while biofeedback treatment may be useful with specific pain disorders and with certain patients, it is more likely to be effective in conjunction with other treatment modalities such as coping-skills training or cognitive restructuring (see below) than as the sole treatment modality.[79] Indeed, it is a frequent ingredient in the comprehensive treatment/rehabilitation packages such as that at Casa Colina Hospital,[80] reviewed towards the end of this chapter.

There is clearly not a simple association between muscle tension, activity and pain,[73] so it is perhaps unsurprising that the efficacy of biofeedback is unclear. At this juncture, more investigation is needed into the role of posture and dynamic movement,[81] into the identification of individual differences in EMG changes in response to different tasks or situations, and into the effect of different postures. It has been remarked[73] that 'More adequately controlled tests of biofeedback are required for assessment of the link between excessive muscle tension and low back pain, as well as for demonstration of the relative effectiveness of this modality.' More specifically, it has been observed[82] that,

> Clearly, further research is needed, using improved methodology, providing outcome data on all levels of behaviour (motor, physiological, subjective), comparing EMG biofeedback to relaxation training and other less expensive treatment approaches, assessing

differential effectiveness of these treatment modalities, and extending the follow-up periods.

This would appear to be a reasonable appraisal of the state of the art as far as the relationship between physiologically focused stress reduction techniques and back pain is concerned.

STRESS REDUCTION II — COGNITIVE APPROACHES

Psychotherapy

Cognitive approaches to pain have now become a major therapeutic focus[40] and can perhaps be construed as a development from the recognition of the importance of attitudes in the outcome of all sorts of medical rehabilitation. The role of attitudes is important in terms of aetiology, compliance with treatment and outcome, and the development of treatment techniques emphasizing the importance of the patient's beliefs and expectations about treatment. Traditionally, psychotherapy has varied from the psychoanalytic approaches (emphasizing the importance of unconscious processes developed at the earliest stages of infancy) to behavioural approaches incorporating detailed appraisal of the patient's current environment.

Recently the development of cognitive modification (or specific techniques designed to produce attitude change) has complicated the picture. As far as pain is concerned, both cognitive and behavioural approaches have had their champions, but as far as back pain specifically is concerned, psychological approaches have tended to focus on strictly behavioural models (often described as operant) or, in the last few years, mixed models with multidimensional approaches and several criteria of outcome. In a sense such distinctions are artificial, since any therapeutic interchange can be construed in a number of different ways, and therapeutic change produced in one modality can be expected to produce change also in other modalities. An attempt will be made nonetheless to describe briefly the more psychodynamic approaches, and continue via a brief review of hypnosis to the more specific cognitive behavioural models. Behavioural approaches will then be reviewed separately.

It is usually considered that psychosomatic patients are especially poor candidates for psycho-

therapy in general and psychoanalysis in particular,[83] and one clinician considered[84] that three-quarters of his psychosomatic patients were unsuitable for intensive, interpretive psychotherapy. It has even been claimed[85] that such patients actually get worse from the psychodynamic process. Motivation of such patients to change therapeutically has been questioned[86] and attempts have been made to elucidate a psychosomatic character pattern.[87] Directly related to motivation for treatment have been the observations that many psychosomatic patients consider psychological conflict as a sign of weak character and emotional problems as synonymous with malingering.[88]

Individual and family psychotherapy are reviewed elsewhere.[83] Group psychotherapy has been advocated as an emotionally less threatening approach to psychotherapy. The group has been described as an excellent medium for making psychosomatic patients aware of their emotions,[89] enabling better information transmission between doctor and patient[90] and producing gains in identification with persons having similar somatic experiences and attitudes.[91] Unfortunately major methodological problems bedevil much such research, and it is difficult, therefore, to have confidence in either the validity of the descriptive system or the clinical importance of the results.

The short-term use of group psychotherapy has been advocated, with particular emphasis on a 'here and now' framework,[92] but such groups differ in frequency, intensity, structure and goals from most groups for chronic pain patients, in which the patient population does not usually have the mental set to become engaged in psychological work.[93] It has been suggested that patients learn to accept such a role much more readily when one of the psychotherapists also functions as an attending medical physician.[94] Many groups, run particularly in chronic pain clinics, have a psychotherapeutic ingredient, although this is frequently not made explicit and groups run as 'stress reduction' or 'problem solving' groups, particularly in in-patient programmes such as those at Swedish Hospital, Seattle, and during the Pain Management Program at St Mary's Hospital, Rochester, are managed by staff with considerable psychotherapeutic skills.[95] Evaluation of psychotherapeutic processes in general is fraught with difficulty. One author[96] has observed:

Short-term didactic therapy is said to provide patients with a different orientation than their habitual chronic invalidism, so that different role concepts develop. In the groups there is little emphasis on individual unconscious motives or on group process. Rather, the emphasis is on rehabilitation goals, ways of achieving these and 'games' or other habits the patient may unwittingly use to sabotage their progress.[. . .] Thus the content of the group's discussion may well be important in maintaining the interest and attention of the patients, but the effect of the therapy may be due more to the learning of adaptive responses by modelling than by the acquisition of cognitive strategies.

Not only is controlled research into psychotherapy (whether individual or group) singularly lacking research into back pain, but major methodological advances in the evaluation of psychotherapy itself may be necessary before adequate evaluation of its contribution to back pain emerges.

Hypnosis

Since its early development, hypnosis has evolved in a number of ways ranging from its use in psychodynamic therapy to its incorporation as a self-control technique in multidisciplinary pain programmes. An interesting history of its early development is presented elsewhere.[97] It has been described as a form of psychotherapy,[64] although much of the experimental work has concentrated on its physiological mechanisms.[98] In the relief of pain, hypnosis has been considered in terms of its effects on sensory pain, suffering and mental anguish,[99] and any adequate evaluation has to consider such distinctions.

There are considerable procedural variations in the technique, ranging from simple direct hypnotic and post-hypnotic suggestions, to indirect suggestions, to elaborate and sophisticated hypnoanalytical techniques, to applications of ego psychology, transactional analysis and behavioural psychology.[100] There are, however, four basic methods of achieving hypnotic pain control:[101]

1. Analgesia or anaesthesia created by suggestion
2. Substitution for a painful sensation of a different, less painful sensation
3. Displacement of the locus of pain to another area of the body (or sometimes even outside the body), and
4. Dissociation of awareness (in an appropriate context).

It has been claimed[102] that hypnoanalysis can help patients distinguish real from imagined pain, but the utility of such a differential diagnosis has been seriously questioned.[15,103] Case descriptions abound,[104-106] but it is proposed in this chapter to limit consideration to studies aiming to clarify the possible mechanisms involved or to evaluate the effectiveness of hypnoanalysis.

Reference is made[107] to neurosurgery under local anaesthesia performed in Texas where subjects were operated on under hypnosis. It is reported that every time the neurosurgeon touched the hippocampus with diathermy, the patient came out of hypnosis. Most experimental work, however, has focused on hynoptic analgesia investigating physiological differences between the response to stimulation with and without hypnotically-induced anaesthesia, frequently using pain threshold and tolerance levels as dependent variables. In an interesting investigation[98] it was demonstrated that hypnotic intervention may in part be a placebo response to be found in most subjects, but with highly hypnotized subjects producing even higher increase in pain threshold and tolerance than a placebo, suggesting that some aspects of the hypnotic procedure may have little to do with hypnotic suggestion per se. It has been stressed, however, that there is probably no general kind of placebo responder, but that difference individuals may respond to different kinds of placebo, e.g. interpersonal placebo such as hypnosis.[108] The issue would seem to merit further investigation.

Hypnotizability is not to be equated with gullibility[108] but may have to do with the demand characteristics of the situation. In an examination of the concept of the 'hidden observer', it was concluded that the experimental results were inconsistent with the notion that 'hidden' reports reflect the intrinsic activity of a 'dissociated state' but suggested in contrast that such 'hidden' reports were a feature of subjects' attempts to conform with their perceived expectations of the experiment.[109]

Reference to the issue of hypnosis in dramatic surgical procedures and with a number of severe pain problems is made elsewhere,[40] but careful studies on back pain specifically are hard to find. Hypnosis was studied in 24 patients with low back pain (5 having been excluded). All had previous surgery, with 75% having had two or more lumbar surgeries. In addition, 84% of the patients were considered to be addicted to or excessively dependent on medication. Of the 20 patients in whom it was possible to induce hypnosis, 16 reported an average of 80% pain relief during the first four sessions, with an average of 70% overall after six sessions.

Results affected a number of outcome measures.[110] Unfortunately no follow-up data are reported and no control groups were employed. Methodological problems in description of the hypnotic procedures are rightly highlighted, but the study can certainly be taken as encouraging. It has been suggested that, whether being used as an anaesthetic or in the relief of side-effects of chemotherapy in oncological pain, hypnosis should be considered as part of the therapeutic regimen rather than as a treatment in its own right;[98,111] and in the context of back pain specifically, it is used most frequently as part of a treatment package.[95]

Theoretical advances in understanding the importance of hypnosis as a self-control technique in back pain depend on an adequate descriptive system for hypnotic procedures, clarity in the description of patients treated, and the incorporation of adequate research designs to enable controlled comparisons with comparable techniques (whether delivered as a single technique or as part of a wider package). Only then will selection of patients likely to benefit and a systematic evaluation of the contribution of hypnosis to the treatment of back pain be possible.

Cognitive therapy

To the extent that in any clinical interview an attempt is made to appraise the patient's perception of the back pain, whether in terms of clinical history or present symptomatology, it could be said that cognitive factors play a part in the treatment or management decision. It has been reported that a psychological stress pattern was initiated by injuries to conscious organisms only, not to unconscious ones.[112] This raises the possibility that the psychological significance of the noxious agent in conjunction with bodily damage is the crucial factor in many diseases.

In a wide-ranging review[40] of the role of cognitive factors in behavioural medicine (within which the authors see such factors as playing a crucial part), cognitive factors are viewed as:

1. Determining the ways in which individuals define health, disease and illness
2. Influencing decisions regarding the utility of engaging in either health-promoting behaviours or risk-related behaviours
3. Determining how individuals respond to symptoms and incapacities
4. Influencing how individuals utilize the health care system, and
5. Contributing directly and indirectly to disease and illness.

In a recent experimental study of ischaemic pain,[113] it has been shown that pain intensity (whether before or after medication) is inversely related to increased cognitive activity on a mathematical task, and a relationship has been demonstrated between pain tolerance (during three experimental stressors) and efficacy of coping strategies. It was shown that not all subjects benefit from self-generated coping tasks, but that those subjects whose tolerance was already high gained further benefit.[114] It has been suggested that many 'unmotivated' patients may in fact have erroneous beliefs about, or expectations of, treatment,[115] and a relationship has been suggested between compliance and belief in relevance of an education and self-care programme for low back pain.[116] It has been shown that influencing thought processes experimentally, in conjunction with an analgesic, can increase the analgesic effect.[117] In a study of the use of alpha-wave biofeedback and hypnotic training for the control of chronic pain, the efficacy of treatment was not a function of alpha-wave activity per se, but a feature of distraction, suggestion, relaxation and a sense of control over the pain.[118]

The role of cognitive factors in a self-management programme for medication reduction in a chronic back pain population has been stressed,[119] and it has also been shown in a number of other clinical studies of low back pain that cognitive factors are important in the outcome of treatment. In one study of an outpatient pain management programme,[120] although significant changes were not produced in pain ratings, general personality traits, anxiety or depression, all patients saw themselves as less seriously ill at the end of the programme, and it has been suggested that efficacy of biofeedback may be found in cognitive rather than sensory dimensions.[65]

The role of psychological assessment in prediction

of outcome of treatment for back pain has been reviewed elsewhere[103] and the role of psychological assessment has been reviewed earlier in this volume. In this part of the review, however, attention will be restricted to cognitive and cognitive-behavioural methods.

Cognitive methods attempt directly to modify thought processes in order to attenuate pain, based on the assumption that a person's 'cognitions' or appraisals of his or her environment are critical determinants of his or her experiences and emotions. Generally they consist of either providing preparatory information about an impending event or training patients in the use of cognitive coping skills or strategies. Preparatory information has been evaluated primarily in the content of aversive physical procedures (e.g. physical examinations or elective surgery),[121-123] and it has been concluded that types of preparatory information may be differentially effective for subjects depending on their 'coping styles' or predispositions.[124]

Cognitive coping strategies have been classified into six main categories[40] which, rather than attempt to alter the appraisal of the situation, aim primarily to divert attention from the pain.

1. *Imaginative inattention* involves concentrating on a mental image incompatible with pain
2. *Imaginative transformation of pain* involves re-interpreting the pain as another sensation, e.g. numbness
3. *Imaginative transformation of context* is self-evident
4. *Focusing attention on physical characteristics of the environment* involves re-directing attention specifically to a particular task using cues from the surroundings
5. *Mental distraction* involves focusing attention on various thoughts without producing a particular image (e.g. mental arithmetic)
6. *Somatization* involves focusing attention, in a dissociative manner, on the part of the body receiving the intense sensation.

It has been suggested that cognitions may lead to anxiety reduction in situations of acute pain, and that cognitive therapy should be designed to cater for differences in the extent to which patients believe either they or the therapists have primary responsibility for effective pain management[53] and that the performance level of back patients during a physically demanding task is not simply a function of actual pain level but a complex interaction between the interpretation of proprioceptive signals and more stable, but unrealistic, expections.[125]

In a recent analogue study[126] it was shown that pain perception can be influenced by attributional strategies which allow negative self-relevant information to be attributed to limitation produced by pain rather than personal failings. It has been shown that chronically ill patients who show signs of the sort of depressive helplessness which is so commonly a feature of the chronic pain patient frequently show signs of personal helplessness in the early months, and that changes in a variety of cognitive factors from the acute to the chronic stage can be demonstrated.[127] Depression in low back pain patients has been shown to be a function of low back pain and cognitive errors, suggesting promise for cognitive therapy, designed to correct such errors, in alleviating depression despite the persistence of pain.[128]

Change in attitudes about pain may be a function of resolving unconscious conflicts (psychodynamic model), reducing the arousal level (physiological model) correcting mistaken beliefs (cognitive model), an effect of reconstructing the patient's environment to produce different effects on pain behaviours, or indeed some combination of these postulated mechanisms.

In one of the few systematic studies of coping strategies in chronic low back pain,[129] three factors were found. They were described as: cognitive coping or suppression, helplessness, and diverting attention. They correlated with emotional and behavioural adjustment to pain, but were unrelated to duration of pain, disability status or history of multiple lumbar surgeries. This study is an example of the careful experimental work needed to elucidate further the nature and specific contribution of cognitions to general treatment outcome.

Few studies, however, exist on the efficacy of cognitive therapy per se. Treatment outcome of migraine was predicted by the reported frequency of use of imagery techniques,[130] and cognitive re-direction strategies in conjunction with relaxation training seem to be useful in the treatment of acute ischaemic pain.[53] In a single case study[131] cognitive relaxation increased constructive activity. Summaries of laboratory studies comparing one cognitive coping strategy with another, and comparing cognitive coping strategies with no treatment and placebo control groups, are presented elsewhere,[40] (Tables 5.3 and 5.2 respectively). They conclude:

> The studies here indicate (1) there is no evidence that subjects who tolerate intense physical stimuli poorly suffer from a deficiency in the number or type of cognitive coping strategies in their repertoires; (2) no one specific category of coping strategies is consistently shown to be more effective than any other; and (3) what appears to distinguish low from high tolerant individuals is their cognitive processes, the 'catastrophising' thoughts and feelings that precede, accompany and follow the aversive situation rather than specific elements of the coping strategies per se.

The few studies on clinical pain seem quite encouraging, if equivocal, but further controlled studies are needed before firmer conclusions regarding the efficacy of particular cognitive methods in isolation are possible.[124] It is not known, for example, whether they are any more powerful than relaxation training given as a unimodal treatment. It is important, however, to consider such methods, since they are an essential ingredient of the cognitive-behavioural methods about to be described and a frequent component of multi dimensional pain programmes to be reviewed later.

Cognitive behavioural therapy

To some extent the distinction between cognitive and cognitive-behavioural therapies is difficult to make, since it is difficult to envisage the delivery of cognitive techniques without at least some prescription for behavioural change. From the theoretical point of view the approaches are quite different, but in practice they differ primarily in terms of degree of emphasis. The basis assumption behind cognitive-behavioural therapy is that sensory, affective, behavioural and cognitive factors all are viewed as contributing to the pain experience. The goal of the approach, therefore, is to alter maladaptive thoughts, feelings and behaviours as well as dysfunctional sensory phenomena. The objective of such treatment is to reduce feelings of helplessness and hopelessness by assisting the patient to gain some control over the pain experience. There are considered to be four major components to treatment:[40]

1. Education about the multidimensional perspective of pain
2. The identification of pain-eliciting and pain-aggravating situations, thoughts and behaviours
3. Stress management via the identification and modification of maladaptive cognitions, and
4. The teaching of coping skills.

The specifics of the therapeutic approach are presented with admirable detail and lucidity elsewhere[40] (chapters 8 to 13), and only an outline will be presented here. A feature of the approach is the linking of assessment with identification of targets for treatment. The initial phase begins before even contacting the patient. Referral sources are informed about the nature and philosophy of the cognitive-behavioural approach to pain management. The patient is also sent a handout, so by the time of arrival he/she is generally acquainted with what to expect. An extremely thorough assessment, involving interview and questionnaires (of various sorts) is then carried out. The 'situational and cognitive-affective analysis' is designed specifically to identify a treatment plan. Additional data may be supplemented by more objective assessment procedures, e.g. using pain diaries, or personality questionnaires.

An important recent study[132] has shown the importance of the spouse's responses in the level of depression reported by patients, and the importance of changing invalidity patterns at home of necessity involves significant others. The role of significant others in assessment is also part of the cognitive-behavioural approach, involving use of spouse-monitoring (e.g. persuading the spouse to use a diary to aid in the assessment of the pain problem) and leading to a joint establishment of goals, with frequently a major reconceptualization of the pain problem (perhaps using an adaptation[133] of the gate-control theory of pain[134,135] to discuss various physical, emotional and cognitive factors which may open or close the gate[40]). The identification of manageable phases of pain completes the assessment proper.

The skills acquisition phase, comprising homework assignment, cue-controlled relaxation, controlled breathing and attention-control techniques (already reviewed earlier in this chapter) lead to the generation of coping ideas, confrontation of the pain problem and self-appraisal. These skills-training techniques are then applied to specific problems such as increasing exercise and activities or to the management of medication, frequently using a graded approach.

A series of 'non-specifics' which influence the effectiveness of such techniques has been identified.[40] Many of these, such as non-compliance, initial resistance to treatment, waiting time and the patients' expectations about or emotional response to the assessment, are well recognized, but perhaps of most interest is their summary of the identification of the treatment elements[136] needed to ensure that patients understand, remember and implement the treatment regimen.

Unfortunately, the majority of studies reviewing such techniques concern headache rather than low back pain.[137] It has been concluded[124] that no definitive statements supporting the consistent efficacy of any of the cognitive and cognitive-behavioural methods for clinical pain control can yet be made, but coping skills per se would seem to merit further attention, with specific research into the application of self-efficacy theory[138] to pain control.

Specific studies on chronic pain patients are few. Biofeedback-assisted cognitive-behavioural group therapy has been found to be superior to structured social support and to no treatment in rheumatoid arthritis.[139] Cognitive-behavioural techniques have been incorporated within a comprehensive in-patient programme for groups of chronic back-pain patients with long-standing problems and poor prognosis, and fairly impressive outcome and follow-up results are reported, although on a limited assessment database.[82] Less positive results have been reported for an out-patient study contrasting cognitive-behavioural therapy and physical therapy.[140] On the other hand, in a well-controlled comparison of group progressive relaxation training, cognitive-behavioural group therapy and a waiting list/attention group, it was found that, at the end of the programme, both treatment groups improved, in contrast to the control group, and the cognitive-behavioural group rated themselves as having improved more in their ability to tolerate pain and participate in normal activities.[57] A postal follow-up at 1–2 years indicated a marked reduction in health care use for patients in both treatments, and the cognitive-behavioural therapy group had improved markedly in the time spent working.

In conclusion, the efficacy of cognitive-behavioural techniques per se in the treatment of back pain is largely undetermined. Problems in methodology and research design have made difficult not only a controlled comparison of such techniques with comparable procedures, but also the identification of the specific value of such approaches within more general treatment packages. Advances in the systematization of the therapeutic procedures[40] in conjunction with the use of imaginative research designs (such as multiple baselines)[56] and powerful statistics[132] will hopefully enable the development and validation of a set of techniques of considerable potential to the chronic back patient.

BEHAVIOURAL APPROACHES

Perhaps the most significant development in psychological approaches to the treatment of pain over the last 15 years has been the advent of behavioural approaches to patient care. In North America, the development of behavioural medicine has been wide-ranging.[96] In the field of pain (and chronic pain in particular), behavioural diagnostic and treatment techniques are now a general feature of the treatment approach, not only of many multidisciplinary pain clinics, but of much rehabilitation for the chronic invalid.[95]

In a sense, changes in behaviour have always been of interest in therapy, but the behavioural approach in general, and the operant approach in particular, lay specific emphasis on producing change in the behavioural manifestations of the pain experience. Rather than changing the inner person (underlying psychopathology or psychodynamic forces) to relieve symptoms, attention is directed specifically at the symptoms themselves, and any generalization of improvement is assumed to benefit the inner person, although this is a secondary or incidental effect.[96] The traditional disease model of pain assumes that symptoms, or indications, of pain are responses to stimuli from underlying pathology; treatment is therefore directed towards the assumed underlying pathology. For much of medicine, and particularly many acute conditions and progressive chronic conditions, such a model has considerable utility, but for other conditions such as chronic intractable benign back pain, the model has limitations.[141]

There are traditionally two types of behavioural model (although, as already discussed, cognitive-behavioural models are a recent development.)

Responses considered to involve automatic involuntary reflex mechanisms have been termed respondent behaviour, while responses involving cognitive function and subject to voluntary control are termed operant behaviour.[142] Recent advances in biofeedback (already reviewed) have called into question the validity of this distinction, in the sense that individuals can learn a degree of control over mechanisms traditionally considered involuntary. Many rehabilitation programmes contain elements of retraining of individual's responses to particular stimuli, but the distinctive feature of most rehabilitation programmes for chronic pain patients is the identification of pain behaviour considered to have come under the influence of the social context in which it is emitted. Positive or negative consequences are considered to increase or decrease the strength of that behaviour and therefore its likelihood of occurrence. Treatment consists in changing the consequences of the behaviour and thereby modifying the behaviour in question. Three steps are considered essential:[142]

1. Precise identification of the behaviours to be modified (i.e. to be increased or decreased)
2. Identification of the reinforcers (the consequences which affect the behaviour), and
3. Programming the environment to achieve the desire behavioural change.

The operant approach

The operant approach differs from the general medical approach in its objective of treatment. For the chronic back patient, the complaint about pain is seen as a problem in its own right, rather than simply the report of a subjective experience. Other typical targets for behavioural modification are requests for analgesics (examples of consulting behaviour), uptime (amount of time spent out of bed during the day), activity levels (assessed in various ways) and other aspects of invalid behaviour. The operant approach thus does not deal directly with pain per se, which is regarded as a private, subjective experience not lending itself to objective measurement or control, but with maladaptive 'pain behaviour'

(which can be thought of as an aspect of invalidism) and 'well behaviour', which comprises behaviours inconsistent with the invalid role and therefore appropriate targets.

A prerequisite for the approach is a behavioural analysis, a form of assessment designed to identify relationships among the behaviours of the patient and of significant others (such as the spouse). The aetiology of the specific pattern of illness behaviour is not of particular interest, although it may provide 'good bets' as far as the selection of new reinforcers or the identification of ingredients of 'well behaviour' are concerned. Childhood factors affecting the adult's repertoire of pain expression are reviewed elsewhere.[103,143,144] The development of chronic invalid patterns is also discussed in detail.[145] Of more concern to the behaviour analyst are the circumstances considered to be maintaining the pain behaviour or invalidism. Frequent consequences of pain and 'illness behaviour' are attention (frequently solicitous) from a doctor and often from the spouse or other family members, rest, 'time out' from stress, medication and financial effects (particularly disability payments or compensation).[146] Variants of all of these are to be found as targets for behaviour modification.

It has been shown recently that abnormal illness behaviour may be related to the amount of failed conservative treatment.[141] The importance of considering iatrogenic factors and the health care delivery system in the planning of treatment will be discussed in the concluding section of this chapter.

Results of treatment using the operant approach specifically are difficult to evaluate, partly because operant conditioning in the management of pain as classically understood and described[145,147,148] is rarely employed on its own. More commonly it represents a general approach which comprises many ingredients and even when employed in the classical manner is open to differing interpretation.[40] A small number of studies, however, have attempted to elucidate specific components of the operant method or attempted to evaluate it specifically. Operant techniques have been used in paraplegia,[149] cerebral palsy[150] and spina bifida,[151] but the first and perhaps most celebrated study on low back pain was from Seattle.[152] The authors systematically manipulated medication, attention and rest as positive reinforcements for non-pain behaviour in a 37-year-old female with an 18-year history of back pain. Medication was provided on a time-contingent rather than a pain-contingent basis (thus weakening the relationship between the complaint of pain and receipt of medication); attention and praise was given for non-pain behaviour, such as increased walking; pain behaviour was ignored; and rest periods were made contingent on increased participation in occupational therapy.

In a later study,[153] following 4–12 weeks in patient treatment and 0–24 weeks out patient treatment, with a follow-up of 5–175 weeks, patients reported less pain, less interference with daily activities, reduction in the use of medication, and decreased 'down time' (time spent reclining). Despite methodological limitations,[154] this study has been enormously influential. A similar approach was adopted in a study of 60 patients at the University of Minnesota,[155] but the apparently impressive results of 74% of patients 'leading normal lives' after treatment are less impressive in view of the rigorous exclusion criteria (e.g. accepting only those significantly motivated to undergo treatment), with the refusal of a significant number of those selected to take part. In fact, the '74%' represent only 19% of the original patients screened over a seven-year period.[154]

There is evidence that feedback alone may significantly affect levels of performance[156,157] and the results of the Seattle study[153] could have been explained by both verbal reinforcement and feedback. A controlled study of the operant treatment of disability due to chronic low back pain demonstrated both verbal reinforcement or visual feedback (graphing) in addition to verbal reinforcement to be superior to both visual feedback alone and to a control condition.[158]

The effectiveness of out-patient group treatment for chronic low back pain was investigated using behavioural treatment and physical therapy (based on traditional rehabilitation therapy designed to improve low back function).[140] The authors had hypothesized differential outcomes on a variety of outcome measures, but the post-treatment results showed general improvement for patients in both groups, with relatively weak support for the differential outcome hypothesis. In a small-out patient controlled study on chronic pain,[55] relaxation training (as a coping skill) and an operant pro-

gramme were superior to both a traditional rehabilitation procedure and a waiting list control. Finally, specific behavioural treatment components within a combined treatment 'package' were examined for four male sufferers of low back pain, using an elegant non-concurrent multiple baseline across subjects.[15] Relaxation training and social reinforcement of increased activity were shown to be necessary ingredients.[56] Functional pain-behavioural analysis training and assertion training, had minimal, if any, effects.

Given the paucity of controlled research into the efficacy of operant methods specifically for low back pain, it is perhaps surprising that they have had such influence. Certainly, immediately the treatment focus shifts from the report of pain specifically as an indicator of underlying physical damage, a whole range of treatment targets becomes available, and coping with pain and the minimization of invalidity become of major concern (which is perhaps not unreasonable, given the level of residual disability and associated distress in the community). A number of multidisciplinary pain programmes (e.g. Department of Rehabilitation Medicine in Seattle) make operant principles explicit and gear the philosophy of the programme to operant objectives. Many others include operant management as one of a number of techniques, which makes it difficult to evaluate the specific contribution of either specific operant procedures or an operant ingredient within a more general approach.

MULTIDISCIPLINARY PAIN PROGRAMMES

Multidisciplinary pain programmes and clinics vary widely in terms of administration, type of patient, funding, operation, philosophy and clinical content.[160] Programmes can be subsumed under the title of 'psychological treatment' to the extent that they employ one or more of the treatment techniques already reviewed in this chapter, or less specifically are directed towards self-learning and self-control programmes delivered within a therapeutic context requiring a large ingredient of self-help in combating the disability accompanying back pain. Such approaches to treatment, with the exception of specific pain reduction or pain control techniques (reviewed above), are perhaps better construed as pain-management techniques rather than treatment per se. To the extent that they produce changes in the patient's view of the disability, and attitude towards his or her future range of possibilities, they can be considered to have rational or cognitive effects. More usually, by encouraging and facilitating behaviour change on the basis of specific didactic teaching, offering the opportunity to extend the boundaries of exercise and movement tolerance, and offering the opportunity for group discussion both with other patients and with staff, the main focus of their therapeutic effect may be the alleviation of the sense of helplessness and hopelessness, variously expressed, which is so characteristic of the chronic back patient. A detailed discussion of the range of such clinics at present in operation, however, is beyond the remit of this chapter. They will be discussed, therefore, only in general terms, on the basis of their contribution to the treatment and management of back pain.

General approach

The general approach is well typified by the Emory Pain Control Center[161] where, among various treatment programmes, is a programme for pain-disabled patients based on contingency management.

> The thrust of the CM programme is cognitive behaviour modification for competent coping in maladaptive situations of existential suffering. The patients are educated to accept the basic idea that chronic pain and impairment of some body functions are not necessarily deterrents from meaningful and self-gratifying lives; through individual and group counselling, they are educated in how to change ways of thinking and acting in order to deal more effectively with their physical and emotional impairments.

A range of specific targets are identified which are achieved through education, specific physiotherapeutic and ergonomic procedures, emotional coping skills and attention to future occupational needs. A minority of programmes have a specifically medical rather than a broadly-based multidisciplinary emphasis,[162] but most are similar to Emory in containing a variety of ingredients[163-165] originating partly in rehabilitation medicine and partly in psychology. The rehabilitation influence can be seen in the design of physiotherapy and mobility programmes, frequently with specific ergonomic advice.

The psychological influence in its purest form is seen in the stress-reduction programmes and the incorporation of individual and group psychotherapy (whether psychodynamic, cognitive, behavioural or cognitive-behavioural), but can be seen also in the behavioural approach to the identification of rehabilitation targets, the application of problem-solving and coping skills, and the adoption of programmes carefully graded in order to build the patient's confidence. Perhaps of widest influence, however, has been the operant approach pioneered at the University of Washington, Seattle[142] and found in a relatively 'uncontaminated' form elsewhere.[166-168]

A number of programmes stress the importance of the psychotherapeutic component,[164] although frequently in the context of what is described as a behaviour modification programme.[161,169] Stress reduction techniques are a particularly important feature of some programmes[170] but are included in almost all.[160] A number of programmes are run as in-patient programmes (usually lasting about three weeks), sometimes with an additional out-patient programme either before or after the in-patient programme, while others are run purely as out-patient programmes. The situation is further complicated by the fact that, although low back pain patients frequently form the largest clinical group, the treatment programme often includes other pain patients, making an overall evaluation of the package specifically for back pain somewhat problematic.

A number of programmes, however, have been designed specifically for back-pain (usually low back) patients. In one study the outcome of broadly-based rehabilitation programmes designed around the theme of self-regulation is reported.[80] Using as outcome criteria both the level of functional physical activity on discharge and restoration to vocational activities, 57 of the 72 chronic back pain patients showed unimpaired physical functioning and 59 successfully resumed activities. In another study[54] the response of 111 chronic low back patients to a comprehensive behavioural treatment programme emphasizing relaxation procedures was examined. Over the course of treatment, significant reductions were obtained on measures of subjective tension, EMG activity and pain. Also, patients who had the best outcome in terms of pain relief were significantly more likely to show improvement in other outcome measures. An 80-week follow-up of 36 low back patients from a multidisciplinary treatment programme demonstrated statistically significant gains in the use of medical resources generally and use of analgesics specifically.[171] Following a comprehensive three-week in-patient package, 15 patients with chronic low back/leg pain showed significant reductions in pain ratings (both sensory and affective), overall distress, overt pain behaviours and use of narcotics, with a concomitant increase in activity levels.[172] In a study of multidisciplinary assessment in chronic low back pain, however, there were fairly equivocal results from the back pain programme.[173]

Few studies of predictors of outcome of psychologically oriented programmes yet exist, but a global measure of distress seems to be more predictive of treatment outcome than patients' reported intensity of pain prior to the programme,[174] illustrating that it is not possible to evaluate outcome without agreed outcome criteria (a topic which will be addressed in the concluding discussion). In a detailed analysis of outcome of a back pain programme it was found that, although 'problem patients' required an average of about 30% more treatment, 86% of all patients were enabled potentially to return to full activity, with 70% actually finding satisfactory employment.[165] Favourable outcome, with significant improvement according to all the test criteria and satisfactory vocational rehabilitation outcome, have also been reported.[175] The authors claim that a 'substantial majority' of patients had been promoted or transferred to better employment within three years of programme completion.

Data from one of the most influential clinics highlight a major problem in rehabilitation of the chronic back patient. In a report of the first 200 patients through the Mayo Clinic Pain Management Program, using a relatively crude measure of outcome (based on improvement in attitude, medication use and physical functioning), the 59% success rate at outcome had fallen to 40% at three months and 25% at one year follow-up.[73] A number of problems in the interpretation of the latter study, however, have been identified.[176]

In a clinic in which at least two-thirds of the patients suffer from chronic low back pain, meaningful therapeutic gains in 75% of patients at 18 months' follow-up are reported.[177] In another study of 100 patients of whom 79% had low back pain, statistically significant decreases in pain intensity and use of medications are reported, with a concomitant increase in activities of daily living, 21 months after an out-patient rehabilitation programme.[139] In an outcome study of 151 patients (including about 40% of patients with back or neck and back pain), a small reduction in pain intensity but a much larger shift towards a positive attitude was documented,[164] and in a follow-up study of 57 patients (of whom 57% had low back pain) significant gains were found at 8 months' follow-up of a multidisciplinary programme, although very low compliance with the prescribed therapeutic regimens was found.[178] Long-term results (5 years) on a small number of chronic-pain patients (of whom a proportion were back patients) showed encouraging improvement in several parameters (although with women improving in disability much more than men).[163] Recently a 37% improvement rate has been claimed in a study of 270 patients (of whom 29% had back pain), but the extent of a psychological component in the programme is unclear.[179]

A number of other studies report varying success rates using varying criteria, but as the clinical composition of the sample is unclear, they will not be reviewed.[120,180-182]

Outcome criteria are many and varied and are but one set of problems bedevilling research into the multidisciplinary pain clinic,[176] but it is perhaps worth drawing the distinction between measures of clinical change in the individual patient and changes in health care use by the patient following discharge. Medication usage and other measures of 'pain behaviour' are frequent targets in behaviourally oriented programmes.[142] In a number of clinics specializing in group therapy (e.g. Mayo Clinic and Swedish Hospital, Seattle), use of the health care system and interactions with health care personnel are specific topics of discussion and are seen as an essential focus for attitudinal, behavioural and emotional change in combating invalidism in chronic back pain patients.[95] Unfortunately, no systematic research appears to have been carried out on this interesting facet of rehabilitation, though it may encompass a critical mechanism for change in the transition from invalidism to successful coping behaviours.

The multidisciplinary pain programme is becoming a well-recognized approach to the management of chronic back pain. Given the duration of the pain problem, spontaneous remission is not to be expected. The results in general are therefore encouraging. (It has been estimated, for example, that a pain programme is cost-effective if 5% of subjects are returned to full employment.)[160] To the extent that the critical therapeutic mechanism may be the belief in the possibility of self-help, it can be argued that the distinction between active and passive forms of treatment is essentially a psychological one. Certainly, specifically focused psychological therapy is now a major ingredient of many multidisciplinary pain programmes, and indirectly may be an important influence in the rehabilitation of many chronic back patients. Delineation of specific psychological mechanisms in the outcome of treatment awaits adequate description of the psychological treatment ingredients themselves and carefully controlled studies with research designs of sufficient precision to be able to disentangle specific from general effects. Methodological studies such as that of Aronoff et al[176] represent a useful beginning.

CONCLUSIONS

The last two decades have seen increasing emphasis placed on psychological factors in the management of chronic back pain, and during the last decade psychological approaches to treatment have become increasingly evident, particularly in multidisciplinary pain clinics. An evaluation of current practice and recent research has highlighted in particular stress reduction techniques and psychotherapies (of various types) directed not so much at the pain experience itself, but at its effects in the form of disability and invalidism. Traditionally, treatment of back pain has used changes in physical status, in reported pain intensity and in return to work as outcome criteria. Psychological studies have demonstrated the importance of distress and other facets of quality of life being of equal significance.

The aims of psychological treatment have therefore frequently been different from more physically-based approaches, and there is evidence that, as far as the patient is concerned, the 'learned helplessness' evident in depressive symptomatology is as much a feature of the resultant disability than of the pain

itself. Coping skills and self-management techniques directed primarily at the 'learned helplessness' seem of considerable promise, particularly for the chronic pain patient who has already reached the end of medical or surgical treatment, or perhaps even earlier, at a stage before full-blown chronicity with its psychological sequelae had developed.

Research is needed, however, into the specificity of the psychological procedures, with appropriate controlled research on comparable therapeutic procedures. Since many of the psychological techniques are delivered within a multidisciplinary package, careful attention to research design and the inclusion of adequate statistical methodology are clearly of major importance. It seems likely at this juncture that the derivation of assessment tools sufficiently sensitive to monitor change and sufficiently broadly based to incorporate assessment of coping strategies and beliefs about control over health is particularly needed.

A 'paradigm' shift is needed in the conceptualization of back pain, with a move from the traditional disease model to a model incorporating aspects of suffering and reaction to pain.[183] The crude differential diagnosis of 'organic' and 'functional' must be replaced with an adequate assessment of both the organic and the psychological components. A move towards a more holistic approach to back pain in no way detracts from the importance of physical methods of treatment, but it makes it imperative that careful attention be paid to a sufficiently broadly based initial assessment to determine the relative importance of various facets of the individual's presenting complaint. A treatment and management plan must then be designed which takes these factors into account. 'Psychology for all' is patently absurd, but as soon as pain persists beyond the expected healing time, a broader assessment is indicated, with back education and psychological training or counselling available at an early stage for those patients showing early signs of excessive disability or distress, or inappropriate illness behaviour.

One final set of observations concerns the health care system and the delivery of health care itself. Recent research[141] has shown that the degree of inappropriate illness is related in part to the amount of previous failed conservative treatment. Doctor--patient communication may be of critical importance in the response to treatment, and compliance with the doctor's recommendation may be crucial in the maintenance of preliminary treatment gains. Much therapeutic endeavour in the multidisciplinary pain programmes for chronic pain patients is directed towards the remedying of inconsistencies in previous treatment and management of the patient. Failed treatment and repeatedly negative investigations maintain the patient in a 'passive' invalid role with little expectation that he or she can influence the course of his or her pain or disability. The simple 'organic–functional' dichotomy may have led to attributions of hypochondriasis or malingering, not only by the medical profession, but also by the patients' family.

The 'mental illness' model is seldom appropriate for the chronic back pain patient. Recognition of the differences among physical disease, mental illness and suffering must be clearly acknowledged and every attempt made not to confuse them. The challenge for the next decade may be to design treatment and management programmes which acknowledge such distinctions while bearing in mind the need for individual programmes based on profile of need. For the chronic back patient at least, it would seem that a multidisciplinary approach to assessment and treatment is essential, and part of the assessment may have to take into account the wider social and occupational context of the chronic pain problem, possibly incorporating more complex models.[184] From the research reviewed, psychological approaches to treatment can be said to have arrived, but much further research is needed to determine their specific contribution to the treatment and management of back pain.

REFERENCES

1   Chabot R D 1911 Differential diagnosis. Saunders, Philadelphia (Cited in Wilfling F J 1981 — see ref 71)
2   Collie J 1913 Malingering and feigned sickness. Boeber, New York
3   Jones A B, Llewellyn J 1917 Malingering or the simulation of disease. Heinemann, London
4   McKendrick A 1912 Malingering and its detection. Livingstone, Edinburgh
5   Gilchrist I C 1976 Psychiatric and social factors related to low-back pain in general practice. Rheum. Rehab. 15: 101–107
6   Gilchrist I C 1983 Different groups of patients with low back pain. Roy. Coll. Gen. Pract. 33: 420–423
7   Thomas M R, Lyttle D 1976 Development of a diagnostic checklist for low back pain patients. Clin. Psychol. 32: 125–129
8   Edwin D H, Pearlson G D, Long D M 1984 Psychiatric symptoms and diagnosis in chronic pain inpatients. IASP 4th World Congress, Seattle
9   Buckelew S P, DeGood D, Schwartz D 1984 Cognitive and somatic aspects of anxiety and depression in pain patients and psychiatric inpatients. IASP 4th World Congress, Seattle
10 Main C J 1983 The modified somatic perception questionnaire. Psychosom. Res. 27: 503–514
11 Sternback R A 1974 Pain patients, traits and treatment. Academic Press, New York
12 Merskey H, Spear F G 1967 The concept of pain. Psychosom. Res. 11: 59–67
13 Pilowsky I, Chapman C R, Bonica J J 1977 Pain, depression and illness behaviour in a pain clinic population. Pain 4: 183–192
14 Pilowsky I, Bassett D L 1982 Pain and depression. Br. J. Psychiat. 141: 30–36
15 Sternbach R A 1978 Clinical aspects of pain. In: Sternbach R A (ed) The psychology of pain. Raven Press, New York
16 Von Knorring L, Perris C, Eisemann M, Eriksson U, Perris H 1983 Pain as a symptom in depressive disorders. II. Relationship to personality traits as assessed by means of KSP. Pain 17: 377–384
17 Von Knorring L 1975 The experience of pain in depressed patients. Neuropsychobiol. 1: 155–165
18 Ward N G, Bloom V L, Friedel R O 1979 The effectiveness of tricyclic antidepressants in the treatment of coexisting pain and depression. Pain 7: 331–341
19 Jenkins D G, Ebbutt A F, Evans C D 1976 Tofranil in the treatment of low back pain. Int. Med. Res. 4: 28–40
20 Alcoff J, Jones E, Rust P, Newman R 1982 Controlled trial of imipramine for chronic low back pain. Journ. Fam. Pract. 14: 841–846
21 Ward N, Bokan J A, Phillips M, Benedetti C, Butler S, Spengler D 1984 Anti-depressants in concomitant chronic back pain and depression: doxepin and desipramine compared. J. Clin. Psychiat. 45: 54–59
22 Benjamin S, Barnes D 1984 Can anaesthetists detect depression in pain patients? IASP 4th World Congress, Seattle
23 Skevington S M 1983 Chronic pain and depression: universal or personal helplessness? Pain 15: 309–317
24 Seligman M E P 1975 Helplessness: on depression, development and death. Freeman, San Francisco
25 Becker J 1977 Affective disorders. General Learning Press, Morriston
26 Bond M R 1980 The suffering of severe intractable pain. In: Kosterlitz H W, Terenius L Y (eds) Pain in society. Chemie, Weinheim, p 53–62
27 Dahlstrom W G, Welsch G S 1960 An MMPI handbook. University of Minneapolis Press, Minneapolis
28 Hanvik L J 1951 MMPI profiles in patients with low back pain. J. Consult. Clin. Psychol. 15: 350–353

29 Pichot P, Perse J, Lekous M O, Dureau J L, Perez C I, Rychewaert A 1972 La personnalité des sujets présentant des douleurs fonctionnelles: valeur de l'Inventair Multiphasique de Personnalité du Minnesota. Revue de Psych. Appliquée 22: 145–172

30 Calsyn D A, Louks J, Freeman C W 1976 The use of the MMPI with chronic low back patients with a mixed diagnosis. J. Clin. Psychol. 32: 532–536

31 Bradley L A, Prieto E J, Hopson L, Prokup C K 1978 Comment on 'Personality organisation as an aspect of back pain in a medical setting'. J. Person. Ass. 42: 573–578

32 Louks J L, Freeman C W, Calsyn D A 1978 Personality organisation as an aspect of back pain in a medical setting. J. Pers. Ass. 42: 152–157

33 Naliboff B D, Cohen M D, Yellen A N 1982 Does the MMPI differentiate chronic illness from chronic pain? Pain 13: 333–341

34 Mandler G, Mandler J M, Uviller E T 1958 Autonomic feedback: the perception of autonomic activity. J. Abnorm. Soc. Psychol. 56: 367–373

35 Lacey J I 1956 The evaluation of autonomic responses. Toward a general solution. Ann. N.Y. Acad. Sci. 67: 123–164

36 Hockersmith V W 1975 Biofeedback applications in chronic back pain disability. Paper presented at the Annual Meeting of the American Psychological Association, Chicago

37 Jacobson E 1962 You must relax, 4th edn. McGraw-Hill, New York

38 Paul G 1966 Insight versus desensitisation in psychotherapy: an experiment in anxiety reduction. Stanford University Press, Stanford

39 Rachman S 1967 Systematic desensitisation. Psych. Bull. 67: 93–103

40 Turk D C, Meichenbaum D, Genest M 1983 Pain and behavioural medicine: a cognitive-behavioural perspective. Guildford Press, New York

41 Lader M H, Mathews A M 1968 A physiological model of phobic anxiety and desensitisation. Beh. Res. Ther. 6: 411–421

42 Van Ergen L F 1971 Psychophysiological aspects of systematic desensitisation: some outstanding issues. Behav. Res. Ther. 9: 65–77

43 Bernstein D A, Borkovec T D 1973 Progressive relaxation training. Research Press, Champaign

44 Turner J A, Chapman C R 1982 Review article: Psychological interventions for chronic pain: a critical review. I. Relaxation training and biofeedback. Pain 12: 1–21

45 Fichtler H, Zimmerman R R 1973 Changes in reported pain from tension headaches. Percept. Mot. Skills 36: 712

46 Tasto D L, Hinkle J E 1973 Muscle relaxation treatment for tension headaches. Behav. Res. Ther. 11: 347–349

47 Warner G, Lance J 1975 Relaxation therapy in migraine and chronic tension headache. Aust. 1: 298–301

48 Cox D J, Freundlich A, Meyer R G 1975 Differential effectiveness of electromyographic feedback, verbal relaxation techniques and medication placebo with tension headaches. J. Consult. Clin. Psychol. 43: 892–898

49 Haynes S, Griffin P, Mooney D, Parise M 1975 Electromyographic feedback and relaxation instructions in the treatment of muscle contraction headaches. Behav. Ther. 6: 672–678

50 Hay K M, Madders J 1971 Migraine treated by relaxation therapy. J. Roy. Coll. Gen. Pract. 21: 664–669

51 Lutker E R 1971 Treatment of migraine by conditioned relaxation: a case study. Behav. Ther. 2: 592–593

52 Raft D, Toomey T, Gregg J M 1979 Behavior modification and haloperidol in chronic facial pain. South Med. Journ. 72: 155–159

53 Clum G A, Luscomb R L, Scott L 1982 Relaxation training and cognitive redirection strategies in the treatment of acute pain. Pain 12: 175–183

54 Keefe F J, Block A R, Williams R B Jnr, Surwit R S 1981 Behavioral treatment of chronic low back pain: clinical outcome and individual differences in pain relief. Pain 11: 221–231

55 Linton S J, Melin L, Stjernlof K 1984 Controlled study of the effects of applied relaxation and operant activity training on chronic pain. IASP 4th World Congress, Seattle

56 Sanders S H 1983 Component analysis of a behavioral treatment program for chronic low-back pain. Behav. Ther. 14: 697–705

57 Turner J A 1982 Comparison of group progressive relaxion training and cognitive-behavioral group therapy for chronic low back pain. J. Consult. Clin. Psychol. 50- 757–765

58 Green E, Walters E D, Murphy G 1969 Feedback technique for deep relaxation. Psychophysiol. 6: 371–378

59 Mills W W, Farrow J T 1981 The transcendental meditation technique and acute experimental pain. Psychosom. Med. 43: 157–164

60 Kabat-Zinn J, Lipworth L, Sellers W, Brew M, Burney R 1984 Reproducibility and four-year follow-up of a training program in mindfulness meditation for the self-regulation of chronic pain. IASP 4th World Congress, Seattle

61 Cram J R, Freeman C W 1984 Specificity of EMG biofeedback in treatment of chronic pain. IASP 4th World Congress, Seattle

62 Cram J R, Steger J C 1983 EMG scanning in the diagnosis of chronic pain. Biofeed. Self-Reg. 8: 229–241

63 Tung A, DeGood D, Tenicela R 1978 Clinical evaluation of biofeedback relaxation training. Pennsylvan. Med. 82: 18–19

64 Freeman C W, Calsyn D A, Paige A B, Haler E M 1980 Biofeedback with low back pain patients. Am. J. Clin. Biofeed. 3: 118–122

65 Flor H, Haag G, Turk D C, Koehler H 1983 Efficacy of EMG biofeedback, pseudotherapy and conventional medical treatment for chronic rheumatic back pain. Pain 17: 21–31

66 Jones A L, Wolf S L 1980 Treating chronic low back pain: EMG biofeedback training during movement. Phys. Ther. 60: 58–63

67 Basmajian J V 1976 Electromyographic investigation of spasticity and muscle spasm. Physiother. (Canada) 62: 319–323

68 Basmajian J V 1978 Cyclobenzaprine hydrochloride effect on skeletal muscle spasm in the lumbar region and neck: two double-blind controlled clinical and laboratory studies. Am. J. Phys. Med. Rehab. 59: 58–63

69 Hirsch C, Ingelmark B E, Miller M 1963 The anatomical basis for low back pain. Acta Orth. Scand. 33: 1–17

70 Simons D G 1975 Muscle pain syndromes — Part 1. Am. J. Phys. Med. 54: 289–311

71 Wilfling F J 1981 Psychophysiological correlates of low-back pain. PhD thesis, University of British Columbia, Vancouver

72 Jayasinghe W J, Harding R H, Anderson J A D, Sweetman B J 1978 An electromyographic investigation of postural fatigue in low-back pain: a preliminary study. Electromyog. Clin. Neurol. 18: 191–198

73 Swanson G H, Cohen M J, Naliboff B D, Schandler S L 1984 Comparison of psychophysiological response patterns during posture and stress tasks in chronic LBP and control subjects. IASP 4th World Congress, Seattle

74 Nouwen A 1983 EMG biofeedback used to reduce standing levels of paraspinal muscle tension in chronic low back pain. Pain 17: 353–360

75 Sherman R A 1984 Relationship between strength of low back muscles' contractions and reported intensity in low back pain. IASP 4th World Congress, Seattle

76 Flor H, Turk D C, Birbaumer N 1984 Paravertebral muscular reactivity during stress exposure in chronic back pain patients. IASP 4th World Congress, Seattle

77 Nigl A J 1981 A comparison of binary and analog EMG feedback techniques in the treatment of low back pain. Am. J. Clin. Biofeed. 4: 25–31

78 Biederman H J 1983 Mechanism of biofeedback in the treatment of chronic back pain: an hypothesis. Psychol. Rep. 53: 1103–1108

79 Turk D C, Meichenbaum D H, Berman W H 1979 Application of biofeedback for the regulation of pain: a critical review. Psychol. Bull. 86: 1322–1338

80 Gottlieb H J, Strite L C, Koller R, Madorsky A, Hockersmith V, Kleeman M, Wagner J 1977 Comprehensive rehabilitation of patients having chronic low-back pain. Arch. Phys. Med. Rehab. 58: 101–108

81 Wolf S L, Nacht M, Kelly J L 1982 EMG feedback training during dynamic movement for low back pain patients. Behav. Ther. 13: 395–406

82 Turk D C, Flor H 1984 Review article: Etiological theories and treatments for chronic back pain. II. Psychological models and interventions. Pain 19: 209–233

83 Karasu T B 1979 Psychotherapy of the medically ill. Am. J. Psychiat. 136: 1–11

84 Wolff H H 1965 The psychotherapeutic approach. In: Hopkins R, Wolff HH (eds) Principles of treatment of psychosomatic disorders. Pergamon Press, London

85 Sifneos P E 1973 Is dynamic psychotherapy contraindicated for a large number of patients with psychosomatic diseases? Psychother. Psychosom. 21: 133–136

86 Sperling M 1952 Psychotherapeutic techniques in psychosomatic medicine. In: Bychowski G, Despert J L (eds) Specialized techniques in psychotherapy. Basic Books, New York

87 Marty P, M'Uzan M, David C 1963 L'investigation psychosomatique. Presses Universitaires de France, Paris

88 Minuchin S, Baker L, Rosman B, Liebman B, Milman L, Todd T C 1975 A conceptual model of psychosomatic illness in children. Arch. Gen. Psychiat. 32: 1031–1038

89 Reckless J, Fauntleroy A 1972 Groups, spouses and hosptialisation as a trial of treatment in psychosomatic illness. Psychosom. 13: 353–357

90 Bilodeau C, Hackett T 1971 Issues raised in a group setting by patients recovering from myocardial infarction. Am. J. Psychiat. 128: 73–78

91 Stein A 1971 Group therapy with psychosomatically ill patients. In: Kaplan H, Sadock B (eds) Comprehensive group psychotherapy. Williams & Wilkins, Baltimore

92 Waxer P A 1977 Short-term group psychotherapy. Int. J. Psychother. 27: 33–41

93 Pinsky J J 1978 Chronic intractable benign pain: a syndrome and its treatment with intensive short-term group psychotherapy. J. Hum. Stress Sept.: 17–21

94 Pinsky J J 1975 Psychodynamics and psychotherapy with chronic intractable pain. In: Crue B L (ed) Pain, research and treatment. Academic Press, New York

95 Main C J 1984 New approaches to the treatment of pain. Unpublished report to the Winston Churchill Memorial Trust

96 Sternbach R A 1980 Psychological techniques in the management of pain. In: Kosterlitz H W, Terenius L Y (eds) Pain and society. Chemie, Weinheim

97 Waxman D 1983 A short history of hypnosis. Psychiat. Pract. June: 30–36

98 Orne M T 1974 Pain suppression by hypnosis and related phenomena. In: Bonica J J et al (eds) Advances in neurology, vol 4. Raven Press, New York

99 Hilgard E, Hilgard J 1975 Hypnosis in the relief of pain. William Kaufmann; Los Altos, California

100 Sacerdote P 1982 Techniques of hypnotic intervention with pain patients. In: Barber J, Adrian C (eds) Psychological approaches to the management of pain. Brunner/Mazel, New York, ch 4

101 Barber J 1982 Incorporating hypnosis in the management of chronic pain. In: Barber J, Adrian C (eds) Psychological approaches to the management of pain. Brunner/Mazel, New York, ch 3

102 Lemmon K W 1983 Chronic low back differentiation of the real and imagined. Med. Hypnoanal. 4: 17–30

103 Main C J 1984 Psychological factors in chronic low back pain. PhD thesis, University of Glasgow

104 Erikson M H 1966 The interspersal hypnotic technique for symptom correction and pain control. Am. J. Clin. Hyp. 8: 198–209

105 Ewin D M 1978 Relieving suffering and pain with hypnosis. Geriatrics, 33: 87–89

106 Schafer D W, Hernandez A 1978 Hypnosis, pain and the context of therapy. Int. J. Clin. Exp. Hypn. 26: 143–153

107 Finer B 1974 Clinical use of hypnosis in pain management. In: Bonica J J et al (eds) Advances in neurology, vol 4. Raven Press, New York, p 573–579

108 Orne M T 1974 Floor discussion: Hypnosis (Moderator W E Fordyce). In: Bonica J J et al (eds) Advances in neurology, vol 4. Raven Press, New York

109 Spanos N P, Hewitt E C 1980 The 'hidden observer' in hypnotic analgesia: discovery or experimental creation. J. Pers. Soc. Psychol. 39: 1–6

110 Crasilneck H B 1979 Hypnosis in the control of chronic low back pain. Am. J. Clin. Hypn. 22: 71–78

111 Reeves J 1982 Hypnotic methods in cancer pain management. Paper presented to the 3rd annual meeting of the American Pain Society, Miami Beach

112 Lazarus R S 1975 The self-regulation of emotion. In: Levi L (ed) Emotions — their parameters and measurement. Raven Press, New York

113 Evans F J 1984 The random number generation task as an objective measure of experimental and clinical pain. IASP 4th World Congress, Seattle

114 Harris G, Rollman G B 1983 The validity of experimental pain measures. Pain 17: 369–376

115 DeGood D E, Schwartz D P, Shutty M S 1984 Factor analysis of patients' responses to a psycho-educational videotape on chronic pain: Can motivation be measured? IASP 4th World Congress, Seattle

116 Kvien T K, Nilsen H, Vik P 1981 Education and self-care of patients with low back pain. Scand. J. Rheum. 10: 318–320

117 Dworkin S F, Chen A C N, Schubert M M, Clark D W 1984 Cognitive modification of pain: information in combination with nitrous oxide. Pain 19: 339–365

118 Melzack R, Perry C 1975 Self-regulation of pain: the use of alpha feedback and hypnotic training for the control of chronic pain. Expt. Neurol. 46: 452–469

119 Alperson B L, Gottlieb H, Hockersmith V, Koller R 1984 Self-management for medication reduction in a chronic back pain population. IASP 4th World Congress, Seattle

120 Large R G 1984 Self-concepts and illness attitudes in chronic pain. A repertory grid study of a pain management programme. IASP 4th World Congress, Seattle

121 Johnson J E, Morrisey J F, Leventhal H 1973 Psychological preparation for an endoscopic examination. Gastro. Endoscop. 19: 180–182

122 Kendall P C, Williams L, Pechacek T F, Graham L E, Shisslak C, Herzoff N 1979 Cognitive-behavioral and patient-education interventions in cardiac catheterization procedures: the Palo Alto medical psychology project. J. Consult. Clin. Psychol. 47: 49–58

123 Langer E L, Janis I L, Wolfer J A 1975 Reduction of psychological stress in surgical patients. J. Exp. Soc. Psychol. 11: 155–165

124 Tan S -Y 1982 Review article· Cognitive and cognitive-behavioral methods for pain control, a selective review. Pain 12: 201–228

125 Schmidt A J M 1984 Effects of cognitive factors on the performance level of chronic low-back (CLBP) patients. IASP 4th World Congress, Seattle

126 Mayerson N, Rhodevalt F 1984 The role of self-serving attributional strategies in pain perception. IASP 4th World Congress, Seattle

127 Skevington S M 1984 The changing beliefs, attributions and expectations of early synovitis patients: a longitudinal study of the effects of chronic pain and hospitalisation. IASP 4th World Congress, Seattle

128 Lefebvre M F 1981 Cognitive distortion and cognitive errors in depressed psychiatric and low back pain patients. J. Consult. Clin. Psychol. 49: 517–525

129 Rosenstiel A K, Keefe F J 1983 The use of coping strategies in chronic low back pain patients: relationship to patient characteristics and current adjustment. Pain 17: 33–44

130 Brown J M 1984 Imagery coping strategies in the treatment of migraine. Pain 18: 157–167

131 Trent J T 1982 Cognitive relaxation as a treatment of chronic pain. A single case experiment. Am. J. Clin. Biofeed. 5: 59–64

132 Turk D C, Kerns R D, Rudy T E 1984 Identifying the links between chronic illness and depression: cognitive-behavioral mediators. Paper presented at the 92nd annual convention of the American Psychological Association, Toronto

133 Karol R L, Doerfler L A, Parker J C, Armentrout D P 1981 A therapist manual for the cognitive-behavioral treatment of chronic pain. JSAS Catalog of Selected Documents in Psychology 11: 15–16

134 Melzack R, Wall P 1970 Psychophysiology of pain. Internat. Anesthesiol. Clin. 8: 3–34

135 Melzack R, Wall P 1965 Pain mechanisms: a new theory. Science 50: 971–979

136 Dunbar J 1980 Adhering to medical advice: a review. Int. J. Ment. Health 9: 70–87

137 Pearce S 1983 A review of cognitive-behavioural methods for the treatment of chronic pain. Journ. Psychosom. Res. 27: 431–440

138 Bandura A 1977 Self-efficacy: toward a unifying theory of behavioral change. Psychol. Rev. 84: 191–215

139 Chapman S L, Brena S F, Bradford L A 1981 Treatment outcome in a chronic pain rehabilitation program. Pain 11: 255–268

140 Cohen M J, Heinrich R L, Naliboff B D, Collins G A, Bonebakker A D 1983 Group outpatient physical and behavioral therapy for chronic low back pain. J. Clin. Psychol. 39: 326–333

141 Waddell G, Bircher M, Finlayson D, Main C J 1984 Symptoms and signs: physical disease or illness behaviour? B.M.J. 289: 739–741

142 Bonica J J, Fordyce W E 1974 Operant conditioning for chronic pain. In: Bonica J J et al (eds) Recent advances in pain: pathophysiology and clinical aspects. p 299–312

143 Craig K D 1978 Social modeling influences on pain. In: Sternbach R A (ed) The psychology of pain. Raven Press, New York, p 73–109

144 Craig K D 1983 Modelling and social learning factors in chronic pain. In: Bonica J J et al (eds) Advances in pain research and therapy, vol 5, p 813–827

145 Fordyce W E 1976 Behavioral methods for chronic pain and illness. Mosby, St Louis

146 Fordyce W E 1974 Pain viewed as learned behavior. In: Bonica J J et al (eds) Advances in neurology, vol 4. Raven Press, New York, p 415–422

147 Fordyce W E 1974 Floor discussion: hypnosis. In: Bonica J J et al (eds) Advances in neurology, vol 4. Raven Press, New York, p 581–582

148 Fordyce W E 1974 Operant conditioning: an approach to chronic pain. In: Current concepts of pain and analgesia. Current Concepts, New York

149 Trotter M, Inman D 1968 The use of positive reinforcement in physical therapy. Phys. Ther. 48: 347–352

150 Rice M, McDaniel M, Denny S 1968 Operant conditioning techniques. Phys. Ther. 48: 342–346

151 Horner R D 1971 Establishing the use of crutches by a mentally retarded spina bifida child. J. App. Behav. Anal. 4: 183–190

152 Fordyce W E, Fowler R S Jnr, Lehmann F J, Delateur B 1968 Some implications of learning in problems of chronic pain. J. Chron. Dis. 21: 179–189

153 Fordyce W E, Fowler R S Jr, Lehmann J F, Delateur B, Sand P, Treischmann R B 1973 Operant

conditioning in the treatment of chronic pain. Arch. Phys. Med. Rehab. 54: 399–408

154   Turk D C, Genest M 1979 Regulation of pain: the application of cognitive and behavioral techniques for prevention and remediation. In: Kendall P C, Hollon S D (eds) Cognitive-behavioral interventions: theory, research and procedures, chap 9, p 287–318

155   Anderson T P, Cole T M, Gullickson G, Hudgens A, Roberts A H 1977 A treatment program by a multidisciplinary team. J. Clin. Orthop. 129: 96–100

156   Bilodeau I, Bilodeau E 1958 Variation of temporal intervals among critical events in five studies of knowledge of results. J. Exp. Psychol. 55: 603–612

157   Underwood B 1966 Experimental psychology. Appleton-Century-Crofts, New York

158   Cairns D, Pasino J A 1977 Comparison of verbal reinforcement and feedback in the operant treatment of disability due to chronic low back pain. Behav. Ther. 8: 621–630

159   Watson P J, Workman E A 1981 The noncurrent multiple-baseline across-individuals design: an extension of a traditional multiple-baseline design. J. Behav. Ther. Exp. Psychiat. 12: 257–259

160   Ng L K Y 1981 New approaches to the treatment of chronic pain: a review of multidisciplinary pain clinics and pain centres, NIDA Res. Monog. Series No 36, Rockville, Maryland

161   Brena S F, Chapman S L, Decker R 1981 Chronic pain as a learned experience: Emory University Pain Control Center. In: New approaches to the treatment of chronic pain: a review of multidisciplinary pain clinics and pain centers, NIDA Res. Monog. Series 36, Rockville, Maryland, p 76–83

162   Long D M 1981 A comprehensive model for the study and therapy of pain: Johns Hopkins pain research and treatment programme. In: Ng L K Y (ed) New approaches to the treatment of chronic pain: a review of multidisciplinary pain clinics and pain centres, p 66–75

163   Carron H, Rowlingson J C 1981 Coordinated out-patient management of chronic pain at the University of Virginia Pain Clinic. In: Ng L K Y (ed) NIDA Res. Monog. Series 36, Rockville, Maryland, p 84–91

164   Crue B L, Pinsky J J 1981 Chronic pain syndrome — four aspects of the problem: New Hope Pain Center and Pain Research Foundation. In: Ng L K Y (ed) NIDA Res. Monog. Series 36. New approaches to the treatment of chronic pain: a review of multidisciplinary pain clinics and pain centers. Rockville, Maryland, p 137–168

165   Rosomoff H L, Green C, Silbret M, Steele R 1981 Pain and low back rehabilitation program at the University of Miami School of Medicine. In: Ng L K Y (ed) New approaches to the treatment of chronic pain: a review of multidisciplinary pain clinics and pain centers. NIDA Res. Monog. Series 36, Rockville, Maryland, p 92–111

166   Cairns D, Thomas L, Mooney V, Pace J B 1976 A comprehensive treatment approach to chronic low back pain. Pain 2: 301–308

167   Roberts A H, Reinhardt L 1980 The behavioral management of chronic pain: long-term follow-up with comparison groups. Pain 8: 151–162

168   Spengler D M 1983 Chronic low back pain: the team approach. Clin. Orth. Rel. Res. 179: 71–76

169   Swanson D W, Swenson W M, Maruta T, McPhee M C 1976 Program for managing chronic pain. I. Program description and characteristics of patients. Mayo Clinic Proc., 51: 401–408

170   Keefe F J, Schapira B, Williams R B, Brown C, Surwit R S 1981 EMG-assisted relaxation training in the management of chronic low back pain. Am. J. Clin. Biofeed. 4: 93–103

171   Newman R I, Seres J L, Yospe L P, Garlington B 1978 Multidisciplinary treatment of chronic pain: long-term follow-up of low-back patients. Pain 4: 283–292

172   Urban B J, France R D, Keefe F J 1984 Comprehensive analysis of multidisciplinary treatment for chronic low back pain. IASP 4th World Congress, Seattle

173   Donovan W H, Dwyer A P, White B W, Batalin N J, Skerritt P W, Bedbrook G M 1981 A multidisciplinary approach to chronic low back pain in Western Australia. Spine 6: 591–597

174   Wharton R N, Yang J C, Clark W C 1984 Psychological distress and outcome of treatment for chronic pain patients. IASP 4th World Congress, Seattle

175   Addison R G 1981 Treatment of chronic pain: The Center for Pain Studies, Rehabilitation Institute of Chicago. In: Ng L K Y (ed) NIDA Res. Monog. Series 36. New approaches to the treatment of chronic pain: a review of multidisciplinary pain clinics and pain centers. Rockville, Maryland, p 12–32

176   Aronoff G M, Evans W O, Kenders P L 1983 Review article: a review of follow-up studies of multi-disciplinary pain units. Pain 16: 1–11

177   Seres J, Painter J R, Newman R I 1981 Multidisciplinary treatment of chronic pain at the Northwest Pain Center. In: Ng L K Y (ed) NIDA Res. Monog. Series 36. New Approaches to the treatment of chronic pain: a review of multidisciplinary pain clinics and pain centers. Rockville, Maryland, p 41–65

178   Lutz R W, Silbret M, Olshan N 1983 Treatment outcome and compliance with therapeutic regimens: long-term follow-up of a multidisciplinary pain program. Pain 17: 301–308

179   Hallett E C, Pilowsky I 1982 The response to treatment in a multidisciplinary pain clinic. Pain 12: 365–374

180   Gottlieb B, Brodey J F, Sewitch T S, Shaw M B, Weiner L L 1984 A one-year follow-up of chronic pain patients treated in an outpatient behavioral program. IASP 4th World Congress, Seattle

181   Khatami M, Rush A J 1982 A one-year follow-up of the multi-modal treatment for chronic pain. Pain 14: 45–52

182   Ross R M, Namerow N S 1984 The evaluation of a chronic pain program: a two-year follow-up study. IASP 4th World Congress, Seattle

183   Waddell G, Main C J, Morris E W, Di Paola M, Gray I C M 1984 Chronic low-back pain, psychologic distress and illness behavior. Spine 9: 209–213

184   Fricton J R 1984 Chronic illness care: an interdisciplinary evaluation and management system for chronic pain based on the biopsychosocial medical model. IASP 4th World Congress, Seattle

Index